# Preformulation in Solid Dosage Form Development

# DRUGS AND THE PHARMACEUTICAL SCIENCES
A Series of Textbooks and Monographs

Executive Editor

**James Swarbrick**
*PharmaceuTech, Inc.*
*Pinehurst, North Carolina*

## Advisory Board

Books are to be returned on or before
the last date below.

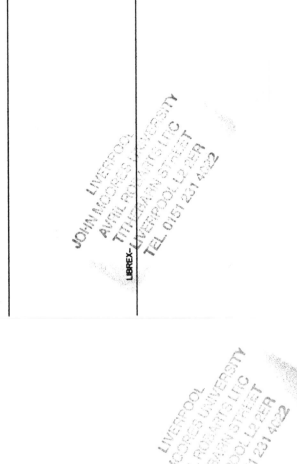

# Preformulation in Solid Dosage Form Development

Edited by

## Moji Christianah Adeyeye
*Duquesne University*
*Pittsburgh, Pennsylvania, USA*

## Harry G. Brittain
*Center for Pharmaceutical Physics*
*Milford, New Jersey, USA*

## informa
healthcare

New York   London

Informa Healthcare USA, Inc.
52 Vanderbilt Avenue
New York, NY 10017

© 2008 by Informa Healthcare USA, Inc.
Informa Healthcare is an Informa business

No claim to original U.S. Government works
Printed in the United States of America on acid-free paper
10 9 8 7 6 5 4 3 2 1

International Standard Book Number-10: 0-8247-5809-9 (Hardcover)
International Standard Book Number-13: 978-0-8247-5809-7 (Hardcover)

---

### Library of Congress Cataloging-in-Publication Data

Preformulation in solid dosage form development / edited by Moji Christianah Adeyeye, Harry G. Brittain.
    p. ; cm. – (Drugs and the pharmaceutical sciences ; 178)
    Includes bibliographical references and index.
    ISBN-13: 978-0-8247-5809-7 (hb : alk. paper)
    ISBN-10: 0-8247-5809-9 (hb : alk. paper)
  1. Solid dosage forms. 2. Drug development. 3. Pharmaceutical chemistry.
  I. Adeyeye, Moji C. II. Brittain, H. G. III. Series.
  [DNLM: 1. Chemistry, Pharmaceutical. 2. Dosage Forms. 3. Pharmaceutical Preparations–chemical synthesis. W1 DR893B v.178 2008 / QV 744 P923 2008]
  RS201.S57P74 2008
  615'.19–dc22                                    2007033181

---

For Corporate Sales and Reprint Permissions call 212-520-2700 or write to:
Sales Department, 52 Vanderbilt Ave., 16th floor, New York, NY 10017.

**Visit the Informa web site at**
**www.informa.com**

**and the Informa Healthcare Web site at**
**www.informahealthcare.com**

# Prefaces

## I

The conception of writing a book on preformulation began many years ago after noticing the dearth of information on characterization of chemical entities and excipients in pharmaceutical drug development while developing lecture notes for the Formulation and Development course that I teach in my school. As a teacher in the "ivory tower," I found this intriguing, knowing that future industry scientists passing through institutions of higher learning need exposure to the basic information as well as current and relevant advances in conducting preformulation research in the industry. During the 1996 American Association of Pharmaceutical Scientists meeting, I brought this up at the preformulation focus group meeting where several colleagues volunteered to contribute chapters toward the making of the book.

The intent of this book is to equip both academia and the pharmaceutical industry with adequate basic and applied principles important to the characterization of drugs, excipients, and products during the preformulation stage in development. The issues of predictability, identification, and product development of drug substances during the preformulation phase and into Phase I clinical trials have been addressed. The relevance of these to setting acceptance criteria (indicative of building quality into the product instead of adding quality) for regulatory purposes has been emphasized. Each chapter has been written with the industry scientist/practitioner and the regulatory authorities in mind so that the book can serve as a handbook and reference text for answering questions or problem solving.

During the evolution of the writing process, several colleagues encouraged me and contributed toward the rationale for writing the book, and these include George Wong and Ivan Santos. I am very grateful for my co-editor, Harry G. Brittain, for his ebullience and encouragement during the making of the book.

*Moji Christianah Adeyeye*

# II

If you ask 20 workers in the pharmaceutical field what is meant by the science of "preformulation," I have no doubt that you will receive 20 different answers. To the early-stage scientist, it represents the process of characterizing a new drug substance, to learn about its properties and tendencies. Working through a pre-planned program of investigational work, scientists obtain a wide range of information. Clearly they cannot learn everything, and in fact, the time and money constraints of modern drug development often dictate that the minimal amount of work is done that will satisfy a regulatory agency. Industrial preformulation groups march through two or three compounds per month, gather the type of data they think will be of use later on, and write a report that they hope will be read by everyone who comes after them in the process.

To the latter-stage scientist, preformulation represents the stage where someone else has profiled a drug candidate to such a degree that he or she has all the information needed to complete the development process. Unfortunately, since this worker has usually had relatively little input into the design of the preformulation studies, it is not a given that the preformulation report will contain all that is really needed. There ordinarily follows a scrambling for new information, or (worse yet) an era of trouble shooting and formulation fixing. Everyone in late-stage development understands that the process is inevitable, but no one has to like it.

In the present volume, Professor Adeyeye and I have tried to outline a program of preformulation that fits better with the modern school of drug development. All of the traditional investigations are contained, but we have tried to look forward through the development process so that appropriate preformulation activities are included in the early work. We equally believe that computational prediction can play an important role in the characterization of drug compounds, and have used the term "preliminary preformulation" to cover such work. It is our hope that we have covered all the topics of importance to preformulation work, and that we have set out a program that can be successfully applied to the majority of drug candidates.

*Harry G. Brittain*

# Contents

*v*

# Contributors

**Moji Christianah Adeyeye**  School of Pharmacy, Duquesne University, Pittsburgh, Pennsylvania, U.S.A.

**Sherif I. Badawy**  Bristol-Myers Squibb Pharmaceutical Research Institute, New Brunswick, New Jersey, U.S.A.

**J. R. Blachére**  Department of Materials Science and Engineering, University of Pittsburgh, Pittsburgh, Pennsylvania, U.S.A.

**Harry G. Brittain**  Center for Pharmaceutical Physics, Milford, New Jersey, U.S.A.

**Charles C. Collins**  College of Pharmacy, East Tennessee State University, Johnson City, Tennessee, U.S.A.

**Robert S. DeWitte**  Advanced Chemistry Development, Inc., Toronto, Ontario, Canada

**Nkere K. Ebube**  Biovail Technologies, Chantilly, Virginia, U.S.A.

**Miriam K. Franchini**  Sanofi-Aventis, Bridgewater, New Jersey, U.S.A.

**Ram N. Gidwani**  Pharmaceutical Consultant, Milford, New Jersey, U.S.A.

**Michel Hachey**  Advanced Chemistry Development, Inc., Toronto, Ontario, Canada

**Munir A. Hussain**  Bristol-Myers Squibb Pharmaceutical Research Institute, New Brunswick, New Jersey, U.S.A.

**Sau Lawrence Lee**  Office of Generic Drugs, United States Food and Drug Administration, Rockville, Maryland, U.S.A.

**Denette K. Murphy**  Bristol-Myers Squibb Company, New Brunswick, New Jersey, U.S.A.

**Shelley Rabel**  ALZA Corporation, Mountain View, California, U.S.A.

**Andre S. Raw**  Office of Generic Drugs, United States Food and Drug Administration, Rockville, Maryland, U.S.A.

**Alan F. Rawle**  Malvern Instruments, Westborough, Massachusetts, U.S.A.

**Stephen Spanton**   GPRD Structural Chemistry, Abbott Laboratories, Abbott Park, Illinois, U.S.A.

**George Wong**   Global R&D Operations, Johnson & Johnson, Skillman, New Jersey, U.S.A.

**Lawrence Yu**   Office of Generic Drugs, United States Food and Drug Administration, Rockville, Maryland, U.S.A.

*Part 1: Introduction*

# 1.1

# Introduction and Overview to the Preformulation Development of Solid Dosage Forms

### Harry G. Brittain

*Center for Pharmaceutical Physics, Milford, New Jersey, U.S.A.*

Once an organic compound has been discovered and shown by one scientific group to have some type of desirable pharmacological activity, it will remain a mere curiosity unless a completely different group of scientists incorporate the compound in a formulation that facilitates its activity. This latter group of investigators constitutes the development effort, and it is their work that turns an interesting compound into an actual drug substance.

Out of the many types of formulations that could be contemplated for a drug substance, the solid oral dose form (i.e., tablets and capsules) continues to be the most important. For this reason, the remainder of the coverage in this volume will center on the development of solid dosage forms, although many of the principles involved will be seen to be applicable to other dosage forms such as liquids, suspensions, emulsions, semisolids, suppositories, and aerosols, to name a few.

Historically, the preformulation stage of drug development has been considered to consist mostly of drug substance profiling, and indeed most of the leading reviews have followed this view (1–6). However, there is far more to the development of drug products than characterization of the active pharmaceutical ingredient, and in its fullest incarnation, preformulation would also extend to studies of drug–excipient compatibilities. At this point, one could simply employ the Edisonian approach of trying all combinations of drugs and excipients to see what would constitute an appropriate formulation, a method that has come to be known today as high-throughput screening. Clearly, it makes more sense to develop profiles of the physical and chemical properties of drug substances and excipients, and to then use this information in order to develop more robust formulations.

For example, while the degree of acidity or basicity of a substance dissolved in an aqueous medium can be adequately defined in terms of pH, comparable expressions for the acidity or basicity of the surface of a solid are more complicated. Such evaluations would be of importance to a preformulation study, as it is known that acidic or basic surfaces of solids can function as catalytic agents. The a priori knowledge regarding the degree of acidity of a surface, or the stoichiometry of binding sites, would be of great use to formulators, and its acquisition would serve to streamline preformulation studies, especially if the body of information was available for the drug substance as well as the excipients intended for its formulation. In the absence of such knowledge, formulators can only assume the existence of certain characteristics of the materials they are working with, and then base their compounding on assumptions rather than hard facts.

The depth of the problem is extremely important, since in a dosage form, under suitable conditions, a drug substance may undergo a variety of interactions or transformations through one or more chemical or physical reactions. The understanding of these solid–solid interactions is highly critical to a successful outcome for the development process, as they can lead to the formation of new impurities, incomplete mass balance, destruction of the dosage form, and changes in physicochemical properties (stability, solubility, dissolution profile, degree of crystallinity, and hygroscopicity). Any or all of these could have a most unfortunate outcome that ultimately results in an inability to obtain successful registration of the drug substance. Hence, the elucidation of possible chemical and/or physical reactions is an absolute requirement to establish the stability of a given dosage form, and an understanding of the plausible range of solid–solid reactions available to a drug substance should be established once a full preformulation study is completed.

After careful evaluation of the current trends and practices in preformulation, and considering where the field ought to be headed, it seemed appropriate to define four areas of activity. These areas roughly follow the chronological sequence of drug development and can be envisioned as beginning with a preliminary preformulation stage, continuing with a program of drug substance profiling and development of the ideal formulation, and concluding with technology transfer steps.

Preliminary preformulation can be thought of as the stage where one may only know the identity and structure of the organic molecule that is proposed to be a drug candidate. Information that can be deduced at this stage is seen to be intrinsic to the drug candidate and is independent of the perturbing influence of physical phases. However, the information can be very valuable as a background that permits one to better understand the solid-state data that will eventually be acquired.

Now that the sophistication of computational programs is reaching the point that one may calculate many of these quantities to an acceptable degree of accuracy, one may use the structural formula of a compound to calculate its ionization constant $(S)$, the pH dependence of its partition coefficient, and its aqueous solubility tendencies. Very often, this information alone can be used to determine whether the free acid or free base form of the compound will have sufficient properties or whether a salt form of the substance might be more appropriate.

As an example, consider ibuprofen (2-(4-isobutylphenyl)propanoic acid) as a potential drug substance. The structure of the molecule is fairly simple (given below), and one would anticipate the important physical chemistry to be dominated by the chemistry of the carboxylate group. Using the PhysChem program [sourced from Advanced Chemistry Development (ACD)], the $pK_a$ value of the carboxylate group can be calculated to be $4.41 \pm 0.01$. Although this $pK_a$ value is not exactly equal to the reported ionization constant that was determined to be in the range of 4.5 to 4.6 by potentiometric titration in mixed organic/aqueous solvent systems (7), the number is sufficiently close to reality so that it may be used to deduce other important properties of the molecule.

The next step in the computational process would be to calculate the partition coefficient and the pH dependence of the distribution coefficient. For ibuprofen, the ACD program calculates the octanol/water partition coefficient to be $\log P = 3.72 \pm 0.23$, indicating that the compound is expected to be substantially hydrophobic in its neutral form. As might be anticipated, the carboxylate group of ibuprofen yields a strong pH dependence in the distribution coefficient, as shown in Figure 1. The calculation indicates that while ibuprofen is predicted to be hydrophobic at low pH, it is also predicted to be hydrophilic at high pH once the carboxylate group becomes ionized.

It is a fundamental precept of solubility theory that hydrophilic compounds should exhibit good solubility in aqueous media. As shown in Figure 2, the calculated pH dependence of solubility is consistent with this prediction, with the compound being predicted to be highly soluble above pH 7.

By performing these simple calculations, one would reach the conclusion that ibuprofen would be best developed as a base addition salt to

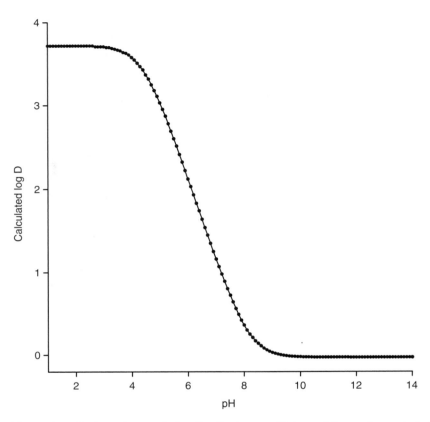

**Figure 1** pH dependence of the distribution coefficient of ibuprofen, calculated using the PhysChem program from Advanced Chemistry Development.

maximize its aqueous solubility. If this decision was made, then the next step would entail prediction of an appropriate salt form. Fortunately, the ionization constants for potential salt formers can be calculated with relative ease. It is relatively easy to show that for the reaction of ibuprofen free acid (H-ibu) with a basic substance (B) to yield the salt $(HB^+)(ibu^-)$,

$$H\text{-ibu} + B \rightleftharpoons HB^+ + ibu^- \tag{1}$$

the value for the salt formation constant $(K_s)$,

$$K_s = \frac{[ibu^-][HB^+]}{[H\text{-ibu}][B]} \tag{2}$$

is given by (8)

$$K_s = K_a K_b / K_w \tag{3}$$

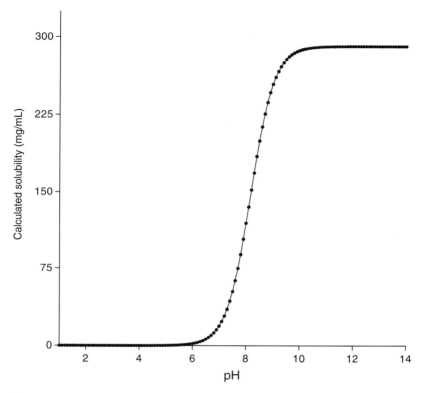

**Figure 2** pH dependence of the aqueous solubility of ibuprofen, calculated using the PhysChem program from Advanced Chemistry Development.

In Equation 3, $K_a$ is the ionization constant expression for the free acid, $K_b$ is the ionization constant expression for the free base, and $K_w$ is the autoionization constant of water. When converted to the Sørensen scale, Eq. 3 becomes

$$pK_s = pK_a + pK_b - pK_w \qquad (4)$$

The value of Equations 3 and 4 becomes evident when we see that they can be used to make rapid deductions regarding the strength of a particular salt species. Suppose one were contemplating forming a salt between ibuprofen (whose $pK_a$ value was calculated to be 4.41) and a base having a $pK_a$ value of 9.45: For the base, it would follow that the $pK_b$ would equal 4.55, and since $pK_w$ equals 14.0 at 25°C, the $pK_s$ of the salt would equal $-5.04$ and $K_s$ would equal approximately 109,650. A reaction characterized by an equilibrium constant of this magnitude would clearly go to completion, and one would predict that the salt in question would be formed without difficulty. Once the range of acceptable acidic salt formers has been determined, one only needs to consult the various compilations of pharmaceutically acceptable acids (9,10) to specify the list of salts that would be actually prepared in the laboratory.

The ability to calculate $\log(K_s)$ values can be of great value in designing the scope of a salt-selection study in that it can be used to select potential salt-forming agents solely on the basis of their ionization constant values. If one accepts the definition of an appropriate salt as one whose degree of formation equals 99% or higher, then one would only attempt to form ibuprofen salts with bases whose $pK_a$ values were sufficiently high, so as to guarantee the required degree of reaction. Assuming a 1:1 stoichiometry, one may use the quadratic equation to solve for the degree of dissociation associated with salts having various $K_s$ values. The equations have been solved analytically, and as shown in Figure 3, for ibuprofen, one finds that the critical $pK$ exceeds 8.41. For example, the formation of sodium or potassium salts (for which $pK_a$ is approximately 14) is obvious, as would be the formation of salts with arginine ($pK_a = 9.59$), lysine ($pK_a = 9.48$), ethanolamine ($pK_a = 9.16$), diethanolamine ($pK_a = 8.71$), and erbumine ($pK_a = 10.68$).

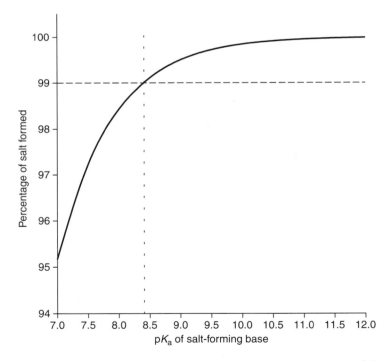

**Figure 3** Degree of salt formation calculated for the reaction of ibuprofen with basic substances of varying $pK$ values; note that the 99% formation criterion interacts with the curve at a $pK_a$ value of 8.41.

At this point in the preformulation process, it becomes necessary to go into the laboratory and begin to perform the experimentation that will ultimately lead to the selection of the drug candidate in its proper solid-state form. To illustrate the process, we will continue with the ibuprofen example, where it has already been established that the formation of a salt form of the drug substance should lead to enhanced solubility and hence dissolution rate. Ibuprofen represents an interesting situation in that it contains one center of dissymmetry, and hence the free acid is capable of being obtained either as a racemic mixture or as one of the separated enantiomers. The physical properties of these forms are quite different, exhibiting different crystal structures, melting points, and degrees of aqueous solubility (7).

Ibuprofen readily forms salts with tromethamine (2-amino-2-(hydro-xymethyl)propane-1,3-diol), and the X-ray powder diffraction patterns of the tromethamine:(S)-ibuprofen and tromethamine:(RS)-ibuprofen salts are shown in Figure 4. One is immediately struck by the strong similarities in the diffraction patterns, which identifies the tromethamine salts as belonging to

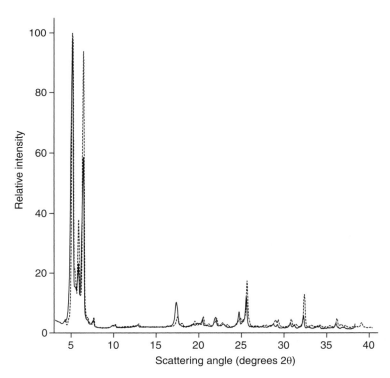

**Figure 4** X-ray powder diffraction patterns of the tromethamine salts with (S)-ibuprofen (*solid trace*) and (RS)-ibuprofen (*dashed trace*).

a conglomerate system. In a conglomerate, the different enantiomers of the solid substance crystallize in different crystals, so that the observed diffraction patterns of the separated enantiomers and the racemic mixture are the same (11).

Optical photomicrographs of the tromethamine salts with (*S*)-ibuprofen and (*RS*)-ibuprofen are shown in Figure 5. It was found that the particles of both salts were obtained in the form of thin flat plates, but the edges were poorly defined. The crystals of both salts exhibited strong birefringence, which would be consistent with the high degree of crystallinity observed in the X-ray diffraction studies.

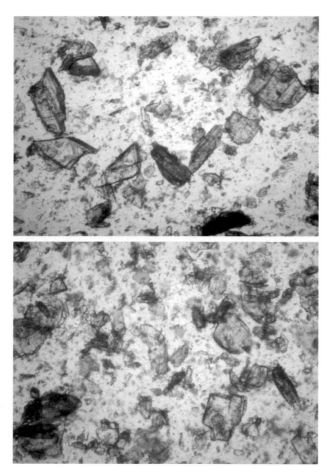

**Figure 5** Optical photomicrographs of the tromethamine salts with (*S*)-ibuprofen (*top*) and (*RS*)-ibuprofen (*bottom*). Both images were taken at a magnification of 40×.

The structural equivalence (i.e., conglomerate nature) of the tromethamine salts with (*S*)-ibuprofen and (*RS*)-ibuprofen is further indicated in the equivalence of their other physical properties. The differential scanning calorimetry thermograms of the salts (Fig. 6) are effectively the same, with the (*S*)-ibuprofen salt exhibiting a melting endotherm at 158.4°C (enthalpy of fusion equal to 159.1 J/g) and the (*RS*)-ibuprofen salt having a melting endotherm of 158.9°C (enthalpy of fusion equal to 160.2 J/g). It is to be noted that these fusion characteristics represent a vast improvement over those of the parent free acids, where (*S*)-ibuprofen was found to exhibit a melting endotherm at 58.8°C (enthalpy of fusion equal to 67.9 J/g) and (*RS*)-ibuprofen exhibited a melting endotherm of 77.3°C (enthalpy of fusion equal to 77.9 J/g).

Since the crystal structures of the (*S*)-ibuprofen:tromethamine and (*RS*)-ibuprofen:tromethamine salts are effectively the same, one would anticipate that the respective solid-state spectra would also be equivalent. This is evident in the fingerprint region of the infrared absorption spectra in Figure 7 and in the Raman spectra in Figure 8. It is clear that the

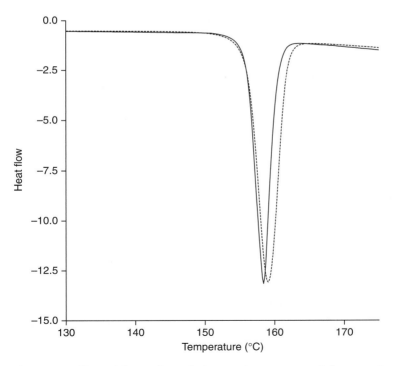

**Figure 6**  Differential scanning calorimetry thermograms of the tromethamine salts with (*S*)-ibuprofen (*solid trace*) and (*RS*)-ibuprofen (*dashed trace*).

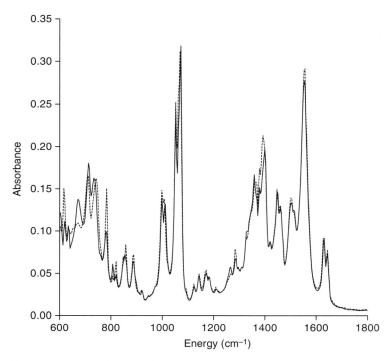

**Figure 7** Infrared absorption spectra of the tromethamine salts with (*S*)-ibuprofen (*solid trace*) and (*RS*)-ibuprofen (*dashed trace*), obtained using the attenuated total reflectance sampling mode. Spectra are shown for the fingerprint region only.

tromethamine salt prepared from the enantiomerically pure and racemic free acids could not be differentiated on the basis of their solid-state spectra.

Although the frequencies of individual group vibrations as measured using either infrared absorption spectroscopy or Raman scattering must always be the same for a given compound, the difference in the nature of the selection rules governing the infrared absorption and Raman scattering processes often leads to differences in the relative intensities, which makes the respective spectra appear to be different (12). This has been illustrated in Figure 9, where one may note the apparent nonequivalence of the infrared absorption spectrum and the Raman spectrum of the (*S*)-ibuprofen:tromethamine salt. Generally, symmetric vibrations will have the most intensity in a Raman spectrum, and the nonsymmetric vibrations will tend to tolerate the infrared absorption spectrum. Hence, it is prudent to obtain both types of vibrational spectra for a compound under development in order to build up a database of characteristics that may prove to be useful during the study of drug–excipient interactions.

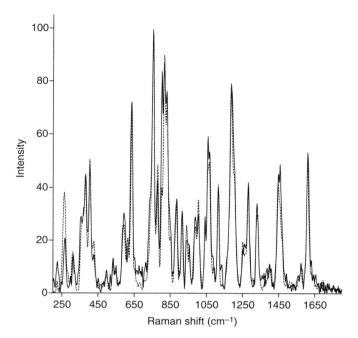

**Figure 8** Raman spectra of the tromethamine salts with (*S*)-ibuprofen (*solid trace*) and (*RS*)-ibuprofen (*dashed trace*), obtained using the attenuated total reflectance sampling mode. Spectra are shown for the fingerprint region only.

The solubility of (*RS*)-ibuprofen free acid has been reported to be less than 0.1 mg/mL, but the aqueous solubilities of the tromethamine salts with (*RS*)-ibuprofen and (*S*)-ibuprofen were found to exceed 100 mg/mL. Given their high degree of solubility in water, and their superior physical characteristics (as evidenced by the thermal analysis results), it follows that if one were given a choice, one would naturally choose to develop one of the tromethamine salts rather than the free acid.

Once the form of the drug substance has been chosen, the next stage in the preformulation program would entail the study of how the compound interacts with excipients of interest. Excipients are naturally chosen on their functional basis, properties that are essential to the release of the drug substance from the dosage form. For a solid dosage form designed to rapidly release the drug substance upon contact with a fluid, one normally seeks a formulation where there are no physical or chemical interactions between the various components. For solid dosage forms, an interaction usually is considered to represent a bad situation, since the quality and stability of the formulation will ordinarily be adversely affected.

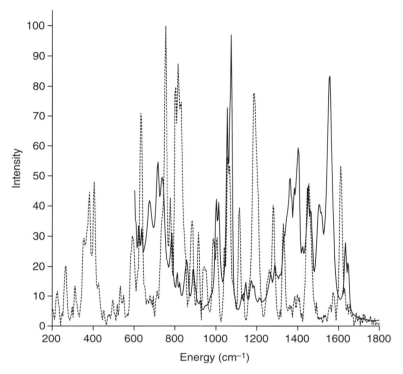

**Figure 9** Infrared absorption spectrum (*solid trace*) and Raman spectrum (*dashed trace*) of the (*S*)-ibuprofen:tromethamine salt. The spectra have been normalized so that the most intense peaks have a relative intensity of 100. Spectra are shown for the fingerprint region only.

A number of reviews have been published that cover the scope of potential solid-state reactions, but in general, one may find what one needs to know in Refs. 13 and 14 and in the other chapters in this book.

One convenient classification for solid-state reactions specifies the natures of the phases involved. For example, the reactions between solids and gases may involve the interaction of the solid substance with water vapor (either sorption or desorption), or with oxygen or other gases. The solid–gas reaction may result in a phase transformation, typically causing the formation of a hydrate or a solvate crystal form. Reactions between solids and liquids can result in hydrolysis of the drug substance [see, for example, the work reported in Ref. 15 on aspirin formulations] or in other acid–base chemistry, or in extreme cases, they may result in the solubilization of the components involved. One must always monitor whether a phase transformation takes place when a liquid interacts with a solid, as solution-mediated phase transformations are well known.

There are also a number of solid–solid reactions that are possible. Among these are association processes, such as those observed in dispersions of indomethacin and polyvinylpyrrolidone (16). One may encounter adsorption reactions, as was noted in the adsorption of ketotifen on Ac-Di-Sol (17). Drug substances may become solubilized in one of the other components, demonstrated, for example, by the existence of a complete phase diagram for the quinine–phenobarbital system (18). The well-known Maillard reaction of lactose with amines can be typified by the addition reaction of fluoxetine with spray-dried lactose (19). Desolvation reactions are frequently studied using spectroscopic techniques, such as the use of near-infrared spectroscopy to monitor the loss of isopropyl alcohol from loracarbef solvatomorphs (20). There are many physical and chemical techniques suitable for the study of drug decomposition in formulations, but one of the more creative methods entails the correlation of quantitative color parameters with and drug content in formulations of flucloxin (21). Of course, one must always remember the possibility of phase transformations in solids, and the number of solid-state phase changes that have been published is very large.

To evaluate the compatibility between drug substance and excipients, one will blend the API with excipients at levels that are realistic with respect to the proposed formulation. For example, if a lubricant is to be used at the 0.5% level in a formulation, the evaluation of a 50% substance–excipient mixture would not be appropriate. Each blend is then stored under an appropriate set of accelerated stress conditions (typically elevated temperature and humidity) and subsequently tested for drug substance quality after an appropriate equilibration period.

The purity and impurity profiling is ordinarily conducted using a chromatographic procedure, while the physical characteristics are normally followed by means of the appropriate physical analysis methodology. The methodologies suitable for the study of chemical compatibilities include high-performance liquid chromatography (HPLC), capillary electrophoresis, gas chromatography (GC), mass spectrometry (especially coupled with GC or HPLC), nuclear magnetic resonance, and vibrational spectroscopy. The methodologies suitable for the study of physical compatibilities include microscopy (either optical or scanning electron), X-ray powder diffraction, thermal analysis (typically differential scanning calorimetry and thermogravimetry), ultraviolet/visible or near-infrared diffuse reflectance spectroscopy, solid-state nuclear magnetic resonance, and solid-state vibrational spectroscopy. The technology to be used during this phase is determined by the nature of the problem, but ordinarily, the correct approach entails a multidisciplinary use of methodology where the optimal tools are selected to obtain the information of interest.

The main goal during this latter stage of preformulation development is to discover and study the formulation(s) that will be used during the Phase 1 and Phase 2 clinical studies. These formulations should not only suit their intended purpose, but also lead the way to the eventual Phase 3 formulation.

Once a few trial formulations of the drug substance have been developed, and tablets or capsules prepared from these, dissolution testing can be taken up in the evaluation studies. Most studies are conducted using the batch dissolution method, where the analyzed concentration of a well-stirred solution is taken as being representative of the entire volume of the dissolution medium. In a dissolution profile of a good formulation, the analyte concentration will increase from its initial zero value until a limiting concentration is attained that indicates full dissolution of the drug substance.

A simple use of dissolution testing as a means of formulation optimization is shown in Figure 10, which contains dissolution profiles of two prototype tablet formulations prepared using the (S)-ibuprofen:tromethamine salt as the drug substance. It was found that only partial dissolution of the

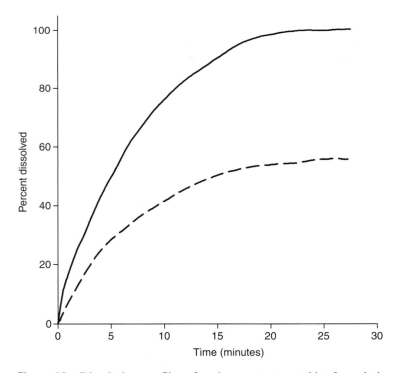

**Figure 10**   Dissolution profiles of various prototype tablet formulations prepared using (S)-ibuprofen:tromethamine salt as the drug substance. Profiles are shown for a formulation consisting of 25% API and 75% microcrystalline cellulose (*solid trace*), and a formulation consisting of 25% API, 65% microcrystalline cellulose, and 10% sodium starch glycolate. *Abbreviation*: API, active pharmaceutical ingredient.

salt could be obtained for a formulation consisting of 25% API and 75% microcrystalline cellulose, but that full dissolution could be obtained from a formulation consisting of 25% API, 65% microcrystalline cellulose, and 10% sodium starch glycolate. These observations seem to indicate not only the existence of a drug–excipient interaction between the (S)-ibuprofen:tromethamine salt and the microcrystalline cellulose, but also that the inclusion of a disintegrant in the formulation can serve to mitigate this effect.

At the conclusion of the second phase of the preformulation work, one should have developed a catalog of the plausible solid-state reactions accessible to the drug substance. Any concerns that developed during this work should receive a degree of attention that is roughly proportional to their likelihood of actually being encountered, making it essential that the studies are performed at appropriate concentration levels. Clearly, since the scope of possible solid–solid reactions encompasses both chemical and physical interactions, it follows that both types need to be studied by an appropriate methodology. Although real-time data would be preferable, in the absence of such data, the use of accelerated studies can greatly expedite matters.

No matter how good or thorough the preformulation program has been, there is no doubt that the work is wasted unless the technology can be transferred to the next stage. This accumulated body of knowledge will enable formulation scientists to build upon what was learned, and will enable them to use the catalog of drug–excipient interactions to avoid additional formulation changes doomed to failure. The physical and the chemical methods of characterization developed during preformulation will be of equal interest to the analytical scientists, who generally use this information to optimize existing methods and develop new ones.

Every organization develops its own models for this technology-transfer process, but there is usually no better method than to collect everything that was learned in one or more preformulation reports. Such documentation may even be filed with a new drug application at some point, should that possibility develop.

The various topics outlined in this brief introduction and overview of the preformulation development of solid dosage forms will be expounded in the following chapters.

## REFERENCES

1. Fiese EF, Hagen TA. Preformulation (chap. 8). In: Lachman L, Lieberman HA, Kanig JL, eds. Theory and Practice of Industrial Pharmacy. Philadelphia: Lea & Febiger, 1986, pp. 171–96.
2. Wells JI, Aulton ME. Preformulation (chap. 13). In: Aulton ME, ed. Pharmaceutics: The Science of Dosage Form Design. Edinburgh: Churchill Livingstone, 1988, pp. 223–53.

3.  Wadke DA, Serajuddin ATM, Jacobson H. Preformulation testing (chap. 1). In: Lieberman HA, Lachman L, Schwartz JB, eds. Pharmaceutical Dosage Forms, 2nd ed., vol. 1. New York: Marcel Dekker, 1989, pp. 1–73.

4.  Carstensen JT. Preformulation (chap. 9). In: Carstensen JT, Rhodes CT, eds. Drug Stability, 3rd ed. New York: Marcel Dekker, 2000, pp. 237–60.

5.  Carstensen JT. Preformulation (chap. 7). In: Banker GS, Rhodes CT, eds. Modern Pharmaceutics, 4th ed. New York: Marcel Dekker, 2002, pp. 167–85.

6.  Ando HY, Radebaugh GW. Property-based drug design and preformulation (chap. 38). In: Hendrickson R, ed. Remington: The Science and Practice of Pharmacy, 21st edn. Philadelphia: Lippincott Williams & Wilkins, 2005, pp. 720–44.

7.  Higgins JD, Gilmor TP, Martellucci SA, Bruce RD, Brittain HG. Ibuprofen (chap. 6). In: HG Brittain, ed. Analytical Profiles of Drug Substances and Excipients, vol. 27, San Diego: Academic Press, 2001, pp. 265–300.

8.  Brittain HG. Strategy for the prediction and selection of drug substance salt forms. Pharm Tech 2007; 31(10):78–88.

9.  Anderson BD, Flora KP. Preparation of water-soluble compounds through salt formation (chap. 34). In: Wermuth CG, ed. The Practice of Medicinal Chemistry. New York: Academic Press, 1996, pp. 739–54.

10. Stahl PH, Wermuth CG. Handbook of Pharmaceutical Salts. Weinheim: Wiley-VCH, 2002.

11. Jacques J, Collet A, Wilen SH. Enantiomers, Racemates, and Resolutions. New York: John Wiley & Sons, 1981, pp. 43–81.

12. Brittain HG. Molecular motion and vibrational spectroscopy (chap. 7). In: Brittain HG, ed. Spectroscopy of Pharmaceutical Solids. New York: Taylor & Francis, 2006, pp. 205–33.

13. Monkhouse DC, Van Campen L. Solid State Reactions—Theoretical and Experimental Aspects. Drug Dev Indust Pharm 1984; 10:1175–276.

14. Byrn SR, Pfeiffer RR, Stowell JG. Solid-State Chemistry of Drugs, 2nd ed. West Lafayette: SSCI Inc., 1999.

15. Carstensen JT. Effect of moisture on the stability of solid dosage forms. Drug Dev Indust Pharm 1988; 14:1927–69.

16. Taylor LS, Zografi G. Spectroscopic characterization of interactions between PVP and indomethacin in amorphous molecular dispersions. Pharm Res 1997; 14:1691–98.

17. Al-Nimry SS, Assaf SM, Jalal IM, Najib NM. Adsorption of ketoifen onto some pharmaceutical excipients. Int J Pharm 1997; 149:115–21.

18. Guillory JK, Hwang SC, Lach JL. Interactions between pharmaceutical compounds by thermal methods. J Pharm Sci 1969; 58:301–8.

19. Wirth DD, Baertschi SW, Johnson RA, et al. Maillard reaction of lactose and fluoxetine hydrochloride, a secondary amine. J Pharm Sci 1998; 87:31–9.

20. Forbes RA, McGarvey BM, Smith DR. Measurement of residual isopropyl alcohol in loracarbef by near-infrared reflectance spectroscopy. Anal Chem 1999; 71:1232–9.

21. Stark G, Fawcett JP, Tucker IG, Weatherall IL. Instrumental evaluation of color of solid dosage forms during stability testing. Int J Pharm 1996; 143: 93–100.

*Part 2: Preliminary Preformulation*

# 2.1

# Accelerating the Course of Preliminary Preformulation Through Prediction of Molecular Physical Properties and Integrated Analytical Data Management

**Robert S. DeWitte and Michel Hachey**
*Advanced Chemistry Development, Inc., Toronto, Ontario, Canada*

**Harry G. Brittain**
*Center for Pharmaceutical Physics, Milford, New Jersey, U.S.A.*

## INTRODUCTION

Preformulation research is the necessary step that takes place between drug discovery and clinical development. In this vital phase of drug development, the physicochemical profile of the active pharmaceutical ingredient is determined and then used to plan the course of subsequent activities. One important activity is to plan a schedule of crystallization conditions in order to maximize the likelihood of finding polymorphs or solvatomorphs, since different crystal forms will likely exhibit different solution characteristics that may be either harmful or helpful toward a particular formulation.

Another important activity is to select excipients that enable the drug substance to be administered with its intended efficacy. Preformulation can therefore be described as the step that deals with the acquisition of data on the drug compound and its excipients, which are then analyzed or processed into information (properties and tendencies), and ultimately transformed (modeled) into knowledge in the form of a recommended formulation. The area of preliminary-preformulation represents the scope of activities that facilitate the design of preformulation studies and is often theoretical in nature.

Although conventional computers cannot match the creativity of the human mind in recognizing, associating, and interpreting data, they can assist scientists by organizing and reducing huge amounts of data to information or knowledge. In the context of preformulation, computers can enhance the consistency and speed of decision making, free experts from tedious tasks, retain the organization's expertise in a readily maintainable form, and provide knowledge for some specific problem. Computers make desirable outcomes possible through three principal capabilities: (*i*) effective data management, (*ii*) information generation and reporting, and (*iii*) prediction.

*Effective data management.* Preformulation scientists can benefit from a data management system owing to the wide range and large amount of data generated in their daily work programs. Consider, for example, that the preformulation scientist's interest in analytical data spans the standard spectroscopic techniques used by organic chemists (such as infrared absorption, Raman spectroscopy, and nuclear magnetic resonance), as well as traditional solid-state characterization techniques (such as X-ray diffraction and thermal analysis). Unless an analytical data management system (ADMS) is used, the late-stage preformulation scientist will not necessarily receive all of the information that has been measured during the conduct of early-stage investigations, or in the associated reports.

*Information generation and reporting.* A good data management system not only stores data, but also directly analyzes and processes this data into information, which can extend beyond the constraints of a particular technique or chemical property. Information can generally be defined as the relational connection between the data that provides meaning. In other words, it is an answer to a question. Generally, the more connections that can be made, the better equipped one becomes to answer questions. However, the ability to generate intelligent links between chemical structures, properties, and analytical data requires more than a simple relational database. It is highly desirable that the links be active rather than passive. For example, to find all previous reports and database entries related to a particular compound, one may execute a structure search if a real active structure object is used in the data file as opposed to a passive image of the structure. Since reports are the embodiment of answers to questions, flexible publication tools are a necessary facet of an information system for preformulation.

*Prediction.* Last, but not least, the ability of computers to find and exploit patterns in collected data and information yields direct knowledge, such as the ability to predict certain chemical or spectral behaviors from a structure. Because vast amounts of information on physicochemical properties already exist in the literature, models can be built that allow one to predict with good accuracy various physical properties (such as log $P$, $pK_a$, log $D$, and solubility) from the chemical structure. The computer's ability to generate these properties in a short amount of time provides inexpensive, rapid, useful, and early insight into the various preformulation issues that may be encountered. In addition, this early insight allows one to design better experiments at the onset that minimize the amount of work required to satisfy regulatory authorities.

In this chapter, we will introduce two practical methods whereby software can be used to accelerate the pace of preformulation research. The concept of preliminary preformulation is easy to state: to know everything that can be known before beginning a preformulation study. Therefore, we will first review the prediction of the physicochemical properties. Second, we will provide an overview of the advantages of an integrated ADMS and the computational tools that form intelligent links between chemical structures and analytical data to enable an efficient increase of laboratory throughput and information dissemination.

## PREDICT BEFORE YOU MEASURE

"Look before you leap into the unknown" is a common maxim that most would agree is good advice. To a large degree, the art and science of measuring thermodynamic properties can be accelerated when one has clear expectations. For example, it is possible to minimize the number of buffer solutions needed to explore the entire pH profile for the log $D$ or the solubility of a compound by choosing several pH values over regions of change, and fewer pH values along plateau areas. Some of the key questions, for a given compound, are the following: Where are the ionization centers that give rise to the various $pK_a$ values, and what is the effect of these on the intrinsic solubility? How many of the predicted ionized forms would be relevant to the formulation of the drug, or to its bioavailability? Armed with this proto-information, the researcher can select experimental conditions that give precise, useful, and timely measurements when the experiment is performed for the first time.

One can gain access to this preliminary information either by conducting screening measurements or by predicting the properties. In certain cases (such as titration studies), the screening measurements are straightforward, but in others (such as pH profiles), they involve a great deal of tedious experimentation. In general, predictive methods can be extremely straightforward; and as long as they are sufficiently accurate, predictions can provide immediate insight into the physical chemistry of the compound and aid in the design of appropriate experimentation. As a bonus, prediction may also provide a degree of understanding that is not readily extractable from the experiment. For example, measuring an accurate $pK_a$ value will not automatically indicate the molecular site of the ionization, whereas the predictive software would provide that assignment.

## Predictive Methods for Molecular Properties

Lipophilicity, $pK_a$, and aqueous solubility, among others, may be regarded as additive constitutive properties. Such properties are derived from the sum of the intrinsic properties of atoms or functional groups within the molecule, and constitutive properties depend on the structural arrangement of the atoms within the molecule. The full description of these algorithms and their theoretical foundations is beyond the scope of this chapter, and has been published elsewhere (1,2). However, it is appropriate to illustrate the computational approach through a summarization of the approaches used by Advanced Chemistry Development (ACD)/Labs in its predictive software programs.

### Calculation of Log *P*

The octanol–water partition coefficient is widely used as an estimation of the relative lipophilicity of a given compound. The log *P* algorithm used by ACD/Labs is based on the well-characterized log *P* contributions of separate atoms, structural fragments, and intramolecular interactions between different fragments. The basis of the ACD/log *P* approach for the prediction of log *P* can be described with reference to the following equation:

$$\log P = \sum f_n + \sum F_m \tag{1}$$

where *f* denotes atomic or fragmental increments, and *F* denotes correction factors. Figure 1 illustrates the fragments and interactions used in the log *P* calculation for a tautomeric form of sildenafil.

Using experimental data and a step-regression technique, simple compounds were studied on a class-by-class basis to derive the *f* and *F* parameters, and then more complex compounds were studied to derive further fragmental and interaction constants. This process was repeated until the most complex compounds had been used to define the entire listing of fragment increments and interaction patterns. In all cases, fragments were defined by applying the principle of the isolating carbon, a procedure that has been described elsewhere (1). It is important to note, however, that the *f* and *F* parameters so produced can be modeled by fundamental physical organic considerations.

Figure 2 shows the composition of the training set used in the calculation of log *P*, and Figure 3 shows the performance of the log *P* calculations against the BioByte Starlist of log *P* measurements. In the comparison of predicted and known log *P* values (for nearly 11,000 experimental values), the correlation was characterized by an $R^2$ parameter of 0.958 and an average error of only 0.213.

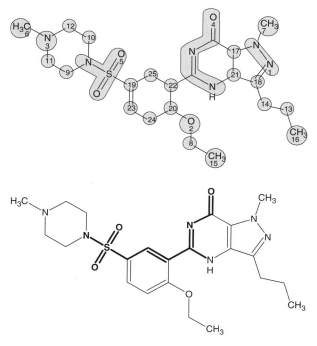

**Figure 1** Log *P* fragments and interactions for a tautomeric form of sildenafil. (*Top*) The fragments recognized according to the principle of isolating carbons are shaded. (*Bottom*) The aromatic interaction between two of the fragments. In this case the chain length is three (carbons 19-25-22).

## Calculation of p$K_a$

The general structure of the algorithm used in the prediction of ionization constants is one of classification, followed by a linear free energy (Hammett equation) relationship. The method uses sigma constants as descriptors of the electron withdrawal and/or donation potency of substituents electronically connected to the ionization center. When more than one ionization center is present in the compound of interest, the researcher must first identify all the separate transitions and their corresponding approximate p$K_a$ values in order to discover the correct sequence of ionizations. When two or more p$K_a$ values are similar in magnitude, multiple scenarios must be considered in order to understand the perturbing influence of one reaction on another. Doing so will serve to define the observable transitions, as well as the specific ionic form of the acid and conjugate base before and after ionization.

These specific ionic structures define the form of the Hammett equation that should be applied, and/or the appropriate sigma constants to be

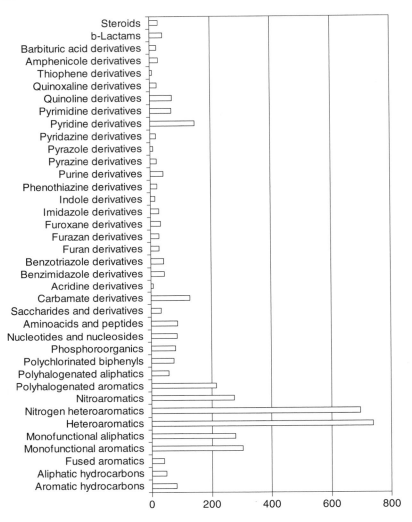

**Figure 2**  Composition of the training set used in the calculation of log *P* values.

used within the equations. The classes, sigma parameters, and Hammett equations were derived by a study of nearly 16,000 compounds having over 30,000 $pK_a$ values. The composition of this training set is given in Figure 4, and the correlation between the predicted $pK_a$ values associated with over 12,000 compounds with corresponding entries from the BioByte Masterfile is shown in Figure 5. The latter comparison of predicted $pK_a$ parameters for more than 12,000 experimental values was characterized by an $R^2$ parameter of 0.992 and an average error of 0.54.

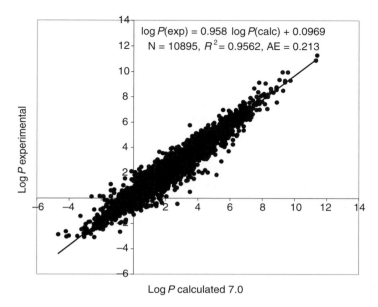

$$\log P(\text{exp}) = 0.958 \log P(\text{calc}) + 0.0969$$
$$N = 10895, R^2 = 0.9562, AE = 0.213$$

Log *P* calculated 7.0

**Figure 3** Correlation of the ACD/Labs method for calculation of log *P* against the BioByte Starlist of log *P* measurements.

## Calculation of Log *D*

The prediction of distribution coefficients (expressed as log *D*) is performed through an evaluation of the system of multiple equilibria associated with all possible ionic forms that would exist in solution at a specified pH value, and the partitioning of each ionic form between water and octanol. Each ionic form partitions with a different effective log *P\**. These log *P\** values are derived from the log *P* value (which is specifically defined only for the neutral form of the compound) by the addition of specific offset parameters that depend on where the charge is localized on the compound. These offset parameters were derived by studying the log *D* profiles of multiprotic compounds. As a means of illustration, Table 1 shows the log *P* correction factors corresponding to the ionic forms (i.e., microspecies) existing in the two-phase system that is used for the calculation of log *D* for albuterol.

The accuracy of log *D* predictions through the ACD/Labs algorithm depends on the accuracy of the pertinent log *P* calculation, as well as how close the pH is to one of the $pK_a$ values of the compound. If $|pH - pK_a| < 2$, the accuracy of the $pK_a$ term can have a large nonlinear effect on the accuracy of the log *D*. If the pH is such that the compound is nearly completely ionized, the accuracy will partially depend on the correction increments such as those in Table 1.

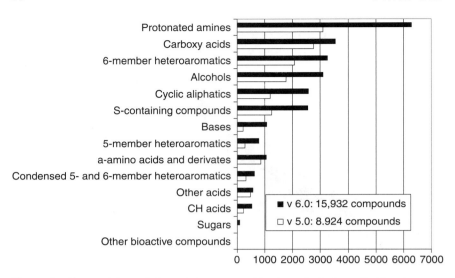

**Figure 4**   Composition of the training set used in the calculation of p$K_a$ values.

## Calculation of Solubility

The models built into the calculation of solubility are designed to be linear combinations of slowly varying physical functions, with at least an "ansatz" justifying their inclusion (i.e., one can construct a phenomenological defense of the resulting model). Where statistics allow, the models also contain a number of specific fragmental contributions. The resulting form of the models is therefore:

$$\log S = \alpha \log P + \beta MW + \gamma MV + \delta BP + \varepsilon HydBond + \zeta FRBonds$$
$$+ \eta Polariz + \lambda nd_{20} + \mu \Sigma Frg + \nu T_m + \text{constant} \qquad (2)$$

where $\log S$ is the intrinsic solubility, mol/L (logarithmic scale); $\log P$ is the octanol–water distribution ratio for partially dissociated compounds (logarithmic scale); MW is the molecular weight*; MV is the McGowan (3) molecular volume*; BP is the boiling point at 760 torr*; HydBond is the hydrogen bond parameter: $\exp(-(NA + ND))$; NA is the number of H-bond acceptors; ND is the number of H-bond donors (in some tables it is specified as exp $(-DA)$*); DA is the sum of hydrogen donors and hydrogen acceptors*; FRBonds is the number of free rotatable bonds*; Polariz is the polarizability*; $nd_{20}$ is the refraction index*; $\Sigma Frg$ is the sum of fragmental increments; and $T_m$ is the melting point (°C).

The parameters marked by an asterisk were calculated from the chemical structure of the molecule using ACD/PhysChem software. Experimental values of $\log S$ and $\log P$ were used to search for the best correlation equations.

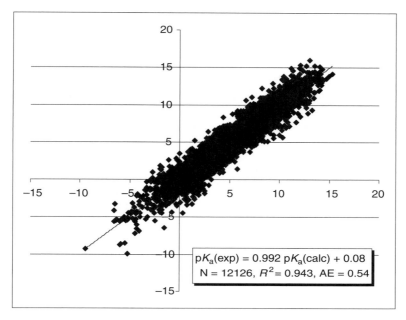

**Figure 5** Correlation of the ACD/Labs method for calculation of $pK_a$ against the BioByte Starlist of log $P$ measurements.

While models were built using the intrinsic solubilities culled from literature and database sources according to Equation 2, the prediction algorithm was implemented with the augmented formula shown in Equation 3 to allow computation of the pH dependence of the solubility, in which,

**Table 1** Log $P$ Correction Increments for Different Charge Locations Within the Multiple Ionic Forms Used in Calculating the Log $D$ of Albuterol

| | |
|---|---|
| *Monoanions* | |
| Charge on O or S near aromatic | −3.15 |
| Charge on O or S near aliphatic | −4.10 |
| | |
| *Monocations* | |
| Charge not near aromatic | −3.10 |
| *Zwitterions* | |
| Zwitterionic correction | −2.50 |
| | |
| *Other charged forms* | |
| Summing charge −1 | −3.5 |
| Summing charge −2 | −4.5 |
| Summing charge −3 | −6.1 |

$$\log S(\mathrm{pH}) = \alpha \log D + \beta \mathrm{MW} + \gamma \mathrm{MV} + \delta \mathrm{BP} + \varepsilon \mathrm{HydBond} + \zeta \mathrm{FRBonds}$$
$$+ \eta \mathrm{Polariz} + \lambda \mathrm{nd}_{20} + \mu \Sigma \mathrm{Frg} + \nu T_{\mathrm{m}} + \mathrm{constant} \qquad (3)$$

where $\log D$ is the octanol–water distribution ratio for partially dissociated compounds (logarithmic scale).

The composition of this training set is given in Figure 6, and results from prediction are given in Figure 7. The comparison with the $\log S$ of over 2000 compounds was characterized by an $R^2$ parameter of 0.87.

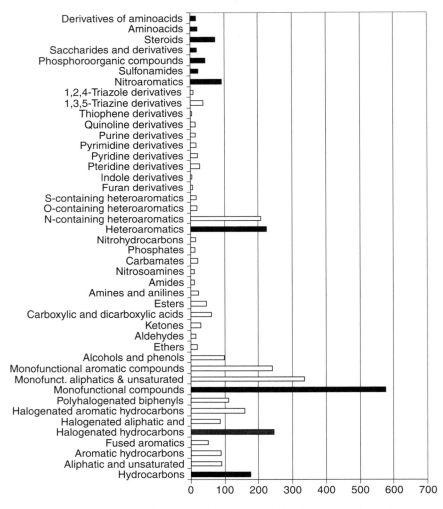

**Figure 6** Composition of the training set used in the prediction of aqueous solubility. The black bars indicate the major classes of compounds covered, and the white bars that precede these indicate subclasses.

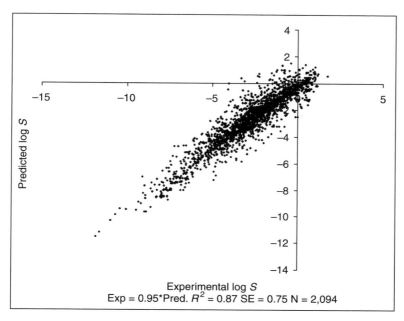

**Figure 7** Correlation of the ACD/Labs method for calculation of log *S* versus experimental values for a set of 2094 compounds.

## How ACD/Labs Software Presents Predictive Results

As an example of the computational approach, the use of ACD/Labs predictive software will be employed. Figures 8 through 11 show screen images obtained for the results of calculations performed to predict the molecular physical properties of Indinavir, an antiviral compound. These calculations only required a few minutes on a laptop computer. It is therefore feasible, and highly informative, to calculate the fundamental properties of a new compound and use the predicted values to design experiments before performing any actual lab experiments.

## ANALYTICAL DATA MANAGEMENT IN PREFORMULATION

Starting with the predicted and existing knowledge about the active ingredient, the preformulation group initiates a number of experimental studies that generate a large amount of new data designed to create as complete a knowledge base as possible. The first sequence of studies entails crystallization and environmental exposure conditions in an attempt to obtain quantities of all polymorphs and solvatomorphs of the compound. These products are usually characterized by X-ray powder diffraction (XRPD),

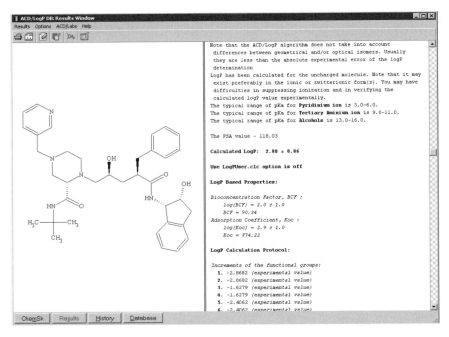

**Figure 8**   Results of log *P* calculation with ACD/log *P* DB. Log *P* is reported, along with statistical uncertainty. In addition, the entire computational protocol is explained, so that the scientist can understand how the summary value was attained and make an independent judgment about his or her degree of trust in the result.

thermal analysis, and at least one solid-state spectroscopic technique. This process ends with identifying the chosen form that will be the subject of continued development.

Once the desired form of the active ingredient is chosen, mixtures of the active ingredient with suitable excipients are subjected to a battery of stress conditions. These stress conditions are designed to reveal possible changes or reactions in the mixtures that indicate the existence of distinct physical or chemical interactions. The stability of these samples is monitored through a variety of techniques including chromatography, optical spectroscopy, XRPD, and traditional solid-state spectroscopy.

It is clear that even if considers just these two programs of study, one would be dealing with a great deal of information, involving a number of laboratories and scientific groups. One of the main challenges in the heterogeneous preformulation environment is ensuring that the various scientists can take advantage of all previous experimental results derived from a variety of prior research activities. For instance, the knowledge base prediction software discussed in the section titled "Predict Before You

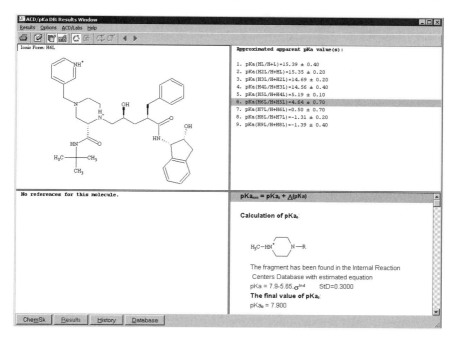

**Figure 9** Although indinavir has nine ionization centers, only two of them are of physiological importance. These two basic ionize sequentially, so that calculation of the second basic center must take into account the fact that one substituent is charged. This and other calculation details are explained in the protocol listed in the bottom right pane.

Measure" is in fact a striking example of literature results being applied directly to preformulation problems.

Unfortunately, despite the best efforts at making complete reports, exchanging data within a laboratory or organization may be much more difficult than obtaining information from the literature, since there is often no convenient local knowledge base. It is not a given that the late-stage preformulation scientist will be provided with all the required information by the early-stage colleagues. One important question to be considered is how much time is spent trying to find information that was omitted in early reports? Then, if the information cannot be found, how much time must be expended to repeat the experiment? Finally, is the insight from previous studies used to design better experiments in cases where new information, troubleshooting, or formulation fixing are required? It is clear that development without optimization of information archiving and transfer is highly inefficient.

This section will use the ACD/Labs' ADMS to illustrate how one may use a platform for capturing data, tracking information, comparing

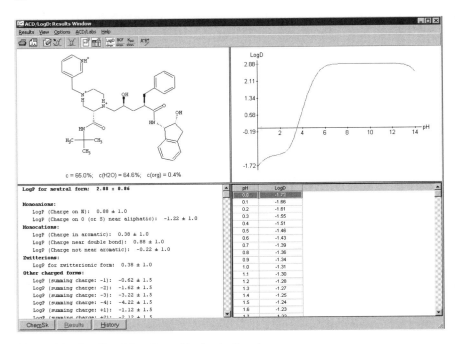

**Figure 10** Predicted log *D* profile for indinavir.

data to the spectral signatures of the active ingredients, and using the comparisons to deduce robust formulations, as well as to prepare comprehensive reports.

## An Integrated ADMS

First, data from the multidisciplinary mix of instruments and techniques must be captured or entered into the system. Ideally, this data is directly loaded with import filters capable of reading the raw instrument file format, public format, or generic ASCII-type formats. The ACD/Labs ADMS, for example, offers on average 17 different import filters per module, and permits batch imports if a large amount of data is collected. Since these data formats are often common to more than one instrument, this system provides easy data capture for a wide number of instruments.

Figure 12 shows the conceptual organization of this suite of programs designed to provide a comprehensive ADMS, which includes support for the mainstream analytical technologies. Each rectangular box represents a computational module, and the boxes together form a complete suite of expert tools for analyzing and processing chromatograms, one-dimensional and two-dimensional nuclear magnetic resonance spectra, mass spectra (including

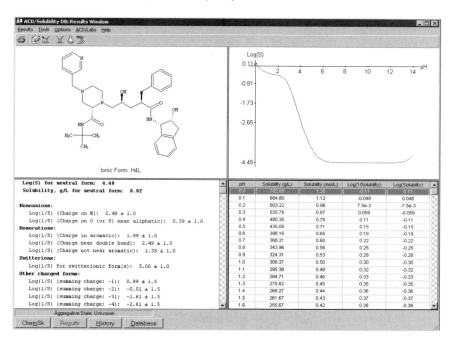

**Figure 11**   Predicted pH profile of aqueous solubility for indinavir.

liquid chromatography–mass spectrometry and gas chromatography–mass spectrometry), optical spectroscopy (including Raman, infrared, near-infrared, ultraviolet-visible, circular dichroism, and ellipsometry), and other analytical curves [including thermogravimetric analysis (TGA), differential scanning calorimetry (DSC), and XRPD]. The processing and analysis of data and conversion to information can be performed manually, interactively, or automatically in a batch-like macro. If desired, common preprocessing and analysis tasks can be performed as part of the data-capture process. The results are displayed graphically, in tabular form, or as data entries, whichever is appropriate. The inclusion of a generic module to handle analytical curves that are not captured by the common spectroscopic, spectrometric, and separation categories is important, and permits the handling of thermal analysis methods, X-ray diffraction data, etc.

The Curve Manager module is designed to provide a flexible data-handling package for any type of $x$–$y$ data plot. It includes built-in generic tools (e.g., differentiation, smoothing, baseline, integration) as well as custom tool-building capabilities. For example, a transform function allows the user to specify a formula to linearize the response, normalize the curve, or even do something as simple as converting units on an axis (e.g., changing the $x$-axis of an XRPD pattern from scattering angles to interplanar distances). Together, these six modules provide a sufficiently broad coverage of analytical techniques to support most preformulation endeavors.

In Figure 12, the processor boxes are enclosed in rounded rectangles to indicate a common interface that provides consistent visualization, storage, retrieval, reporting, and, to some degree, universal analysis and processing functions. For example, the interface includes a built-in structure-drawing package and database-searching tools. The structure-drawing package is a key component, since it provides the intelligent chemical structure objects that are used in the prediction engines, as well as for characterizing the analytical data stored in the ADMS. It is possible to attach a structure to a record, and then use a command to populate the record with the predicted physicochemical properties for that compound (requires the corresponding predictor engine). At the same time, the chemical structure object enables advanced searches based on structure, substructure, structural similarity, and Markush representation. Using the chemical structure of the active ingredient provides a rallying point around which the properties and analytical data can be organized in a chemically meaningful way. This software system facilitates the reduction of the paper trail and can increase data access through the shared database.

Continuing the exploration of Figure 12, we observe that the dark connecting lines join the different modules to one another, indicating that these are all linked. Further, the lines connect the modules to various commercial databases of reference spectra and to user-created databases of analytical data, ensuring persistent storage of information. The ADMS supports local databases (Spec DB Flat) and optionally may also support enterprise-scale databases (Spec DB SQL) through Oracle technology. The ADMS allows the user to make complex searches of multiple databases simultaneously with a combination of logical (Boolean), comparison, and containment operators (in range). This means that a scientist gains real-time access to the information in the database through a variety of different search strategies, whether it is stored locally or at remote sites.

Finally, templates and macros can be designed to automate the production of professional reports in standard electronic formats. The printing template allows customization of the report, and can include multiple techniques, the chemical structure, the analytical data, and more. In the following sections, specific examples will be given of the system described above.

## Measuring Physicochemical Properties

After the prediction and experiment planning work is performed, specific measurements will be made, and the results of these become critical pieces of the overall preformulation study. Shown in Figure 13 are different views of this type of data, captured from the RefinementPro™ software, which

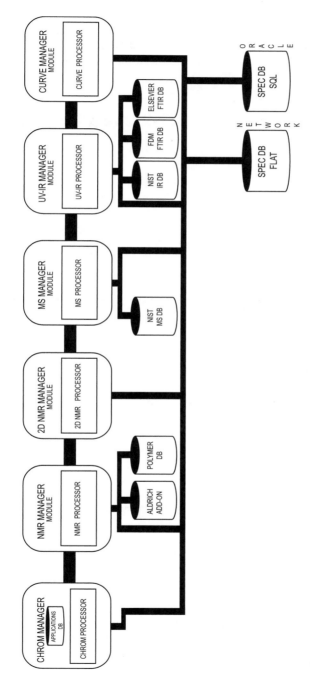

**Figure 12** A schematic of the ACD/Lab's Analytical Data Management system that spans all of the major analytical techniques, and provides for the capture, interpretation, and management of other techniques.

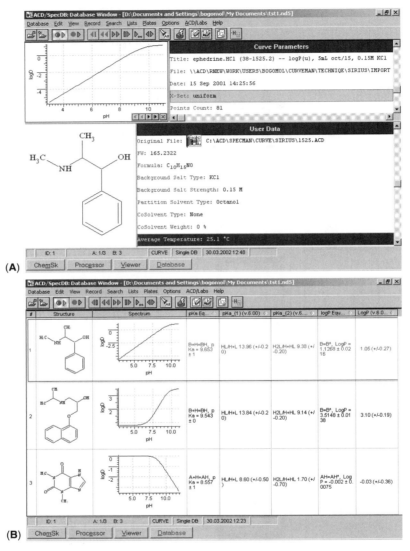

**Figure 13** Capturing the results of measurements of log *D* versus pH profiles from the Sirius RefinementPro™ software, which accompanies their instruments for p$K_a$ and log *D* determination. The images are screens from ACD/Curve Manager showing one record in detail (**A**) and summary information from several records in a table view (**B**). ACD/Curve Manager is able to directly read the output from the RefinementPro software and allows the user to attach the chemical structure, the key experimental parameters, and several additional important pieces of information that the user defines (these might include compound ID numbers, notebook number references, scientist name, and other critical observations).

accompanies the popular Sirius instrument for log *D* evaluation. The simulated log *D* profile generated using this software represents the result of hours of lab work, but is readily accessible to investigators having search access privileges on ADMS. If a large database of these profiles is built-up over time, then structure similarity searches may also provide hits that are sufficiently close to give some early insight into the expected behavior.

## Differential Scanning Calorimetry

Among other things, DSC is used to obtain information regarding the thermally induced phase transitions characteristic of a sample and to measure the enthalpy content of these transitions. DSC plays an essential role in assessing whether the thermal properties of a given sample are similar to, or qualitatively distinct from, another sample. It is used to help determine the occurrence of polymorphism, drug–excipient compatibility, moisture content, glass transitions, melting points, and freeze-drying optimization, and in purity studies and the study of liposomes. Applied to an ensemble of crystals from a variety of crystallization conditions, DSC thermograms can often be used to distinguish multiple polymorphs from one another.

Figure 14 illustrates the manipulation of DSC thermograms within the ADMS. The peaks were picked automatically, and the peak area range was selected interactively. Note that the chemical structure representation supports two-dimensional polymeric drawing conventions, if necessary.

## X-Ray Powder Diffraction

XRPD is used as the primary means to establish the crystallography of a sample and is able to provide a necessary unique fingerprint of the solid form of different solids. To illustrate the use of databasing, Figure 15 shows the results of peak picking for an XRPD spectrum of sucrose, as well as the corresponding infrared and Raman spectra. The example shows that it is easy to deal simultaneously with complementary data obtained using different techniques.

## Thermogravimetric Analysis

TGA is used as an adjunct during preformulation research, providing a considerable amount of support to the many studies conducted during this phase of development. TGA is used to measure the degree of mass lost by a sample during a programmed heating profile and is used to provide insight into important factors such as hygroscopicity, glass transition, volatility, sublimation capability, decomposition, and thermo-oxidative degradations. It is common to differentiate a thermogram with respect to time in order to more effectively distinguish the rates of loss at each step.

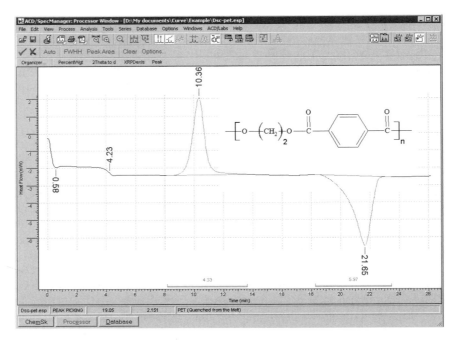

**Figure 14**  Differential scanning calorimetry results for a polyethylene terephthalate polymer. The peak minima and maxima were picked using the auto-peak-picking function. The area between curve and baseline has been integrated.

The analysis of TGA thermograms requires the ability to differentiate the scan, to measure *y*-axis distances between points, and to transform the axis from absolute weight loss to percent weight loss. As illustrated in Figure 16, all of these capabilities can be found, or set up, within the ADMS.

**Other Techniques**

It is critical to realize that the techniques highlighted in the previous sections do not represent the complete gamut of techniques normally applied in preformulation research. In addition, workers in the field also make use of optical spectroscopy, liquid chromatography, mass spectrometry, and solid-state nuclear magnetic resonance to obtain important information for the complete characterization of the properties of a sample in solution, in solid form, or in conjunction with excipients. It is beyond the scope of this review to completely describe these capacities of the ADMS, but the interested reader is referred to information at their web site (4), as well as the links contained therein.

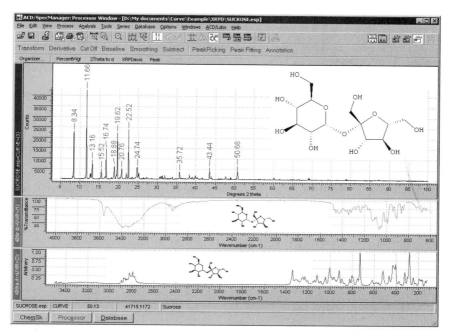

**Figure 15** The X-ray powder diffraction spectrum captured within ACD/Curve Manager, with peaks picked and labeled. The infrared and Raman spectrum of sucrose are tiled in the same display and processing interface.

## Reporting

At the completion of a comprehensive characterization program conducted on an active ingredient in conjunction with its excipients and various solid forms, the resulting interpretations must be compiled into various reports. Without a comprehensive ADMS, preparing such a report can involve days of tedious manipulation in various independent software programs followed by graphic format conversions (where possible) to consolidate the results. Often, such electronic means are not even possible, and specialized printouts must be appended to the report.

The comprehensive ADMS described in this review carries with it a sophisticated report template generation scheme that allows one to specify the page layout of all data elements captured within. In this manner, one can standardize reporting and, through the use of macro commands, automatically generate reports. These reports can be exported in Adobe Acrobat (PDF) and/or Microsoft Word formats, allowing them to be shared and stored electronically. An example is shown in Figure 17.

Since the report is searchable by the chemical structures contained within it, they can in this case be characterized as dynamic in character, as

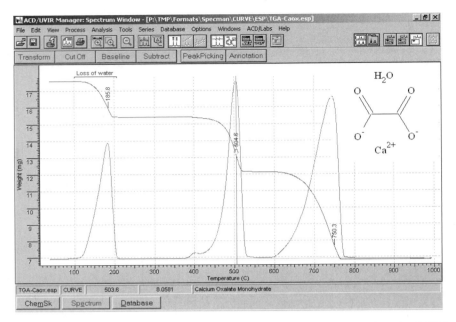

**Figure 16** Thermogravimetric analysis of calcium oxalate monohydrate in ACD/ Curve Manager along with the differentiated thermal analysis curve processed from it.

opposed to being merely static in nature. An important feature of the search capabilities is that searches are not confined to just the ADMS. One can search electronic files containing a specific structure in Microsoft Word, Excel, or PowerPoint, Adobe Acrobat, ACD/ChemSketch, in the chemical table format data files (SDfiles, molfiles, etc.), as well as in ACD/Labs databases, whether they are from the predictor or from the ADMS.

## CONCLUSIONS

Some of the most time-consuming aspects of a preformulation study can be greatly streamlined by using molecular prediction software and advanced experiment-processing tools that are united in a common database architecture (i.e., automated report generation). This chapter outlined how prediction tools can be used to generate physicochemical predictions that minimize the number of experiments needed in preformulation, as well as provide insight into the chemical behavior. Then, the impact of an integrated ADMS was discussed in terms of its ability to provide real-time access to data and to form information links between properties, analytical data, and chemical structures. These links could then be exploited to provide as complete a report as possible.

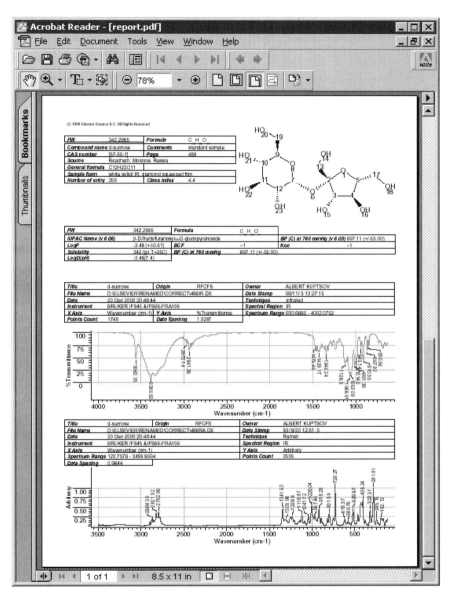

**Figure 17** An example of a multitechnique report with spectra and instrument parameters, including predicted physicochemical data and searchable chemical structure.

## REFERENCES

1.  DeWitte RS. Prediction of molecular physical properties. In: Borchardt RT, Middaugh CR, eds. Biotechnology: Pharmaceutical Aspects, vol. 2. Pharmaceutical Profiling in Drug Discovery for Lead Selection. Arlington, VA: AAPS Press, 2003.
2.  McGowan JC, Mellors A. Molecular Volumes in Chemistry and Biology: Applications Including Partitioning and Toxicity. Chichester: Ellis Harwood, 1986.
3.  Petrauskas AA, Kolovanov EA. Perspect Drug Discov Design 2000; 19:1–19.
4.  www.acdlabs.com/products.

# 2.2

# Prediction of Crystallographic Characteristics

Stephen Spanton

*GPRD Structural Chemistry, Abbott Laboratories, Abbott Park, Illinois, U.S.A.*

## INTRODUCTION

The crystal form of a compound gives rise to both physical and chemical properties that are unique to that crystal form. The physical properties are crystal habit, melting point, solubility, rate of desolvation, color, and mechanical properties. The chemical stability of a compound is a function of its crystal form. The understanding of these properties is important in the development of a compound for use in a wide range of applications.

Computational methods can extract additional structural information from X-ray data and provide the basis for understanding the physical and chemical properties of a crystal form. There are computational methods for obtaining the atomic coordinates from single-crystal X-ray data and X-ray powder diffraction (XPD) data. The solution of single-crystal X-ray data sets is a well-established technique, and there are a number of software packages available that can be used to obtain the solution (1,2). The use of these methods is well established and will not be discussed further. The ability to obtain atomic coordinates from XPD data has been developed over the last several years, and there are now several packages that provide these computational methods.

Once the atomic coordinates of a crystal form have been determined, they can then be used to predict the properties of the crystal form. The theoretical XPD pattern can be calculated from the atomic coordinates. An experimental powder pattern can then be analyzed against the theoretical XPD pattern for preferred orientation, purity of the crystal form, and the average shape of the sample (3). The morphology of the crystal form can be predicted by several methods. An investigation of the fastest growing faces can provide information that will lead to the development of a custom additive that will bind to the crystal face, causing a modification of the morphology (4).

## CRYSTAL STRUCTURE DETERMINATION OF XPD

There are numerous situations where suitable crystals cannot be obtained for single-crystal X-ray analysis (5,6). The growing of high-quality single crystals typically requires slow growing conditions where the degree of super saturation is low. Bulk materials are generally crystallized in a rapid process where there is a high degree of supersaturation that leads to a metastable crystal form (kinetic control). If the compound exhibits multiple crystal forms, then the thermodynamically more stable polymorphs will typically be created in the slow crystallizations. Therefore, it may not be possible to obtain suitable single crystals of these kinetic products for single-crystal X-ray analysis.

There is a range of quality of crystals in bulk material, which is the result of crystallization conditions and the polymorphic form. The XPD pattern will show the crystal quality and will determine which technique can be used to solve for the three-dimensional structure. Figure 1 shows a representation of the different degrees of crystal quality and the resulting diffraction patterns. The highest-quality crystals result in single crystals that are suitable for single-crystal X-ray analysis. With the introduction of charge-coupled device (CCD) area detectors, the crystal size needed for routine single-crystal X-ray analysis is down to about ~0.4 mm. The next quality of samples produce XPD patterns that have well-resolved lines and have good intensity out to 35°2. These patterns may be indexed and provide sufficient peaks that their structures may be determined with powder solution methods. The third category of samples produces low-quality patterns that do not index or provide few peaks.

The structures of these materials can sometimes be determined by polymorph prediction software.

## DIRECT SOLUTIONS

Solving a good-quality XPD pattern for the three-dimensional coordinates is possible with the development of software packages such as Powder Solve (7,8), Dash (9,10), Endeavour (11), and Espoir (12).

Solving good-quality XPD patterns has several steps, as shown in Figure 2. The success of the subsequent steps is dependent on the data and decisions made in the previous steps. Therefore, care should be taken at each step. The steps of the process are sample preparation, data collection, determination of the unit cell, refinement of unit cell and powder pattern parameters, determination of space group, building the model, solution search, and structure refinement. The example that will be discussed is a metastable intermediate between a solvate and the thermodynamically most

## Types of XPD data

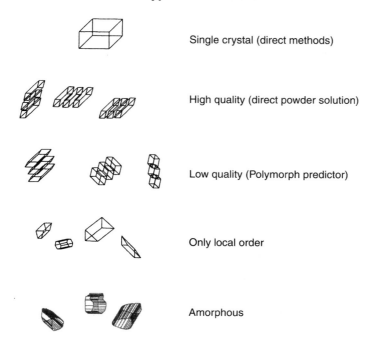

Single crystal (direct methods)

High quality (direct powder solution)

Low quality (Polymorph predictor)

Only local order

Amorphous

**Figure 1** Solid materials can have different states of crystallinity. The techniques used to extract information and build models are highly dependent on crystallinity.

stable form (13). Clarithromycin (Fig. 3) can be crystallized as an ethanol solvate, form 0. This solvate rapidly loses ethanol to form a stable non-solvate, form 1. Upon heating to about 80°C, form 1 is converted to form 2. Form 2 is the most thermodynamically stable form. The structures of form 0 and form 2 have been solved with standard single-crystal analysis. The unit cell parameters are listed in Table 1.

The preparation of the sample for XPD data collection is important to ensure that no preferred orientation or large single crystals are present. These conditions are necessary to ensure that the data does not have any systematic errors in the measured intensity.

Microscopic examination of the powder with a polarized light micro-scope can reveal information about the purity of the phase and sample pre-paration necessary. Many solvates are unstable and will readily lose solvent and convert to another crystal form. This transformation results in a loss of crystallinity and can produce a metastable crystal form that cannot be pro-duced directly. Therefore, the crystals should be observed before removal from the crystallization medium and then again after they are removed from

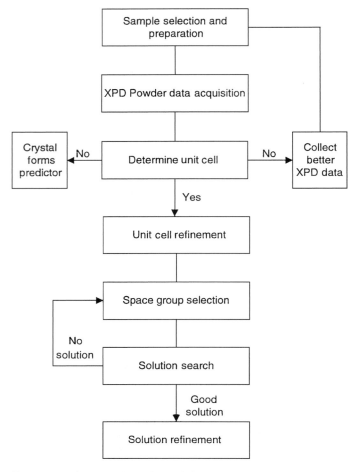

**Figure 2**  The workflow for solving a high-quality XPD pattern for its crystal structure. *Abbreviation*: XPD, X-ray powder diffraction.

the crystallization medium for changes indicating a loss of solvent. The presence of crystals with different habits can indicate that there is more than one crystal form present. If the crystal habit is either plates or needles, when the sample is packed into the sample holder, there will be a preferred orientation of the crystals. The sample can be ground to produce a more uniform powder. Care must be taken with any sample preparation method to prevent changes in the crystal form due to the preparation conditions.

There are a number of different systems that can be used for data collection. The conventional laboratory XPD system is the most commonly available instrument. These systems have good resolution, but have the lowest sensitivity of the systems and are not designed to reduce preferred

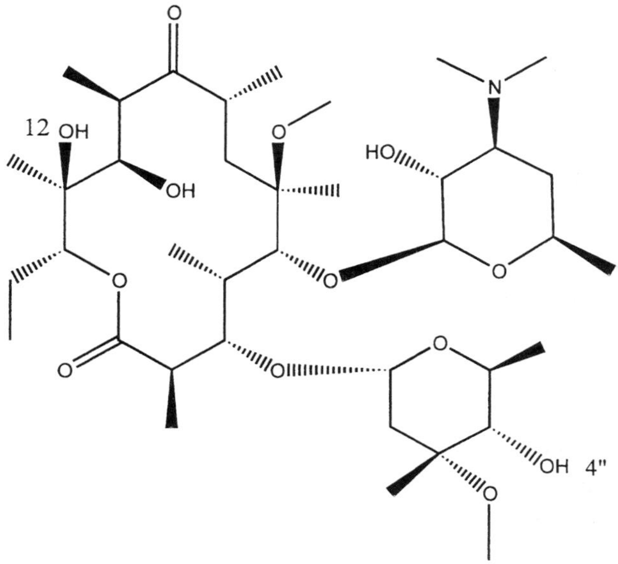

**Figure 3** The chemical structure of clarithromycin.

orientation. Area detectors are available for the collection of XPD using conventional laboratory X-ray sources (14,15). These systems have the limitation that there can be no exit filter or monochromator. As a result, there is no method of filtering out X-ray fluorescence. There are synchrotron beam lines that have powder diffraction systems. Synchrotron XPD systems

**Table 1** Unit Cell Parameters for Clarithromycin Forms as Determined by Single-Crystal X-Ray or XPD Analysis

|  | Form 0 | Form 1 | Form 2 |
|---|---|---|---|
| Crystal class | Orthorhombic | Orthorhombic | Orthorhombic |
| Space group | $P_{2_12_12_1}$ | $P_{2_12_12_1}$ | $P_{2_12_12_1}$ |
| Unit cell length | $a = 14.65190$ | $a = 34.0517(9)$ | $a = 20.134(1)$ |
|  | $b = 38.99639$ | $b = 14.3597(1)$ | $b = 23.945(2)$ |
|  | $c = 8.866700$ | $c = 8.6862(1)$ | $c = 8.840(2)$ |
| Unit cell angles | $\alpha = \beta = \gamma = 90°$ | $\alpha = \beta = \gamma = 90°$ | $\alpha = \beta = \gamma = 90°$ |
| Molecules in unit cell | 4 | 4 | 4 |
| Cell volume | 5066(7) | 4246 | 4272(1) |
| Density | 1.04 | 1.17 | 1.17 |

*Abbreviation*: XPD, X-ray powder diffraction.

have the highest resolution and sensitivity among the three systems. Each type of system has its own set of requirements on how the data needs to be collected for optimum results. The indexing of the XPD needs high-resolution data, and the intensity measurements need the highest sensitivity. For indexing the XPD pattern, the data should be collected with the highest resolution possible so that accurate peak positions can be determined. To improve the resolution, on conventional laboratory XPD systems, the slit width is reduced. This results in a decrease in the sensitivity. A second XPD pattern should be collected with a wider slit width and extended counting times. If there are other known crystal forms of the compound, the XPD pattern should be reviewed for the presence of crystal forms. The difference in the powder patterns collected with the different techniques can be seen in Figure 4.

The next step in the process is the determination of the unit cell. The peak positions in the XPD pattern must be determined. Approximately 25 peaks need to be determined. The peak positions are used to determine possible unit cells. There are a number of indexing applications that are

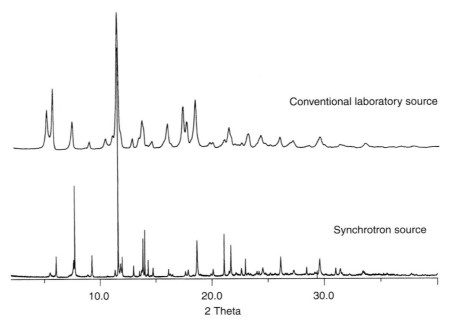

**Figure 4**  A comparison of XPD patterns of clarithromycin collected with a conventional laboratory diffractometer and with a synchrotron diffractometer. *Abbreviation*: XPD, X-ray powder diffraction.

available for indexing powder patterns such as DICVOL (16), TREOR (17), or X-Cell (18). The indexing results should be reviewed to make sure that most of the peaks are indexed and for the presence of a reasonable unit cell volume. A reasonable volume range can be determined by multiplying the number of nonhydrogen atoms by 18 A for the lower limit and by 20 A for the upper limit. A careful review of the peaks may show that there are different peak shapes; this can indicate that the sample is not a single phase. Try selecting only those peaks that have similar peak shapes. A second problem can be that the XPD pattern exhibits a preferred orientation or a short crystallographic axis that will cause a zone of reflections to be underrepresented in the XPD pattern. In this case, the X-Cell application will search for zones and refine the two-dimensional cell parameters. The remaining cell parameters will be determined from the peaks that were not assigned to the initial zone.

Many attempts to crystallize clarithromycin in form 1 failed to produce crystals suitable for single-crystal analysis. The next approach was to use the XPD pattern to solve for the structure. The indexing programs mentioned above were unable to find a reasonable solution from the conventional laboratory XPD system. An XPD pattern obtained on a synchrotron system (19) was indexed with DICVOL. The solutions with the highest figure of merit were monoclinic and orthorhombic crystal systems (Table 2). Both of these solutions have reasonable volumes, and the cell lengths are consistent with the other crystal forms in this transformation pathway. In the first trial, the orthorhombic cell was selected because both the other forms are orthorhombic.

In the next step, the unit cell parameters, data parameters, and sample parameters should be refined. The unit cell parameters are the unit cell lengths and angles that are not fixed by the crystal lattice. The data collection parameter is the zero point error or the sample height misalignment. The sample parameters are the background, peak shape, particle size, and sample strain. The space group used during this refinement phase should be one that does not have any systemic absences. The *R* factor is a measure of the fit between the parameters and the experimental XPD pattern. If there is a large baseline offset, then removing just the offset will result in a small *R*

**Table 2** The Top Indexing Result for the Synchrotron Data on Form 1 Using DICVOL

| FOM | System | $A$ | $B$ | $C$ | $\alpha$ | $\beta$ | $\gamma$ | Volume |
|------|-------------|----------|----------|----------|--------|--------|--------|---------|
| 19.9 | Monoclinic | 34.06453 | 8.68500 | 14.35463 | 90.000 | 90.034 | 90.000 | 4246.82 |
| 19.0 | Orthorhombic | 34.06747 | 14.36450 | 8.68449 | 90.000 | 90.000 | 90.000 | 4249.86 |

*Abbreviation*: FOM, figure of merit.

factor. This baseline contribution does not represent the fitting of experimental data to the unit cell and peak shape. Therefore, it is better to use the $R$ factor without the baseline correction component. The result of this process is a peak list of $H\ K\ L$ and intensity.

The synchrotron XPD pattern for clarithromycin form 1 showed different peak shapes for different classes of reflections. The peak shape anisotropy was refined as crystal lattice strain parameter. The lattice strain was greatest along the $A$ axis, as shown in Figure 5. From both the conventional laboratory data and the synchrotron data, there is evidence of a second crystal form in the powder patterns, shown by the presence of peaks that are not indexed. These peaks can be assigned to peaks in form 2.

The next step is the determination of the space group. The list of $H\ K\ L$ values is reviewed for the presence of systematic absences. The international tables provide a listing of systematic absences for each of the space groups. The data from the XPD pattern is often limited, and an unambiguous assignment of the space group is not possible. A second method is to refine

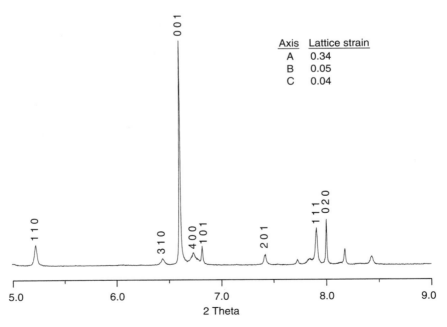

**Figure 5**  XPD peak shape analysis. The peaks that have a component for the *a*-axis are broadened, indicating more disorder along this axis. *Abbreviation*: XPD, X-ray powder diffraction.

**Table 3** The Refinement of Form 1 Against Possible Orthorhombic Space Groups

| | | |
|---|---|---|
| $P_{222}$ | 18.80 | 12.52 |
| $P_{222_1}$ | 31.81 | 18.76 |
| $P_{22_12}$ (a-bc) | 18.81 | 12.52 |
| $P_{2_122}$ | 18.98 | 12.59 |
| $P_{22_12}$ (bca) | 18.81 | 12.52 |
| $P_{2_12_12}$ | 18.98 | 12.59 |
| $P_{2_122_1}$ (a-cb) | 31.91 | 18.83 |
| $P_{2_122_1}$ (c-ab) | 31.82 | 18.67 |
| $P_{22_12_1}$ (bca) | 31.91 | 18.83 |
| $P_{2_12_12_1}$ | 31.92 | 18.83 |

The groups with the lower $R$ values represent space groups with systematic absences that are consistent with the XPD pattern.
*Abbreviation*: XPD, X-ray powder diffraction.

the XPD pattern against all the possible space groups. The possible space groups for this phase are those that have the lowest $R$ factors.

The form 1 powder pattern was refined against each of the different settings in each of the space groups (16–19). The results shown in Table 3 indicate that there are five possible settings. The space group $P_{2_12_12}$ was chosen for the first trial because it has the highest symmetry among the space groups and is closest to the space group of both the starting and the final crystal form.

The time required for the structure search is dependent on the number of degrees of freedom. The model will have three degrees of translational freedom, three degrees of rotational freedom for each molecule, and internal torsional rotation. The next step is preparing a model of the chemical structure having the minimum degrees of freedom that accurately represents the molecule. If other crystal forms have been solved for this compound, these structures can be used as starting models. The Cambridge Structure Database (CSD) (20) should be searched for related structural fragments.

If the degrees of freedom are too large, then some of the bond rotations may be restricted to one or a few values. The bonds in the molecule are reviewed to determine which one can have free rotation. If a bond has restricted rotation, a search of the CSD will provide a most probable torsional angle. These bonds can then be restricted to one of the most probable torsional angles. If the structure cannot be solved, then the other possible torsional angles need to be used in the XPD solution application. An example of a less common torsional angle conformation in the most stable crystal form can be found in the second crystal form of Norvir (Fig. 6) (21). This crystal form shows a carbamate

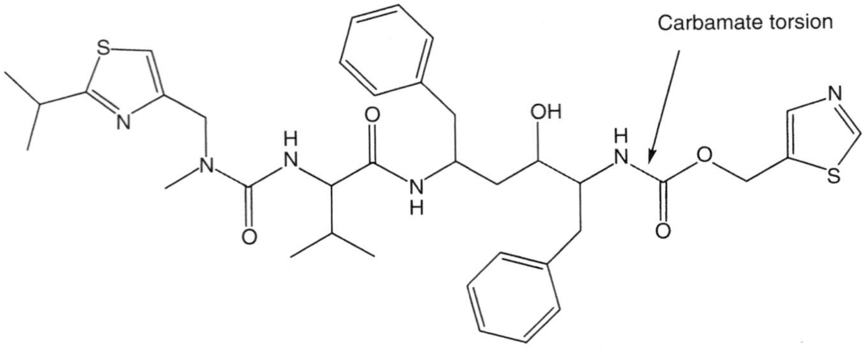

| Torsion angle | Form I | Form II |
|---|---|---|
| Carbamate bond | −178 (trans) | −8 (cis) |

**Figure 6** The more stable crystal form has a *cis* carbamate bond. This example illustrates the need for care in the selection of bond for fix geometry during the solution phase.

bond torsional angle that has a low frequency of occurrence in the CSD as shown in Figure 7.

The model for the clarithromycin form 1 was taken for the X-ray structure of the thermodynamically most stable form. The bonds between the 14-member macrocycle and the sugar moieties are allowed to rotate. This gave a model with ten degrees of freedom (three translational, three rotational, and four torsional).

The Monte Carlo/simulated annealing is then run to determine if a possible structure can be found in the selected space group. The process is repeated for each possible space group.

Powder Solve found a chemically reasonable solution in space group $P2_12_12$. The hydrogen-bonding network that is present in the ethanoate solvate, form 0 (Fig. 8) and form 2 (Fig. 9), was also present in form 1 (Fig. 10). The only intermolecular hydrogen bond is between the 12 alcohol and the 4" alcohol. The crystal symmetry is preserved along the *B* and *C* crystallographic axis in going from the ethanol solvate to form 1. This also provides an explanation for the increased lattice strain along the *A* axis.

The final step is to refine the structure against the powder pattern. At this point, additional degrees of freedom can be allowed.

## PREDICTION OF POLYMORPH

If the XPD pattern cannot be solved directly because of poor quality, an alternative approach is to use a crystal form prediction tool. The theoretical

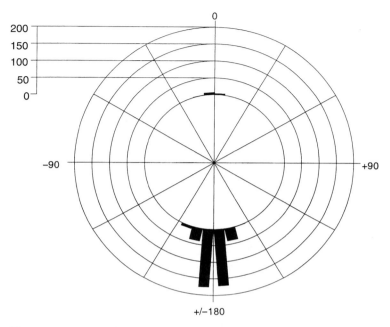

**Figure 7** The distribution of acyclic carbamate torsional angles from the CSD. *Abbreviation*: CSD, Cambridge Structure Database.

XPD pattern can then be compared with the experimental pattern to determine which crystal form fits the experimental data. The steps that are involved in determining a potential crystal structure using a polymorph prediction method are shown on Figure 11. The example that will be presented is the determination of a crystal form of Terazosin (Fig. 12) [Frank Leusen (Accelrys) and John Bauer (Abbott), unpublished results] for which there are only low-resolution powder patterns. Two single-crystal X-ray structures are known. From the single-crystal X-ray structures, it is known that there is disorder in the furan ring.

The first step for crystal form prediction is the creation of the molecular model. The prediction method is a computationally intense application. Therefore, it is necessary to limit the number of degrees of freedom. If a crystal structure is known for the compound, its coordinates can be used as the starting point for building the model. An important part of this process is selecting the best force fields. One method of testing the force field is to refine a known crystal form of the compound and determine if the force field changes the conformation of the structure.

The second step is the prediction of possible polymorphs. The polymorph prediction often results in a large number of structures with reasonable intermolecular interactions and similar energies. The next step is the

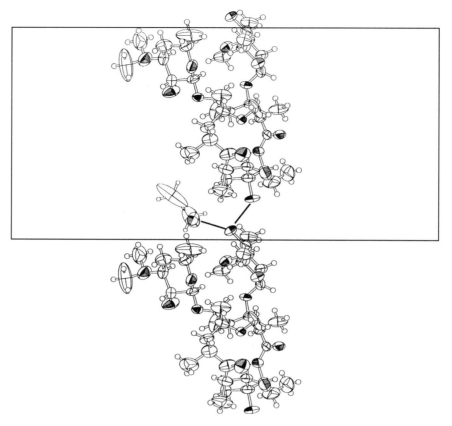

**Figure 8**   The X-ray crystal structure for clarithromycin form 0. The packing view is looking down *C* axis. This form is an ethanol solvate.

comparison of the experimental powder pattern with those calculated from the different possible solutions.

   In the example of terazosin, a match was found between one of the predicted polymorphs and the experimental XPD pattern. The structure of the crystal form is shown in Figure 13. The experimental XPD pattern and that calculated from the predicted structure show a good correlation (Fig. 14). The quality of this pattern would not have allowed the approach of solving the powder pattern for the structure more directly.

   The prediction of polymorphs can be used to determine what possible polymorphs could be formed without comparison to experimental data. This experiment can provide an understanding of the different packing arrangements possible and intramolecular bonding. The resulting crystal forms can be assessed by the calculation of properties to determine if the

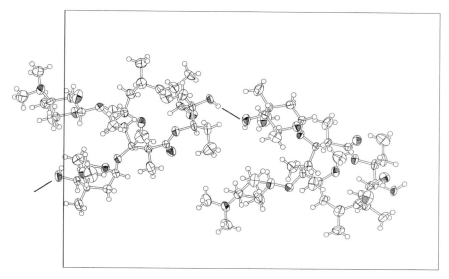

**Figure 9** The X-ray crystal structure for clarithromycin form 2. The packing view is looking down the *C* axis. This form is the most stable form.

predicted result represents viable forms (22). Possible polymorphs can be eliminated because they have predicted low growth rates and plate-like morphology, or the crystal form is not predicted to be mechanically stable. This is one tool for assessing whether other crystal forms are available for this compound. Polymorph prediction alone should not be used to make a final decision about the number of polymorphs that are possible for a system.

## PREDICTION OF MORPHOLOGY

The morphology of a sample influences its manufacturing and stability because of its shape and exposed crystal surfaces. The shape of the crystals determine the degree of difficulty in operations such as filtration from solution, how freely the solid flows, and how tightly the solid packs during storage. The different faces of a crystal expose different functional groups to the external environment. For example, the morphology of Norvir shows that the fastest growing faces, those with the smallest surface area, are those perpendicular to the hydrogen bonding direction in the crystal form (Fig. 15). The fastest growing surfaces are more hydrophilic than the other surfaces of the crystal. Changes in morphology between different batches of material can therefore lead to different chemical reactivities by changing the ratio of functional groups that are exposed (23,24). The observed

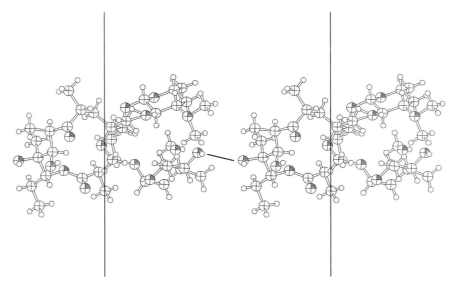

**Figure 10** The Powder Solve solution for clarithromycin form 1. This packing view is looking down the *C* axis. This form is a metastable form between the solvate the most stable form.

morphology of a sample is controlled by crystallization factors such as the degree of supersaturation, viscosity of the crystallization medium, number of nucleation sites, rate of mixing, temperature, and rate of crystallization (25). There are several methods for the calculation of morphology: Bravais Friedel Donnay Harker (BFDH), attachment energy, surface energy, and Hartman-Perdok method. The applications Cerius2, MARVIN (26,27), HABIT (28), ORIENT (29), and FASELIFT can be used to predict the morphology from a single-crystal structure.

The BFDH method is based on the crystal lattice parameters and symmetry. This method does not use the energetics of the crystal system. The basis of this calculation is that for an *H K L* plane, the center-to-face distance is inversely related to the plane spacing.

The attachment energy method (30) assumes that the growth rate of a crystal surface is proportional to the attachment energy of the growth slice to the surface. The attachment energy is the energy that is released when a growth slice is attached to the growing crystal surface. A second component of this method uses the intermolecular forces to define periodic bonding chains (PBCs). Stable growth planes are defined as those planes that contain two-dimensional connection nets of PBCs. This method requires a model of the intermolecular potential. There are a number of force fields that are

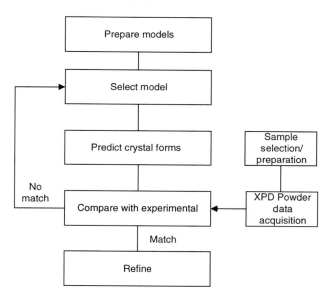

**Figure 11** The workflow for solving a low-quality XPD pattern for its crystal structure. *Abbreviation*: XPD, X-ray powder diffraction.

parameterized for organic molecules. The selected force field should be validated for use with the model. One validation method for the force field is to refine the lattice parameters of the crystal structure. The change in lattice parameters should be less than 3% for a good model (31). The morphology for E-caprolactam, hexamethylene tetramine, B-succinic acid, urea, and pentaerythritol has been calculated using five different force fields and

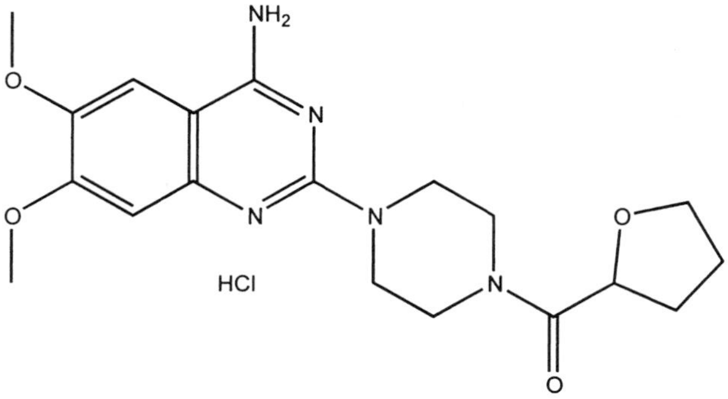

**Figure 12** The chemical structure for terazosin.

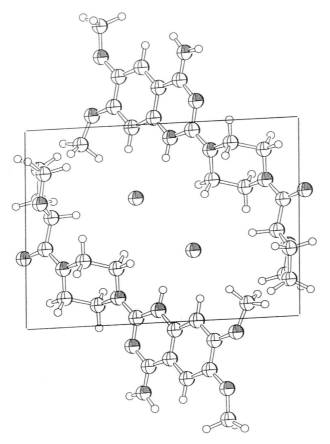

**Figure 13**   The crystal structure generated by the polymorph predictor.

compared to the experimental and BFDH morphologies (32). For example, the calculated morphology for B-succinic acid showed that none of the methods exactly reproduced the experimental morphology (Fig. 16). The lack of agreement between the experimental and calculated morphology may be due to limitations on the assumption of the attachment energy model.

The equilibrium morphology method is based on calculating the surface free energy for each of the relevant faces. The surface free energy is defined as the energy difference between the molecules on the surface compared to molecules in the bulk crystal. A comparison of the experimental and calculated morphology of form A and B of 1,3-di(cyclopropylmethyl)-8-aminoxanthine shows that the BFDH and attachment energy

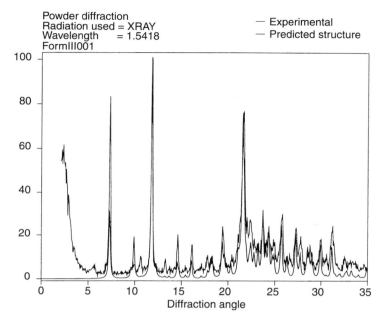

**Figure 14** A comparison between the experimental powder pattern for terazosin form 3 and that calculated for the predicated structure.

give better agreement with the experimentally observed morphology than the equilibrium method (33).

## AVERAGE CRYSTAL SHAPE

The different faces of a crystal have differences in properties such as chemical reactivity and dissolution rates because different functional groups are present at the different surfaces. An average crystal shape can be obtained from XPD patterns (collected to maintain the preferred orientation) and the theoretical pattern. The theoretical powder pattern is generated from the single-crystal X-ray data. The change in intensity of each peak from its theoretical value is calculated. These intensity differences are then used to construct an "average" crystal shape for the samples (4).

## VOID VOLUME IN CRYSTALS

The calculation of the void volume and the determination of hydrogen bonding in solvated crystals can lead to an understanding of the rate of

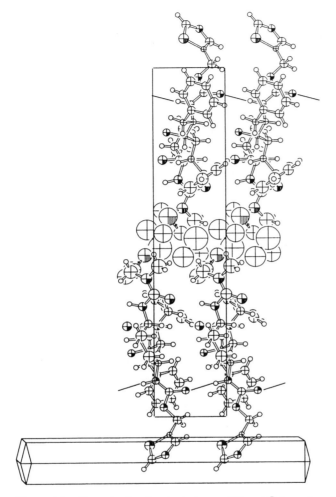

**Figure 15**   The calculated morphology of Norvir® form 1 and its the relationship to the crystal structure. The smallest surfaces of the crystal are those that grow the fastest. In this example, the hydrogen bond donor and acceptors are exposed at these faces.

desolvation. If the solvent participates in a linked hydrogen bond network, then loss of the solvent typically results in a major change in the crystal structure. In the clarithromycin example presented earlier, the hydrogen bonding of the solvent was not a direct participant in a hydrogen bond network. The void volume that would be present if the solvent was removed from this crystal forms channels that run parallel to the longest

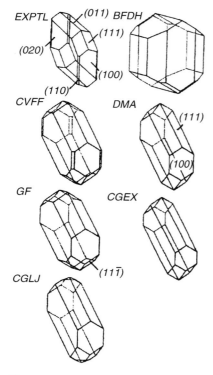

**Figure 16** The predicated morphology of 13-succinic acid using different force fields by the attachment energy method. *Source*: Courtesy of Dr. Sarah Price.

dimension of the crystal morphology (Fig. 17). A typical behavior of these types of crystal systems is that the solvent is lost through the smallest crystal surfaces. This behavior is easily observed with hot stage microscopy of the crystal immersed in oil.

If the void volumes created by removing the solvent do not form channels in the crystals, then the rate of solvent lost would be lower, because there is no direct path for the solvent to escape from the crystal.

## CONCLUSION

There are a growing number of computational tools that can be used to extend our understanding of crystalline systems. The more experimental data that can be integrated into the calculations, the closer the models will be to predicating the correct structures and properties. Changes to the development process can be made more easily and for less expense, the earlier in the process that the solid-state chemistry of a system is understood.

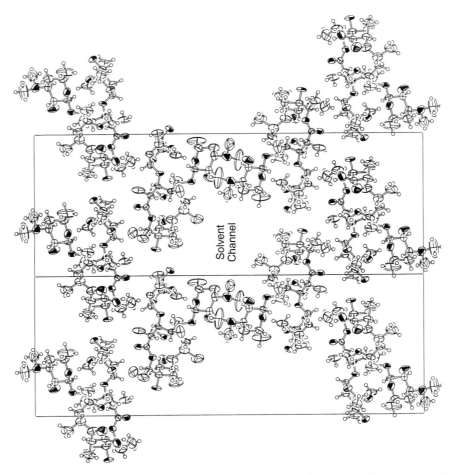

Solvent
Channel

**Figure 17**   The solvent channels present in clarithromycin form 0. The presence of the solvent channels explain the rapid loss of solvent from this crystal form.

## ACKNOWLEDGMENT

I would like to thank Rodger Henry for discussion of the analysis and insights that he provided into the structural analysis.

## REFERENCES

1.   SHELXS, Sheldrick GM, Kruger C, Goddard R. Crystallographic Computing, vol. 3. Oxford: Oxford University Press, 1985, pp. 175–89.
2.   teXsan. Crystallographic Software Package Rigaku/MSC. www.rigakumsc.com.

3. Morris K, Schlam R, Cao W, Short M. Determination of average crystallite shape by X-ray diffraction and computational methods. J Phar Sci 2000; 89: 1432–42.

4. Karfunkel HR, Rohde B, Leusen FJ, Gdanita RJ, Rihs G. J Comp Chem 1993; 14: 1125–35.

5. Stephenson G. Structure determination from conventional powder diffraction data: application to hydrates, hydrochloride salts, and metastable polymorphs. J Pharm Sci 2000; 89:958–66.

6. Sacchetti M, Varlashkin P, Long S, Lancaster R. Crystal structure prediction for eniluracil. J Pharm Sci 2001; 90:1049–55.

7. Powder Solve, Accelrys, www.accelrys.com.

8. Engel GE, Wilke S, König O, Harris KDM, Leusen FJJ. Powder solve a complete package for crystal structure solution from powder diffraction patterns. J Appl Cryst 1999; 32:1169–79.

9. Dash, CCDC Software Limited, Cambridge, UK.

10. Dinnebier R, Sieger P, Nar H, Shankland K, David W. Structural characterization of three crystalline modifications of telmisartan by single crystal and high-resolution X-ray powder diffraction. J Pharm Sci 2000; 89: 1465–79.

11. Putz H, Shon JC, Jansen M. Combined method for ab initio structure solution from powder diffraction data. J Appl Cryst 1999; 32:864–70.

12. Espoir, Mileur M, Le Bail A, University of Lemans. www.cristal.org/sdpd/espoir/

13. US Patent 5,858,986, "Crystal Form I of Clarithromycin".

14. D8 Discover with GADDS from Bruker AXS, www.bruker-axs.com.

15. X'Celerator from Philips, www.analytical.philips.com.

16. Boulfif A, Louer D. Indexing of powder diffraction patterns for low-symmetry lattices by the successive dichotomy method. J Appl Cryst 1991; 24:987–93.

17. Eriksson L, Westdahl M. TREOR, a semi-exhaustive trail-and-error powder indexing program for all symmetries. J Appl Cryst 1985; 18:367–70.

18. Accelyris Inc., www.accelrys.com.

19. COMCAT beam line, Argonne National Laboratories.

20. Cambridge Crystallographic Data Centre, Cambridge, United Kingdom.

21. Bauer J, Spanton S, Henry R, Quick I, Dziki W, Porter W, Morris J. Ritonavir: an extraordinary example of conformational polymorphism. Pharm Res 2001; 18(6):859–66.

22. Beyer T, Day O, Price S. The prediction, morphology, and mechanical properties of the polymorphs of paracetamol. J Am Chem Soc 2001; 123: 5086–94.

23. Muster T, Prestide C. Face specific surface properties of pharmaceutical crystals. J Pharm Sci 2002; 91:1432–44.

24. Brittain HG, ed. Polymorphism in Pharmaceutical Solids. New York: Marcel Dekker, 1999; pp. 1–34, 279–330.

25. Rodriguez-Hormedo N, Murphy D. Significance of controlling crystallization mechanisms and kinetics in pharmaceutical systems. J Pharm Sci 1999; 88(7): 651–60.

26. Rohl AL, Gay DH. J Cryst Growth 1996; 166:84–90.

27. Gay DH, Rohl A. MARVIN: A new computer code for studying surfaces and interfaces and its application to calculating the crystal morphologies of corundum and zircon. Chem Soc Faraday Trans 1995; 91:925–36.

28. Clyclesdale G, Docherty R, Robert JJ. J Comput Phys Commun 1991; 64: 311–28.

29. Stone AJ, Dullweber A, Engkvist O, et al, Orient: A program for studying interactions between molecules, version 4.5. University of Cambridge 2002; Enquiries to A.J. Stone.

30. Hartman P, Perdok WG. Acta Crystallogr 1954; 8:49–52.

31. Coombes DS, Price SL, Willock DJ, Leslie M. J Phys Chem 1996; 100:7352–60.

32. Brunsteiner M, Price SL. Morphologies of organic crystals: sensitivity of attachment energy predictions to the model intermolecular potential. Crystal Growth Design 2001; 1(6):447–53.

33. Coombes DS, Catlow CR, Gale JD, Herdy MI, Saunders MR. Theoretical and experimental investigations on the morphology of pharmaceutical crystals. J Pharm Sci 2001; 91(7):1652–8.

# 2.3

# Salt Selection for Pharmaceutical Compounds

### Sherif I. Badawy

*Bristol-Myers Squibb Pharmaceutical Research Institute, New Brunswick, New Jersey, U.S.A.*

### Miriam K. Franchini

*Sanofi-Aventis, Bridgewater, New Jersey, U.S.A.*

### Munir A. Hussain

*Bristol-Myers Squibb Pharmaceutical Research Institute, New Brunswick, New Jersey, U.S.A.*

## INTRODUCTION

It has been estimated that 40% of new drug molecules suffer from poor aqueous solubility. In polar compounds, low solubility may be due to strong intermolecular electrostatic attraction and/or hydrogen bonding, while the low aqueous solubility of hydrophobic and lipophilic compounds is usually attributed to an unfavorable free energy of solvation by water. In the case of hydrophobic compounds, these may additionally be poorly soluble in oils, which may make formulation much more challenging than for lipophilic compounds, which may be solubilized by oily vehicles. If a drug molecule possesses an ionizable group, one way of improving the aqueous solubility of polar, hydrophobic, or lipophilic compounds is by salt formation. In some cases such as in taste masking, for controlled release, to improve chemical stability, or lymphatic targeting, it may be desirable to decrease the aqueous solubility. Judicious choice of the proper counterion can help accomplish these goals.

## SOLUBILITY CONSIDERATIONS

### Solubility of Salts

The concentration of an ionizable compound in solution is the sum of the concentration of the ionized and unionized species. For example, the solubility of a weak base can be represented as follows:

$$S_T = [BH^+] + [B] \tag{1}$$

where $S_T$ is the total concentration in a saturated solution, $[BH^+]$ is the concentration of the protonated form, and $[B]$ is the concentration of the free base in the saturated solution. The solubility of an acidic compound is expressed by a similar equation. The ratio of the two species is determined by the pH of the solution according to the Henderson–Hasselbach equation (Eq. 5):

$$[BH^+] \rightleftharpoons [B][H^\pm] \tag{2}$$

$$K_a = [B][H^+]/[BH^+] \tag{3}$$

$$-\log K_a = pK_a = -\log[B] - \log[H^+] + \log[BH^+] \tag{4}$$

$$pK_a = pH - \log[B]/[BH^+] \tag{5}$$

where $K_a$ is the ionization constant of the conjugate acid for the compound of interest, $pK_a$ is $-(\log K_a)$, and pH is $-(\log[H^+])$.

The solubility limit for the compound is reached when the concentration of either the ionized or the unionized species attains saturation. Thus, at high pH values, the solubility is limited by the unionized species. When this limit is reached, the solid in equilibrium with the solution is the free base, and the concentration of the ionized species is well below saturation. As the pH is decreased, the total solubility increases as the concentration of the ionized form increases according to Eq. 5. This will continue until a certain pH, usually referred to as the pH of maximum solubility, or $pH_{max}$, is reached. Solubility at $pH_{max}$ is determined by both the base and the counterion, where the concentration of the ionized form reaches saturation as well. The solubility of the ionized form is reached when the solubility product ($K_{sp}$) is exceeded. The solubility product of a salt $BH_mA_n$ is described as follows (1):

$$BH_mA_n(\text{solid}) \rightarrow mBH^{n+} + nA^{m-} \tag{6}$$

$$K_{sp} = [BH^{n+}]^m [A^{m-}]^n \tag{7}$$

where $[A^{m-}]$ is the counterion concentration. As the pH decreases further, the concentration of the free base in solution is reduced and is no longer at saturation. Thus, at pH values below $pH_{max}$, compound solubility is determined by the solubility of the ionized form of the drug. The $pH_{max}$ of a base can be expressed by the following equation (2):

$$pH_{max} = pK_a + \log(S_0/\sqrt{K_{sp}}) \tag{8}$$

where $S_0$ is the solubility of the unionized form.

The solubility product depends not only on the nature of the compound itself but also on the counterion. Thus, different salts for the same compound would possess different values for the solubility product depending on the counterion. For a basic compound, solubility would be determined by the solubility product only when the final solution pH is lower than $pH_{max}$. Above $pH_{max}$, the solubility is limited by that of the free base. As a result, the solid in equilibrium with a saturated solution would be the free base rather than the salt, regardless of the form added initially to the solvent. It is noteworthy that the solid in equilibrium with a saturated solution is determined by solution pH relative to $pH_{max}$, regardless of the $pK_a$ of the compound. It is therefore possible to have the free base in equilibrium with the solution even though the solution pH may be significantly lower than the $pK_a$, as long as the pH is still higher than $pH_{max}$. Consider the case of a salt of a weakly basic drug and the counterion of a weak acid. When such a salt is added to water, the pH of the solution is approximated by (3)

$$pH = 1/2(pK_a(base) + pK_a(acid)) \tag{9}$$

Thus, for a given base and a series of acid-derived counterions, the pH of the salt solution will decrease as the $pK_a$ of the acid decreases. If the resulting pH is higher than $pH_{max}$, the free base will precipitate, and the solubility value will be determined by that of the free base regardless of the counterion. The "true" solubility of the salt, which is determined by the solubility product, can be determined by estimating the solubility at $pH_{max}$ from the pH solubility profile of the compound and then subtracting the solubility of the free form from the estimated solubility at $pH_{max}$.

## Factors Affecting Salt Solubility

The counterion of a pharmaceutical salt has a significant effect on its solubility. The counterion can influence both the "true" and "apparent" solubility of a salt as described in the previous section. The counterion affects the pH of the solution resulting from the dissolution of the salt as described in Equation 9. For a basic compound, the solution pH would be lower for a salt with a counterion derived from a stronger acid. The lower pH in this case can result in a higher "apparent" solubility of the salt compared to a salt with a counterion derived from a weaker acid. Although the effect of counterions on pH may not be significant in dilute and well-buffered solutions of the salt, it may have an important effect in other cases. For example, the effect of the counterion on the micro-environmental pH during dissolution can greatly impact the dissolution rate of a salt.

The effect of counterion on the "true" solubility of a salt is manifested through its effect on the solubility product. The enthalpy change of solution is determined by the net balance between the heat of fusion and the sum of the heats of hydration of the compound and of the counterion. Salt solubility would decrease with the increase in the heat of fusion (lattice energy) and would increase by the increase in heats of hydration for the anion and the cation.

The lattice energy is usually related to the melting point of a crystalline material. The increase in melting point for a salt is hence expected to decrease the solubility as predicted by the equation,

$$\ln X_{\text{ideal}} = -(1/T - 1/T_{\text{m}})\Delta H/R \tag{10}$$

where $X_{\text{ideal}}$ is the ideal solubility, $\Delta H$ is the molar heat of fusion, $T$ is the absolute temperature, $T_{\text{m}}$ is the melting point, and $R$ is the gas constant. Agharkar et al. studied the solubility of a number of salts for the antimalarial drug $\alpha$-(2-piperidyl)-3,6-bis(trifluoromethyl)-9-phenanthrenemathanol (5). They attributed the lower solubility of the hydrochloride and sulfate salts (at least in part) to their higher melting point compared to the lactate and 2-hydroxyethane-1-sulfonate salts. The solubility of a series of ammonium salts of flurbiprofen was inversely related to the melting point of the salt (6).

The melting point for a series of salts of a compound usually correlates with that of the conjugate acid or base from which the counterion is derived. The melting point of a series of salts for UK-47880 increased by the increase in the melting point of the conjugate acid (7). Salts of UK-47880 derived from the higher-melting-point aromatic sulfonic or hydroxycarboxylic acids showed higher melting points compared to those derived from the lower-melting-point long-chain aliphatic acids. The planar aromatic acids are more capable of closer packing in the crystal lattice compared to the aliphatic acids with long flexible chains, which results in a higher melting point for the former acids and their salts.

Aqueous solubility therefore increases as the interaction between the counterion and water is enhanced. The energy of hydration would increase with the increased hydrophilicity of the counterion and higher tendency of the counterion to form hydrogen bonds with water. For example, the higher solubility of the digluconate salt of chlorhexidine compared to the lactate salt was attributed, at least partly, to the higher degree of hydroxylation of the gluconate counterion, which enhances the capability of the counterion to interact with the solvent, resulting in a higher energy of hydration.

Hydrophobic acids, such as pamoic acid, usually form salts that are poorly water soluble due to the low hydration energy for the counterion. The hydration energy of the salt also increases with the increase in the charge and the decrease of the size of the counterion. It is noteworthy that factors that increase the hydration energy can also result in a higher lattice energy. The increase in the energy of hydration of the counterion for a given compound, therefore, does not necessarily result in increased solubility, since it may be associated with an increased melting point. In this case, the net effect on solubility depends on the balance of these two opposing factors. As a result, Chowhan found no trend relating the counterion and solubility for a series of alkali and alkali earth metal salts of organic carboxylic acids (8).

Certain fatty acid counterions such as laurate and stearate may be specifically chosen to reduce solubility for the purpose of taste-masking bitter drugs such as gatifloxacin, prepared as the stearate salt for pediatric formulations (9), and erythromycin estolate, where the salt form has one-twelfth the solubility of the free base (10), or to improve stability, or both, as in the case of the erythromycin salts (11). Poorly water-soluble fatty acid salt forms of drugs may show an improvement in bioavailability compared to the free form or the water-soluble salt form of the drug if the undissociated salt form is taken up by the lymph. Targeting the more slowly circulating lymphatic system can result in prolonged blood levels (12).

## STABILITY CONSIDERATIONS

Salt form can play an important role in determining the stability of a pharmaceutical compound. Different salt forms may have different stability characteristics. Salt stability can be related to factors such as melting point, solubility, hygroscopicity, and microenvironmental pH.

Aqueous suspensions of poorly water-soluble salt forms of drugs are one way of stabilizing drugs prone to hydrolysis, e.g., chlortetracycline. The process for producing a stable chlortetracycline suspension was developed at Lederle Laboratories between 1951 and 1954. The HCl and free base forms of the drug were very unstable in aqueous solution, but an extremely stable suspension in water could be obtained from the practically insoluble calcium salt. The process produced the stoichiometric (1:1) calcium salt (or complex) as a wet cake of amorphous solid, which was then suspended in suitable aqueous vehicles, with the resultant suspension having a pH of ~7.5. Stability was acceptable for at least two years, and the formulation was ~80% as bioavailable as the HCl salt formulated as a capsule. Identification of this salt form and its formulation helped Lederle to assume a competitive position in the marketplace (13).

In the late 1950s, erythromycin estolate, the poorly soluble estolate salt form of erythromycin was found to be very stable in suspension, which was also a more palatable dosage form than a solution (11).

## Hygroscopicity

The ability of a solid material to pick up moisture is usually associated with decreased chemical stability. Water enhances degradation by acting as a reactant in hydrolytic reactions or by acting as a medium that provides increased reactivity. Earlier reports described the water present in a predominantly crystalline solid as forming an adsorbed layer of free moisture around the solid particles. This adsorbed moisture layer resembles bulk water, and the active ingredient can dissolve in such a layer where it would be more reactive compared to the solid crystals (14). Another proposed model describes the water as being absorbed in amorphous regions and in areas of crystal defects. The water in these regions acts as a plasticizer that enhances molecular mobility and hence increases the rate of chemical and physical changes (15). Since regions of molecular disorder have higher tendency to pick up moisture, the concentration of water in these regions is typically much higher than the average moisture content in a solid system. This creates reactive "hot spots" and tends to magnify the destabilizing effect of water.

The counterion usually has a pronounced effect on the moisture-uptake properties of a salt. The moisture-uptake tendency of a salt is usually higher for the more hydrophilic counterions. Hydrochloride salts in particular have been often reported as being hygroscopic (7), which can in some cases limit their utility in solid dosage forms. Also, from the authors' experience, potassium salts tend to be less hygroscopic than sodium salts. Penicillin G potassium, for example, was much less hygroscopic than penicillin G sodium (16). Potassium salts, however, tend to have an unpleasant metallic taste (16).

## Microenvironmental pH

The stability of compounds that degrade via pH-dependent pathways is usually dependent on the microenvironmental pH of the solid system. Although the concept of pH does not apply to solids, the term "microenvironmental pH" has been loosely used to describe hydrogen ion activity in noncrystalline regions such as adsorbed water layers or water-plasticized amorphous domains. The deleterious effect of water on stability is largely dependent on the microenvironmental pH for compounds with pH-dependent stability. The microenvironmental pH of a solid is typically related to the pH of solution formed when the solid is dissolved in water. Salts of a weak base formed using a counterion derived from a strong acid (e.g., inorganic acid salts) will have a low microenvironmental pH, which can be deleterious to acid labile compounds. This destabilizing effect will be more pronounced if the salt is hygroscopic and hence would have a high concentration of acidic moisture.

On the other hand, organic salts of such weak bases would provide a less acidic microenvironmental pH, which may be more stable. Eq. 9 can be used to estimate the microenvironmental pH of a salt of a weak acid and a weak base. The microenvironmental pH thus increases as the $pK_a$ of the conjugate acid of the counterion increases. Selecting a counterion that provides a micro-environmental pH that approximates as closely as possible the pH of maximum stability can therefore maximize stability. The mesylate salt of a prodrug for a glycoprotein IIb/IIIa receptor antagonist was more stable in solid dosage forms than the acetate salt, which was attributed to the more favorable microenvironmental pH provided by the mesylate salt (17).


## BIOAVAILABILITY CONSIDERATIONS

Generally speaking, different salt forms of the same drug rarely differ pharmacologically, unless the dose is sufficiently high such as to render the counterion toxic or pharmacologically active (18). Rather, the onset and intensity of the drug plasma concentration is that which may be considerably different between different salt forms, as well as between a salt and its free acid or free base. If the improvement in bioavailability of the drug is significant, certain pharmacological responses may be elicited as a result.

Although it is not possible to accurately predict the magnitude or direction of the response, there do appear to be some general trends. For example, making a salt form of a free acid may not be advantageous if the salt rapidly converts to the less soluble and potentially less bioavailable free acid form in the stomach milieu. However, if the free acid precipitates as very fine and/or amorphous particles with a greater surface area compared to a formulation administered as the free acid, dissolution and bioavailability may be enhanced. In the case of iopanoic acid and its sodium salt, the sodium salt immediately precipitated in gastric fluid to a very fine suspension of the free acid, which was much more rapidly dissolved and absorbed than the free acid. For this drug, the improvement in bioavailability resulted in toxicity (19) that was unrelated to the counterion itself.

Although oral administration of a salt form of an acid may result in rapid transformation and precipitation of the free acid, the use of a salt form of an acid for targeted delivery to the intestine, e.g., in an enteric-coated formulation, may result in higher bioavailability. The reason is that the rate of dissolution of the salt is typically much higher than the corresponding free form, even though the equilibrium solubilities at a particular pH are the same. This may be attributed to a decrease in the contact angle between the dissolving solid and the solution in the case of the salt, leading to improved wetting. The more rapid dissolution of a series of sodium salts compared to the free acid is illustrated in Table 1.

Frequently, merely delaying the conversion to the free form can result in a significant improvement in onset and/or bioavailability. The "hang" time prior to "crashing out" to the equilibrium solubility of the free form will be affected by bulk pH, temperature, agitation, and the self-buffering effect the dissolving form has on the microenvironmental pH of the diffusion boundary layer (21). The precipitation kinetics of the free form can be slowed down by the addition of a buffer modifier or crystallization inhibitor such as polyvinylpyrrolidone in the formulation to help delay conversion to the less-soluble free form.

Quite often, the plasma concentration versus time area under the curve of a free form and its salt may be similar, but the salt form may show a more rapid onset, owing to its faster rate of dissolution. For example, the extent of absorption of ibuprofen lysinate (1025 mg, powder for oral suspension) was found to be the same as an equivalent dose of the free acid (600 mg effervescent granules), when compared in a two-way crossover design in 24 healthy volunteers. However, the $C_{max}$ for ibuprofen was higher, and the onset of the lysinate formulation was significantly faster, the lysinate having a $T_{max}$ of 0.54 versus 1.75 hours for the free acid (22). Similar results were obtained by other investigators from a 400 mg dose (23).

In the case of the weak base erythromycin, the lauryl sulfate salt, also known as estolate, has been repeatedly reported to demonstrate greater bioavailability than the ethylsuccinate salt, even when dosed as a suspension at 1000 mg, such that a lower dose and less-frequent dosing is required with the estolate (24). Erythromycin estolate, with a $pK_a$ of 6.9 for erythromycin, is the salt of a strong hydrophobic acid, lauryl sulfuric acid, and remains undissolved and protected from hydrolysis in the stomach (11). Lauryl

**Table 1**  Dissolution Rate ($mg/100 \, min/cm^2$) of Some Weak Acids and Their Sodium Salts as a Function of pH

|  |  | Dissolution rate | | | | | |
|---|---|---|---|---|---|---|---|
|  |  | At pH 1.5 | | At pH 6.8 | | At pH 9.0 | |
|  | $pK_a$ | Free acid | Na salt | Free acid | Na salt | Free acid | Na salt |
| Salicylic acid | 3.0 | 1.7 | 1870 | 27 | 2500 | 53 | 2400 |
| Benzoic acid | 4.2 | 2.1 | 980 | 14 | 1770 | 28 | 1600 |
| Sulfathiazole | 7.3 | <0.1 | 550 | 0.5 | 810 | 8.5 | 1300 |
| Phenobarbital | 7.4 | 0.24 | 200 | 1.2 | 820 | 22 | 1430 |

*Source*: From Ref. 20.

sulfate contains 12 carbons in a straight chain and is amphiphilic, which may render it more permeable through membranes or result in lymphatic targeting (25).

In the case of propranolol, a drug subject to first-pass metabolism, the hydrophobic laurate counterion was selected in order to reduce the aqueous solubility and dissolution rate, thereby sustaining its release. When tested in dogs, the laurate salt resulted in improved bioavailability compared to the hydrochloride salt in immediate- and sustained-release formulations, as illustrated in Table 2. This is unusual in that ordinarily, if a drug is susceptible to metabolism, an increase, not a decrease, in solubility will lead to improved bioavailability, owing to saturation of the metabolic enzymes. This may be a case where the lipophilic counterion did not dissociate at stomach pH, leading to lymphatic targeting of the poorly water soluble ion pair.

Low blood levels obtained from salt forms are not necessarily an indication of poor absorption, and may indicate rapid uptake by tissue, organ, tumor, or the lymph. For example, it was discovered that by converting streptomycin, neomycin, viomycin, and streptothricin to macromolecular salts, these antibiotics could be targeted at the slowly circulating lymphatic system, which has an affinity for macromolecules and colloidal particles. Macromolecular salts were prepared from polyacrylic acids, sulfonic and phosphorylated polysaccharides, and polyuronic derivatives. Parenteral administration resulted in low, but prolonged, blood levels and high lymph levels (26).

In the case of halofantrine, the poorly lipid-soluble hydrochloride salt is much more water soluble than the highly lipid-soluble free base, the free base having a solubility of ~50 mg/mL in triglyceride lipids and a calculated log $P$ of 8.5. The solubility of the HCl salt in long-chain triglyceride lipids was found to be less than 1 mg/mL, and thus it was not considered to be a substrate for lymphatic transport. After postprandial administration of the hydrochloride salt, a 12-fold increase in oral bioavailability was observed in

**Table 2** Pharmacokinetic Parameters for Immediate and Controlled Release Formulations of Propranolol HCl or Laurate Salts after Oral Administration to Dog Mean ± Standard Error

|  | 40 mg HCl salt, immediate-release formulation | 80 mg HCl salt, sustained-release marketed formulation | 80 mg (HCl equivalents) laurate salt |
|---|---|---|---|
| $C_{max}$ (ng/mL) | 34.8 ± 4.0 | 18.7 ± 0.7 | 151 ± 28 |
| $T_{max}$ (hr) | 1.1 ± 0.4 | 4.7 ± 1.4 | 1.8 ± 0.5 |
| Bioavailability (%) | 7.2 ± 0.3 | 9.4 ± 1.0 | 17.9 ± 2.5 |

*Source*: From Ref. 12.

beagle dogs, and a threefold increase was observed in humans. At first, this was attributed to enhanced drug dissolution and solubilization in the bile salt secretion induced by the fed state. However, when the lymph was examined, it was found to account for 47% of the 100-mg administered dose, similar to the 54% observed when the free base was administered. In the absence of food, lymphatic transport of the free base only accounted for 1.3% of the administered dose. The extensive intestinal lymphatic transport observed in the presence of food was achieved due to the rapid conversion of the hydrochloride to the free base at the elevated pH levels induced by the fed state (27).

## SURFACE TENSION CONSIDERATIONS

The surface activity and self-association behavior of a salt can affect its solubility and bioavailability. Supersaturation in the region of $pH_{max}$ has been frequently observed and is thought to be due to self-association and a self-buffering effect, which can delay the onset of nucleation to the free or salt form. The degree of supersaturation at $pH_{max}$ has been reported to be as high as four times the equilibrium solubility of the salt form (28).

The nature of the counterion has been known to affect the self-association of drug molecules in solution. For example, the apparent critical micelle concentration (CMC) of chlorhexidine digluconate is 6.6 mM, while that of the corresponding diacetate salt is 10.5 mM. (29). Additionally, a correlation was observed between the absorption rate constant and the surface tension of various pH 2 buffer salt solutions used to administer tetracycline free base ($pK_{a1} = 3.3$); those solutions with the lowest surface tension showed the best absorption (30). A similar correlation between surface tension and absorption was reported for dextromethorphan administered in various buffer salt solutions (31). More recently, a drug-induced decrease in surface tension at the membrane surface was proposed to be the reason for an increase in colonic permeability as fluvastatin drug concentration was increased (32).

For some drugs, an increase in aqueous solubility afforded by particular salt forms results in high-enough drug concentrations to allow self-association, which may result in improved bioavailability. For example, in the case of nicardipine, the surface tension of the hydrochloride salt in water was lower than corresponding concentrations of the phosphate salt of the drug in water. However, the solubility of the phosphate salt in water was 10-fold greater, such that at concentrations above 5 mg/mL, the solubility limit of the HCl salt, the phosphate salt self-associated (33).

In the case of DuP 747, the methanesulfonic acid form, having an aqueous solubility of ~60 mg/mL and a melting point of 210°C, was able to self-associate and was more soluble than the HCl form in water, which had a solubility of only 3 mg/mL and a melting point of 232°C. As observed with nicardipine, although the solubility of the hydrochloride was not sufficient for self-association, a slightly greater surface tension lowering effect was observed for the HCl salt at preassociation concentrations than for the phosphate salt of nicardipine or the methanesulfonate salt of DuP 747 (34).

In some cases, the solubility of the salt form of a drug has been found to be higher than the free form in a cosolvent system such as propylene glycol and water. Although this phenomenon must be ascertained by experimentation, the solubilization of a salt form of a drug in a cosolvent may allow for higher solution concentrations than either a free form in a cosolvent or a salt form in an aqueous system (35).

## MANUFACTURABILITY CONSIDERATIONS

The decision of whether to develop a salt form or a free form of a drug must also include the cost and feasibility of making the desired form. The feasibility and ease of crystallization of a salt form could be an important factor in the salt selection decision. Since the crystallization process serves the important purpose of purifying a drug substance, a salt form with a higher degree of crystallinity will be preferred from the chemical processing perspective. A less-crystalline salt form may not readily provide the desired chemical purity and could require extensive effort and cost to develop a robust crystallization process. In some cases, however, the most bioavailable form is developed, and appropriate manufacturing and storage conditions are implemented to minimize degradation and conversion to another form.

Another approach is to prepare the form that is most convenient from a chemical processing point of view, and convert to the desired form during product manufacture. For example, the solubility of nicardipine hydrochloride is only 4.5 mg/mL, but when added to solutions of 5 M acetate or propionate, solubilities of 68 and 270 mg/mL, respectively, may be achieved due to complexation. Nicardipine hydrochloride is reasonably easy to prepare, but the acetate, propionate, and butyrate salts cannot be isolated easily (33). Thus, one approach for the preparation of an IV injectable formulation of nifedipine would be to manufacture the hydrochloride salt and form one of the carboxylate complexes in situ, by adding the appropriate buffer solution to the hydrochloride salt. Such an approach was described for in situ preparation of salts/complexes of a rebeccamycin analog (36) in order to provide a ready-to-use solution from the poorly soluble free base. Interestingly, this work was initiated because while early development lots of the rebeccamycin hydrochloride salt formed solutions in water, scale-up GMP. lots, of slightly greater purity, formed gels. The salt selection process revealed that certain molar quantities of counterions such as citrate were required to form a solution of the free base, and that control of pH alone was not sufficient to prevent gelling.

   More recently, conversion of a highly stable benzenesulfonate form (bulk drug substance form) to the less stable but highly soluble and more bioavailable hydrochloride salt was accomplished by a single-step nanofiltration process in which counterions were exchanged during the final stages of pharmaceutical processing of drug product. This allowed indefinite storage at room temperature of the drug substance, while providing the most optimum form in the dosage unit (37).

   In some cases, conversion to a salt form may not be for solubility or bioavailability considerations, but rather for ease of processing. For example, some drugs cannot be isolated as their free acids or bases, and only crystallize as certain salt forms (or vice versa). Some forms may have a melting point that is too low to allow for the unit operations required to make a solid dosage form and may be ruled out. Additionally, if a solid dosage form is to be coated or wet granulated, too high a solubility can result in manufacturing problems such as pitting of the tablet during coating or uncontrolled agglomeration of the wet mass in wet granulation. The number of polymorphs or hydrates a certain salt possesses may also influence the decision not to pursue a particular salt form, for fear of partial or complete conversion during processing and/or storage of the drug product. For example, for anhydrous drug forms that need to be wet granulated, formation of the hydrate during wet granulation can lead to dissolution and bioavailability issues. On the flip side, it is possible to dehydrate during the drying step, which may lead to unstable amorphous forms of the drug. In situ monitoring by, e.g., near-infrared detection has been used to monitor form changes during the milling and drying operations.

## GENERAL CONSIDERATIONS

Rapid onset is particularly important for the analgesic or antipyretic classes, but for chronically dosed drugs or very potent drugs, an improvement in onset may not be required or even desired. The decision to investigate salt forms should be driven by the intended use and properties of the drug, such as the $pK_a$, which will influence the selection of counterions used to make salts and the propensity of the salt form to disproportionate.

   Weak acids such as benzoic and acetic acid would not be expected to form salts with weakly basic amine drugs having $pK_a$ values less than 4; in these instances, strong mineral acids such as HCl ($pK_a = -6.1$), $H_2SO_4$ ($pK_a = -3.0$), or methanesulfonic acid ($pK_a = -1.2$) would have to be used for salt formation. This concept is illustrated by erythromycin, whereby salts made from weak acids such as acetic, formic, and phosphoric acids are easily disproportionated to the free base, in some cases, by merely drying under vacuum, whereas stronger acids such as sulfamic and sulfuric acids form stable salts (38).

Generally, potassium and sodium salts of acidic compounds are more soluble than polyvalent salts, such as calcium salts, which may result in improved bioavailability.

The hydrochloride salt of an amine is one of the most widely used salt forms, owing to its low cost and safety, as well as the low mass of the hydrochloride entity, which becomes important for high-dose drugs. For strong bases, these are reasonably stable, but hydrochloride salts of very weak amines will be more easily displaced at slightly elevated temperatures and/or humidity, liberating HCl gas. A decrease in the chloride content of the hydrochloride salt of the antifungal compound, X-7801, was observed upon heating at temperatures well below its melting point (39). Hydrochloride salts, which are hydrophilic, also tend to be more hygroscopic than other salt forms (7).

Hydrochloride salts may also result in lower-than-expected solubility in the stomach due to the high concentration of chloride ions in the stomach. This results in a shift in the equilibrium toward lower solubility, as predicted by the law of mass action, also known as the common ion effect (Eq. 6) (2,5,40–42). Similarly, dilution of a salt form (7) with normal saline (0.9% NaCl) may result in precipitation of the less soluble hydrochloride salt (43).

An alternative to the hydrochloride salt is the methanesulfonate, or mesylate, salt, which can often provide aqueous solubilities significantly higher than the free base or hydrochloride salt form (5,34). For example, methanesulfonic acid has a relatively low $pK_a$ ($\sim-1$) and low volatility and therefore provides much more stable salts than hydrochloric acid for weak amines due to the potential loss of hydrochloric acid as a gas.

For DMP 728 (aka XL118), a zwitterionic cyclic peptide, the zwitterion had an aqueous solubility of 5.4 mg/mL, while the benzenesulfonate, sulfate, and mesylate salts had solubilities of 5, 50, and 73.5 mg/mL, respectively, in water. The initial water content of these forms was ~1.2% for the mesylate, 6% for the benzene sulfonate, ~15% for the zwitterion, and ~17% for the sulfate. After storage at 85% relative humidity for 21 days, none of the three salt forms showed a change in water content from the initial, whereas the zwitterion was hygroscopic and took up ~5% water over the test period. Therefore, the mesylate, having the lowest intrinsic water content and the highest aqueous solubility, was selected for development (44).

Depending on the $pH_{max}$ and $pK_a$ of the drug, the mesylate salt may rapidly convert to the free form even in an acidic environment such as the stomach; however, if the hang-time of the salt in solution can be prolonged, improved bioavailability can result (45). For example, it is possible to use the highly soluble mesylate form in a modified-release formulation, as suggested for carvedilol. The mesylate form of carvedilol, a free base with one $pK_a$ of 7.6, was found to have a solubility in water of about

8.5 mg/mL compared to 5 microgram/mL for the free base and 1.65 mg/mL for the hydrochloride salt. A maximum solubility of ~0.2 mg/mL is noted for the free base between pH 4 and 5, and at acidic pH of 1 to 4, the solubility is limited by the solubility of the protonated form or its salt formed in situ. The solubility of the hydrochloride salt formed in situ in simulated gastric fluid is less soluble than carvedilol itself, and the mesylate rapidly converts to this form in simulated gastric fluid. However, if the mesylate is contained in an enteric-coated core, it will be released in the intestine, where it does not undergo significant disproportionation to the free base. Such an approach could result in improved bioavailability. The mesylate also provides for the development of injectable formulations, again because at plasma pH, this salt form would not disproportionate (46).

## SUMMARY OF SALT SELECTION CONSIDERATIONS

Factors that influence salt selection include drug dose and route of administration, the half-life, the desired clinical onset and duration of action, drug substance manufacturability considerations, the solubility at stomach pH (1 to 4) and intestinal pH (6 to 8), the rate of precipitation of the free form from a salt solution, the pH range over which the precipitation occurs, and the form of the precipitate (gel, particles, polymorph, particle size) (47).

Most companies perform salt screening to select salt forms that have the appropriate physicochemical attributes such as crystallinity, low hygroscopicity, melting point, dissolution rate, solubility, and stability. Bioavailability considerations must also be integrated into the decision process. Various integrated approaches may be used to screen and select the appropriate salt form for development (4,7,16,45,48–55). Quite often, these approaches require a cross-departmental team including those who will synthesize the salt forms and those who will evaluate the physicochemical properties such as crystallinity, molar ratio, polymorphs and hydrates, physical and chemical stability including hygroscopicity, solubility, and morphology; excipient compatibility, processability, including good flow properties, and yield also factor into the decision making. Additionally, for high-dose drugs, the size of the counterion may limit the choices of salts to those that do not add excessive weight, so as to keep the final dosage form to a reasonable size. Physical properties such as compactibility and bulk density may also be important factors in choosing a salt form for high-dose drugs.

The first step in salt selection must involve the determination that the drug possesses ionizable groups that can be manipulated under the conditions necessary to make salt forms. As these often involve a pH-adjustment step in an aqueous or nonaqueous environment, the ability to make the salts will be affected by the stability of the drug under these conditions, as the drug may possess other functional groups that may undergo a reaction during the process. Salts of bases must be made from a conjugate acid having a $pK_a$ less than the $pK_a$ of the basic center of the drug. Thus, if the $pK_a$ of the base is around 2, salt formation will be restricted to strong acids such as the mineral and sulfonic acids, whereas a higher $pK_a$ will allow a broader selection. A similar argument holds for salts of acids.

Salt selection is usually done early in the development process, when the availability of drug substance may be limited. In such cases, the selection process may be dictated by timeline and drug-supply constraints. With the advent of computers, liquid handlers, and robotics, however, it is possible to screen for many different salt forms with a limited amount of drug substance, and several companies are available to specifically screen for salts under a contract. Generally, it is advisable to patent as many forms as is practical, but since switching salt forms may involve additional toxicology and pharmacokinetic testing, it is advisable to perform a thorough salt screening process as early as possible in the development process, preferably before or during phases I and II.

## REFERENCES

1. Connors K. A Textbook of Pharmaceutical Analysis, 3rd ed., chaps. 1–3. New York: John Wiley and Sons, 1982.
2. Bogardus J, Blackwood RK. Solubility of doxycycline in aqueous solution. J Pharm Sci 1979; 68(2):188–94.
3. Martin A, Swarbrick J, Cammarata A. Physical Pharmacy: Physical and Chemical Principles in the Pharmaceutical Sciences, 3rd ed. Philadelphia, PA: Lea and Febiger, 1983, p. 205.
4. Anderson BD, Flora KP. Preparation of water-soluble compounds through salt formation (chap. 34). In: Wermuth CG, ed. The Practice of Medicinal Chemistry. New York: Academic Press, 1996.
5. Agharkar S, Lindenbaum S, Higuchi T. Enhancement of solubility of drug salts by hydrophilic counterions: properties of organic salts of an antimalarial drug. J Pharm Sci 1976; 65(5):747–9.
6. Anderson BD, Conradi RA. Predictive relationships in the water solubility of salts of a non-steroidal anti-inflammatory drug. J Pharm Sci 1985; 74(8): 815–20.
7. Gould PL. Salt selection of basic drugs. Int J Pharm 1986; 33:201–217.
8. Chowhan ZT. pH-solubility profiles of organic carboxylic acids and their salts. J Pharm Sci 1978; 67(9):1257–60.
9. US Patent 6,589,955B2. Raghavan KS, Ranadive SA, Bembeneck KS, et al. Pediatric Formulation of Gatifloxacin, July 8, 2003.
10. Jones PH, Rowley EK, Weiss AL, Bishop DL, Chun AHC. Insoluble erythromycin salts. J Pharm Sci 1969; 58(3):337–9.
11. Stephens VC, Conine JW, Murphy HW. Esters of erythromycin IV, alkyl sulfate salts. J Am Pharm Assoc 1959; 48(11):620–2.

12. Aungst BJ, Hussain MA. Sustained propranolol delivery and increased oral bioavailability in dogs given a propranolol laurate salt. Pharm Res 1992; 9(11): 1507–9.
13. Personal communication.
14. Carstensen JT. Effect of moisture on the stability of solid dosage forms. Drug Develop Ind Pharm 1988; 14(14):1927–69.
15. Ahlneck C, Zografi G. The molecular basis of moisture effects on the physical and chemical stability of drugs in the solid state. Int J Pharm 1990; 62:87–95.
16. Berge SM, Bighley LD, Monkhouse D. Pharmaceutical salts. J Pharm Sci 1977; 66(1):1–19.
17. Badawy SIF. Effect of salt form on chemical stability of an ester prodrug of a glycoprotein IIb/IIIa receptor antagonist in solid dosage forms. Int J Pharm 2001; 223:81–7.
18. Kondritzer A, Ellin RI, Edberg LJ. Investigation of methyl pyridini4um-2-aldoxime salts. J Pharm Sci 1961; 50(2):109–12.
19. Peterhoff R. Acta Radiol 1958; 46:719.
20. Martin A, Swarbrick J, Cammarata A. Physical Pharmacy: Physical and Chemical Principles in the Pharmaceutical Sciences, 3rd ed. Philadelphia, PA: Lea and Febiger, 1983, p. 578.
21. Serajuddin ATM, Jarowski CI. Effect of diffusion layer pH and solubility on the dissolution rate of pharmaceutical bases and their hydrochloride salts 1: phenazopyridine. J Pharm Sci 1985; 74(2):142–7.
22. Portoles A, Vargas E, Garcia M, Terleira A, Rovira M, Caturla MC, Moreno A. Comparative single-dose bioavailability study of two oral formulations of ibuprofen in healthy volunteers. Clin Drug Invest 2001; 21(5):383–9.
23. Schettler T, Paris S, Pellett M, Kidner S, Wilkinson D. Comparative pharmacokinetics of two fast-dissolving oral ibuprofen formulations and a regular-release ibuprofen tablet in healthy volunteers. Clin Drug Invest 2001; 21(1):73–8.
24. Potthast H, Schug B, Elze M, Schwerdtle R, Blume H. Comparison of bioavailability of erythromycin estolate and erythromycin ethylsuccinate suspensions after oral multiple-dose administration. Pharmazie 1995; 50:56–60.
25. Charman WN, Stella VJ. Lymphatic Transport of Drugs. Boca Raton, FL: CRC Press, 1992.
26. Malek P, Kolc J, Herold M, Hoffman J. Antibiotics Annual 1957–1958. New York, NY: Medical Encyclopedia 1958:546.
27. Khoo SM, Prankerd RJ, Edwards GA, Porter CJH, Charman WN. A physicochemical basis for the extensive intestinal lymphatic transport of a poorly lipid soluble antimalarial, halofantrine hydrochloride, after postprandial administration to dogs. J Pharm Sci 2002; 91(3):647–59.
28. Ledwidge MT, Corrigan OI. Effects of surface active characteristics and solid state forms on the pH solubility profiles of drug-salt systems. Int J Pharm 1998; 174:187–200.
29. Heard DD, Ashworth RW. The colloidal properties of chlorhexidine and its interaction with some macromolecules. J Pharm Pharmacol 1968; 20:505–12.
30. Perrin JH, Vallner JJ. The effect of the anion on the absorption of tetracycline from the rat stomach. J Pharm Pharmacol 1970; 22:758–62.

31. Fiese G, Perrin J. J Pharm Sci 1969; 58:599–601.

32. Lindahl A, Persson B, Ungell A, Lennernas H. Pharm Res 1999; 16:97–102.

33. Maurin MB, Rowe SM, Koval CA, Hussain MA. Solubilization of nicardipine hydrochloride via complexation and salt formation. J Pharm Sci 1994; 83(10): 1418–20.

34. Hussain MA, Wu LS, Koval C, Hurwitz AR. Parenteral formulation of the kappa agonist analgesic, DuP 747, via micellar solubilization. Pharm Res 1992; 9(6):750–2.

35. Rubino JT, Thomas E. Influence of solvent composition on the solubilities and solid-state properties of the sodium salts of some drugs. Int J Pharm 1990; 65: 141–5.

36. EP0397147 A2 Stable solutions of rebeccamycin analog and preparation thereof. Venkataram UV, Franchini MK, Bogardus JB (November 1990).

37. Antonucci V, Yen D, Kelly J, et al. Development of a nanofiltration process to improve the stability of a novel anti-MSRA carbapenem drug candidate. J Pharm Sci 2002; 91(4):923–32.

38. Stephens VC, Conine JW, Murphy HW. Esters of erythromycin IV, alkyl sulfate salts. J Am Pharm Assoc 1959; 48(11):620–2.

39. Maurin MB, Addicks WJ, Rowe SM, Hogan R. Physical chemical properties of alpha styryl carbinol antifungal agents. Pharm Res 1993; 10(2): 309–12.

40. Anderson JR, Pitman IH. Solubility and dissolution rate studies of ergotamine tartrate. J Pharm Sci 1980; 69(7):832–5.

41. Miyazaki S, Oshiba M, Nadai T. Precaution on use of hydrochloride salts in pharmaceutical formulations. J Pharm Sci 1981; 70:594–5.

42. Serajuddin AT, Sheen PC, Augustine MA. Common ion effect on solubility and dissolution rate of the sodium salt of an organic acid. J Pharm Pharmacol 1987; 39(8):587–91.

43. Raghavan KS, Nemeth GA, Gray DB, Hussain MA. Solubility enhancement of a bisnaphthalimide tumoricidal agent, DMP 840 through Complexation. Pharm Dev Tech 1996; 1:231–8.

44. Maurin MB, Rowe SM, Rockwell A, Foris CM, Hussain MA. Characterization of the salts of a cyclic RGD peptide. Pharm Res 1996; 13:481–4.

45. Engel GL, Farid NA, Faul MM, Richardson LA, Winneroski LL. Salt form selection and characterization of LY333531 Mesylate monohydrate. Int J 6Pharm 2000; 198(2):239–47.

46. WO 01/35958 A1. Franchini MK, Venkatesh GM. Carvedilol methanesulfonate. Publication date May 25, 2001.

47. Bogardus JB. Salt Form or Free Species: Making the Right Decision. AAPS Workshop on Chemical and Physical Form Selection of Drug Candidates. Arlington, VA, April 2002.

48. Morris KR, Fakes MG, Thakur AB, et al. An integrated approach to the selection of optimal salt form for a new drug candidate. Int J Pharm 1994; 105: 209–17.

49. Cotton ML, Lamarche P, Motola S, Vadas EB. L-649,923-selection of an appropriate salt form and preparation of a stable oral formulation. Int J Pharm 1994; 109:237–49.

50. Gu L, Huynh O, Becker A, Peters S, Chu N, et al. Preformulation selection of a proper salt for a weak acid-base (RS-82856)-a new positive inotropic agent. Drug Dev Ind Pharm 1987; 13(3):437–48.
51. Senior N. Some observations on the formulation and properties of chlorhexidine. J Soc Cosmet Chem 1973; 24:259–78.
52. Tong WQ, Whitesall G. In situ salt screening—a useful technique for discovery support and preformulation studies. Pharm Dev Tech 1998; 3(2):215–23.
53. Gu L, Strickley RG. Preformulation salt selection—physical property comparisons of the tris(hydroxymethyl)aminomethane (THAM) salts of four analgesic/anti-inflammatory agents with the sodium salts and the free acids. Pharm Res 1987; 4:255–7.
54. Graffner C, Johansson ME, Nicklasson M, Nyqvist H. Preformulation studies in a drug development program for tablet formulations. J Pharm Sci 1985; 74(1): 16–20.
55. Stahl PH, Wermuth CG, eds. Handbook of Pharmaceutical Salts, Properties, Selection, and Use. Weinheim: Wiley-VCH, 2002.

# 2.4

# Intelligent Preformulation Design and Predictions Using Artificial Neural Networks

### Nkere K. Ebube
*Biovail Technologies, Chantilly, Virginia, U.S.A.*

## INTRODUCTION

The ultimate goal of a formulation scientist, whether in the pharmaceutical, agrochemical, or specialty chemical industry, is to develop a stable product that would retain its desirable physical and chemical properties throughout the shelf-life of the product (1). The desired product attributes could include one or more of the following: improved bioavailability, enhanced disintegration time, controlled or retarded drug release, and improved solubility, tensile strength, crystallinity, or hydrophobicity. Often times, achieving these goals can be quite challenging, and sometimes very elusive.

The majority of pharmaceutical companies and research institutions rely on the expertise of more experienced formulators to fabricate stable products with the desired attributes. These formulation scientists sometimes utilize various mathematical or statistical models to predict the best formula that would yield a product with predetermined characteristics (2,3). Although these approaches appear logical, they are usually expensive and could require extensive experimental design, considerable amount of resources, time, and importantly good luck. Also, the use of statistical or mathematical models can be limiting and cumbersome, particularly when the desired product characteristics are influenced in a complex manner by multiple formulation and processing factors.

In the present day competitive environment fueled by pressures to reduce health-care costs, companies continuously strive to control the market share and profit in order to remain successful (4,5). The ability of a

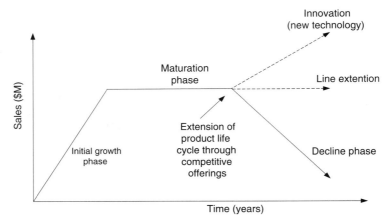

**Figure 1**   Typical life cycle for a pharmaceutical dosage form.

firm to innovate and sustain a competitive advantage on a regular basis guarantees its superiority in the market place (6). In general, a product's life is limited, as indicated, by its sales volume and profitability. A product's life cycle is typically characterized by periods of initial growth, maturation, decline, and obsolescence (Fig. 1) (1). During the growth phase through the maturation phases, firms begin to seek ways to extend the life of their products by changing the formulation, packaging, or physical appearance to enhance consumer appeal. As a result, firms are under enormous pressure to develop and successfully launch new products periodically in order to maintain their competitive edge. Therefore, the search for an effective and less expensive tool to predict dosage form performance or desirable material characteristics over the shelf-life of the product is warranted.

   Preformulation studies at an early stage in the development of a drug product aim at identifying suitable combinations of active pharmaceutical ingredients (API), excipients, and processes required to formulate a stable dosage form. Regulatory constraints or corporate policy on inactive ingredient usage can influence the selection of ideal excipients. The formulation scientist must have specific knowledge of the properties of the drug(s) and excipients, as well as an understanding of all possible interactions between them in order to design a formulation with acceptable physical and chemical stability. For a new active ingredient, an extensive characterization of its physicochemical properties such as solubility, permeability, partition coefficient, polymorphism, melting point, molecular weight, deformation behavior, etc., is needed for effective formulation design.

   Dosage form performance and product stability can also be affected by the processing conditions. An understanding of the complex relationship between the formulation, processing variables, and dosage form performance is pivotal to accelerating drug development. Formulation scientists have relied on their expertise and several years of experience to tackle this fundamental challenge. This knowledge is often lost when the formulator retires or moves to another company. Neural computing technology is capable of solving problems involving complex pattern recognition and can be a useful tool to capture and retain such knowledge or expertise (7).

## BACKGROUND

Dosage form attributes or performance is determined not only by the composition and ratios of the various ingredients, but also by the processing conditions. Although the relationship between ingredient levels, processing conditions, and product performance may be known anecdotally, rarely can they be precisely quantified (1). Quantitative prediction of a system's behavior from basic physical and chemical principles is often difficult, particularly when the formulation development process is performed in a multidimensional design space (7). This applies to both simple oral tablets and complex parenteral or controlled-release devices.

Intelligent preformulation design involves the use of artificial intelligence to study, discern, and understand complex relationships between formulation and processing variables in order to predict dosage form performance. The ultimate goal is to develop a stable, reproducible, and cost-effective product utilizing symbolic, nonalgorithmic, "nonperishable," easy-to-duplicate problem-solving tool. This involves extensive simulation work and generation of predictive models that are utilized to derive responses that compares well with actual values. Scientific knowledge and expertise derived from artificial intelligence can be captured in a documented form and are available to all.

Artificial intelligence is a rapidly emerging field of knowledge discovery and data-mining science, which stemmed from recent advances in the fields of computer technology, neuroscience, and applied mathematics (7). Artificial neural networks (ANNs) and neurofuzzy logic are two commonly used technologies in pharmaceutical product development to identify and learn correlative patterns between input and output data pairs (8). A prior understanding of the underlying process or phenomena under study, although quite helpful, is not required when using artificial intelligence to solve product-development problems.

## ARTIFICIAL INTELLIGENCE

### Expert System

The terms "expert system" and "knowledge-based system" have been used interchangeably. Arguably, the difference is in the source of the information—in expert systems, the input knowledge is acquired through human experts, whereas in knowledge-based systems, the information is acquired through nonhuman sources, e.g., databases.

An expert system has been defined as a computer program based on knowledge of human experts that is integrated in a knowledge base and utilized to solve problems that normally require a human expert (9). It requires at least three components—an interface, a monitor, and a keyboard—to facilitate communication between the user and the system. Knowledge in any domain takes the form of facts and heuristics. It can be developed using conventional computer languages or special purpose languages, or with the assistance of development shells or toolkits, e.g., PASCAL, PROLOG, and SMALLTALK.

Product Formulation Expert System (PFES, Logica UK Ltd) was presumably the first operational expert system developed from a concerted effort by various researchers in government agencies and private sectors between 1985 and 1987 (9). This system is generic in nature and consists of a decision support framework that comprises a task level with a distant problem-solving step required for creating a formulation, and a physical level that contains specific knowledge about the properties of the ingredients and processes involved (10).

The Cadila System developed by Cadila Laboratories (Ahmedabad, India) has been used to develop the tablet formulation of certain actives based on their physical properties (e.g., solubility, hygroscopicity), chemical properties (e.g., functional groups), and interrelated biological properties (e.g., dissolution rate). This system identifies compatible formulation composition, as well as the optimal proportions of the ingredients required to achieve the desired dosage form profiles. The Cadila System is written in PROLOG and is menu driven. Other notable expert systems include the Sanofi System (for formulating hard gelatin capsules), Capsugel System (for hard gelatin capsules), and the Galenical System (for developing aerosols, tablets, capsules, and IV injections) (9,11,12).

The advantages of the expert system include accuracy of decision making and problem solving, increased competitive edge, improved risk management, increased revenue, decreased cost, and increased profitability (13).

## Neural Networks

The term "neural networks" is not uniquely defined because of the existence of different network types and models. In general, neural networks or ANNs are mathematical algorithms that seek to emulate the interconnected structures of the human brain and its ability to learn (14,15). It is a mathematical model of the brain that works through pattern recognition. It has been demonstrated that the human brain is by far superior to a digital computer at many tasks. Some of the outstanding features of the brain that are desirable in ANN systems include their being (16)

- Flexible—can adjust easily to a new environment by learning about it
- Highly parallel
- Small and compact
- Robust and fault tolerant
- Capable of dealing with fuzzy, probabilistic, noisy, or inconsistent patterns.

The only task at which the computer outperforms the human brain is in simple arithmetic. Although the ANN is not biologically realistic in details, it is inspired by knowledge derived from neuroscience. It attempts to model the networks of real neurons in the human brain. A schematic diagram of a typical neuron is shown in Figure 2.

A typical nerve cell consists of four distinct parts: (a) dendrites—accept inputs; (b) soma—process the inputs; (c) axons—convert the processed inputs into outputs; and (d) synapses—the electrochemical contact

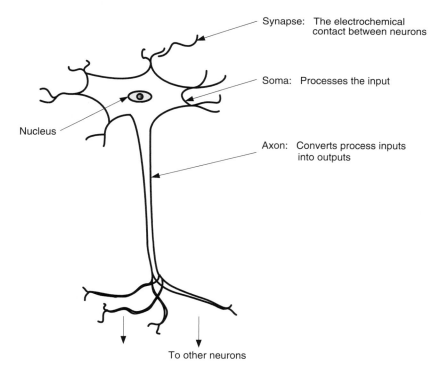

**Figure 2**   Schematic diagram of a simple neuron.

between neurons. The biological neuron receives inputs from other sources, combines them in some way, performs a generally nonlinear operation on the results, and then outputs the final result (15). The transmission of a signal at a synapse is a complex chemical process and involves specific transmitter substances released at the synaptic junction. Thus, the electrical potential at the receiving cell can be raised or lowered. When the potential reaches a threshold, an action potential is transmitted along the axon, and the cell is said to have "fired." This is followed by a refractory period—a wait period before the cell can fire again.

The biological neurons are structurally more complex than the simplified artificial neurons that culminate into the neural networks (15). McCulloch and Pitts (16) were the first to propose a simple model of a neuron as a binary threshold unit. Studies by Hebb (17), Frank Rosenblatt (18), Werbos (19), and Hopefield (20) further improved this simplistic network. In 1986, Hinton and Sejnowski (21) constructed formulations using stochastic networks. Hussain et al. (7) published the first article on the application of neural computing in pharmaceutical product development.

The basic processing unit of a neural network is the neuron. It can take one or more inputs and convert them into an output via a processing element. Each input unit is associated with a weight that defines its significance. The neuron computes the sum of the weights from each input through a summation function and calculates an output. This output is further modified via a transfer or activation function before being forwarded to another neuron (22). An example of a basic artificial neuron (feed forward system) is presented in Figure 3.

For a standard neural network such as a single-unit perceptron, the relationship between the input, $x = (x_1...x_p)$, and the output, $y$, is represented by a multiple linear regression model as shown in the following equation (23):

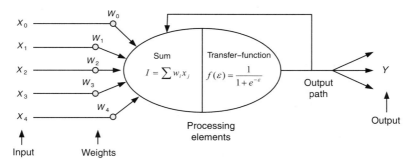

**Figure 3** A simple artificial neuron. *Source*: Adapted from Ref. 15.

$$y = w_0 + \sum_{j=1}^{p} w_j x_j \tag{1}$$

$w_0$ is a bias term and $w_j$, $j = 1 \ldots p$, represent connection weights, which are also called connection strengths or connectivities.

The ANNs are generally characterized by the network architecture, transfer function, and learning paradigm (24). The network may consist of a simple feed forward or multilayer perceptrons, depending on the complexity of the architecture and update rule. The most widely used neural network for pharmaceutical and biomedical applications is the multilayer back-propagation neural network. It is ideal for generating general purpose, flexible, and nonlinear models that can predict desired response values with a high degree of accuracy. It is also capable of handling complicated non-linear patterns.

### Neural Network Architecture

A neural network can consist of many neurons, and the method by which the neurons are organized is termed the "network architecture." The neural network architecture shows the connections between the individual pro-cessing element and its counterparts in other layers. In general, the neural network architecture consists of the input layer, the hidden layer, and the output layer. The input layer consists of one or more input nodes that distribute the input to the hidden layer nodes. Each node in the input layer can represent an independent variable. The nodes in the hidden layer per-form a weighted summation of the inputs followed by a nonlinear trans-formation. The hidden layer can consist of one or more layers of parallel nodes, which provide input to the output layer. The number of hidden layer nodes in a network can be critical to the network performance (24). If the hidden layer has few nodes, the network will lack the power it needs to classify patterns in the data. On the other hand, if the hidden layer has too many nodes, patterns will be memorized. Memorization limits the network's ability to generalize; though a model with a perfect fit is obtained, the ability to interpolate is diminished. Typically, memorization occurs when the number of hidden layer nodes equals the number of facts (input–output set) used to train the network. Kolmogorov's theorem predicts that twice the number of input nodes plus one is enough hidden nodes to compute any arbitrary continuous function (25). It is usually a good strategy to start with this assumption initially, and reduce the number of nodes until a satisfactory model is obtained.

The output layer consists of one or more nodes, which represent the response variables. In a classical sense, the output layer can also perform nonlinear transformation, but for calibration purposes. An example of the neural network architecture is shown in Figure 4.

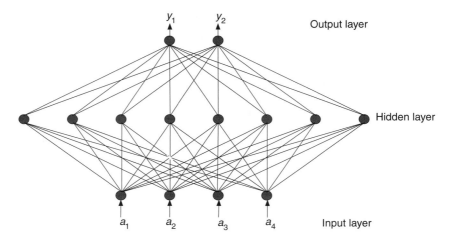

**Figure 4** Architecture for artificial neural networks ($a_1-a_4$ are inputs, and $y_1$ and $y_2$ represent response factors).

### Transfer Function

The transfer function computes the output value of the node based on the total value of its input. It can scale the output or control its value via a threshold. Examples of some commonly used transfer functions are sigmoid, sine, and hyperbolic tangent. The sigmoid function is the most widely used transfer function in back-propagation neural networks (Fig. 5) (15,24). The sigmoid function output from each node is given by the following (26):

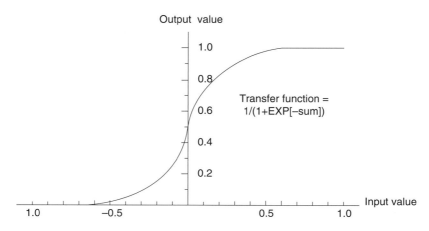

**Figure 5** Sigmoid transfer function.

$$f(\Sigma) = \frac{1}{1 + e^{-\Sigma}} \tag{2}$$

where $\Sigma$ is the sum of the inputs to the node. The output is usually limited to values between 0 and 1. This sigmoidal normalization process provides for nonlinear outputs and prevents domination or overload effects in the network that can result from a single large input value (24). The sigmoid activation function also has the advantage of facilitating rapid network learning.

### Training Paradigm

ANNs have the ability to "learn" during the training process, whereby they are presented with a sequence of stimuli and a set of expected responses. During the training phase, the information that is passed from one processing element to another is contained within a set of weights (7). The training begins by randomly assigning weights for each node interconnection and bias term. These weights, which are adjustable during successive iterations or computational sweeps through the network, are determined by minimizing the sum of the squares of the deviations between the experimental and network output values. Thus, new interconnect weights are computed to reduce the total error until a minimum total error value is attained (7):

$$\omega_{ji}^{n+1} = \omega_{ji}^{n} \beta \left( \delta_i O_j \right) + \alpha \left( \omega_{ji}^{n} - \omega_{ji}^{n-1} \right) \tag{3}$$

where $\omega_{ji}$ represents the adjustable weight connecting element $i$ to element $j$, $O_j$ is the output from the element, $\alpha$ is the momentum factor, $\beta$ is the learning rate, $n$ is the number of iterations, and $\delta$ is the error signal from the previous processing element.

The learning rate is a multiplication factor that can be adjusted to speed-up the learning process. It also determines the magnitude of successive weight change. Increasing the learning rate enhances the process. If the learning rate is too high, it results in drastic weight changes and the inability of the network to converge at an optimal solution set or learn effectively. On the other hand, if the learning rate is too low, the network will be caught in a local minimum, and the learning process is slowed down. The momentum factor is a proportionality constant that has the effect of smoothing weight-change oscillation during the optimization process, and is also important for accelerating the learning process.

The error signal for the process element $i$ of the output layer is given by (7)

$$\delta_i = (T_i - O_i) f(I_i) \tag{4}$$

and that for the processing element $j$ in the hidden layer by (7)

$$\delta_i = f(I_i) \sum_k (\delta_k \omega_{ik}) \tag{5}$$

where $T_i$ is the target value, $f(I_i)$ is the first derivative of the transfer function with respect to $I_i$, $\delta_k$ is the error signal of the element $k$ in the hidden layer, and $\omega_{ik}$ is the weight between node $i$ and node $k$.

A trained neural network is expected to recall and generalize well. However, the ability to generalize can be determined by evaluating how well the network classifies data outside the training set. This is called cross-validation, and the data used for this purpose is called cross-validation set. The training error decreases monotonically during training, whereas the cross-validation error usually reaches a minimum early in training, when the training error is still decreasing. The training error is not a reliable indicator of the network's ability to generalize; one must monitor the cross-validation error separately (27). The cross-validation error can be determined by the following relationship (27):

$$\delta_{cv} = \left[ \left(\frac{1}{N}\right) \Sigma_i (T - A)^2 \right]^{0.5} \tag{6}$$

where $\delta_{cv}$ is the cross-validation error, $N$ is the number of cases or facts in the data, $T$ is the target output, and $A$ is the network output ($0 < A < 1$). The optimal training cycle for a predictive network is one that corresponds to the cross-validation error.

### Supervised and Unsupervised Learning

There are two approaches by which the neural networks can learn—supervised and unsupervised. In supervised learning, the network is presented with a pair of one or more input and output variables, and the resulting outputs are compared with the desired outputs. The network computes and propagates the error back through the system, adjusts weights, and attempts again to generate an output. This process continues over several iterations until a desired output is computed with minimal error, and training is stopped. The set of data that enables the training is referred to as the "training set." The current commercial software contain integrated systems to monitor the training and also to determine how well the network converges on its ability to accurately predict the response variables. Ideally, the network must be presented with sufficient data to facilitate complete learning. As indicated previously, in order to ensure that the network does not memorize, the neural network model must be cross-validated. The network must have appropriate algorithms for the adaptive feedback required for adjusting weights during training. When the desired neural network model is generated, the training set can be frozen or turned into a hardware for routine analysis.

In unsupervised learning, the network is provided with a set of input and output variables with no feedback on what the outputs mean or whether they are correct or not. In other words, a set of data is provided to the network and there is no teacher. The network must discover for itself patterns, features, regularities, correlations, or categories in the input data and establish codes for them in the output (28). The type of pattern that an unsupervised learning network detects depends on the architecture. The network uses one or more of the following self-organization or adaptation techniques—data clustering, principal component analysis, encoding, feature mapping, prototyping, and familiarity (28). At the present time, unsupervised learning is not well understood. Tuevo Kohonen of Helsinki University of Technology is one of the leading researchers in this area, and his research in three-dimensional mapping and topological ordering is showing promise for a more powerful self-learning network in the future (29–33).

A vast majority of neural networks utilize supervised training. The unsupervised training is typically used for initial screening and characterization of inputs. Hybrid networks have been developed that combine supervised and unsupervised learning (34). The independent variables in a hybrid network are the input layer, and the principal components of the independent variables are the hidden, unsupervised layer. The predicted values from regressing the dependent variables on the principal components are the supervised output (35). An example of a hybrid network is the counterpropagation network—it has a rapid learning ability, uses cluster analysis, and is effective for discontinuous regression functions.

## Genetic Algorithm

Genetic algorithms are optimization techniques based on the concept of biological evolution. It is an attempt to mimic the evolutionary process by which biological systems self-organize and adapt (22). Initially, the network selects possible candidate solutions for a given task, and after the first round, if no optimum solution is found, further generation of potential solutions is produced by selecting those judged to be superior using certain fitness criteria and through crossover operations. These random changes mimic mating and reproduction or mutation in biological systems. As in evolution, the population will evolve slowly, and only the fittest (i.e., best solutions) survive and are carried forward. Eventually, following numerous attempts, an optimum solution is identified. The operating principle is based on logic and mathematics derived from the schema theorem (i.e., good solutions proliferate).

The advantages of genetic algorithms include the following: they have the ability to find global minima/maxima, are rapid and efficient, are effective optimization tools, are stochastic, and are not susceptible to the initial starting point. They have been successfully integrated with neural networks (CAD/Chem Custom Formulation Software, AI Ware, Cleveland, OH), whereby the formulation is modeled using the neural network and then optimized using a genetic algorithm (22,36).

## Fuzzy Logic

Lotfi Zadeh of the University of Berkeley, California, introduced fuzzy logic in the 1960s as a means to model the uncertainties of natural language (37). It is a problem-solving control system implemented in a software or hardware that mimics human control logic. It is inherently robust and flexible, and does not require precise or noise-free inputs. It is ideal for nonlinear systems that would otherwise be difficult or impossible to model mathematically (38). Modeling can be performed with a minimum number of input and output data pairs; however, the system complexity increases rapidly with increase in the data set.

A fuzzy expert system exists and it is composed of a series of fuzzy membership functions and rules (different from Boolean logic) that are used to reason about or model complex data. Similarly, Rowe and Colbourn have evaluated a neurofuzzy logic system for modeling pharmaceutical formulations (8). Unlike for neural networks, the linguistic rules for neurofuzzy logic can be generated from the models, thus minimizing the illusion or conception as a black box.

Shao et al. have demonstrated the use of both neural networks and neurofuzzy logic in modeling tablet formulations (39). Both data-mining technologies were successfully applied in predicting tensile strength, disintegration, and in vitro dissolution from a tablet formulation. The quality of the models was assessed based on ANOVA statistics. Models generated by neurofuzzy logic in general gave lower $R^2$ values, because the models were simpler. Also, the poor prediction of both the friability and the capping response was attributed to the scatter in the experimental data.

In general, Shao et al. showed that the ANN models were better than those generated by neurofuzzy logic in terms of ANOVA statistics (39). This may be attributed to the fact that "the 'FormRules' is designed to be a 'parsimonious' model, pruning out extraneous variables so as to make the rules as intelligible as possible." Therefore, some detailed information is usually sacrificed during training.

An important feature of fuzzy logic is that it is capable of generating the rules of the type IF (condition 1) AND (condition 2) AND (condition 3) THEN (result), with the associated confidence level (8,39).

## APPLICATIONS OF ANNs IN PREFORMULATION STUDIES

ANNs have been extensively applied in biomedical and pharmaceutical sciences (26,40–45). Earlier applications include prediction of adverse drug reactions, epidemiology, diagnosis of various disease states, image processing, speech recognition, prediction of amino acid sequence, and qualitative structure–activity relationships.

Recent advances in drug delivery science and technologies have resulted in the fabrication of very complex, often times multicomponent, dosage forms using considerably complicated processes. Retaining leadership and competitive advantages in the global market arena requires that firms develop products more efficiently and flawlessly the first time, and get to the market fast. These firms can no longer rely only on the experience of the formulation scientists or the use of traditional statistical or mathematical physics models to develop products, which become cumbersome when the number of formulations and process variables are increased considerably. ANN has emerged as a promising tool to speed-up the pharmaceutical product-development process due to its flexibility and ability to model complex nonlinear data with multiple variables.

Until recently, there have been limited attempts to use neural networks in preformulation designs and the prediction of performance of dosage forms. However, the possibility of such applications is now being realized.

## Data-Driven Modeling

ANNs, e.g., multilayer perceptron networks, can be used to generate data-driven models that predict desired dosage form response from a pair of input–output data. For pharmaceutical formulations, the input can be the ingredients, their amounts, and any processing condition, whereas the outputs represent the response observed when the inputs are systematically varied. For a controlled-release formulation, the input can be the polymeric composition, and the output might be the percent drug released at a specific time period (46) and/or corresponding pharmacokinetic properties such as $T_{max}$, $C_{max}$, and/or area under the curve (AUC). For an immediate-release formulation, the input can be ingredients, particle size of API, blend time, and/or the level of lubricant used, and the output might be tablet hardness, disintegration time, friability, and/or percent drug dissolved.

Ideally, it is better to start with input data that represent low and high design boundaries and generate corresponding responses or outputs. The input–output data pairs are presented to the network, which weighs the inputs and sums them up, and then applies a smoothening function to produce an output (47). The network identifies cause and effect relationships in the data presented to generate the initial model. The model is used to predict an output, which is compared with a known response, and the weights adjusted based on the difference between the actual and predicted values in order to improve the fit of the model to the real data. To ensure that the model is predictive, it is validated with a pair of input–output data that has not been previously exposed to the network.

The predicted response is compared to the desired output, and if the values are considerably different, they are incorporated into the training set, and a new model is generated. Again, the model is used to generate the required inputs necessary to produce the desired output. The predicted optimal formulation is fabricated and evaluated, and the actual response is compared with the predicted values. This process is carried out iteratively until a value of the predicted response factor that matches closely that of the experimental value is obtained. The error associated with the model usually gets smaller and better as the number of training sets is increased.

The data-driven modeling approach does not require any prior assumptions (e.g., linearity) between the inputs and outputs. The network copes quite well with complex multidimensional problems in which many input variables exist.

## Classical Case Studies

Pharmaceutical applications of ANNs have been extensively investigated. Initial studies focused on establishing whether neural networks can be used successfully, as well as ascertaining their particular strengths and weaknesses in formulation development (7,22,43–45,47,48). Contemporary focus has shifted to exploring their utility as a preformulation tool (49,50), as well as combining neural networks with other techniques, e.g., expert systems, and genetic algorithms (51,52).

Neural networks can develop cause and effect relationships readily, thus facilitating the development of models capable of predicting dosage form performance. Recent advances in drug delivery technologies, and increasing consumer and/or regulatory demands specify certain unique dosage form properties, which increases the complexity of formulation development. It becomes even more difficult for the researcher or formulation scientist when some of the desired properties conflict with each other; e.g., a dosage form specification requiring very hard tablets that disintegrate in a few seconds (47). In such instances, traditional search techniques that rely on gradient descent methods cannot identify the local optimum; these require a combination with evolutionary computing algorithms. Some classical examples of the use of intelligent hybrid systems, neurofuzzy logic systems, and other conventional systems as a preformulation tool have been reported in the literature (4,7,9,49). Examples of selected case studies will be presented.

### Case Study 1: Neural Network Modeling in Drug Delivery Systems (47)

The objectives of this study were to determine the contributions of functional groups of a series of enhancers on skin permeability, and also to develop predictive neural network models to correlate skin flux with chain length of the enhancers containing aliphatic chains. This study allowed the screening of a variety of structurally different new enhancers for their ability to improve permeability through the skin, without performing as many experiments as would otherwise be required (53).

For the neural network analysis involving the prediction of the cumulative amount of drug released, the inputs were drug concentrations, diffusion length, and time. The output was the cumulative amount of drug released. The neural network modeling was based on the back-propagation paradigm, and the neural network architecture consisted of two hidden layers containing 10 and 20 neurons. The neural network simulation on the effects of drug concentration and diffusion length on the cumulative amount of drug released is shown in Figures 6 and 7.

For correlating the structural properties of the enhancers to their functions, the inputs were the type and number of all the chemical constituents of the enhancers, e.g., number of methyl groups, double bonds, aromatic rings. The response variable was the skin flux. Figure 8 shows the effect of changes in the aliphatic chain length of the enhancer on skin flux.

This study demonstrated the utility of ANNs for initial screening of a series of new permeation enhancers, as well as for correlating changes in their structural properties to in vitro performance.

### Case Study 2: Multiobjective Simultaneous Optimization Technique based on an ANN in Sustained-Release Formulations (54)

The majority of pharmaceutical formulations consist of multiple ingredients, and often times require the measurement of multiple responses in order to

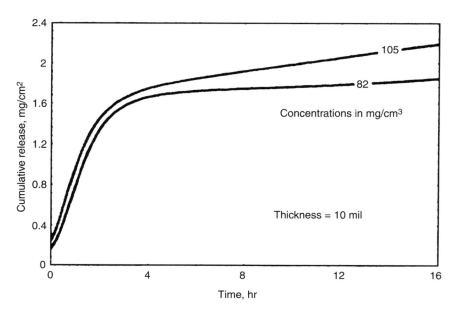

**Figure 6** Neural network simulation of the effect of nicotine concentration on the cumulative release per unit area at constant diffusion length. *Source*: From Ref. 53.

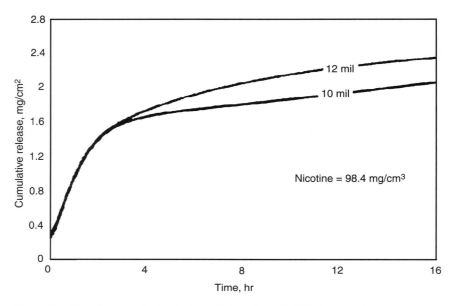

**Figure 7** Neural network simulation of the effect of diffusion length on the cumulative release per unit area at constant nicotine concentration. *Source*: From Ref. 53.

evaluate dosage form performance. The use of quantitative approaches for formulation design to provide an understanding of the real relationship between causal factors and individual pharmaceutical responses is difficult. This is even more complicated when multiple-objective optimization is required, particularly because an optimal formulation for a particular response may not be desirable for other needed characteristics.

Response surface methods have been applied to predict pharmaceutical responses based on the second-order polynomial equation (PNE); however, its

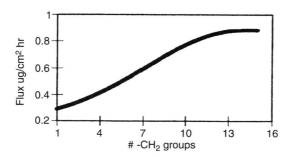

**Figure 8** Neural network simulation of the effect of enhancer aliphatic chain length on skin flux. *Source*: From Ref. 53.

use is limited to a very low level, resulting in poor estimation of the optimal formulation. Therefore, this study evaluated a novel optimization method based on ANNs that involves the application to a formulation design of a sustained-release tablet containing Trapidil for the treatment of angina pectoris (54).

Eighteen trapidil tablet formulations containing microcrystalline cellulose (MCC), hydroxypropyl methylcellulose (HPMC), and magnesium stearate were developed based on a 3-factor spherical second-order composite experimental design. The amounts of MCC and HPMC and the compression pressures were selected as causal factors, whereas the levels of the active and lubricant were fixed. In vitro release profiles of trapidil at pH 1.2 and 6.8 were determined, and the rate constant, $k$, and release exponent, $n$, calculated accordingly (55). A neural network analysis was performed using a program based on the Kalman filter algorithm. The three causal factors mentioned above were used as the input layer, whereas the output layer consisted of four response variables—$k_1$ and $n_1$ (derived from dissolution profiles performed at pH 1.2) and $k_2$ and $n_2$ (derived from release profiles at pH 6.8). A set of training data consisting of a pair of input and output variables was used to train the network, as well as to determine the optimal ANN structure (56). Another data set was used for validating the ability of the network to predict the responses. The normalized error (NE) between the predicted and experimental response was used as a parameter for selecting the optimal ANN structure (54):

$$NE = \left[ \sum \left\{ \frac{FP_i - F_i}{F_i} \right\}^2 \right]^{1/2} \tag{7}$$

where $F_i$ and $FP_i$ represent actual and predicted values of the responses, respectively. The optimal network structure required to obtain an excellent prediction of the response variables consisted of five hidden layer nodes and 300 iterations. The NE value obtained with the ANN was 0.496, whereas a value of 0.562 was achieved using a second–order PNE.

Nonlinear relationships between the causal factors and the release parameters were represented well with the response surfaces of ANN, whereas the PNE exhibited relatively plane surfaces for both parameters $k$ and $n$ (54). The optimization of trapidil sustained-release tablet formulations was performed according to the generalized distance function method (57):

$$S = \left[ \sum \left\{ \frac{FD_i - FO_i}{SD_i} \right\}^2 \right]^{1/2} \tag{8}$$

where $S$ is the distance function generalized by the standard deviation $SD_i$ of observed values for each response variable. $FD_i$ is the ideal value of each response and $FO_i$ is the predicted value. The simultaneous optimum can be estimated by minimizing $S$ under the restriction of the experimental region (54,57). The ANN model facilitated the prediction of the optimal Trapidil formulations, with a good correlation between the experimental and predicted dissolution profiles. Therefore, findings from this study demonstrated that a multiobjective optimization technique incorporating ANN is quite useful for optimizing pharmaceutical formulations when predictions of pharmaceutical responses based on PNE are limited to low levels.

Case Study 3: Preformulation Studies and Characterization of
the Physicochemical Properties of Amorphous Polymers
Using ANN (49)

During the past two decades, polymers that swell in aqueous medium have been extensively used for the preparation of oral sustained-release dosage forms. For a matrix-type device (e.g., a tablet dosage form) in which the drug(s) is distributed as solid particles within the polymer, the polymer swells upon contact with an aqueous medium and forms a gel layer, which then retards drug release. One of the important limitations of this type of device is dose dumping, which is mainly facilitated by the inability of the matrix polymer(s) to hydrate rapidly to form a gel layer around the dosage form to regulate drug release. This may result in the release of a high dose of the drug(s) initially prior to the gel layer formation to retard drug release. This problem could be overcome by the use of a rapidly hydrating polymer that would form a gel layer of desirable consistency and hence drug-release profile. The process of screening or selecting an ideal polymer or polymer matrix that will provide a target drug-release profile is expensive and may involve extensive preformulation studies or hydration experiments. ANNs can identify and learn correlative patterns between input and output data pairs and thus show a good potential as a preformulation tool to characterize polymeric matrices. Therefore, the purpose of this study was to explore the utility of ANNs as a preformulation tool to determine the physicochemical properties of amorphous polymers, e.g., the hydration characteristics, glass transition temperatures, and rheological properties. The water sorption characteristics of the amorphous polymers and their various blends were expressed in terms of percent water uptake, and the latter was determined by the gravimetric method.

Water uptake by amorphous polymers is mainly determined by the total mass of the solid, and it is independent of the specific surface area (58). The dissolved water in the amorphous polymer acts as a plasticizer to greatly increase the free volume of the solid by reducing hydrogen bonding between adjoining molecules of the solid, and consequently reduces the glass transition temperature of the solid. The glass transition temperature of the solid is progressively reduced as more water is dissolved into the solid. The change in the polymer from the glassy state (below $T_g$) to the rubbery state (above $T_g$) is accompanied by changes in the viscoelastic properties of the polymer. This certainly has a strong implication with regard to modeling the drug release for a polymeric matrix delivery system. A detailed description of the experimental design and the ANN analysis has been described elsewhere (49). A segment of the data derived from this study are presented to illustrate the utility of ANN in preformulation development.

For this study, the neural network simulator, CAD/Chem, based on the delta back-propagation paradigm, was used. The ANNs software was trained with sets of experimental data consisting of different polymer blends with known water-uptake profiles, glass transition temperatures, and viscosity values. A set of similar data, not initially exposed to the ANNs, was used to validate the ability of the ANNs to recognize patterns. The composition of the matrix polymer, training set, and validation data used for the ANNs analysis of the polymer hydration data is shown in Table 1A; and Table 1B shows the correlation matrix. The latter illustrates that the mechanism of hydration of the different polymers varies for each polymer.

The results of this investigation indicate that the ANNs accurately predicted the water uptake (Fig. 9), glass transition temperatures, and viscosities of different amorphous polymers and their physical blends with a low percentage of error (0–8%) of prediction (Tables 2–6). The ANNs also showed good correlation between the water uptake and changes in the glass transition temperatures of the polymers. This study demonstrated the potential of the ANNs as a preformulation tool to evaluate the characteristics of amorphous polymers. This is particularly relevant when designing sustained-release formulations that require the use of a fast-hydrating polymer matrix.

## Case Study 4: Optimization of Pharmaceutical Unit Processes and Prediction of In Vitro Acetaminophen Release Using ANN (59)

Pharmaceutical unit processes are series of operations used to produce desired results, e.g., comminution, mixing, drying, compaction. The target response may include good flow characteristics, compressibility, batch-to-batch reproducibility, hardness, friability, target drug-release profile, or ease of scale-up. Proper design and development of the scale-up process is desirable in order to reduce the time to market and allow for more rapid commercialization of a product.

Most of the pharmaceutical unit operations such as mixing and compaction require powder movement. For this reason, flowability of pharmaceutical powders is of critical importance for achieving target weight of solid dosage forms, good content uniformity, and a desired in vitro drug-release profile. It is a well-known fact that processing can influence the functional behavior of powders and hence the final dosage form performance.

**Table 1A**   Composition of Matrix Polymer, Training and Validation Data Used for the ANNs Analysis of the Polymer Hydration Data

| Expt. no. | Matrix polymer composition[a] | | | | Mean percent water uptake | | | | |
|---|---|---|---|---|---|---|---|---|---|
| | K4M | PVP | Na ALG | CARGN | Hydration time = 15 (min) | Hydration time = 30 (min) | Hydration time = 60 (min) | Hydration time = 120 (min) | Hydration time = 240 (min) |
| *Training set* | | | | | | | | | |
| 1 | 1.00 | 0.00 | 0.00 | 0.00 | 61 | 90 | 192 | 283 | 388 |
| 2 | 0.00 | 1.00 | 0.00 | 0.00 | 116 | 196 | 272 | 309 | 370 |
| 3 | 0.00 | 0.00 | 1.00 | 0.00 | 49 | 87 | 195 | 480 | 695 |
| 4 | 0.00 | 0.00 | 0.00 | 1.00 | 95 | 115 | 159 | 219 | 335 |
| 5 | 0.50 | 0.50 | 0.00 | 0.00 | 79 | 98 | 136 | 196 | 302 |
| 6 | 0.50 | 0.00 | 0.50 | 0.00 | 64 | 123 | 171 | 368 | 751 |
| 7 | 0.50 | 0.00 | 0.00 | 0.50 | 96 | 136 | 174 | 235 | 349 |
| 8 | 0.00 | 0.50 | 0.50 | 0.00 | 62 | 100 | 191 | 442 | 718 |
| 9 | 0.00 | 0.50 | 0.00 | 0.50 | 85 | 132 | 188 | 277 | 418 |
| 10 | 0.00 | 0.00 | 0.50 | 0.50 | 93 | 121 | 188 | 306 | 680 |
| 11 | 0.33 | 0.33 | 0.33 | 0.00 | 96 | 137 | 179 | 235 | 349 |

| | | | | | | | | |
|---|---|---|---|---|---|---|---|---|
| 12 | 0.33 | 0.33 | 0.00 | 0.33 | 71 | 97 | 139 | 198 | 511 |
| 13 | 0.33 | 0.00 | 0.33 | 0.33 | 78 | 104 | 146 | 235 | 476 |
| 14 | 0.00 | 0.33 | 0.33 | 0.33 | 95 | 119 | 201 | 447 | 688 |
| 15 | 0.25 | 0.25 | 0.25 | 0.25 | 73 | 100 | 143 | 227 | 449 |
| *Validation set* | | | | | | | | |
| 1 | 0.05 | 0.20 | 0.45 | 0.30 | 87 | 108 | 196 | 373 | 733 |
| 2 | 0.60 | 0.00 | 0.00 | 0.40 | 88 | 118 | 159 | 219 | 355 |
| 3 | 0.25 | 0.00 | 0.00 | 0.75 | 85 | 126 | 174 | 239 | 374 |
| 4 | 0.25 | 0.00 | 0.75 | 0.00 | 56 | 98 | 195 | 435 | 711 |
| 5 | 0.00 | 0.25 | 0.75 | 0.00 | 60 | 105 | 192 | 455 | 688 |
| 6 | 0.25 | 0.75 | 0.00 | 0.00 | 93 | 135 | 193 | 278 | 351 |
| 7 | 0.00 | 0.00 | 0.75 | 0.25 | 66 | 104 | 195 | 423 | 731 |
| 8 | 0.00 | 0.75 | 0.25 | 0.00 | 91 | 156 | 224 | 358 | 426 |
| 9 | 0.75 | 0.00 | 0.00 | 0.25 | 74 | 101 | 169 | 219 | 361 |

[a] Represents fraction of each polymer in the matrix.

*Abbreviations*: ANN, artificial neural network; Na ALG, sodium alginate; PVP, poly(vinylpyrrolidone); CARGN, carrageenan.

**Table 1B**   Correlation Matrix Obtained from the Polymer Hydration Data

| Hydration time (min) | Correlation for percent water uptake for | | | |
| --- | --- | --- | --- | --- |
|  | K4M | PVP | Na ALG | Carrageenan |
| 15 | −0.13 | 0.31 | −0.30 | 0.43 |
| 30 | −0.08 | 0.26 | −0.04 | 0.27 |
| 60 | −0.39 | 0.18 | 0.31 | −0.15 |
| 120 | −0.33 | 0.01 | 0.67 | −0.24 |
| 240 | −0.19 | −0.09 | 0.78 | −0.11 |

*Abbreviations*: ALG, alginate; PVP, polyvinylpyrro.

Lubricants such as magnesium stearate and Pruv® have been widely used to improve the flow characteristics and compressibility of poorly compressible drugs such as acetaminophen. Low concentrations of the lubricants are usually blended with the drug(s) and directly compressible excipients such as Avicel® or granules in order to produce tablets. Variations in the mixing time of powder blends can alter the characteristics of the powder and consequently the final dosage form.

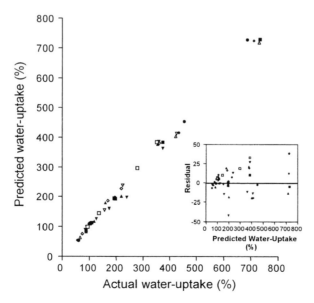

**Figure 9**   Comparison of actual versus predicted water uptake (%) for polymeric matrix contained in the validation set. *Insert*: Plot of residual versus predicted water uptake (%). *Source*: From Ref. 49.

**Table 2** Comparison of Predicted and Actual Glass Transition Temperatures ($T_g$) of HPMC at Different Relative Humidities and Water Contents

| Relative humidity | Eq. water content (g/100 g polymer) | Glass transition temperature | | | | |
| | | Actual[a] | | Predicted[b] (ANNs) | $R^2$ | Error (%) |
| | | Mean | SD | | | |
|---|---|---|---|---|---|---|
| 0.113 | 0.8901 | 495.9 | 3.76 | 496.2 | 91.9 | 0.06 |
| 0.324 | 1.9621 | 499.5 | 1.91 | 490.6 | 97.5 | 1.78 |
| 0.560 | 3.4687 | 476.1 | 5.23 | 481.5 | 93.9 | 1.13 |
| 0.679 | 5.4834 | 466.7 | 6.53 | 466.5 | 90.6 | 0.43 |
| 0.836 | 12.1438 | 445.7 | 1.01 | 463.6 | 97.9 | 4.02 |

[a] Experimental $T_g$ values were previously determined (43).
[b] Predicted $T_g$ by ANNs.
*Abbreviations*: ANN, artificial neural network; HPMC, hydroxypropylmethyl cellulose.

Therefore, optimization of pharmaceutical unit processes is important for achieving target product profiles, and it involves the identification of critical process parameters and optimal ranges required to obtain a target response. This process is usually very tedious and requires extensive preformulation work. The goal of this study was to utilize ANNs to optimize pharmaceutical unit operations such as mixing of powders, compression of the powder blends into tablets, and evaluation of the in vitro drug release from the tablets using acetaminophen as a model drug.

**Table 3** Comparison of Predicted and Actual Glass Transition Temperatures ($T_g$) of HPC at Different Relative Humidities and Water Contents

| Relative humidity | Eq. water content (g/100 g polymer) | Glass transition temperature | | | | |
| | | Actual[a] | | Predicted[b] (ANNs) | $R^2$ | Error (%) |
| | | Mean | SD | | | |
|---|---|---|---|---|---|---|
| 0.113 | 0.6707 | 517.3 | 0.00 | 517.3 | 99.7 | 0.06 |
| 0.324 | 1.5878 | 509.6 | 3.43 | 508.3 | 93.8 | 0.26 |
| 0.560 | 3.0814 | 488.5 | 5.74 | 495.2 | 86.2 | 1.37 |
| 0.679 | 4.4492 | 486.1 | 3.07 | 482.6 | 84.4 | ·0.72 |
| 0.836 | 11.1348 | 453.3 | 2.51 | 482.7 | 98.9 | 6.49 |

[a] Experimental $T_g$ values were previously determined (43).
[b] Predicted $T_g$ by ANNs.
*Abbreviations*: NN, artificial neural network; HPC, hydroxypropyl cellulose.

**Table 4**  Comparison of Predicted and Actual Glass Transition Temperatures ($T_g$) of PVP at Different Relative Humidities and Water Contents

| Relative humidity | Eq. water content (g/100 g polymer) | Glass transition temperature | | | | |
| | | Actual[a] | | Predicted[b] (ANNs) | $R^2$ | Error (%) |
| | | Mean | SD | | | |
|---|---|---|---|---|---|---|
| 0.113 | 2.0784 | 482.5 | 5.77 | 464.9 | 99.1 | 3.65 |
| 0.324 | 8.0405 | 463.6 | 2.12 | 468.8 | 85.3 | 1.12 |
| 0.560 | 16.3652 | 453.6 | 2.86 | 453.1 | 90.6 | 0.11 |
| 0.679 | 21.7768 | 449.0 | 1.07 | 449.9 | 97.2 | 0.20 |
| 0.836 | 34.0355 | 447.9 | 1.56 | 447.9 | 99.8 | 0.00 |

[a] Experimental $T_g$ values were previously determined (43).
[b] Predicted $T_g$ by ANNs.
*Abbreviations*: ANN, artificial neural network; PVP, polyvinylpyrrolidone.

The drug, acetaminophen, was blended with either Avicel PH 101 or PH 103 and a fixed level of the lubricant (magnesium stearate or sodium stearyl fumarate, Pruv® NF at 0.5%, 0.75%, or 1%) for 2, 5, and 10 minutes. The physical properties of the powder blends were evaluated, e.g., bulk and tap densities, angle of repose, and particle distribution and morphology using standard techniques. The powder blends were compressed into 300 mg tablets using a 38-station Elizabeth-Hata HP 438 MSU instrumented press with 3/8 inch concave tooling. The average compression

**Table 5**  Comparison of Actual and Predicted Viscosity of 2% Polymer Solution Consisting of Physical Mixtures of HPMC and HPC

| HPMC | HPC | Viscosity (cps) | | | | |
| | | Actual[a] | | Predicted[b] (ANNs) | $R^2$ | Error (%) |
| | | Mean | SD | | | |
|---|---|---|---|---|---|---|
| 1.00 | 1.00 | 561 | 0 | 1144 | 99.6 | 103.90 |
| 1.33 | 0.66 | 1240 | 26 | 1227 | 91.5 | 1.05 |
| 1.50 | 0.50 | 1820 | 6 | 1827 | 99.9 | 0.39 |
| 1.60 | 0.40 | 2310 | 6 | 2309 | 96.7 | 0.04 |
| 1.66 | 0.33 | 2620 | 6 | 2441 | 99.8 | 6.83 |

[a] Experimental viscosity values were previously determined (43).
[b] Predicted viscosity values by ANNs.
*Abbreviations*: ANN, artificial neural network; HPC, hydroxypropyl cellulose; HPMC, hydroxypropylmethyl cellulose.

**Table 6** Comparison of Actual and Predicted Viscosity of 2% HPMC Solutions at Different Temperatures

| | Viscosity (cps) | | | | |
| | Actual[a] | | Predicted[b] | | |
| Temperature (°C) | Mean | SD | (ANNs) | $R^2$ | Error (%) |
| --- | --- | --- | --- | --- | --- |
| 25 | 4400 | 101 | 4032 | 99.6 | 8.36 |
| 31 | 3670 | 71 | 3638 | 85.7 | 0.87 |
| 37 | 2920 | 17 | 2942 | 93.6 | 0.75 |
| 43 | 2360 | 53 | 2381 | 90.7 | 0.89 |
| 50 | 1890 | 66 | 2173 | 99.7 | 14.90 |

[a] Experimental viscosity values were previously determined (43).
[b] Predicted viscosity values by ANNs.
*Abbreviations*: ANN, artificial neural network; HPMC, hydroxypropylmethyl cellulose.

force was 1.3 tons, which achieved a tablet hardness of 4 to 9 KP. The tablets were evaluated for in vitro dissolution using USP apparatus II (Vankel) at 37 ± 0.5°C and 100 rpm.

The neural network analysis was performed using the ANN simulator, CAD/Chem version 5.0 (Computer Associate, Cleveland, OH). The ANN model was developed using optimized software variables. The composition of the training set and the validation set is shown in Table 7. For predicting the flow properties of the powder blend, the input consisted of the formulation and process variables (Avicel, lubricant, and mixing time), and the outputs were angle of repose and Carr's Index. Comparisons of the actual versus predicted angle of repose are shown in Figures 10 and 11.

The physical properties of the tablets were predicted using the formulation and process variables, as the input and the output consisted of tablet hardness and friability. Comparisons of the actual versus predicted tablet hardness and friability are shown in Figures 12 and 13 respectively. The ANN model also predicted the in vitro release of acetaminophen at one, three, five, and seven minutes. A comparison of the actual versus predicted drug release is shown in Figure 14. The inset shows the residual, which is indicative of the accuracy of prediction.

The ANN predicted the flow properties of various powder blends, physical properties of the tablet, and in vitro drug release from the compressed tablets with good accuracy ($R^2 \geq 80–99\%$). Changes in the mixing time did not considerably affect the powder flow properties, tablet characteristics, and drug release in vitro. Tablet hardness increased when Pruv was used as a lubricant instead of magnesium stearate.

ANNs show good promise for use in the optimization of pharmaceutical unit operations. The results of this work are particularly relevant as

**Table 7** Composition of Training Set and Validation Set Used for ANN Analysis of Various Pharmaceutical Unit Operations

| Form[a] | Ingredients (mg) | | | | | Tablet weight (mg) |
|---|---|---|---|---|---|---|
| | APAP | MgSt. | Pruv | AV[b]PH 101 | AV[b]PH 101 | |
| *Training set* | | | | | | |
| 1 | 100 | 1.50[c] | 0.00 | 198.50 | 0.00 | 300 |
| 2 | 100 | 3.00[d] | 0.00 | 197.00 | 0.00 | 300 |
| 3 | 100 | 1.50 | 0.00 | 1.00 | 198.50 | 300 |
| 4 | 100 | 3.00 | 0.00 | 0.00 | 197.00 | 300 |
| 5 | 100 | 0.00 | 1.50 | 198.50 | 0.00 | 300 |
| 6 | 100 | 0.00 | 3.00 | 197.00 | 0.00 | 300 |
| 7 | 100 | 0.00 | 1.50 | 0.00 | 198.50 | 300 |
| 8 | 100 | 0.00 | 3.00 | 0.00 | 197.00 | 300 |
| *Validation set* | | | | | | |
| 9 | 100 | 2.25[e] | 0.00 | 197.75 | 0.00 | 300 |
| 10 | 100 | 2.25[e] | 0.00 | 0.00 | 197.25 | 300 |
| 11 | 100 | 0.00 | 2.25[e] | 197.25 | 0.00 | 300 |
| 12 | 100 | 0.00 | 2.25[e] | 0.00 | 197.25 | 300 |

[a] Formulation.
[b] Avicel®.
[c] Represents 0.5% lubricant.
[d] Represents 1.0% lubricant.
[e] Represent 0.75% lubricant.
*Abbreviations*: ANN, artificial neural network; APAP, acetaminophen.

they can be extended to the examination of formulations and process parameters that influence scale-up of pharmaceutical unit processes.

## Limitations

Several articles have been published on the applications of ANNs and its utility in pharmaceutical product development (7). This extensive application stems from its flexibility, ability to learn from limited historical unstructured data and model with nonlinear and discontinuous functions (ideal for adaptive modeling), and ease of automation.

Despite this promising evolution of novel modeling philosophy, neural networks are not useful in illustrating the mechanistic nature of the correlation established between variables (43). It still requires a sound understanding of scientific principles to effectively and efficiently interpret the data generated using the neural network; otherwise, it becomes a black box.

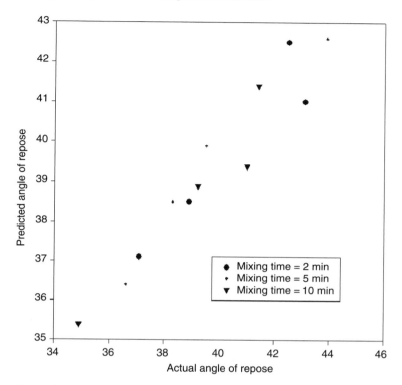

**Figure 10**   Comparison of the actual versus predicted angle of repose of powder blends at different mixing time: 2, 5, and 10 minutes.

Depending on the neural network simulator used, a correlation matrix can be generated that if carefully interpreted can provide valuable insight into the important formulation and process variables that affect dosage form performance. This information can be useful to achieve optimal product profiles with minimal experimentation.

Another limitation of the ANNs is that there are no set rules and guidelines for selecting the number of hidden layer nodes, number of training iterations, and preprocessing of data (40). As indicated earlier, Kolmogorov's theorem predicts that twice the number of input nodes plus one is enough hidden nodes to compute any arbitrary continuous function (25). When developing an ANN model, it is usually a good strategy to start with this assumption initially and reduce the number of nodes until a satisfactory model is obtained.

The predictor set of variables used in the neural network model may not adequately provide information for predicting target responses. Therefore, additional independent variables might be needed for the neural

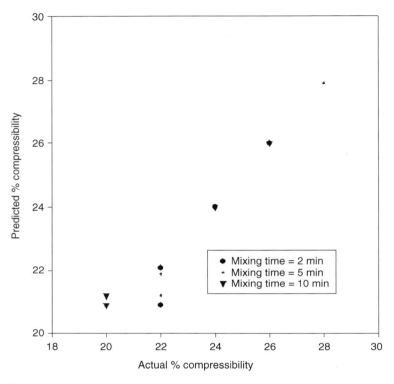

**Figure 11**   Comparison of the actual versus predicted percent compressibility of powder blends at different mixing time: 2, 5, and 10 minutes.

network model to predict some dependent variables (60). The addition of these factors to the ANN model will result in better prediction.

The quality and scatter of the data set used to train the network can affect the ability of the neural network model to generalize and accurately predict the response factors. The application of experimental design, sometimes, may prove useful for generating good quality data to train the network. Also, additional formulation data may contain the characteristic pattern of the test formulation and can improve the ANN model and facilitate the recognition of elusive patterns (60).

Ebube et al. have demonstrated that the prediction of responses outside the range of a data set exposed to the network may result in the poor prediction of the response variables (46). Optimization of the software variables, such as the number of hidden layer nodes and the number of training iterations, is important for achieving good predictions, and results in a network with improved forecasting capabilities.

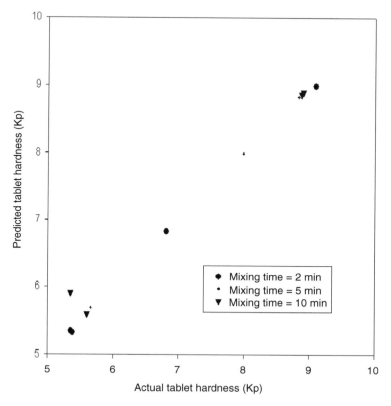

**Figure 12**  Comparison of the actual versus predicted tablet hardness for various formulations (mixing time: 2, 5, and 10 minutes).


## Future Prospects

Neural networks and genetic algorithms constitute two rapidly emerging technologies in the field of knowledge discovery in databases and data-mining (22). Contemporarily, attempts have been made to develop hybrid systems utilizing fuzzy logic and expert systems. These new "intelligent machines" are more robust and faster, and exhibit profound capabilities to model ordinarily impossible data.

The hybrid network combines supervised and unsupervised learning. For this system, the independent variables are the input layer, and the principal components of the independent variables are the hidden, unsupervised layer. The predicted values from regressing the dependent variables on the principal components are the supervised output layer (35). A detailed description of an intelligent hybrid system developed for hard gelatin capsule formulation development has been described elsewhere (4). It has the

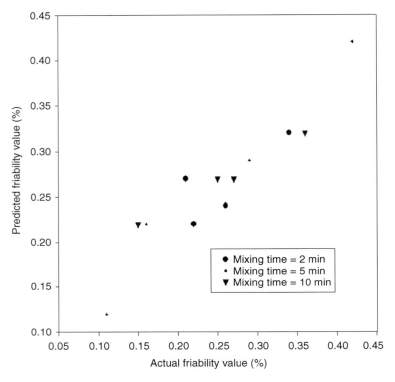

**Figure 13** Comparison of the actual versus predicted tablet friability for various formulations (mixing time: 2, 5, and 10 minutes).

strengths of both ANN and expert systems, with the limitations of both systems minimized.

## CONCLUSIONS

The ANN methodology is historically based on the attempt to model the way the biological brain processes data (45). ANNs provide a real alternative to the polynomial regression method to model nonlinear relationships. The ANN models are distribution free and do not require all variables to be continuous. They are quite suitable for simulation and optimization of pharmaceutical systems, and minimize the need to perform additional experiments.

In spite of some of the limitations of ANNs, they have proven to be a powerful tool for preformulation studies and the development of pharmaceutical dosage forms. The emergence of intelligent hybrid systems will further help formulation scientists to speed-up product development, as well

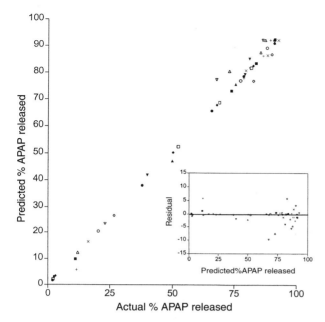

**Figure 14** Comparison of the actual versus predicted (%) APAP released (*insert*: residual). *Abbreviation*: APAP, acetaminophen.

as keep pace with both the number and the complexity of new therapeutic substances and drug delivery systems.

## REFERENCES

1. Rowe RC, Roberts RJ. Intelligent Software for Product Formulation. London: Taylor & Francis, 1998, pp. 1–25.
2. Fonner DE Jr, Buck R, Banker GS. Mathematical optimization techniques in drug product design and process analysis. J Pharm Sci 1970; 59:1587–96.
3. Johnson AD, Anderson VL, Peck GE. A statistical approach for the development of an oral controlled release matrix tablet. Pharm Res 1990; 7: 1092–7.
4. Guo M, Kalra G, Wilson W, Peng Y, Augsburger LL. A prototype intelligent hybrid system for hard gelatin capsule formulation development. Pharm Technol 2002; 26(9):44–60.
5. Thieme RJ, Song M, Calantone RJ, Marinova D. Artificial neural network decision support systems for new product development project selection. J Market Res 2000; 37(4):499–514.
6. Porter ME. Competitive Advantage: Creating and Sustaining Superior Performance. New York: The Free Press, 1985.
7. Hussain AS, Yu X, Johnson RD. Application of neural computing in pharmaceutical product development. Pharm Res 1991; 8(10):1248–52.

8. Rowe RC, Colbourn EA. Pharma Visions 2002 (Spring Issue):4–7.
9. Rowe RC, Roberts RJ. Artificial intelligence in pharmaceutical product formulation: knowledge-based and expert systems. PSIT 1998; 1(4).
10. Turner J. Product formulation expert system. Manuf Intell 1991; (9):12–14.
11. Lai S, et al. An expert system to aid the development of capsule formulations. Pharm Technol Eur 1996; 8(9):60–8.
12. Bateman SD, Verlin J, Russo M, Guillot M, Laughlin SM. The development of a capsule formulation knowledge-based system. Pharm Tech 1996; 20(3): 174–84.
13. Thomas M. Manuf Intell 1991; (7):6–8.
14. Walczak B, Wegscheider W. Non-linear modeling of chemical data by combinations of linear and neural net methods. Anal Chem Acta 1993; 283: 508–17.
15. Anderson D, McNeill G. Artificial neural networks technology, a DACS state-of-the-art report. Kaman Sciences Corporation, NY, 1992.
16. McCulloch WS, Pitts W. A logical calculus of ideas immanent in nervous activity. Bulletin of Mathematical Biophysics 1943; 5:115–33. Reprinted in Anderson and Rosenfeld 1988.
17. Hebb DO. The Organization of Behavior. New York: Wiley 1949. Reprinted in Anderson and Rosenfeld 1988.
18. Rosenblatt F. Principles of Neurodynamics. New York: Spartan 1962.
19. Werbos P. Beyond regression: new tools for prediction and analysis in behavioral sciences. Ph.D. Thesis, Harvard University 1974.
20. Hopfield JJ. Neural networks and physical systems with emergent collective computational abilities. Proceedings of the National Academy of Sciences, USA 79, 2554–2558 (1982).
21. Hinton GE, Sejnowski TJ. Learning and relearning in Boltzmann machines. In Parallel Distributed Processing: Explorations in the Microstructure of Cognition, Vol 1. Cambridge Massachusetts: MIT Press 1986, pp. 282–317.
22. Rowe RC, Roberts RJ. Artificial intelligence in pharmaceutical product formulation: neural computing and emerging technologies. PSIT 1998; 1(5): 200–5.
23. Cheng B, Titterington DM. Neural networks: a review from a statistical perspective. Statist Sci 1994; 9(1):1–30 (reprint).
24. Randall J. Introduction to backpropagation neural network computation. Pharm Res 1993; 10(2): 165–70.
25. Hecht-Nielsen R. Kolmogorov's mapping neural network existence theorem. In: Proc. First IEEE Int. Joint Conf. Neural Networks, San Diego, CA, June 21–24, 1987, pp. III-II–III-14.
26. Alvager T, Smith TJ, Vijay F. The use of artificial neural networks in biomedical technologies: an introduction. Biomed Instrum Technol 1994; July/August: 315–22.
27. Astion ML, Wener MH, Thomas RG, Hunder GG, Block DA. Overtraining in neural networks that interpret clinical data. Clin Chem 1993; 39(9): 1998–2004.
28. Hertz J, Krogh A, Palmer RG, eds. Introduction to the Theory of Neural Computation. California: Addison-Wesley, 1991, pp. 197–216.

29. Kohonen T. An adaptive associative memory principle. IEEE Trans Comp 1974; C-23:444–5.
30. Kohonen T. Self-organized formation of topologically correct feature maps. Biol Cyber 1982; 43:59–69.
31. Kohonen T. Self-Organization and Associative Memory, 3rd edn. Berlin: Springer-Verlag, 1989.
32. Kohonen T, Barna G, Chrisley R. Statistical pattern recognition with neural networks: benchmarking studies. In: IEEE International Conference on Neural Networks, San Diego, 1988. New York: IEEE, 1988, vol. 1, pp. 61–8.
33. Kohonen T, Mäkisara, Saramäki T. Phonotopic maps—insightful representation of phonological features for speech recognition. In: Proceedings of the Seventh International Conference on Pattern Recognition, Montreal, 1984. New York: IEEE, 1984, pp. 182–5.
34. Myer RH. Classical and Modern Regression with Applications. Boston: Duxburry Press, 1986.
35. Sarle WS. Neural networks and statistical models. In: Proceedings of the 19th Annual SAS Users Group International Conference, April 1994.
36. Colbourn EA. In: Rowe RC, Roberts RJ, eds. Intelligent Software for Product Formulation. New York: Taylor and Francis, 1998, pp. 77–94.
37. Zadeh L. Fuzzy sets. Inform Control 1965; 8:338–53.
38. Bezdek JC. Fuzzy models...what are they, and why? IEEE Trans Fuzzy Systems 1993; 1(1):1–6.
39. Shao Q, Rowe RC, York P, Colbourn E. A comparison of two data mining technologies in the modeling of tablet formulation. In: Proceedings from AAPS Annual Conference, Salt Lake City, Utah, October 2003.
40. Hussain AS, Johnson RD, Vachharajani NN, Ritschel WA. Feasibility of developing a neural network for prediction of human pharmacokinetic parameters from animal data. Pharm Res 1993; 19(3):466–9.
41. Alvager T, Smith TJ, Vijai F. Neural network applications for analysis of adverse drug reactions. Biomed Instrum Technol 1993; September/October: 408–11.
42. Maclin PS, Dempsey J. How to improve a neural network for early detection of hepatic cancer. Cancer Lett 1994; 77:95–101.
43. Achanta AS, Kowalski JG, Rhodes CT. Artificial neural networks: implications for the pharmaceutical sciences. Drug Dev Ind Pharm 1995; 21: 119.
44. Takayama K, Fujikawa M, Nagai T. Artificial neural network as a novel method to optimize pharmaceutical formulations. Pharm Res 1999; 16:1.
45. Bourquin J, Schmidli H, van Hoogevest P, Leuenberger H. Application of artificial neural networks (ANN) in the development of solid dosage forms. Pharm Dev Technol 1997; 2(2):111–21.
46. Ebube NK, McCall T, Chen Y, Meyer MC. Relating formulation variables to in vitro dissolution using an artificial neural networks. Pharm Dev Technol 1997; 2(3):1–8.
47. Colbourn EA, Rowe RC. Neural computing boost formulation productivity, Pharm Technol IT innovations Supp 2003; 22–5.

48. Turkoglu M, Ozarslan R, Sakr A. Artificial neural network analysis of a direct compression tableting study. Eur J Pharm Biopharm 1995; 41:315–22.
49. Ebube NK, Owusu-Ababio G, Adeyeye CM. Preformulation studies and non-destructive characterization of the physicochemical properties of amorphous polymers using artificial neural networks. Int J Pharm 2000; 196:27–35.
50. Gasperlin M. Viscosity prediction of lipophilic semisolid emulsion systems by neural network modeling. Int J Pharm 2000; 196:37–50.
51. Agatonovic-Kustrin S, Alany RG. Role of genetic algorithms and artificial neural networks in predicting the phase behavior of colloidal delivery systems. Pharm Res 2001; 18:1049–55.
52. Colbourn EA, Rowe RC. Modeling and optimization of a tablet formulation using neural networks and genetic algorithms. Pharm Technol Eur 1996; 8(9): 46–55.
53. Kurnik RT, Shah K, Ma X. Neural network modeling in drug delivery systems. Proc Int Symp Control Release Bioact Mater 1995; 22:368–9.
54. Takahara J, Takayama K, Nagai T. Multi-objective simultaneous optimization technique based on artificial neural network in sustained release formulations. J Control Rel 1997; 49:11–20.
55. Ford I, Rubinstein MH, McCaul F, Hogan JE, Edgar PJ. Importance of drug type, tablet shape and added diluents on drug release kinetics from hydroxypropyl methylcellulose matrix tablets. Int J Pharm 1987; 40:223–34.
56. Jha BK, Tambe SS, Kulkarni BD. Estimating diffusion coefficients of a micella system using an artificial neural network. J Colloid Interf Sci 1995; 170:392–8.
57. Khuri I, Conlon M. Simultaneous optimization of multiple responses represented by polynomial regression functions. Technometrics 1981; 23: 363–75.
58. Zografi G. States of water associated with solids. Drug Dev Ind Pharm 1988; 14:1905–26.
59. Ebube NK, Adeyeye CM. In: Proceedings of the AAPS Annual Meeting, Boston, MA, Nov 1997.
60. Kesavan JG, Peck GE. Pharmaceutical granulation and tablet formulation using neural networks. Pharm Dev Technol 1996; 1(4):391–404.

*Part 3: Profiling the Drug Substance*

# 3.1

# Developing a Profile of the Active Pharmaceutical Ingredient

**Harry G. Brittain**

*Center for Pharmaceutical Physics, Milford, New Jersey, U.S.A.*

## INTRODUCTION

The essential component of a solid dose form is, of course, the active pharmaceutical ingredient (API), and most drug substances are still administered via the solid dose form (1). It is a truism that one cannot develop such a dosage form without determining the scope of excipients that might be used in the formulation; but before one can begin to comprehend the scope of these studies, one must first catalog and understand the chemical and physical properties of the bulk drug substance. The acquisition of a sufficiently detailed body of information regarding the properties of an API allows a formulator to set up drug–excipient compatibility studies, rationally design formulations, and ultimately cope with unanticipated crises.

Systematic approaches to the chemical physical characterization of pharmaceutical substances have been outlined in the context of preformulation programs (2–6), with particular attention being paid to the drug stability (7), analytical testing (8,9), and physical property aspects of the API (10,11). Equally important are studies of the crystallographic state of the drug substance, and how these effects translate into properties of pharmaceutical utility (12–14). It is now accepted that the properties of a given drug substance are to be thoroughly investigated early during the stages of development, and the results of these investigations included in the Chemistry, Manufacturing, and Control section of a New Drug Application.

At the outset of the API characterization program, certain items of general information need to be established. Very often, all the information that proceeds out of the basic chemical and pharmacological studies is the identity of the active ingredient, which therefore should be subject to specification of the proper nomenclature. This will include the systematic chemical name and a nonproprietary name if one has been identified and approved by the United States Adopted Name Council (USAN) and WHO. One would have the knowledge of the empirical formula, the molecular weight, the CAS number, and the molecular structural formula. When the compound contains one or more centers of dissymmetry, the absolute configuration of the active enantiomer or diastereomer should be determined.

To illustrate the principles of API profiling through example, a case study profile of benzene-carboxylic acid (commonly known as benzoic acid) will be developed. The rational for developing this compound would originate in its antibacterial and antifungal properties, and in its ability to act as a preservative in pharmaceutical formulations (15). The empirical formula of this compound is $C_7H_6O_2$, the molecular weight is 122.121, the CAS number is 68-85-0, and the molecular structural formula is

The elemental composition is calculated as carbon $= 68.85\%$, hydrogen $= 4.95\%$, and oxygen $= 26.20\%$. The compound possesses no centers of dissymmetry and is therefore incapable of exhibiting optical activity.

This information constitutes the starting place for an API profiling program. It may be noted that the most extensive compilation of drug substance profiles can be found in the *Profiles* series that began in 1972, with volumes being published on an annual basis since then (16–18), and the contents of these profiles can be used to develop the scope of profiles of new drug substances. These topics will be developed in great detail in succeeding chapters of this book, but it is first appropriate to provide an overview as to how one would go about developing a profile of the drug substance that contains all of the information required to move the API along its development timeline.

## PHYSICAL CHARACTERISTICS OF THE API

### Solution-Phase Properties

Since many drug substances contain functional groups that can be classified as being either weak acids or weak bases, one of the most important characteristics of a drug substance (and frequently one of the earliest obtained) is its pattern of ionization constants. This type of discussion is usually derived from the 1923 definitions of J.N. Brønsted and T.M. Lowry, where an acid is a substance capable of donating a proton to another substance, such as water:

$$HA + H_2O \leftrightarrow H_3O^+ + A^- \tag{1}$$

The acidic substance (HA) that originally donated the proton becomes the conjugate base ($A^-$) of that substance, since the conjugate base could conceivably accept a proton from an even stronger acid than the original substance. One can write the equilibrium constant expression corresponding to Equation 1 as

$$K_C = \frac{[H_3O^+][A^-]}{[HA][H_2O]} \tag{2}$$

But since $[H_2O]$ is a constant, one can collect the constants on the left-hand side of the equation to derive the acid ionization constant expression:

$$K_A = \frac{[H_3O^+][A^-]}{[HA]} \tag{3}$$

And, of course, one can define $pK_A$ as

$$pK_A = -\log(K_A) \tag{4}$$

A strong acid is a substance that reacts completely with water, so that the acid ionization constant defined in Equation 3 is effectively infinite. This situation can only be achieved if the conjugate base of the strong acid is very weak. A weak acid will be characterized by an acid ionization constant that is considerably less than unity, so that the position of equilibrium in the reaction represented in Equation 1 favors the existence of unreacted free acid.

A discussion of the ionic equilibria associated with basic substances exactly parallels that just made for acidic substances. A base is a substance capable of accepting a proton donated by another substance, such as water:

$$B + H_2O \leftrightarrow BH^+ + OH^- \tag{5}$$

The basic substance (B) that originally accepted the proton becomes the conjugate acid ($BH^+$) of that substance, since the conjugate acid could conceivably donate a proton to an even stronger base than the original substance. Working through a parallel analysis, one can derive the base ionization constant expression:

$$K_B = \frac{[BH^+][OH^-]}{[B]} \tag{6}$$

and p$K_B$ is defined as

$$pK_B = -\log(K_B) \tag{7}$$

A strong base will react completely with water, so that the base ionization constant defined in Equation 6 is effectively infinite, and this requires that the conjugate acid of the strong base be very weak. A weak base will be characterized by a base ionization constant that is considerably less than unity, so that the position of equilibrium in the reaction represented in Equation 5 favors the existence of unreacted free base.

Finally, it is not difficult to show that for conjugate acid–base pairs

$$K_w = K_A K_B \tag{8}$$

or that

$$pK_w = pK_A + pK_B \tag{9}$$

Another useful expression can be derived by taking the negative logarithm of Equation 3 and obtaining the equation usually attributed to Henderson and Hasselbach:

$$pH = pK_A + \log\left(\frac{A^-}{HA}\right) \tag{10}$$

One of the consequences of Eq. 10 is that when the concentrations of a weak acid and its conjugate base are equal (i.e., $[HA] = [A^-]$), then the pH of the solution would equal the p$K_A$ value of the weak acid.

Returning to the case study of benzoic acid, when the determination is made at a temperature of 25°C, the single carboxylic acid group is characterized by a p$K_A$ value of 4.19, which is equivalent to $K_A = 6.40 \times 10^{-5}$ (19). From these values, one would deduce that the acid form would be the predominate species in solutions where the pH was less than 4.2, and that the anionic form would be the predominate species in solutions where the pH exceeded 4.2.

Knowledge of the ionization constants of a drug substance is of extreme importance in profiling its properties. Since cell membranes are more permeable to the nonionized forms of drug substances, the state of ionization of an API is important to its absorption in the body. Since the pH of body fluids varies with position in the gastrointestinal tract (e.g., pH $\approx$ 1.2 in the stomach, and pH $\approx$ 6.8 in the intestine), drug substances that are weak acids or weak bases will undergo greater or lesser degrees of absorption in the different organs.

The absorption of a drug substance is frequently considered in terms of its ability to penetrate the membrane barriers of cells. Owing to the greater lipid solubility of nonionized forms and to the highly charged nature of the cell membrane that interacts strongly with charged ionic species, the uncharged drug substances are frequently the most efficiently absorbed forms. In addition, charged ionic forms of an API are invariably solvated, and the larger dimensions of these solvated ions present additional difficulties to their absorption. For these reasons, scientists often determine the degree to which a drug substance will partition between water and a model organic phase such as octanol.

The stability of drug substances frequently depends strongly on the degree of ionization, so that evaluation of the pH stability profile is an essential task within the scope of preformulation studies. Knowing the pH conditions under which a given compound will be stable is of vital importance to the chemists seeking to develop methods of synthesis, to analytical scientists seeking to develop methods for analysis, and to formulators seeking to develop a stable drug product. Typically, the preformulation scientist will prepare solutions of the drug substance in a variety of buffer systems and will then determine the amount of drug substance remaining after a predefined storage period. However, for the information to be useful, the investigator will also need to verify that the buffer itself does not have an effect on the observed reactions.

It is also well established that the solubility of a compound containing one or more ionizable functional groups is usually a strong function of the pH of the dissolving aqueous medium. The graphical representation of these qualities is known as the pH–solubility profile. Generally the solubility of a free acid is much less than the solubility of its ionized form, while the solubility of a free base is usually much less than the solubility of its protonated form. For molecules containing more than one ionizable functional group, the pH dependence of the aqueous solubility can be fairly complicated.

The aqueous solubility of benzoic acid has been reported as 3.4 mg/mL (20), classifying it as being slightly soluble according to the United States Pharmacopeia (USP) solubility system. Sodium benzoate, on the other hand, exhibits an aqueous solubility of 555.6 mg/mL, or freely soluble according to the USP system. The low solubility of the acid form and the high solubility of its anionic form would suggest that it would be prudent to develop the salt of benzoic acid with a base to maximize its bioavailability. Having knowledge of the $pK_A$ value, and of the solubilities of the acid and its sodium salt, enables a calculation of the pH dependence of the aqueous solubility, and these data are plotted in Figure 1. It has also been reported that the aqueous solubility of benzoic acid is strongly dependent on pH (20), with the values plotted in Figure 2 exhibit the classic behavior of a solute characterized by an endothermic heat of solution.

From the pH dependence of the solubility of benzoic acid, one would predict that the substance would be more soluble in nonpolar solvent systems than in polar systems. This prediction is borne out by the

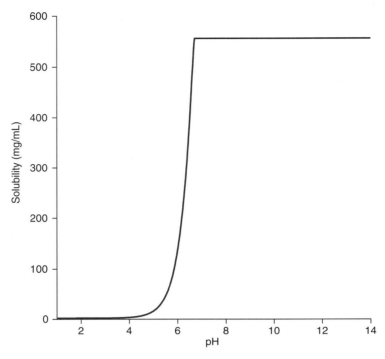

**Figure 1**   Calculated pH dependence of the aqueous solubility of benzoic acid.

octanol– water partition coefficient, where a value of log $P$ equal to 1.9 has been reported (20).

   Not only does the ionization of benzoic acid affect its aqueous solubility, but the process is also manifested in the ultraviolet absorption spectrum. Figure 3 shows the UV spectra obtained for a 5 μg/mL solution of benzoic acid in methanol (i.e., the protonated form) and for the same concentration of substance dissolved in 0.1N sodium hydroxide solution (i.e., the ionized form). The spectrum of the protonated form is dominated by the peak at 228 nm (molar absorptivity = 11,900 L/mole), while the analogous peak of the ionized form is slightly blue-shifted to 225 nm and is significantly less intense (molar absorptivity = 8640 L/mole).

## Solid-State Properties

The first evaluation of the solid-state properties of an API should entail study of the morphology of its component crystals, since it is well known that the shape of crystals will exert a strong influence over the micromeritic properties of the substance (21–23). In addition, one can quickly obtain a

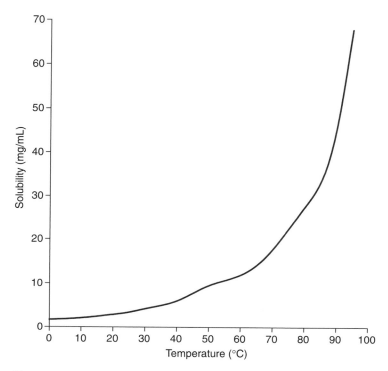

**Figure 2** Temperature dependence of the aqueous solubility of benzoic acid. *Source*: Plotted from data provided in Ref. 20.

visualization of the average particle size and even estimations as to how variable the crystal size might be. Furthermore, the use of polarizing optics enables one to evaluate the relative degree of crystallinity inherent to the material, and for well-formed crystals it is even possible to obtain crystallographic information as well.

The component particles of the benzoic acid example were imaged using polarizing light microscopy and, as shown in Figure 4, are seen to exist as columnar to tabular type particles. When viewed between crossed polarizing optics, the component crystals exhibit moderately strong birefringence, which can be transformed into a higher order through the use of quartz quarter-wave plates. When the substance is crystallized under accelerated conditions, one obtains needle-like morphologies for the crystals rather than the columnar morphology shown in Figure 4.

Although there is no doubt that the ultimate proof of crystal structure is obtained using single crystal X-ray diffraction methods, it is equally true that powder diffraction represents the technique of choice for rapid evaluations of the crystal form of an API. The technique is eminently suited to

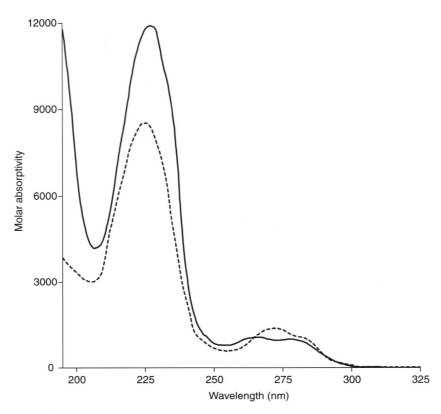

**Figure 3** Ultraviolet absorption spectra of 5 µg/mL solutions of benzoic acid dissolved in methanol (*solid trace*) and in 0.1N sodium hydroxide solution (*dashed trace*).

establish only the polymorphic identify of an isolated solid, and X-ray powder diffraction (XRPD) is the predominant tool for the study of poly-crystalline materials (24–28). To measure a powder pattern, a randomly oriented sample is prepared so as to expose all the planes of a sample and irradiated with monochromatic X-ray radiation. The XRPD pattern consists of a series of peaks detected at characteristic scattering angles (measured in degrees 2θ), and these angles and their relative intensities constitute a definition of the crystal form.

For example, the XRPD pattern of benzoic acid is shown in Figure 5. One may define this particular crystal form by the angles of the five most intense scattering peaks, namely 8.15, 10.21, 16.24, 17.20, and 21.67 degrees 2θ. Through use of the Bragg equation

$$nz\lambda = 2d\sin\theta \tag{11}$$

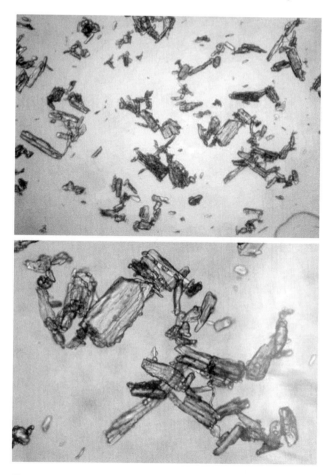

**Figure 4**  Morphology of benzoic acid crystals, obtained using optical microscopy at magnifications of 40 × (*upper photo*) and 100 × (*lower photo*).

one may calculate the distances between the planes in the crystal generating these lines (the $d$-spacings) from knowledge of the scattering angles and the wavelength of the incident beam ($\lambda$). For the benzoic acid example, the calculated $d$-spacings for the five most intense scattering peaks, namely 10.840, 8.657, 5.453, 5.151, and 4.098 Å, actually constitute a better definition of this particular crystal form.

Thermal analysis methods are defined as those techniques in which a property of an analyte is determined as a function of an externally applied temperature, where one seeks to understand the scope of physical and chemical changes that may take place in a heated sample. Thermal reactions

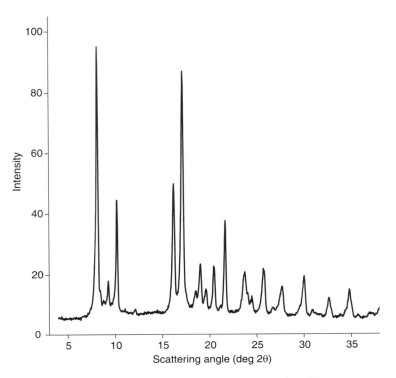

**Figure 5**  X-ray powder diffraction pattern of benzoic acid.

can be endothermic (melting, boiling, sublimation, vaporization, desolvation, solid–solid phase transitions, chemical degradation, etc.) or exothermic (crystallization, oxidative decomposition, etc.) in nature, and their cataloging represents a powerful tool for substance characterization (29–32). For characterization of drug substances in the context of a preformulation program, differential scanning calorimetry (DSC) and thermogravimetry (TG) are probably the most useful techniques. However, the use of thermal microscopy should not be discounted, especially in the characterization of polymorphic systems.

In the DSC method, the sample and reference materials are maintained at the same temperature, and the heat flow required to keep the equality in temperature is measured. DSC plots are therefore obtained as the differential rate of heating (in units of W/sec, cal/sec, or J/sec) against temperature (33). The area under a DSC peak is directly proportional to the heat absorbed or evolved by the thermal event, and integration of these peak areas yields the heat of reaction (in units of cal/sec g or J/sec g).

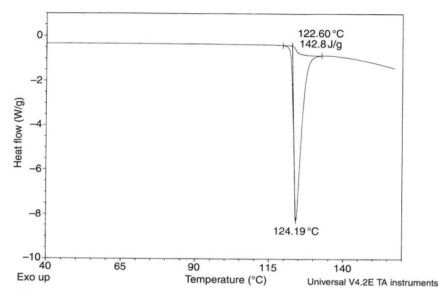

**Figure 6** Differential scanning calorimetry thermogram of benzoic acid, obtained at a heating rate of 10°C/min.

The DSC thermogram of benzoic acid is shown in Figure 6 and is seen to consist entirely of an endothermic transition associated with the melting phase transition of the compound. No thermal events were observed at the lower temperatures that would be indicative of the existence of a solvatomorphic crystal form. Under the conditions of measurement, the melting endothermic transition is characterized by an onset temperature of 121.9°C, a peak maximum of 123.7°C, and an enthalpy of fusion equal to 138.9 J/g.

TG is a measure of the thermally induced weight loss of a material as a function of the applied temperature (34) and is obviously restricted to transitions that involve either a gain or a loss of mass. For these reasons, TG analysis is most commonly used to study desolvation processes and compound decomposition and represents an appropriate method to quantitatively determine the total volatile content present in a small quantity of solid. During a typical preformulation program, TG analysis facilitates distinction between solvatomorphs and anhydrous forms of the materials isolated during screening studies.

The TG thermogram of benzoic acid indicates that the compound does not undergo any weight loss until it is heated to the point of its exothermic decomposition, demonstrating its anhydrous nature. In order to evaluate the possibility hygroscopicity of the compound, one would expose samples to varying degrees of relative humidity, and then use TG to determine the degree of water gain. Owing to its inherent kinetic nature, skillful manipulation of heating rate profiles in TG analysis can serve to identify different solvate types in certain systems.

In addition to the crystallographic and thermal characterization of drug substances, there is no doubt that spectroscopic methods of analysis form an essential part of the overall characterization program. Vibrational spectroscopy (infrared absorption or Raman scattering) contains information about the motions of functional groups in the solid (35) and is often reflective of specific structural differences between different crystal forms.

One of the two main techniques used to measure the vibrational spectrum of a drug substance is infrared absorption spectroscopy, now almost universally obtained using Fourier transform technology (the FTIR method), since this approach minimizes transmission and beam attenuation problems. The technique is highly useful in the profiling of bulk drug substance characterization and, through the use of structure–spectra correlation tables, has found extensive application in structure elucidation. In addition, when the energies of molecular vibrational modes are altered as a result of the structural differences inherent to polymorphs and solvatomorphs, vibrational spectroscopy can play an important role in solid-state characterization studies (36–41). Continuing with the profiling example, the solid-state infrared absorption spectrum of benzoic acid (obtained using the attenuated total reflectance method of sampling) is shown in Figure 7.

As discussed above, the energies of pattern of molecular vibrations inherent to a drug substance may fruitfully be studied using Raman spectroscopy, which detects the vibrational modes through a polarizability mechanism rather than an electric dipole mechanism (37–40,42–44). The inelastically scattered radiation can be observed at lower frequencies (the Stokes lines) and at higher frequencies (the anti-Stokes lines) relative to the frequency of the excitation laser, with the observed energy differences corresponding to the vibrational transition frequencies of the analyzed system. As an illustrative example, the Raman spectrum of benzoic acid is shown in Figure 8.

Although both infrared absorption and Raman scattering yield information on the energies of the same vibrational bands, the different selection rules governing the band intensities for each type of spectroscopy can be exploited to obtain a deeper understanding of the origins of the observed bands, even in the absence of their full assignment. For the low-symmetry structures that characterize molecules of pharmaceutical interest, every vibrational mode will be active in both infrared absorption and Raman scattering spectroscopies. However, the relative intensities of a given vibrational mode will generally differ when that vibration is observed by either infrared absorption or Raman spectroscopy. In general, symmetric vibrations and nonpolar groups tend to yield the most intense Raman scattering bands, while antisymmetric vibrations and polar groups usually

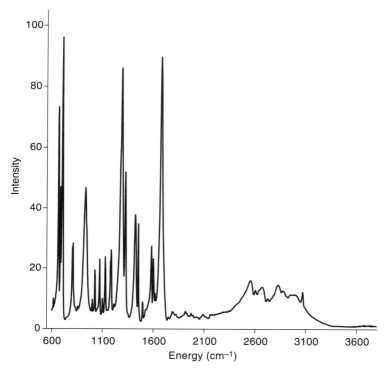

**Figure 7** Infrared absorption spectrum of benzoic acid, obtained using the attenuated total reflectance method of sampling.

yield the most intense infrared absorption bands. This has been illustrated in Figure 9 for the benzoic acid example.

One technique that is becoming increasingly important for the characterization of materials is that of solid-state nuclear magnetic resonance (NMR) spectroscopy (45), and the application of this methodology to topics of pharmaceutical interest has been amply demonstrated (46–48). Although any nucleus that can be studied in the solution phase can also be studied in the solid state, most of the work has focused on $^{13}C$ studies. The solid-state NMR spectrum of benzoic acid is shown in Figure 10, which is seen to consist of resonance bands associated with the carbon atoms in the aromatic nucleus and the carbon atom of the carboxylic acid group.

As mentioned in the case of vibrational spectroscopy, the ability of solid-state NMR to differentiate between a system of polymorphs and a system of solvatomorphs requires that individual nuclei exist in nonequivalent magnetic environments within the two crystal structures. If the structural variations do not lead to a magnetic nonequivalence for a given

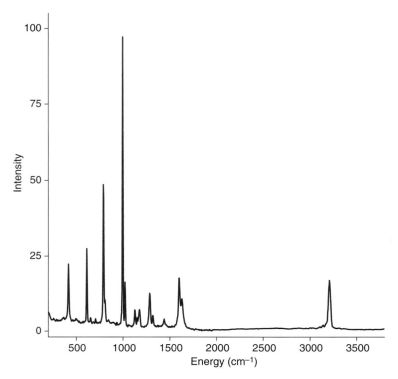

**Figure 8**   Raman spectrum of benzoic acid within the fingerprint vibrational region.

nucleus, then the resonance obtained for the nucleus will not differ. Powerful as the technique has proven to be, one must remember that the ultimate arbiter of polymorphism is crystallography, and not spectroscopy.

At the preformulation stage, it is usually appropriate to obtain the mass spectrum (MS) of the compound under study, as the combination of MS detection with either liquid or gas chromatographic separation techniques can yield extremely useful analytical methods for the quantitation of substance in body fluids. For example, Clarke's handbook (49) lists the principal MS peaks of benzoic acid as being observed at $m/z$ values of 105, 77, 51, 122, 50, 39, 74, and 76, and the text provides a copy of the mass spectrum itself.

## CHEMICAL CHARACTERISTICS OF THE API

### Analytical Methodology and Validation

Development of analytical methods is an essential part of the profiling of an API. Generally, one is interested at this stage in methods for the

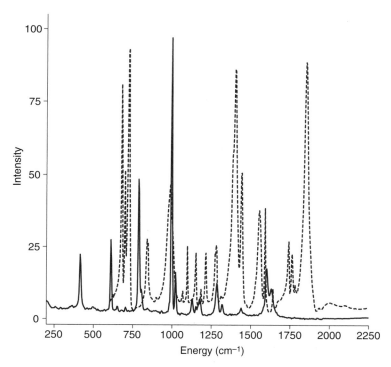

**Figure 9** Overlay of the Raman spectrum (*solid trace*) and infrared absorption spectrum (*dashed trace*) of benzoic acid within the fingerprint vibrational region.

identification and assay of the drug substance and in methods for deducing its profile of impurities. At the earliest state of development, it is most convenient and rapid to develop methods of chemical analysis that are either titrimetric or chromatographic in nature. However, if the methods are to be sufficiently reliable, they must be validated to an appropriate degree. The degree of validation will generally be less than that expected for later-stage work, but still must prove the quality of the method.

In USP 28, general test < 1225 > contains the overall guidelines for method validation and provides a summary of the particular performance parameters required for various types of assay methods (50). Category I assays are those developed for the quantitation of major components of bulk drug substances or active ingredients (including preservatives) in finished pharmaceutical products. Category II assays are those that are used for the determination of impurities in bulk drug substances or degradation products in finished pharmaceutical products and can include either quantitative assays or limit tests. Methods belonging to category III are used to determine performance characteristics (such as dissolution profile, disintegration time, rate of drug release, etc.) of a drug substance or dosage

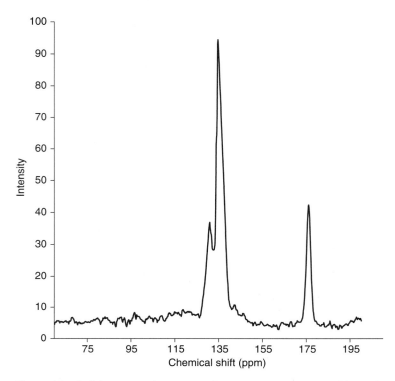

**Figure 10** Solid-state nuclear magnetic resonance spectrum of benzoic acid.

form. For analytical methodology suitable for preformulation studies, the procedure should be validated as to its precision, accuracy, specificity, limits of detection and quantitation, linearity, and range.

The precision of an analytical procedure expresses the closeness of agreement between a series of results obtained from the multiple sampling of the same homogeneous sample under the exact conditions required for performance of the method. This quantity is normally expressed in terms of the relative standard deviation measured during the multiple series of measurements. To evaluate the precision of an analytical method, one assays a sufficient number of aliquots of a homogenous sample so as to be able to calculate a statistically valid estimate of the relative standard deviation. Assays used to establish the method precision should be independent analyses of samples that have been carried through the complete analytical procedure from sample preparation to final test result.

The accuracy of an analytical procedure expresses the closeness of agreement between the value found using the assay and the value that is accepted either as a conventional true value or as an accepted reference value. As such, it is a measure of the exactness of the analytical method.

Accuracy is expressed as the percent recovery by the assay of a known quantity of analyte spiked into a sample matrix. The accuracy of an analytical procedure is properly determined by applying the procedure to samples, or to mixtures of excipients (i.e., a suitable placebo), to which known amounts of analyte have been added. The analyte should be spiked into the matrix at concentration values that span the anticipated end result, and spiking levels of 50%, 75%, 100%, 125%, and 150% of the expected concentration are appropriate. The accuracy is calculated from the test results as the percent of analyte recovered by the assay.

Specificity is the ability to assess the analyte unequivocally in the presence of components that might be expected to be present. It is therefore a measure of the degree of interference (or absence thereof) in the analysis of complex sample mixtures. Specificity is expressed as the degree of bias of test results obtained through the analysis of samples containing added impurities, degradation products, related chemical compounds, or placebo ingredients, when compared to analogous results obtained without the added substances. The specificity of an analytical procedure is obtained through the analysis of a sample or samples containing potentially interfering species, and demonstrating the ability of the method to yield reliable information even in the presence of these species. This sample is prepared by spiking possible interfering species (process impurities, degradation products, or related chemical compounds) into a typical sample matrix, and demonstrating that the method is capable of their differentiation.

The degree of specificity associated with a given analytical procedure is especially important for assay methods used to demonstrate the stability of drug substances or drug products. Such assay methods must be shown to be capable for the detection and quantitation of any compound that may be present in the sample, whether these originate from processing or whether they result from a degradation pathway. During the development of the analytical procedure, the analyst will vary a sufficient number of experimental conditions so as to prove that the method in question is capable of totally resolving any impurity that might be present in the sample. Analysts also stress drug substances and drug products to intentionally produce potential reaction products and then prove that the method is capable of identifying and quantitating these substances as well.

The linearity of an analytical procedure is its ability to yield test results that are directly proportional to the concentration of an analyte in samples within a given range. Linearity is expressed in terms of the variance around the slope of the line (calculated using standard linear regression) from test results obtained through the analysis of samples containing varying concentrations of analyte. The slope of the regression line provides the mathematical relationship between the test results and the analyte concentration, and the $y$-intercept is an estimation of any potential bias in the assay method.

The limit of detection of an analytical procedure is the lowest amount of analyte in a sample that can be reported to be present (detected) with a given limit of confidence using the specified experimental procedure. Similarly, the limit of quantitation of an analytical procedure is the lowest amount of analyte in a sample that can be quantitatively determined with acceptable precision and accuracy when using the specified experimental procedure. Both quantities are expressed in units of concentration. The limits of detection and quantitation of an analytical procedure are determined by analyzing a number of low concentration samples. The concentration of these samples (two or three in number) should span the lowest quarter of the range established during the linearity study. Each sample is assayed six times, and the standard deviation of the analyte response is calculated. The standard deviation values are then averaged to deduce the mean standard deviation associated with the analytical procedure within the lowest quarter of the method range. This mean standard deviation is then divided by the slope of the calibration curve to yield an estimate of the noise associated with the assay method. The value deduced for the assay noise multiplied by a factor of 3 is taken as the estimate of the detection limit, and the quantitation limit is estimated as the assay noise value multiplied by a factor of 10.

During the preformulation stage of development, a lot of drug substances are typically undergoing biotesting in animals, and therefore the assay (and impurity) methods of analysis need to be validated to the appropriate degree. The compendial requirements for such validation have been discussed in detail (51,52).

## Methods for Identification of an API

As the title indicates, an identification test is any procedure that can be used to differentiate the API from all other substances, including structurally related compounds. In the very earliest stages of work, one can use the retention time of an API as measured using thin-layer chromatography or high-pressure liquid chromatography for identification purposes. Alternatively, when the molecule of interest contains a suitable range of functional groups, one can develop either spot tests or colorimetric procedures to serve as identity tests.

For example, the current USP monograph for benzoic acid specifies the performance of two tests for the identification of this substance (53). The procedure begins with the preparation of a saturated solution of benzoic acid in water, which is filtered twice to remove any undissolved solid. The filtrate is divided into two portions, and to one of these the analyst adds ferric chloride test solution. The positive reaction consists of the formation of a salmon-colored precipitate. To a separate 10-mL portion of the filtrate, the analyst adds 1 mL of 7N sulfuric acid and cools the mixture. The positive reaction consists of the formation of a white precipitate after about 10 minutes, and the analyst must demonstrate that this precipitate is soluble in ether.

However, infrared absorption spectroscopy probably represents the most useful method for identity testing, as the spectra of even closely related compounds are usually sufficiently different. For example, the FTIR spectra of benzoic acid, sodium benzoate, and the tromethamine salt of benzoic acid (obtained using attenuated total reflectance sampling) are shown in Figure 11. The acid is readily differentiated from the salts on the basis of its carbonyl band absorbance at $1678 \, cm^{-1}$, a feature totally lacking in the spectra of the salts. Differentiation of the two salts from each other is slightly more difficult, but the difference in absorption bands in the $725 \, cm^{-1}$ and the $1025 \, cm^{-1}$ regions suffices for identification purposes.

## Methods for Determining the Purity of an API

There is invariably a need to develop an assay method for the drug substance in the preformulation stage of its drug development, namely since one often needs to verify the quality of the substance after it has been subjected

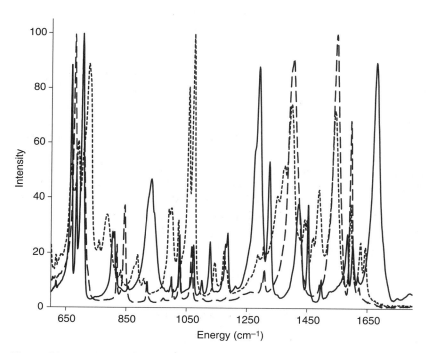

**Figure 11** Overlay of the fingerprint region infrared absorption spectra of benzoic acid (*solid trace*), sodium benzoate (*short-dashed trace*), and tromethammonium benzoate (*long-dashed trace*).

to one or more of the profiling techniques mentioned in preceding sections. There is, of course, an extremely wide range of technology to choose from when setting up an assay method, and workers can develop methods of analysis based on titrimetric, electrochemical, spectroscopic, or chromatographic principles (54).

However, at the preformulation stage, it is often the simplest method that suffices for the assay determination. Whenever a drug substance contains an acidic or basic function, one should consider the development of a titration method. It is not widely appreciated that titrimetric methods of analysis often achieve superior degrees of accuracy and precision when compared to chromatographic methods, and the simplicity of a titrimetric method coupled with its ease of development makes such methodology highly useful in preformulation studies. The endpoint of a titration can be determined visually using colorimetric indicators, but titration to a potentiometric endpoint will generally yield more reliable results (55).

For example, the USP contains a titrimetric method for the assay of benzoic acid (53). One dissolves approximately 500 mg of substance that has been accurately weighed in 25 mL of ethanol that had been previously neutralized with 0.1N sodium hydroxide solution. A few drops of phenolphthalein indicator test solution are added, and the resulting solution is titrated with standardized 0.1N sodium hydroxide to the first sustainable pink color. Each milliliter of 0.1N sodium hydroxide used in the titration is equivalent to 12.21 mg of benzoic acid.

However, when one is seeking to determine the assay of a substance in a matrix of substances having acidic or basic functional groups, titrimetry will not suffice and one would have to combine a separation method with the quantification step. For example, the separation of a mixture of substituted benzoic acids on three different column types ($C_8$, phenyl, and cyano) has been investigated as a function of the mobile phase composition (56). It was learned that the parameters of the method could be varied to maximize the analysis of the desired component. Such systematic studies are of great value in zeroing in on the appropriate method for determination of the content of a drug substance in the presence of structurally related process impurities. The subject of suitable high performance liquid chromatography columns has been discussed in depth (57), and the general topic of chiral separations of enantiomers and diastereomers has also been treated (58).

## Methods for Determining the Impurity Profile of an API

Since forced-degradation studies of an API are routinely performed during preformulation, it is also appropriate to develop methods suitable for determining the impurities and degradants in the drug substance (59). It is at this stage that workers often move into chromatographic methods of analysis, but there are still other methods that may be suitable at this stage in development. For example, the USP monograph for benzoic acid specifies tests for readily carbonizable substances and readily oxidizable substances that are based on classical wet chemical procedures (53).

Analytical methods used to evaluate the impurities in a lot of drug substances during preformulation will usually be concentrated on process impurities (substances remaining in the API at the completion of its synthesis), residual solvents (remnants of the solvents used during synthesis of the API), and degradants (substances formed in the API as a result of environmental stress). More formalized definitions can be found in the USP general chapter on impurities in compendial articles (60).

The concept of process impurities can be discussed by considering various methods for the preparation of benzoic acid (61). Toluene will produce benzoic acid when heated with strong oxidizing agents.

For benzoic acid produced by this route, the residual level of toluene or any of the oxidizing reagents would require detection and quantitation. The presence of an oxygen atom in the side chain greatly facilitates reaction with the oxidizing agent.

For this reaction, the residual amount of acetophenone would require detection and quantitation.

Benzoic acid may also be produced by the hydrolysis of aromatic halides and subsequent reaction of the intermediates.

and

The first reaction would require detection and quantitation of the initial benzyl chloride and benzyl alcohol intermediate, while the second reaction would require detection and quantitation of the initial benzotrichloride and orthobenzoic acid intermediate.

Benzoic acid is capable of undergoing a number of reactions that result in its degradation, but only two have any possible pharmaceutical significance. One of these is the formation of an ester by reaction in an acidic environment with an alcohol such as ethanol.

The second is salt formation between benzoic acid and a basic substance such as tromethamine.

The first reaction would require detection and quantitation of the ethyl benzoate ester, while the second reaction would require detection and quantitation of the tromethammonium benzoate salt.

## STABILITY OF THE API

During the sequence of preformulation studies, the stability of the API is evaluated, with this work being conducted in both the solid-state and the solution phases. Samples are stored under appropriate stressful environmental conditions so as to identify any circumstances that would lead to degradation of the API. Examples of suitable stress would include increased temperature, elevated relative humidity, the presence of oxidizing agents, and exposure to high intensity light. Samples are withdrawn from the bulk at definite time intervals and analyzed by both physical and chemical methods that had already been shown to be stability-indicating.

The most common guideline for stability studies specifies a long-term condition characterized by a temperature of $25 \pm 2°C$ and a relative humidity of $60 \pm 5\%$, and an accelerated test condition characterized by a temperature of $40 \pm 2°C$ and a relative humidity of $75 \pm 5\%$. In general test $<1150>$, the USP defines the mean kinetic temperature as the single calculate temperature at which the total amount of degradation over a particular period is equal to the sum of the individual degradations that would occur at various temperatures (62). This parameter may be considered as representing an isothermal storage temperature that simulates the nonisothermal effects of storage temperature variation. Additional information regarding the stability structures can be obtained from the guidelines of the United States Food and Drug Administration.

## Solid-State Stability

Although the conduct of stability studies in the solid state is a required practice in industry, the principles underlying solid-state reactivity have not been reviewed as extensively as one might think. Reviews of appropriate topics have been published (63–65), and Carstensen has contributed two entire volumes that contain sections having particular significance to the question of stability of drug substances in the solid state (7,116).

A key determinant in the kinetics of a solid-state decomposition is the particle size of the degrading particles since the reaction will begin at the exterior of the particle and then proceed in a linear manner through the interior (66). The reactions can rarely be described using a completely linear model, and the four reaction profiles identified for thermal decompositions are illustrated in Figure 12. Most of the reaction profiles are sigmoidal in nature, with the typical profiles in Figure 12 suggesting these to be autocatalytic in nature. For some substances, the induction time period can be short or even nonexistent. Not illustrated is the instance when the compound decomposition proceeds by a sequence of reactions (such as the evolution of gas followed by substance decomposition), and in that case the reaction profile will appear to be biphasic in nature.

For systems of pharmaceutical interest, one is usually only interested in understanding the kinetics associated with the first 5% to 10% of the decomposition in order to assign a shelf life to the API. For this reason, and given the similarity in reaction profiles at the earliest time limits, Carstensen has suggested that one use first-order kinetics to analyze such decomposition data and to determine the activation energy associated with the reaction (64). In practice, one would attempt to plot the data according to zero-order and first-order kinetics and use the relationship that provides the best statistical fit in order to calculate rate constants for the reaction.

To illustrate the kinetic approach, we will consider the thermally induced degradation of a substance. The rate of the reaction can be determined by following either the disappearance over time of the reactant substance or the appearance of the degradant over time. If the initial concentration of substance is $C_0$, and if it is determined that after an elapsed time of $t_i$ that the concentration of reacted substance is $C_i$, then the rate of disappearance of the starting material ($dC/dt$) would therefore be given by

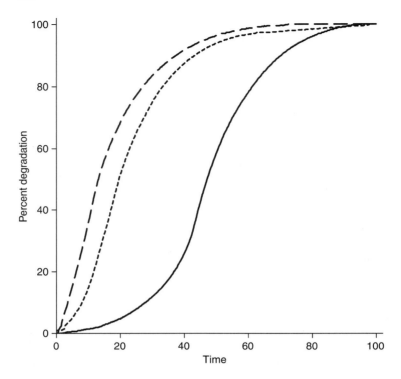

**Figure 12**   Typical reaction profiles associated with the thermal decomposition of solids. *Source*: Adapted from Ref. 66.

$$-\frac{\mathrm{d}C}{\mathrm{d}t} = \frac{-\mathrm{d}(C_0 - C_i)}{\mathrm{d}t} \tag{12}$$

Defining the amount of substance remaining at a time of $C_i$ as

$$R = C_0 - C_i \tag{13}$$

then the rate of the reaction can also be written as

$$-\frac{\mathrm{d}c}{\mathrm{d}t} = \frac{\mathrm{d}R}{\mathrm{d}t} \tag{14}$$

As long as the rate of the reaction is proportional to the concentration of reactant substance, one can introduce a constant of proportionality (known as the rate constant) to yield

$$-\frac{\mathrm{d}c}{\mathrm{d}t} = \frac{\mathrm{d}R}{\mathrm{d}t} = k_1[C] \tag{15}$$

Since the rate of the reaction is proportional to the concentration [C] raised to the first power, Equation 15 is said to describe first-order reaction kinetics, and $k_1$ is the first-order rate constant. Integration of Equation 15 and noting the limit that R must equal zero at $t = 0$, after rearrangement one obtains the linear relation

$$t = \frac{2.303 \log(C_i)}{k_1} - \frac{2.303 \log(R)}{k_1} \tag{16}$$

According to Eq. 16, a plot of the logarithm of substance remaining against time will be linear if the reaction follows first-order kinetics. The slope of the line equals $(-2.303/k_1)$, the intercept equals $(2.303 \log(C_i)/k_1)$, making it trivial to numerically solve for $k_1$. One may also calculate that the time for half of the substance to decompose (i.e., the half-life, or $t_{1/2}$, of the reaction) is given by

$$t_{1/2} = \frac{0.693}{k_1} \tag{17}$$

For reactions taking place in the solid state, one often finds that the kinetics do not follow the simple first-order relationship, and that the reaction rates are independent of the amount of starting material. Such reactions instead follow zero-order kinetics where the rate is constant, and the rate equation simplifies to

$$-\frac{dC}{dt} = \frac{dR}{dt} = k_0 \tag{18}$$

where $k_0$ is the zero-order rate constant. Through integration of Equation 18 and noting the limit that C must equal zero at $t = 0$, one obtains the relation

$$R = k_0 t \tag{19}$$

For an authentic zero-order reaction, a plot of the amount of substance remaining against time yields a linear relationship having a slope equal to $k_0$ and an intercept of zero.

The rates of chemical reactions are often strongly dependent on temperature, and the measurement of rate constants at different temperatures enables one to determine the activation energy of the reaction. As long as there is no change in reaction mechanism, or in the reaction order, the temperature dependence in measured rate constants is given by the Arrhenius equation:

$$\log(k) = \log(A) - \frac{E_a}{2.303RT} \tag{20}$$

where $E_a$ is the activation energy, A is a constant known as the frequency factor, R is the gas constant, and T is the absolute temperature. When $\log(k)$ is plotted against $1/T$, the slope of the linear relationship equals $(E_a/2.303R)$.

The thermally induced decomposition of a number of benzoic acid derivatives in the solid state has been investigated as a function isothermal heating temperature (67). For example, when heated at a temperature of 185°C, 4-hydroxybenzoic acid slowly decomposed with the evolution of carbon dioxide:

$$HO-C_6H_4-COOH \rightarrow HO-C_6H_5 + CO_2$$

Interpreting the kinetics of this reaction was complicated by the fact that the phenol product was a liquid at the reaction temperature, and its presence could not be detected until the headspace of the reaction vessel had become saturated. Ultimately, the data were interpreted assuming the existence of two decomposition mechanisms, one consisting of degradation of the solid, and the other consisting of degradation of a liquid phase.

## Solution-Phase Stability

Drug substances are frequently administered in a dissolved state early in development, and it is therefore critical to establish the conditions under which one can obtain a stable solution. Primarily carried out in aqueous media, such work will entail studies on the effect of pH, temperature, and potential dissolved solutes on the stability of the API.

Probably the most important sequence of solution-phase stability studies concerns development of the pH–stability profile, and the protocol can be designed so that the effect of temperature is factored in. Typically, the preformulation scientist will prepare solutions of the drug substance in a variety of buffer systems and will then determine the amount of drug substance remaining after a predefined storage period. However, for the information to be useful, the investigator will also need to verify that the buffer itself does not have an effect on the observed reactions.

The study reported by Zhou and Notari on the kinetics of ceftazidime degradation in aqueous solutions can be viewed as a suitable template for the design of such work (68). First-order rate constants were determined for the hydrolysis of this compound at several pH values and at several temperatures. The kinetics were separated into buffer-independent and buffer-dependent contributions, and the temperature dependence in these is used to calculate the activation energy of the degradation using the Arrhenius equation. Rate constants for the decomposition of ceftazidime constants were determined as a function of pH, temperature, and buffer by combining the pH–rate expression with the buffer contributions calculated from the buffer catalytic constants and the temperature dependencies. These equations and their parameter values were able to calculate over 90% of the 104 experimentally determined rate constants with errors less than 10%.

Aqueous solutions of benzoic acid are very stable, although it has been reported that autoclaving a 0.125 M solution at 200°C results in a slight decomposition and gas formation (69). Marked formation of benzene and carbon dioxide was reported to take place when solutions were heated within the range of 300°C to 350°C.

## CONCLUDING REMARKS

The comprehensive profiling of drug substances is probably the most essential aspect of the pharmaceutical development of that substance. There is no doubt that compilation of a comprehensive catalog of physical and chemical data, analytical methods, routes of compound preparation, and degradation pathways is a crucial task. Among the numerous important items that need to be determined, one can list acid or base ionization constants, solubility in aqueous and nonaqueous solvents, pH dependence of solubility, partition coefficient profile, hygroscopicity, and the possible occurrence of multiple polymorphs and solvatomorphs.

Certainly, studies of the solid-state and solution-phase stability associated with the drug substance are of great importance. It is essential to establish a catalog of the plausible solid-state reactions accessible to a drug substance. Since the scope of possible solid–solid reactions encompasses both chemical and physical interactions, both types will need to be studied by appropriate methodologies. Workers must consider solid–gas reactions (such as sorption or evolution of water vapor, interactions with oxygen, and phase transformations caused by interaction with vapors), solid–liquid reactions (such as hydrolysis, acid–base chemistry, solubilization, or phase transformations caused by interaction with liquids), and solid–solid reactions (such as association, adsorption, solubilization, addition, desolvation, decomposition, and phase transformations caused by interaction with other solids).

There is no doubt that comprehensive profiling of an API takes a great deal of time, which may not be available in the pressure-packed environment of modern industrial development. However, history has demonstrated time and time again that neglect of good science early during preformulation often leads to the occurrence of significant problems during later development stages, and some of these problems can prove to be fatal to the ultimate registration of the drug substance. Clearly, a balance must be struck between the need for the acquisition of scientific knowledge and the financial bottom line of the company, and hopefully the proper degree of API profiling can be fit into this compromise.

## REFERENCES

1.  Byrn SR, Pfeiffer RR, Stowell JG. Solid State Chemistry of Drugs, 2nd ed. West Lafayette, IN: SSCI Inc., 1999.
2.  Fiese EF, Hagen TA. Preformulation. In: Lachman L, Lieberman HA, Kanig JL, eds. The Theory and Practice of Industrial Pharmacy, 3rd ed. Philadelphia: Lea and Febiger, 1986:171–96.

3. Wells JI. Pharmaceutical Preformulation: The Physicochemical Properties of Drug Substances. New York: Halsted Press, 1988.
4. Wadke DA, Serajuddin ATM, Jacobson H. Preformulation testing. In: Lieberman HA, Lachman L, Schwartz JB, eds. Pharmaceutical Dosage Forms: Tablets, 2nd ed. New York: Marcel Dekker, 1989:1–73.
5. Carstensen JT. Pharmaceutical Preformulation. Boca Raton: CRC Press, 1998.
6. Gibson M. Pharmaceutical Preformulation and Formulation. Boca Raton: CRC Press, 2001.
7. Carstensen JT, Rhodes CT. Drug Stability: Principles and Practices, 3rd ed. New York: Marcel Dekker, 2000.
8. Ahuja S, Scypinski S. Handbook of Modern Pharmaceutical Analysis. San Diego: Academic Press, 2001.
9. Ohannesian L, Streeter AJ. Handbook of Pharmaceutical Analysis. New York: Marcel Dekker, 2002.
10. Brittain HG. Physical Characterization of Pharmaceutical Solids. New York: Marcel Dekker, 1994.
11. Carstensen JT. Advanced Pharmaceutical Solids. New York: Marcel Dekker, 2001.
12. Brittain HG. Polymorphism in Pharmaceutical Solids. New York: Marcel Dekker, 1999.
13. Bernstein J. Polymorphism in Molecular Crystals. Oxford: Clarendon Press, 2002.
14. Stahl PH, Wermuth CG. Handbook of Pharmaceutical Salts. Weinheim: Wiley-VCH, 2002.
15. Merck Index entry for benzoic acid.
16. Florey K, ed. Analytical Profiles of Drug Substances, Vols. 1–20. New York: Academic Press, 1972–1991.
17. Brittain HG, ed. Analytical Profiles of Drug Substances and Excipients. Vols. 21–29. San Diego: Academic Press, 1992–2002.
18. Brittain HG, ed. Profiles of Drug Substances, Excipients, and Related Methodology. Vols. 30–32. Amsterdam: Elsevier/Academic Press, 2003–2005.
19. Martell AE, Smith RM. Critical Stability Constants, Vol. 3. New York: Plenum Press, 1977:16.
20. Budavari S. The Merck Index, 12th ed. Whitehouse Station: Merck Co., 1996, entry 1122 for benzoic acid and entry 8725 for sodium benzoate.
21. McCrone WC, McCrone LB, Delly JG. Polarized Light Microscopy. Ann Arbor, MI: Ann Arbor Science Publishers, 1978.
22. Rochow TG, Rochow EG. An Introduction to Microscopy by Means of Light, Electrons, X-Rays, or Ultrasound. New York: Plenum Press, 1978.
23. Newman AW, Brittain HG. Particle morphology: optical and electron microscopies. In: Brittain HG, ed. Physical Characterization of Pharmaceutical Solids. New York: Marcel Dekker, 1995:127–56.
24. Klug HP, Alexander LE. X-Ray Diffraction Procedures for Polycrystalline and Amorphous Materials, 2nd ed. New York: Wiley, 1974.
25. Suryanarayanan R. X-ray powder diffractometry. In: Brittain HG, ed. Physical Characterization of Pharmaceutical Solids. New York: Marcel Dekker, 1995:199–216.
26. Chung FH, Smith DK. Industrial Applications of X-Ray Diffraction. New York: Marcel Dekker, 2000.

27. Brittain HG. X-ray diffraction of pharmaceutical materials. In: Brittain HG, ed. Profiles of Drug Substances, Excipients, and Related Methodology. Amsterdam: Elsevier Academic Press, 2003:273–319.

28. Blachére JR, Brittain HG. X-ray diffraction methods for the characterization of solid pharmaceutical materials. In: Adeyeye CM, Brittain HG, eds. Preformulation. New York: Taylor and Francis.

29. Giron D. J Pharm Biomed Anal 1986; 4:755.

30. Ford JL, Timmins P. Pharmaceutical Thermal Analysis. Chichester: Ellis Horwood, 1989.

31. McCauley JA, Brittain HG. Thermal methods of analysis. In: Brittain HG, ed. Physical Characterization of Pharmaceutical Solids. New York: Marcel Dekker, 1995:223–51.

32. Michael Maurin, et al. Thermal analysis and calorimetric methods for the characterization of new crystal forms. In: Adeyeye CM, Brittain HG, eds. Preformulation, New York: Informa 2008; 279–321.

33. Dollimore D. Thermoanalytical instrumentation and applications. In: Ewing GW, ed. Analytical Instrumentation Handbook, 2nd ed. Marcel Dekker, New York, 1997:947–1005.

34. Keattch CJ, Dollimore D. Introduction to Thermogravimetry, 2nd ed. London: Heyden, 1975.

35. Brittain HG. Molecular motion and vibrational spectroscopy. In: Brittain HG, ed. Spectroscopy of Pharmaceutical Solids. Boca Raton: Taylor and Francis, 2006:205–33.

36. Markovich RJ, Pidgeon C. Pharm Res 1991; 8:663.

37. Bugay DE, Williams AC. Vibrational spectroscopy. In: Brittain HG, ed. Physical Characterization of Pharmaceutical Solids. New York: Marcel Dekker, 1995: 59–91.

38. Bugay D. Pharm Res 1993; 10:317.

39. Threlfall TL. Analyst 1995; 120:2435.

40. Brittain HG. J Pharm Sci 1997; 86:405.

41. Bugay DE, Brittain HG. Infrared absorption spectroscopy. In: Brittain HG, ed. Spectroscopy of Pharmaceutical Solids. Boca Raton: Taylor and Francis, 2006: 23–269.

42. Grasselli JG, Snavely MK, Bulkin BJ. Chemical Applications of Raman Spectroscopy. New York: Wiley, 1981.

43. Lewis IR, Edwards HGM. Handbook of Raman Spectroscopy. New York: Marcel Dekker, 2001.

44. Bugay DE, Brittain HG. Raman spectroscopy. In: Brittain HG, ed. Spectroscopy of Pharmaceutical Solids. Boca Raton: Taylor and Francis, 2006:271–312.

45. Fyfe CA. Solid State NMR for Chemists. Guelph: CFC Press, 1983.

46. Bugay DE. Pharm Res 1993; 10:317.

47. Bugay DE. Magnetic resonance spectrometry. In: Brittain HG, ed. Physical Characterization of Pharmaceutical Solids. New York: Marcel Dekker, 1995; 93–125.

48. Medek A. Solid-state nuclear magnetic resonance spectrometry. In: Brittain HG, ed. Spectroscopy of Pharmaceutical Solids. Boca Raton: Taylor and Francis, 2006:413–557.

49.   Moffat AC, Osselton MD, Widdop B. Clarke's Analysis of Drugs and Poisons, Vol. 2. London: Pharmaceutical Press, 2004:686.

50.   General Test <1225>. Validation of compendial methods. United States Pharmacopoeia, 29th ed. Rockville, MD: United States Pharmacopoeial Convention, 2006:3050–3.

51.   Riley CM, Rosanske TW. Development and Validation of Analytical Methods. New York: Pergamon Press, 1996.

52.   Miller JM, Crowther JB. Development Analytical Chemistry in a GMP Environment. New York: Wiley, 2000.

53.   Benzoic Acid. United States Pharmacopoeia, 29th ed. Rockville, MD: United States Pharmacopoeial Convention, 2006:254.

54.   Cazes J. Ewing's Analytical Instrumentation Handbook, 3rd ed. New York: Marcel Dekker, 2005.

55.   Serjeant EP. Potentiometry and Potentiometric Titrations. New York: Wiley, 1984.

56.   Snyder LR, Kirkland JJ, Glajch JL. Practical HPLC Method Development. New York: Wiley, 1997:260–3.

57.   Neue UD. HPLC Columns, New York: Wiley-VCH, 1997.

58.   Ahuja S. Chiral Separations: Applications and Technology. American Chemical Society: Washington, DC, 1997.

59.   Ahuja S. Impurities Evaluation of Pharmaceuticals. New York: Marcel Dekker, 1998.

60.   General Test <1086>. Impurities in official articles. United States Pharmacopoeia, 29th ed. Rockville, MD: United States Pharmacopoeial Convention, 2006:2920–3.

61.   Brewster RQ, McEwen WE. Organic Chemistry, 3rd ed. Englewood Cliffs, NJ: Prentice-Hall, 1961:651–2.

62.   General Test <1150>. Pharmaceutical stability. United States Pharmacopoeia, 29th ed. Rockville, MD: United States Pharmacopoeial Convention, 2006: 2994–5.

63.   Garrett ER. Kinetics and mechanisms in stability of drugs. Advances in Pharmaceutical Sciences, Vol. 2. London: Academic Press, 1967:1–94.

64.   Carstensen JT. J Pharm Sci 1974; 63:1.

65.   Byrn SR, Pfeiffer RR, Stowell JG. Introduction to the solid-state chemistry of drugs. Solid State Chemistry of Drugs, 2nd ed. West Lafayette, IN: SSCI Inc., 1999:1–43.

66.   Jacobs PWM, Tompkins FC. Classification and theory of solid reactions. In: Garner WE, ed. Chemistry of the Solid State. London: Butterworths Scientific Publications, 1955:184–212.

67.   Carstensen JT, Musa MN. J Pharm Sci 1972; 61:1112.

68.   Zhou M, Notari RE. J Pharm Sci 1995; 84:534.

69.   Indrayanto G, Cyahrani A, Mugihardjo, et al. Benzoic acid. In: Brittain HG, ed. Analytical Profiles of Drug Substances and Excipients, Vol. 26. San Diego: Academic Press, 1999:1–46.

# 3.2

# Particle Morphology and Characterization in Preformulation

**Alan F. Rawle**

*Malvern Instruments, Westborough, Massachusetts, U.S.A.*

## INTRODUCTION

Particle shape and size play a fundamental role in determining both primary and bulk powder and suspension properties. There are a number of techniques, both qualitative and quantitative, that can be used to characterize materials and use these properties to predict the behavior of the materials in formulations or for quality control purposes. This chapter explores the various particle size and morphological properties that can be measured and the variety of techniques used in this characterization.

The answer to the question "Why?" is too infrequently tackled within particle size measurement and the reasons for the determination forgotten or ignored. Heywood (1), in the closing speech at the first major particle size congress in 1966, expressed this unwillingness to look further than the end of one's nose:

"However, it must be realised that particle size analysis is not an objective in itself but is a means to an end, the end being the correlation of powder properties with some process of manufacture, usage or preparation."

Thus we need to examine the real scientific reasons behind taking the particular measurement that we will be attempting. Are we concerned with bulk particle or powder properties such as flowability, viscosity, filter blockage, tendency to agglomerate ("balling"), dusting tendency, etc., or is our measurement related to primary particle properties such as dissolution rate, e.g., Noyes-Whitney equation (2), chemical reactivity, moisture absorption, gas absorption? If, as too often, the answer to the question

"Why?" is "Because my boss says so" or "For QA," then we must take time out to go back and explore the real reasons or the measurement itself becomes meaningless. It can be noted at this stage that the energies found in any particle size "dispersion" unit, wet or dry, are considerably higher than can be found in any conventional plant processing conditions. Thus, if we have a problem related to inability of a powder to flow, such as blockage in a silo, then it is ridiculous to try to correlate this to a primary dispersed size achieved by either high ($\Delta$) pressures in a dry unit or sonication to stability in a wet particle size measurement.

In the pharmaceutical scenario, we may be trying to relate our particle properties to dissolution rate to obtain a handle on how quickly an oral formulation is likely to act or trying to relate the numbers to drug entry to the nasal cavity or lungs. Shape characterization is vital here as different crystal faces dissolve at different rates and delivery into the lungs is markedly different for rounded as compared to needle-like particles. At the preformulation stage, we may want to identify the techniques we would need to use further down the line in production in order to produce a formulation with the desired efficacy in line with optimized and economic production techniques.

A little time at the start thinking through the answers to the question "Why?" will pay dividends further down the particle size and morphology road. On this journey, the following text will provide the basic knowledge needed but this will not make the reader an expert. Indeed the author is still an open-minded learner in this field. In the words (3) of Chris Leslie (referring to violin making): "These are the basics for a lifetime's improvement."

Hopefully we will not be giving the reader enough information to get him/her into serious trouble!

## THE FUNDAMENTAL PARTICLE SIZE CONUNDRUM

Hindsight is a wonderful ally and it may seem obvious to state that a particle is a three-dimensional entity. We may easily accept that any image of a particle is only a two-dimensional representation of the same particle. However, the next stage of accepting that any particle sizing technique provides only a one-dimensional descriptor of the particle becomes virtually impossible to accept or understand. However, it is this dimensional reduction (to absurdity?) that all particle characterization techniques must battle with. This is because single numbers are desired for process control and specification purposes. In these days of computer hindered design, then it may be possible or even desirable to describe a particle with a large number of parameters but this will be too many degrees of freedom for the production or quality control manager. It is generally the case especially for regulatory bodies such as the FDA that control and specification revolve around a single number and the accepted tolerances on this selected number.

## THE EQUIVALENT SPHERE

All particle sizing techniques measure some one-dimensional property of the particle (e.g., weight, volume, settling rate, projected area, minimum sieve aperture through which the particle will fall) and relate this to a spherical particle of the same property as that of our irregular particle (4). This then allows a single number ("equivalent spherical diameter") to be reported. It is clear that for a cylinder, only two numbers are required to specify the particle exactly (height and diameter) and for a cuboid (e.g., a matchbox), three numbers (length, breadth, height) are required. Thus a single number obtained from any particle sizing technique cannot be used to fully specify the material and some form of imaging of the particle is required and essential in order to obtain an understanding for the shape of the material. This finds expression in USP General Test <766> (5): "For irregularly shaped particles, characterization of particle size must include information on particle shape." Thus shape and size go together like strawberries and cream.

The end result of this link between size and shape is that we have a number of correct one-dimensional answers as to the particle size of a single three-dimensional particle. We also have a number of one-dimensional "answers" taken from two-dimensional information of the "size" of the particle when imaged (Figs. 1 and 2).

We thus have the seemingly unbelievable situation in Figure 1 above that we have seven different but all correct answers for the reported size of the indicated irregular particle. The two important consequences of this for irregular particles are the following:

■ Different techniques will measure different properties of the particle and will thus generate different answers. Therefore there are a whole gamut of international standards on particle size measurement, reflecting the different techniques of measurement. Result emulation (sometimes called "shape correction") is not advisable as it will identically map the two results obtained by the two different techniques, with the big assumption that the two samples offered to the two techniques are identical in both particulate composition (sampling) and dispersion. Should the sample change markedly (e.g., introduction of enormous particles from some production disaster. A good example is a wrench falling into a powder), then this result emulation cannot be obviously now valid (a real wrench in the works!) as these large particles were never emulated.

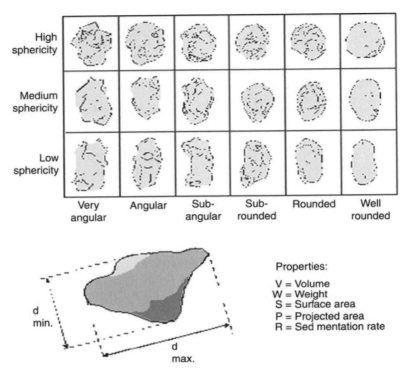

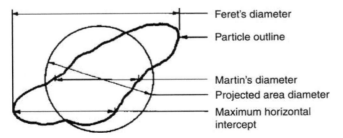

**Figure 1** Particle shape descriptions and most commonly used one-dimensional descriptors. *Source*: Adapted from Ref. 28.

■ Different techniques can only be compared by the use of spherical particles—only for these particles should identical answers (the "true" diameter of the spheres) be obtained. The corollary to this consequence

**Figure 2** Most frequently used image analysis diameters. *Source*: Adapted from Ref. 38.

is that particle size standards should be spherical in order that there is no dispute as to the size of the particle. Nonspherical particles can be characterized with one technique and should read the same on this particular technique but necessarily the same with other techniques. A good example of this is the irregular quartz standard BCR66 produced within the European Economic Community. This material has been thoroughly characterized by sedimentation in the range 0.5 to 2.5 μm roughly. Thus it is a good test of sedimentation equipment. Laser diffraction will read a much larger result as particles in this size range do not strictly behave as predicted by Stokes' law. They do not settle in a straight line due to Brownian motion and have a bigger drag on them than an equivalent spherical volume particle (the sphere compresses the most volume or mass into any shape). Thus the particles will be measured larger on laser diffraction equipment, which is measuring volumes of particles (in the derived sense—actually scattering is mapped to identical scattering behavior in the same way that sedimentation has measured settling rate and not "size"). Indeed, agreement between techniques on such a system would be suspicious. Again we must exercise caution as the preparative technique may have induced errors. In the early 1960s, spherical monodisperse particle size "standards" were characterized by electron microscopy and found to have a median diameter exactly half that expected and to be extremely broad in distribution. Puzzled researchers soon realized that this was a consequence of dispersing the particles in epoxy resin and microtoming to produce thin sections. A nice distribution of spheres had been produced by slicing through all diameters of the sphere from "0" units in diameter to the expected size with a preponderance of slices tending toward the $d/2$ value.

Let us take an easy (at least for mathematicians!) example of a set of cylinders on different heights but with the same radii and calculate how these would appear in terms of equivalent volume and equivalent surface (Table 1).

Note that $d_v$ falls much more rapidly than $d_{sa}$ for this system because $d_v \propto V^{1/3}$ but $d_{sa} \propto SA^{1/2}$. This again shows how the sphere packs in more material than any other shape. As volume considers the amount of material any particle possesses, it is desirable that any technique should at least generate this as first reported diameter and then report the particular diameter that the technique is measuring (6).

## FUNDAMENTAL MEASURES OF CENTRAL TENDENCY

For a non-mathematician, it may have been easier to title this section "Averages" but we will see shortly why this is likely to be ambiguous.

**Table 1**  Equivalent Volume and Surface Area of Various Cylinders of Constant Diameter

| Size of cylinder | | | | | | |
|---|---|---|---|---|---|---|
| Height | Diameter | Aspect ratio | Volume | Surface area | $d_v$ | $d_{sa}$ |
| 400 | 20 | 20:1 | 125663.6 | 25796.38 | 62.14 | 90.62 |
| 200 | 20 | 10:1 | 62831.8 | 13212.78 | 49.32 | 64.85 |
| 100 | 20 | 5:1 | 31415.9 | 6920.98 | 39.15 | 46.94 |
| 40 | 20 | 2:1 | 12566.36 | 3145.9 | 28.84 | 31.64 |
| 20 | 20 | 1:1 | 6283.18 | 1887.54 | 22.89 | 24.51 |
| 10 | 20 | 1:2 | 3141.59 | 1258.36 | 18.17 | 20.01 |
| 4 | 20 | 1:5 | 1256.636 | 880.852 | 13.39 | 16.74 |
| 2 | 20 | 1:10 | 628.318 | 755.016 | 10.63 | 15.50 |
| 1 | 20 | 1:20 | 314.159 | 692.098 | 8.43 | 14.84 |
| 0.4 | 20 | 1:50 | 125.6636 | 654.3472 | 6.21 | 14.43 |

*Abbreviations*: $d_v$, equivalent spherical diameter by volume (= mass when constant density); $d_{sa}$, equivalent spherical diameter by surface area.

Consider a simple system consisting of three spherical particles of diameters 1, 2, and 3 units, respectively. It is likely that the statistician would want the average of the system, which they may call the mean size. What would this average be? The most likely answer to be shouted out in a class new to particle size is 2. This is a value that anyone without time-share on a neuron can fathom out the origin: $(1 + 2 + 3)/3 = 2.00$.

This is the value that would probably be isolated by simple microscopy on the system—add up all the diameters of the measured particles and divide by the number of particles, thus obtaining the average value 2.00. As the mean contains the number of particles in the system, it is referred to as a number mean. As the numerator in the equation contains diameter terms expressed as simple lengths, this is called a number-length mean diameter, $d_{nl}$. This is a bit of a mouthful, so one mathematical shorthand for reducing this mouthful is to note that there are no diameter terms on the denominator of the equation but diameter terms (lengths) to the power 1 in the numerator—a D[1,0] is thus generated.

However, consider the following scenarios:

- The dissolution rate of a material is governed amongst other parameters by the surface area of the material—the more the surface area, the more rapid the dissolution rate.
- The catalytic activity of a substance is governed by the surface area exposed to the reactants. More finely divided metals, e.g., Raney nickel, speed up the hydrogenation of fats. Indeed, chemical reactions, in general, are speeded up by having finer constituents—gunpowder being a prime example.

- The hydration rate of cement (yet another chemical reaction) is related to the surface area (usually expressed in Blaine units) of the cement.
- The burning rate of fuels is governed by the rate at which oxygen can get to the surface of the fuel. Too large a particle and coke formation results from too slow a burn, whilst finely divided fuel is explosive (the internal combustion engine), as can be all finely divided oxidizable materials.

Thus we may wish to consider calculating an average based on the surface areas of the three particles. We have a slightly more complicated calculation. The surface areas are calculated by taking the squares of the diameters (because SA of a sphere is $4\pi r^2$). We then calculate an average surface area by dividing by the number of particles. Taking the square root of this average recovers an average diameter by surface area: $[(1^2 + 2^2 + 3^2)/3]^{0.5} = 2.16$.

For those of you wondering what has happened to the $\pi$'s (rather than the pies), the same answer will be obtained by the more complicated and tedious route. A little thought will show that one first multiplies by the $\pi$'s to get surface areas and then divides by them again when the diameter is recovered.

The above average diameter is again a number mean as the number of particles appears in the equation. It is though a number-surface area diameter, $d_{ns}$; and in the simplest mathematical shorthand, D[2,0]. This could be the first mean isolated by an image analysis technique by scanning a beam of light (laser or white) across a photograph and processing the particle to recover the equivalent spherical surface area.

The unwary may not consider the next step! He/she may be a chemical engineer considering pumping fluids around a plant or weighing materials that are to be sold or value added to them in the process. This individual may therefore consider averaging the particles on the basis of volume or weight/mass. Volumes or masses are obtained by cubing the diameters, averaging for an average volume or mass, and taking a cube root to recover an average diameter: $[(1^3 + 2^3 + 3^3)/3]^{1/3} = 2.29$.

For reasons already stated, this is a number-weight or number-volume mean, $d_{nv}$, more conveniently expressed as D[3,0]. An electrozone-sensing instrument may measure the volumes of particles and divide by the number of particles to obtain such a mean.

It should be noted at this stage that there is an international (ISO) norm (9) that recommends alternative ways of showing the above means. For example, the D[1,0] shown above can be represented as: $x_{1,0} = D_{1,0} = M_{1,0} = M_{-2,3}/M_{-3,3}$.

Although more mathematically correct for the pedants, it is less easy to understand from the simplistic forms first proposed by Mugele and Evans (although now there is ASTM E2578) and which we have derived above (7).

Other common statistical ways of looking at the central tendency of any distribution are the following:

- Median: this is the point at which exactly half (50%) of the distribution lies above and exactly half (50%) below. Normally we would specify which type of distribution we are dealing with by the appropriate suffix, e.g., D[v,0.5] for a volume median.
- Mode: this is the most common or frequent point in the distribution, "the summit of the mountain."

## THE MOMENT MEANS

We now need to take a journey in which the reader must have some faith or wishes to delve deeper into a textbook such as Allen's (8) or ISO9276-2 (9). The simple number means shown above possess one major difficulty and that is that they contain the number of particles. A simple calculation will show that 1 g of $SiO_2$ ($\rho = 2.5$) will contain around $750 \times 10^6$ particles at 10 μm size and around $750 \times 10^9$ particles when 1 μm in size. It is generally a difficult technical task to count such huge numbers of particles. Particle counters generally deal with very small numbers of particles and this will be discussed further in a later section. At this stage, only the example of Federal Standard 209D [we will ignore the metric (per)version at this stage] will be quoted. This requires for a class 100 clean room that no more than 100 particles of 0.5 μm and above are present in a cubic foot of air. This equates to ppb (usually accepted to be $10^{-9}$ nowadays). So particle counters are equipped to deal with very low levels of particles, whereas particle size analyzers are equipped to measure powders, suspensions, emulsion, etc., in raw form (albeit at high dilutions too).

The problem of having to deal with huge unfeasible quantities of particles is dealt with statistically in particle size analysis by what are known as the moment means, the two most commonly encountered being the following:

- The surface area moment mean or Sauter mean diameter calculated as D [3,2] for the ASTM (E2578) method of displaying particle moments. For our three-sphere system, the calculation is thus: $D[3,2] = (1^3 + 2^3 + 3^3)/(1^2 + 2^2 + 3^2) = 2.57$.
- The volume or mass moment mean less commonly known as the De Brouckere mean calculated as follows for our three-sphere system: $D[4,3] = (1^4 + 2^4 + 3^4)/(1^3 + 2^3 + 3^3)$.

The big advantage of the above means is that they do not involve the need to know the total number of particles in the system in order that particle statistics can be calculated. Laser diffraction which in the Mie deconvolution of the scattering intensity–angle measurement considers total volumes of particles on an ensemble basis will thus usually extract the D[4,3] at an early stage. The laser diffraction instrument does not therefore need to know or calculate the total numbers of particles present in size classes.

The disadvantage for the student of particle size analysis is that these means seem less easily understood than the number means present in the preceding section. They arise from considering the frequency plot of surface area or volume diameters and the centre of gravity or moment of inertia of such a distribution. The average weighted diameters represent the abscissa of the centre of gravity of the relevant frequency distribution. This is the point at which the entire distribution will rotate freely. As a moment of inertia involves an extra term (force = mass × distance), then in the particle size analysis an extra diameter term gets introduced. Thus surface area ($\alpha d^2$) "moves up" to a $d^3$ and a mass or volume ($\alpha d^3$) moves up to the fourth power of the diameter. At this stage, it is better just to accept these mean diameters; the pedant can consult the literature for more rigorous treatments.

So where are we now? For our seemingly simple system containing only three spheres, we have these mean or average diameters:

$$D[1,0] = \frac{1+2+3}{3} = 2$$

$$D[2,0] = \left(\frac{1^2+2^2+3^2}{3}\right)^{0.5} = 2.19 \quad (= d_{ns})$$

$$D[3,0] = \left(\frac{1^3+2^3+3^3}{3}\right)^{1/3} = 2.26 \quad (= d_{nv})$$

$$D[3,2] = \left(\frac{1^3+2^3+3^3}{1^2+2^2+3^2}\right) = 2.57 \quad (= d_{sv})$$

$$D[4,3] = \left(\frac{1^4+2^4+3^4}{1^3+2^3+3^3}\right) = 2.72 \quad (= d_{mv})$$

Note how as we progress up the scale from number through surface and then to volume, the values of the means increase. Although this may seem confusing at this stage, this increase is a clue as to when such means should be employed.

It is possible (mathematically, at least) to convert between the various means listed above, but it is usually desirable not to do so. The conversions are known as the Hatch-Choate transformations (10) and rely on the assumption of the data being log-normal and mapping parallel lines to this data (8). Errors in converting number to volume will be increased markedly as volume is proportional to the cube of diameter. It is always best to rely on the fundamental output of any instrument type rather than try to bend it to simulate another technique or type of result.

## WHICH MEAN IS THE MEANEST?

Or which mean should we use? The three-sphere system was obviously too complicated for the average manager; so let us consider a more simple system consisting of only two spheres of diameters 1 and 10 units, respectively. We will change the rules slightly and assume that these are particles of gold. The simplest number means consider each particle as equivalent (equal weighting but maybe this is a confusing term in this context) and equally important from a statistical point of view:

$$D[1,0] = (1 + 10)/2 = 5.50.$$

Now if we have a choice of which particle we would rather have, then most would opt for the larger diameter particle as this contains more mass of gold and is thus worth financially more. It can be easily seen that this larger particle has a mass of $10^3$ or 1000 units and constitutes 1000/1001 parts of the complete system. The volume moment mean expresses this well:

$$D[4,3] = (1^4 + 10^4)/(1^3 + 10^3) = 9.991.$$

It tells us where the mass of the system is located and is thus treating the larger particle as "more important" (we can see why higher weighting now sounds confusing) from a statistical perspective.

Perhaps another example illustrates this better. The most common difficulty encountered in particle size is the difference between number means (usually obtained by a microscopical technique) and a weight- or volume-based technique (e.g., sieves or light scattering). Because the eye cannot judge volumes or masses in the same way as numbers we tend to feel that "seeing is believing" and this clouds our statistical judgment on the many occasions when mass or volumes are required as opposed to numbers of particles. The example below is that of artificial objects in space classified by scientists on the basis of size from the largest (satellites and rocket motors) to the smallest (flakes of paint, dust, etc.) (Table 2).

If this represented a gold mine, then we would want to collect the 7000 easy nuggets rather than the dust in the system. To design a spacesuit though would require protection against the many tiny objects, the larger satellites being easy to avoid (one would think).

The person with a headache does not request 4.3 billion particles of paracetamol from the pharmacist. Likewise the supplier of titanium dioxide to the paint industry supplies tons rather than numbers of particles. Mass balances combined with particle size data on mine classifier circuits in order

**Table 2** Volume–Number Relationship for Man-made Objects in Space

| Size (cm) | Number of objects | Percentage by number | Percentage by mass | Percentage by $/£/€ |
|---|---|---|---|---|
| 10–1000 | 7,000 | 0.2 | 99.96 | 99.96 |
| 1–10 | 17,500 | 0.5 | 0.03 | 0.03 |
| 0.1–1 | 3,500,000 | 99.3 | 0.01 | 0.01 |

Number mean ~0.6 cm; mass mean ~500 cm.
*Source*: Adapted and recalculated from article in *New Scientist* (13 October 1991).

to generate Tromp plots (classifier efficiency curves) are exactly that—masses not numbers.

Number and volume are also applicable to literature according to a text that the author read in an Indian hotel: "Words should be weighed and not counted." So when do we need to know or count the numbers of particles?

## PARTICLE COUNTING

Particle counting is the basis of a number of techniques, which will merit further discussion in the context of the pharmaceutical industry. These include

- Microscopy (manual or electron)
- Image analysis
- Light obscuration or shadowing techniques for air or liquid applications
- Electrozone sensing

The use of counting is when we wish to know about any of the three C's in a system:

- Concentration
- Contamination
- Cleanliness

We have already seen the small number of permitted particles that need to be counted in air for a class 100 clean room. Indeed for air cleanliness in the semiconductor or pharmaceutical industries according to Fed Stan 209D, we only need to consider particles at one size only (0.5 μm) although intuitively we would realize that the number of particles will increase exponentially as the size decreases. The number of size classes in the first three techniques above is usually very limited. The electrozone sensing device will be treated later in this chapter and is a "special case" of counter. The other pertinent pharmaceutical example is that of parenteral or intravenous fluids as opposed to intralipid emulsions. These parenteral fluids (small or large volume) have BP and USP specifications related to them (11). For example, particles measuring 50 microns or larger can be detected by visual inspection. Specialized equipment is needed to detect particles less than 50 microns in size. The USP 24/NF19 Section <788> sets limits on the number and size of particulates that are permissible in parenteral formulations. This standard seems to be undergoing constant revision, so I am unsure whether the following from Ref. 11 is up to date or not. For large volume parenterals, the limit is not more than 25 particles/mL that are equal to or larger than 10 microns, and not more than 3 particles/mL that are equal to or larger than 25 microns. For small volume parenterals, the limit is 6000 particles/container that are equal to or larger than 10 microns, and not more than 600 particles/container that are equal to or larger than 25 microns (11).

Microscopy has been removed from the pharmacopoeias as a quantitative form of particle sizing. For example, Appendix XIII of BP2000 "Microscope Method" based on Ph. Eur. Method 2.9.21 states "This test is intended to provide a qualitative method for identifying any particles that may be present in a solution." Normally a light obscuration counter is used for particle counting purposes. Using either a laser or white light source the typical range of such a counter used in the pharmaceutical industry is quite limited (e.g., 1–100 µm for liquid, 0.3–10 µm or so for air). It need not do more than this as both BP now and USP call for measurement at 10 and 25 µm for parenterals and 0.5 µm only for air counting (Fed Stan 209D/E). Note the limited range and limited number of size classes that a counter operates with. Also the range of a counter is limited—the larger the size of particle to be counted, the lower the absolute count or concentration can be. Typically a 1 to 100 µm liquid counter cannot deal with more than around 50,000 particles/cm$^3$ of fluid—well below the 1 g of $SiO_2$ particles that would be of no trouble to an ensemble technique such as diffraction.

A particle counter operating on the obscuration or shadowing principle is a secondary form of measurement. A reference standard is delivered through the measurement zone and the response adjusted until the signal sits in the required or "correct" channel. Note that it is quite difficult for standard latex material larger than a micron or so to be nebulized so that it can pass through the measurement zone of an air counter. Furthermore, although the x-axis (size) can be calibrated quite easily, it is another matter to confirm that the absolute count is correct.

So a particle counter will answer the question "How many?"

## PARTICLE SIZE ANALYSIS

A particle size analyzer in contrast to a particle counter is interested in the answer to the question "How much?"[*]:

---

[*] Some languages other than English can seem to deal with this distinction in an apparently superior manner. For example we have in Finnish "Kuinka monta?" (How many?) and "Paljonko?" (How much?).

- How much (volume or weight) material $> x$ μm?
- How much (volume or weight) material $< y$ μm?
- How much material between two size bands?
- Mill efficiency calculations (Tromp curves).
- What is the average size? How has this changed on a quality control chart?
- How much is the value of my material?

These are the situations where we have a powder, emulsion, suspension, or spray and we are concerned with obtaining a particle size distribution. There is a subtle difference between "How many?" and "How much?" and this is not always appreciated by the average purchaser of an instrument. Relating the question back to USP <776> (5), the question "How many?" is answered by either some form of imaging or a light obscuration counter (counting single particles) and the question "How much?" by a laser particle size analyzer (ensemble method) in a modern laboratory.

## METHODS OF PARTICLE SIZE ANALYSIS

We will discuss briefly the most common means of particle size analysis found in the pharmaceutical laboratory: sieves, electrozone sensing, and laser diffraction. BET measurement of powder surface area is extremely valuable, as it will probably correlate to the amount of available surface for dissolution. A back-calculated mean particle size is only inferred with surface area measurements and no distribution obtained; we will only point the reader to the standard text in this field (12) for further details. This is not to belittle surface area measurements—indeed they could be considered to be providing more information in a practical sense (dissolution) than those methods measuring particle size, so to say. But particle sizing is the theme of this script and therefore we must stick to it. Other chapters within this volume will be devoted to the other techniques related to surface area.

### Sieves/Sieving/Sifting/Screening

There are a lot of excellent texts and standards relating to this technique, e.g., Allen (8), Cadle (13) and Wills (14), but the author has gratefully made extensive use of a presentation given by Dominic Rhodes of BNFL at a number of U.K. Royal Society of Chemistry meetings.

Reference texts (15) suggest that this technique has been around since ancient Egyptian times, where along with separating wheat from chaff ("winnowing"), we can see foodstuffs being sifted with sieves made from reeds and holes punched in metal plates. Screening is normally encountered in production environments where separation or rejection/recycling of material is to be made. In the pharmaceutical area, this is likely to be an Alpine Jet Sieve as well as the standard type of screens found in the laboratory. Specifications are often based around a single point (e.g., <0.5% material >38 μm or >99.5% material <38 μm), which as Kaye points out is prone to be exceedingly dangerous (16). He refers to two separate micrographs of ibuprofen made to the "same specification":

"In Figure 3 we show two different ibuprofen powders which both met the specification that *a small amount of residue on a sieve constitutes an adequate definition of the fineness of the product.* The specification made no mention of the shape of the powder grains and the two powders differ enormously in their grain shape subsequently creating large differences in the way that they packed in a storage device and responded to pressure." [*My italics*].

The basis of the separation of particles is around both size and shape, although a weight distribution is usually postulated as the sieved fractions are weighed. Of all techniques, this one, as well as producing a crude particle size distribution, has the advantage that a material can be separated into distinct size classes. For large material (>2 mm/2000 μm), there are no real competitive techniques; although for a single material of known density, counting and weighing can produce a mean size and some form of distribution if every particle is laboriously recorded. Imaging techniques can also be used in this large size area, but again these will not be routinely encountered in the preformulation stage of a pharmaceutical.

Interestingly, there are similarities between sieving and image analysis techniques. Shape is combined with orientation. All these techniques deal with geometrical area or cross-sectional perimeter. With a microscope or image analysis, the object or particle will always present a preferred two-dimensional axis to the direction of view. With sieving, a preferred orientation of particle will be passed by the sieve—this can be a time-dependent process too.

The shape dependence of a screen has been known for many years. To quote a text that will soon celebrate its 100th anniversary (17):

"In considering the results of a sieve analysis, it must be remembered that the particles passing through the sieve are not necessarily round or symmetrical in shape, but may often be needle-like in form, and though they pass through the sieves, they are apt to be larger in bulk than particles retained, which approach the more ideal spherical shape."

The sieve equivalent diameter is defined as the diameter of a sphere that will just pass through the mesh of a particular size of screen. Hence, a particle must have two dimensions less than the sieve gap diameter in order to pass through. Consequently, sieving is often said to size particles according to their second largest dimension, although if the smallest dimension allows penetration of the mesh without falling, it seems that the second smallest dimension would allow the particle passage. Care should be taken with the equivalent sphere concept in sieving as particle length may prevent passage due to stability preventing an end-on orientation. Sieves will not cope well with elongated particles and it is difficult to see what it actually being measured in such a case.

The types of sieve routinely encountered are the following:

- Punched hole or perforated screens normally coping with the larger material and rarely seen in a pharmaceutical laboratory but more common in mining. These can have round or square-shaped holes.
- Wire cloth sieves, which are woven to produce nominally square apertures with a defined tolerance (see later!). These are generally brass or stainless steel although plastic is also available. One should avoid carrying out a heavy metal analysis by AAS or ICP on a screened fraction after screening through metallic sieves!
- Microsieves generally from 150 μm downward (even 1 μm sizes are specified!), but used extensively for wet sieving below 38 μm or so. These are generally made by electroetching nickel alloys in a process identical to that of forming semiconductor components (photoresist, UV expose, develop, etch, strip). In theory, any possible shape could be produced by a different photomask, but again, in reality, square and round holes are the norm. In practical terms for organic materials and water-based systems, these can be a real pain to use, as blockage is common and tightly bound material (agglomerated) resists all attempts to "disperse" it through the screen. At small sizes ultrasonic sieving will considerably speed up the process.

It is common to specify sieves in terms of mesh number (the number of wires per unit length, e.g., inch), but this is ambiguous as a variety of national test standards are in use worldwide:

- ASTM E11
- American Tyler series
- German DIN 4188
- French Standard AFNOR (on a $\sqrt[10]{10}$ separation basis as opposed to the more common $\sqrt[4]{2}$ progression between sizes. The advantage of this is that it gives a 2:1 volume change between adjacent screens rather than a 2:1 change in specific surface area as the BS sieves may be considered having.)
- British Standard BS410 (now replaced by the ISO standard 3310-1:2000. This refers to the metal wire cloth sieves. The −2 and −3 of this standard refer to perforated metal plate and electroformed sheets, respectively.)

The technique is generally of fairly low resolution as a limited number of size classes will usually be determined. It is not the case that large numbers of sieves are stacked on top of one another to form a "nest." Very often only four or five sieves are used, which can make comparison ("result emulation") with other techniques problematic at best.

In terms of accuracy, sieves are calibrated less frequently than they ought to be and at this stage it is useful to examine permitted tolerances for screens of the smallest dimension, which are those to be found routinely in the pharmaceutical laboratory. Taking the set of Tyler mesh sieves from Cadle's text (13), we see that the 37 μm screen (400# in this designation but this would be 38 μm in others) is permitted to have a maximum opening of 90% of the nominal opening if no more than 5% of the holes exceed this value! Thus 70 μm holes would be permitted (37 + 33 = 70 μm) in such a screen. If we sieved long enough on such a screen, 50 μm beads would eventually pass through and could be sized as <37 μm! It should not be necessary to indicate that the same listing states that ±7% is permitted on the average size of hole against the nominal. In practice, though, sieves are made to considerably tighter tolerances than this although the example does show the importance of regularly calibrating the screens in use in the laboratory aside from the possibility of operator-induced damage, which also increases the size of the aperture.

In terms of methodology, dry materials are rarely sieved below 63 μm or so and this is where wet sieving finds its main application. Traditionally the region below 38 μm was (and is) referred to as the "sub-sieve size" region.

Although hand sieving is considered to be the reference point, it is clearly susceptible to difficulties relating to standardization. Thus some mechanical form of assistance (e.g., The Ro-Tap) is preferable and the duration and frequency can be regulated.

The Chairman of the Institution of Mining and Metallurgy speaking in 1903 and quoted by Leschonski in 1977 gave this riposte (18): "Screening is not a scientific means of measurement."

The author disagrees with this statement, but it takes a little care (like all techniques) to understand the basis of this deceptively simple form of measurement and to put it on a scientific and logical platform.

Perhaps the words of Edward Lear's poem "The Jumblies" are appropriate to end on a note of humor, but not intended to be scathing of sieving as a particle sizing technique: "They went to sea in a sieve ..."

## Electrozone Sensing

This is more usually known as the most common instrument utilized by users of this technique: the Coulter counter. Many researchers over the age of 50 or so will have been brought up on this technique, as it was one of the few reputable electronic techniques available in the 1960s and 1970s for particle sizing. First developed by Wallace Coulter in the 1950s for blood-cell counting (after optical methods were found to be problematical!), the technique quickly showed its versatility for large numbers of applications where witchcraft had been the norm before. Even in areas where its use was complicated (e.g., lack of conductivity), researchers found interesting routes to bypass these (e.g., measurement in ethanol + ammonium thiocyanate, $NH_4SCN$).

The principle of measurement is simple. Particles are forced to flow through an aperture or orifice situated between two electrodes (Fig. 3). When the particle traverses the measurement zone, there is a change in voltage, current, resistance, and capacitance, all of which could be measured and used to count and size the particle. The method is a secondary one in that the instrument is calibrated against known NIST-traceable latex standards and all measurements of our material interpolated against these standards. Given its birth just before the time of the Information Age, there is a wealth of literature to be found on practical examples of the technique.

Orifices are available in a variety of sizes and it is recommended that particles are no less than 10% of the aperture size and no more than 30% of the same size for efficient processing. Like most rules this can (and has been) be stretched. This restricts the dynamic range of the system to a maximum of around 100:1, although it is possible to combine analyses from different aperture sizes.

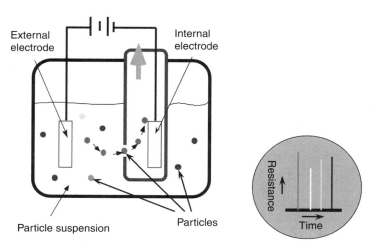

**Figure 3** Principle of the electrical zone sensing method. Particles that are nonconductors are suspended in the electrically conductive diluent. When a particle passes through the aperture during the counting process, the particle decreases the flow of current, increasing the resistance between the electrodes. The resistance causes a voltage change between the electrodes proportional to the volume of the particle.

The main difficulties in using the technique for pharmaceutical usage are

- the solubilities of many pharmaceuticals in aqueous and alcoholic media,
- the broad size range of pharmaceutical preparations leading to blockage of the orifices and slow speed of measurement,
- in emulsion work the 0.9% NaCl electrolyte can promote agglomeration, and
- the inadequate lower size range for a number of formulations.

This is not to be negative against an extremely high-resolution technique capable of dividing a monodisperse latex material into 256 or more size channels. ISO13319 can be consulted for further detail on the method.

In practice though, another electronic technique based on the laws of light scattering has virtually superseded the usage of electrozone sensing for powder, emulsion, and suspension measurement.

## Light Scattering

In this section of the chapter, we shall be referring only to what is commonly called laser diffraction as photon correlation spectroscopy, another light-based technique used exclusively for the sub-100 nm region, is dealt with by another author in this volume. Again we have a technique that appears extremely simple in concept. Indeed, we will break and quote Rose (19):

"I wish now to mention a method of mean size determination which is charming in its simplicity and in the low cost of the apparatus which is but a few shillings, but I am sorry to have to damp enthusiasm at the outset by stating that the method is applicable to but a limited range of materials."
He then goes on to describe classic diffraction.

The principle of measurement is that large particles scatter light into narrow angles (specifically the forward scattering direction) and small particles scatter light into wider angles. A simple helpful (but rough) tool for linking size and diffraction angle is (20): $\theta \sim 35/d$, where $\theta$ is the scattering in degrees and $d$ the size of the particle in microns ($\mu$m).

This formula gives the total extent of scattering—note that one angle does not correspond to one size. This is easily seen by the measurement of the scattering occurring with different sizes of sphere (Fig. 4).

Note the broad scattering occurring with the smallest particle shown and also the secondary scattering arising from passage of light through rather than around the particle. The crude formula shows roughly that as given in Table 3.

Thus small particles need very wide angular detection and conversely large particles will require detectors to be crammed into very small space. Bond pad limitations and crosstalk prevent detectors being spaced closer

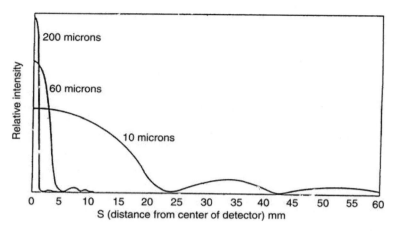

**Figure 4**  Scattering angle and form in relation to different sized spheres.

than around 75 μm for conventional silicon technology. Charge coupled devices (CCDs) operate in a different fashion and permit closer spacing of detectors as these are in an *X–Y* matrix form (see "Image Analysis"). The scope of laser diffraction is given in the ISO 13320-1 document (21) as 0.1 to 3000 μm broadly fitting in with the scattering of particles. At the smaller size, the scattering becomes weak ($I \propto d^6$ or $V^2$ in the Rayleigh region; $d < \lambda/10$ typically). At the larger sizes, the detector has to be mounted so far away from the particles that temperature and vibration compromise the measurement.

The advent of three developments after the writing of Rose's book mentioned above allowed this "simple" technique to become a practical reality: the laser, the silicon slice allowing precise photodetectors to be built, and the computer. This also increased the cost beyond the few shillings that he and some present-day customers envisaged!

**Table 3**  Approximate Range of Scattering Angles for Various Sizes of Particle

| Size of particle (μm) | Approximate total scattering angle (deg) |
|---|---|
| 3000 | 0.012 |
| 1000 | 0.035 |
| 10 | 3.5 |
| 1 | 35 |
| 0.1 | 350 |

Although developed in the 1970s, this method has pushed forward the frontiers of particle size measurement for a number of reasons.

- Flexibility: ability to measure dry, suspensions, emulsions, and even sprays. The latter was the first application of the technique to military jet and diesel engines to optimize the performance.
- Wide range: 0.02 to 2000 μm or better in a single unit. We must be a little suspicious at anything outside the quoted scope stated within ISO 13320-1, but limits are there to test and stretch.
- Rapid: single measurement in 0.001 seconds or quicker. This allows sprays to be "sliced" and huge amounts of interesting information generated.
- Excellent repeatability: integration of many single measurements. A five-second measurement will have 5000 individual measurements registered and integrated.
- No calibration necessary but easy verification. This is sometimes a problem for QA inspectors and users alike, but relates to fundamental, first principle measurements as opposed to secondary or comparative measurements. There is no formal way to "calibrate" a laser diffraction equipment. That is, it does not operate by comparing a signal with that of a known material and adjusting the performance to read the designated value. Rather, if the wavelength of the light is known together with the optical properties of the material and the angular scattering is measured, then the particle size is derived from first principles as the only unknown remaining in the equations linking light scattering with size. However, challenging the equipment with a verifiable material is a regular occurrence to prove performance (within the tolerance of the standard and the manufacturing tolerances) and this is termed verification. As seen earlier, particle size standards (verify the $x$-axis, "$d$") should be both spherical (no debate as to the "size") and polydisperse (verify the $y$-axis, %) to correctly challenge the performance.

The disadvantages must also be seen as well:

- very new in relative terms (mid-1970s), so limited number of formal methods (but now ASTM-1458-92 and ISO 13320-1),
- not applicable to material over 3 mm or so where sieves take over, and
- is an optical technique so the optical properties of materials are required (ISO 13320-1 indicates that when $D < 40\lambda$ (~25 μm for He–Ne laser at 632.8 nm, then the optical properties are essential for accuracy).

The basic layout of a state-of-the-art instrument (Malvern Instruments Mastersizer® 2000) is used as an illustration of the basic construction of a unit (Fig. 5). Operation is usually remarkably and deceptively simple and many users lull themselves into a false sense of security because of this.

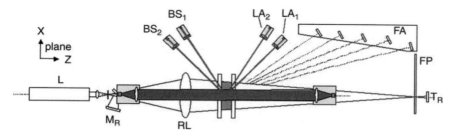

**Figure 5** Schematic outline of a laser diffraction equipment (Malvern Mastersizer® 2000).

Method development is simple for any unknown material. This method development must be carried out before a standard operating procedure (SOP) is formalized or the latter is just a means to getting the wrong result more precisely. Method development follows the guidelines of ISO 13320-1, in particular Section 6.2.3:

- Ensure the equipment has formal traceability by verification with NIST-traceable standards (see Section 6.4 of ISO 13320-1) appropriate to the specific material.
- Ensure that a representative sample of the bulk material is taken—this almost will necessitate the use of a spinning riffler if any material >75 μm is present.
- Dry: pressure–size titration followed by wet to decide on an appropriate pressure (Section 6.2.3.2 of ISO 13320-1) or to reject dry if significant attrition is occurring (like with many organics).
- Wet: before, during, and after sonication in order to obtain a plateau of stability. For organics the formation of a stable dispersion will follow the steps wetting, separation, stabilization. This may need some work with solvents and perhaps surfactants. These are only vehicles in which to circulate the powder (or slurry/suspension, etc.).
- SOP formulated around the stable dispersed region for primary size or against input of minimum energy for bulk size (possibly only one measurement may be possible in the latter if dispersion is occurring in the wet).

The key features of any method must be

- Repeatability
- Reproducibility
- Robustness

These three R's are explored further in Ref. 22 to which the reader is referred. As an illustration, the particle size plots and comparisons involved in method development for an organic compound should be easy to understand without further comment (Figs. 6–9).

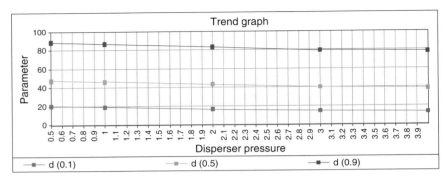

**Figure 6** Dry measurement. Pressure–size titration as per ISO 13320-1 (21).

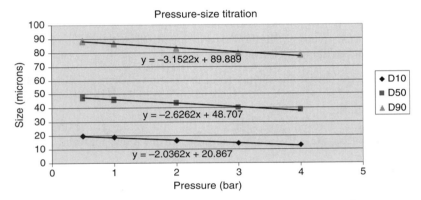

**Figure 7** Dry. Initial check on method. Note slopes $D_{90} > D_{50} > D_{10}$. The magnitude of the slopes ($-2$ to $-3$ mm/bar increased pressure here) indicates little or no attrition, but this needs confirmation by comparison against wet.

Interpretation of the raw angular scattering pattern (intensity–angle plot) can be undertaken with either approximations (Fraunhofer, Anomalous) or more rigorous and exact theories (Mie). For readers who wish to explore the differences between right and wrong in the modern computer age, the Appendix of ISO 13320-1 is recommended.

## PARTICLE MORPHOLOGY

### Setting the Scene

As stated earlier, size and shape cannot be dealt with as separate issues. Hence we need to have some means of visualizing our particles or particulate system in order to get handles on

- the approximate shape of the particles,
- the approximate size,

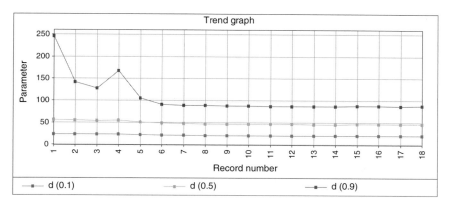

**Figure 8** What pressure do we measure at in Figures 6 and 7? This figure illustrates a wet measurement of the same material with sonication (dispersion) to stability.

- the state of dispersion, and
- the nature of the fundamental particles—whether made from crystallites.

This two-dimensional visualization can be made with microscopy (manual or electron) and made more quantitative with image analysis (at least for the shape aspect of the particles).

The terms used to describe shape in pharmaceutical technology are those common to crystallography and used extensively in other fields (e.g., geology). These terms are encompassed in USP 776 and other definitions (e.g., the old BS standards).

- Equant: approximately equal length, breadth, and height, e.g., a cube or sphere. Such particles may be more robust in terms of attrition than thin particles from which the corners may be fractures.
- Tabular: literally table-like. The thickness of table is less than the length and breadth. This particle will prefer to present the face of the table (length and breadth rather than height) to the visualization technique. If the particles are subject to flow (air or liquid) then they may prefer to align in a preferred manner.
- Plate: thinner than a tabular material.
- Flake: yet thinner than a plate!
- Acicular: needle-like particles whose width and thickness will be similar. These can be rounded (e.g., glass fiber) or formed by growth of preferred crystal faces, so can appear square or rod-like (tetragonal) or hexagonal if ever viewed lengthways. Now we can see why a single descriptor of particle size is impossible. What (single) size is a needle?
- Columnar: column-like. These can be considered to be less of a needle by possessing a larger width and breadth than the acicular system.
- Blade or lath: long thin, blade-like particle (Fig. 10).

4 bar

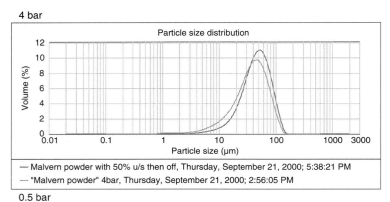

— Malvern powder with 50% u/s then off, Thursday, September 21, 2000; 5:38:21 PM
— "Malvern powder" 4bar, Thursday, September 21, 2000; 2:56:05 PM

0.5 bar

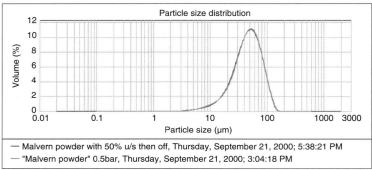

— Malvern powder with 50% u/s then off, Thursday, September 21, 2000; 5:38:21 PM
— "Malvern powder" 0.5bar, Thursday, September 21, 2000; 3:04:18 PM

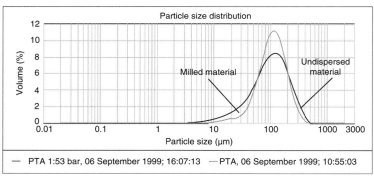

— PTA 1:53 bar, 06 September 1999; 16:07:13    — PTA, 06 September 1999; 10:55:03

**Figure 9** Comparison of wet with dry measurements at 4 and 0.5 bar. Illustration of attrition for another organic material where it is noted that the dry is broadened in comparison to the wet.

Already we can see the qualitative descriptions creeping in! And, therefore, with the possible danger of operator subjectivity.

We can also complicate matters by considering groups of particles and the way that they may preferably associate (aggregate or agglomerate):

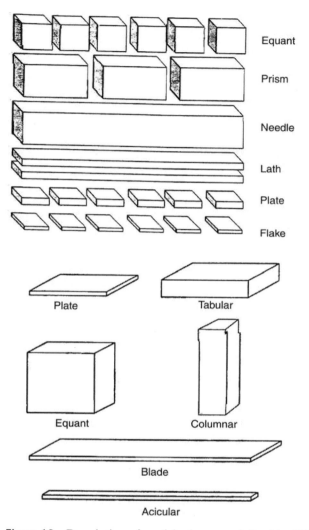

**Figure 10** Description of particle shapes as defined by USP. *Source*: Adapted from Refs. 5, 25.

- lamellar: stacked plates,
- foliated: stacked sheets like a book. Clay minerals can appear in this form,
- spherulitic: radial clusters of needles forming an overall spherical shape. These can sometimes be induced to fracture into triangular or individual needles,
- cemented: large particles set in a matrix. Commonly encountered in soil science where the term conglomerate is also used,

- drusy: coated with smaller particles. This can occur as a result of pseudomorphism (a crystal taking the habit of another crystal usually in such a way that a nonpreferred or unusual structure is observed) or particle–particle attraction.

Even the definitions of aggregation and agglomeration are confused, with USP considering agglomerate "hard" and aggregate "soft" in comparison to ISO and BS (23,24).

We then have to try and make sense of this confusion by placing numbers to quantify the system. Rather like the earlier concepts, we now have a number of diameters to characterize our particles under microscopical or image analysis conditions (seen earlier in Fig. 2 and now defined in Ref. 25):

- length: the longest dimension from edge to edge of a particle oriented parallel to the measurement graticule/scale,
- width: the longest dimension of the particle measured at right angles to the length,
- Feret's diameter: the distance between imaginary parallel lines tangential to the (randomly oriented) particle and perpendicular to the scale, and
- Martin's diameter: length of the particle at the point that divides a particle into two equal projected areas.

Most imaging techniques connected to a computer will calculate/derive these plus other descriptors:

- perimeter diameter: diameter of a circle having the same perimeter as the projected outline of the particle,
- projected area diameter: diameter of the circle having the same area as the projected area of the particle in a stable position, and
- circularity (Fig. 11).

So we have another set of diameters to get our head around—these again are not necessarily related to other diameters we may have obtained by, say, ensemble techniques where all the particles may have random orientations to the measurement direction.

The Pfizer manual on shape and size gives an excellent format to describing a powder sample under a microscope, so I make no apologies for reproducing it in full:

"The description should include

- Description of crystal habit
- Average size of particles (note the maximum size)
- Description of association with other crystals
- Any observations about crystallinity

Circularity and diameter

Circularity = perimeter of circle/perimeter of particle

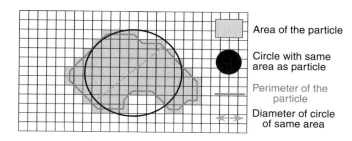

Area of the particle

Circle with same
area as particle

Perimeter of the
particle

Diameter of circle
of same area

Circularity and diameter

Circularity and diameter enable
evaluation of particle shape numerically

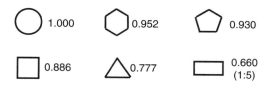

1.000     0.952     0.930

0.886     0.777     0.660
                    (1:5)

Examples of particle shape and their circularity
[Wadell's sphericity]

**Figure 11**  Descriptions of circularity. *Source*: After Ref. 26.

- Photomicrographs (with scale bar and magnification)
- Record of mounting medium used (e.g. silicone oil)
- A note of the microscope used

The manual gives an excellent example together with a micrograph:
"The powder consists of a mixture of laths, plates and needles. The laths and needles range in length from about 50 μm to about 1.5 mm with length to breadth aspect ratios of between 3:1 and 15:1. The plates range in size from about 100 μm to 300 μm across. There are a few agglomerates. Between crossed polarisers, the particles show bright interference colours, which extinguish every 90° of rotation and this indicates that the particles are crystalline. The powder was mounted in silicone oil and examined using a Nikon Labophot microscope." The spelling of "colour" and "polariser" must indicate a UK origin for this manual!

## Microscopy

This is the oldest and most fundamental measurement of particle morphology. There are three possible parts to consider about morphology:

- Surface texture or perhaps roughness. This is the short-order structure that we may observe on the surface of the particle usually only with electron microscopy. Although it is not normally considered to be part of the shape of a particle, it will exert considerable influence on such properties as surface area (and therefore dissolution and gas absorption), settling velocity, and propensity for particles to adhere to one another and to surfaces. Thus bulk properties such as flowability may be affected. Fractal analysis is interesting in this area.
- Roundness. This is on a larger scale than surface texture but smaller than the overall shape of the particle. It reflects how angular or otherwise a particle is. Wadell's definition (26) based on Wentworth's earlier definition (27): roundness, $R$ = average radius of curvature of corners/ radius of largest inscribed circle. This has obvious difficulties in measurement—Wentworth's definition only specified the sharpest corner. Semiqualitative means ("very angular," "sub-rounded," etc.) of assessment are provided in the form of photographs by Powers (28), which form the basis of the diagrams in Figure 1 of this chapter. We note that Powers actually used clay models and not real particles for these qualitative terms. Folk has dealt with assigning class numbers to these (29) ranging from 0 ("perfectly angular") to 6 ("perfectly rounded").
- Sphericity. Again we are back to Wadell (26) who defined sphericity as the ratio between the diameter of the sphere with the same volume of the particle and the diameter of the equivalent surface: $\psi = (d_v/d_s)^2$. This is on a bigger scale than roundness and measures the tendency to form spherical shape of a particle. Defining three linear dimensions of a particle and making a triaxial ellipsoid assumption (makes a change from spherical!) allows sphericity, $\phi$, to be calculated as follows: $\phi = \sqrt[3]{(d_s d_i/d_l^2)}$, where $d_s$, $d_i$, and $d_l$ are the diameters for the smallest, intermediate, and longest dimensions, respectively.

Microscopes can be manual or electron and we need to explore the limitations of both. The first major obstacle to overcome is that of taking a sample that is representative of the bulk. We may at best be looking at milligrams of sample under a manual microscope and maybe picograms or nanograms under an electron microscope. We had better be sure that we are looking at something that relates to our problem!

Going back to our example of $SiO_2$, we may remember that 1 g of a powder containing 1 µm particles would have around $750 \times 10^9$ such particles present. Taking 50,000 particles from such a system even on a random basis samples less than seven millionths of 1% of the sample! And is 1 g all we have of a production lot?

Clearly, if our powder is monodisperse (i.e., every particle the same), then we would only need to take one particle from the bulk for it to be totally representative. Thus the width of the particle size distribution will determine how much sample we need for statistical validity—wider distributions requiring more sample to have adequate numbers of large particles (which dramatically affect the volume or mass distribution) for representative sampling to be assured.

We can calculate the numbers of particles needed in the highest size band for statistical validity at the 1% level as follows: $1/100 = 1/n^{0.5}$, leading to a need for 10,000 particles in the highest size band. The number 10,000 is interesting [although it does not provoke a large entry in the Book of Interesting Numbers (30); in fact it provokes no entry at all in the aforementioned volume] as it is the same number of images (not particles) that NBS stated that was needed for statistical validity in image analysis (31):

"S(tandard error) is proportional to $N^{-1/2}$ where N is the total number of particles measured...This consideration implies that image analysis may require the analysis of on the order of 10,000 images to obtain a satisfactory limit of uncertainty" (p. 718, paragraph 1).

Note the term "images" (i.e., photo- or micrographs) rather than particles. An earlier document from 1954 (32) states that 20,000 particles are needed. All this shows that usually we do not count enough particles for statistical validity and thus the conclusions that we may draw on *particle size* are likely to be qualitative and not quantitative.

Indeed we can crudely calculate (33) the amount of sample required for statistical validity where the top end of the size band is at various points (Table 4).

**Table 4** Calculation of Weight of Sample Required for Statistical Validity at the 1% Level (with Assumptions as Defined)

| $D$ (μm) | Diameter (cm) | Radius (cm) | Density (g/cm$^3$) | Weight in top size fraction (g)[a] | Total weight (g) ( = last column × 100)[b] |
|---|---|---|---|---|---|
| 1 | 0.0001 | 0.00005 | 2.5 | 1.31358E−08 | 1.31358E−06 |
| 10 | 0.001 | 0.0005 | 2.5 | 1.31358E−05 | 0.001313579 |
| 100 | 0.01 | 0.005 | 2.5 | 0.013135792 | 1.313579167 |
| 1,000 | 0.1 | 0.05 | 2.5 | 13.13579167 | 1313.579167 |
| 10,000 | 1 | 0.5 | 2.5 | 13135.79167 | 1313579.167 |
| 200[c] | 0.02 | 0.01 | 3.15 | 0.13240878 | 13.24 |

[a] This is the weight of 10,000 particles; assuming spheres.
[b] This is where 1% of the particles are in the top size band.
[c] This represents a typical cement.
*Source*: From Ref. 33.

More rigorous theoretical solutions are provided by Masuda and Gotoh (34) and enhanced by Wedd (35), but the figures crudely calculated above in Table 4 are in the same ballpark. We note that the old maxim that 75 or 100 μm provided the point at which sampling became the predominant error in particle size analysis is easily understood if a sample size of around 1 g is assumed for many analytical techniques.

So we do not put enough sample in! Let us also examine how small we can see with visible light. The limit of resolution is defined as the minimum distance between two points that permits the objective to reveal the existence of both points.

Abbé's Theory (for axial illumination): $l = \lambda/NA$, where $l$ is the limit of resolution, $\lambda$ the wavelength of illumination, and NA the numerical aperture.

For oblique illumination: $l = \lambda/2NA$, or with Rayleigh's equation: $l = 1.2\lambda/2NA$. These two equations are close enough (only 20% different). We need then a definition of numerical aperture: $NA = i \sin(AA/2)$, where $i$ is the refractive index of the medium (air or immersion fluid) between the objective and substage condenser and AA, the angular aperture, is the angle between the most divergent rays that can pass through the objective to form an image. This indicates why we can get higher magnifications with an immersion lens.

Those given by the equations are theoretical and represent the best case with well-corrected lenses, proper illumination, and high contrast images. NA is normally in the range 0.5 to 1.0, giving a theoretical lower limit of 0.5 μm (NA is usually stated on the lens). Allen states (8, p. 114), "A more realistic size is 0.8 μm with limited accuracy below 3 μm. BS3406 does not recommend optical microscopy for particles smaller than 3 μm."

Small particles become oversized as their size approaches the limit as the diffraction disc produced is larger than the particle (equal area: Fraunhofer Approximation, Mie predicts correctly a maximum for the diffraction considering the volume of the particle). Under dark field illumination can detect particles much smaller than the resolution of light (because they scatter light)—but the apparent size is a disc at the resolution limit of the microscope—so all particles appear to be 0.5 μm in diameter. This is similar state of affairs to that of a condensation nucleus counter, where all particles appear at around 50 nm when the alcohol has condensed on them. Small discs therefore appear to be oversized as we approach the limits of visible light microscopy (Fig. 12).

This has the usual effect of producing a false maximum just above the theoretical limit for optical microscopy. Quoting Heywood [in Lang (32)],

"Dr Brownowski asked if anyone could comment upon automatic star counting methods: although I cannot say what methods were used for this purpose, there was an interesting similarity between star and particle

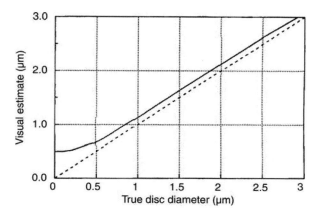

**Figure 12** Oversizing of small discs by optical microscopy. *Source*: From Ref. 8.

counting results when the limit of visibility was approached. Early records of microscopical counts when extended to the extreme limit of resolution, showed a false maximum frequency at a particle size just greater than the lower limit, where it is known that the numerical frequency for normal dusts increases continuously as the particle size decreases. Star counts made by unaided vision about 300 years ago showed a maximum frequency at about 4th magnitude, the limit of such vision being about 6th magnitude. With the aid of telescopes it was easily shown that the numerical frequency of stars increased as the magnitude increased i.e. brightness decreased. The important feature of this comparison was that false effects might be observed if any counting process was worked to the extreme limit of its capabilities."

Fed Stan 209E bases its calculations on particle count increasing exponentially as size decreases. This comment also indicates that the harder we look (e.g., with an electron microscope), the more we see and the tendency to feel that our particulate system is much smaller than it really is, as we are really investigating the "dust" in the system. It is the equal importance attached to each and every single particle in number counting that is both its disadvantage and advantage. The author has been given a white powder (supposedly of ZnO) and told that it was 0.7 nm in size! It is easy to see how taking any microscopy to its limits can produce a false impression of the material. Incidentally, the above sample of ZnO settled to the bottom of a beaker of water in less than one minute.

Once again we must state that microscopy is only a two-dimensional representation of a particle. Also we must be aware that the preparation conditions can alter the sample and that the material will present a preferred axis to the light.

Refractive index is important from a number of points of view. The higher the relative refractive index between particle and the medium that it is sitting in, the better the contrast and features that are observable. Indeed if the particle's refractive index and that of the medium it resides in are identical, then the particle appears invisible (if this not a contradiction!). Putting the particle in different immersion fluids (e.g., Cargille) allows (by means of the Becke lines) the refractive index of the particle to be determined.

Notwithstanding all the above comments, visualization together with the generation of the appropriate micrographs is essential in any particle characterization, but we must be careful with assigning quantitative interpretations to what we see.

Fractal analysis is another possibility here, but the reader should refer to texts by Mandelbrot (36) and Kaye (37) for further information.

Finally we need to consider the magnification that we are using or attempting to use. The tradeoff of high magnification is that the depth of field becomes smaller and smaller. The depth of field is the distance within which the image will appear to be sharp and in focus. The amateur photographer will be well aware of the differences in attempting to focus a picture using a 500 mm lens ("high" magnification) as opposed to using a 24 mm (wide-angle) lens. The latter is "low" magnification—in fact about twice as wide as our normal eye field of vision—usually stated to be 50 mm or so. Thus we could term it 0.5× magnification.

High magnification objective lenses are generally more expensive and need to be brought close to the object to obtain focus. How many of us have crashed such a lens against the microscope slide? The usual rule is to look at the slide and move the objective as close as possible toward the particle and then gradually move the objective away until focus is achieved.

The mathematical description of depth of field is the distance, $D$, the objective can be moved such that a point appears to be a circle having a radius no bigger than $c$: $D = 2c/\tan(AA/2)$.

Thus $D$ depends on the value of $c$ that one is prepared to accept and decreases with decreasing size of the particles. Again a photographic example is useful here. To avoid a long focal range lens becoming too large, a mirror can be placed on the front of the lens to reflect the light back thus halving the length of the lens. Such mirror lenses exhibit the feature that out-of-focus spots appear as rings or donuts. Table 5 (38) shows the effect on depth of field by increasing the magnification.

The image or particle can be brought up against various graticules from the simple "ruler" to those with spots to place over the particles in the hope that projected areas can be isolated by the operator. The literature is full of examples of the differences obtained by trained and untrained operators and those between trained operators. And is it easy to rotate the graticule correctly to obtain a Feret's or Martin's diameter?

**Table 5** Maximum Useful Magnification and the Eyepiece Required for Different Objectives

| Objective magnification | Focal length (mm) | NA | Depth of focus (μm) | Maximum useful magnification | Eyepiece required |
|---|---|---|---|---|---|
| 2.5× | 56 | 0.08 | 50 | 80 | 30× |
| 10× | 16 | 0.25 | 8 | 250 | 25× |
| 20× | 8 | 0.5 | 2 | 500 | 25× |
| 43× | 4 | 0.66 | 1 | 660 | 15× |
| 97× | 2 | 1.25 | 0.4 | 1250 | 10× |

*Note*: NA, numerical aperture; the magnification of the objective lens is calculated by dividing the microscope tube length, usually 160 mm, by the focal length.
*Source*: From Ref. 38.

Last but no means least, we need to consider some aspects of electron microscopy where sample preparation can be vital for correct interpretation. In some cases (e.g., polymers), increasing the magnification too much will start to boil the sample! Again there is the tendency to observe the "interesting" or unusual rather than the representative. Bearing in mind too that $1 \times 100$ μm particle has the same mass as 1 million $\times$ 1 μm particles, if we happen to spot this one in a million particle, then there is the tendency to ignore it and state that it is not typical (which is true on a number basis!). However, it makes up half of the overall mass of the system—it is the proverbial golden nugget!

## Image Analysis

It is quite clear that the techniques described in the previous section can be tedious, long-winded, and prone to operator error and subjectivity. Hence the obvious move to speed things up and automate the process of obtaining information. Hopefully with the computer making the judgments, we should have less chance of being prone to vagaries of the operator. Plus we should be able to scan hundreds, thousands, and even tens of thousands of particles in a considerably quicker mode than by hand. We must therefore be getting closer to statistical validity. However, too with the computer playing a part we have the ability to generate literally hundreds of pieces of information and transformations, so again we must be cautious in sifting the real requirements from those that are ancillary or unnecessary.

There are a number of good texts in the market from the simple and easy, e.g., Refs. 8 and 39, to the more advanced, e.g., Refs. 40 and 42.

The main stages in any image analysis sequence are

- Image acquiring
- Object extraction

- Segmentation
- Calculations

A standard microscope will normally have a CCD camera connected to it via a "T" adaptor and the signal passed to a frame grabber board normally residing in a PC. These frame grabber boards advance every three months in terms of speed and features, and this has spawned almost as many home-built packages as those obtained from companies with a known reputation in the field. The image is usually made visible on a monitor, and large memory requirements (previously handled by optical discs and similar technology) are required. Those with experience of digital photography will appreciate that even a single modest picture of $2048 \times 1024$ picture elements (pixels) takes over 2 MB of memory for black and white only. This will be trebled at a minimum for color use, although the latter still finds less usage

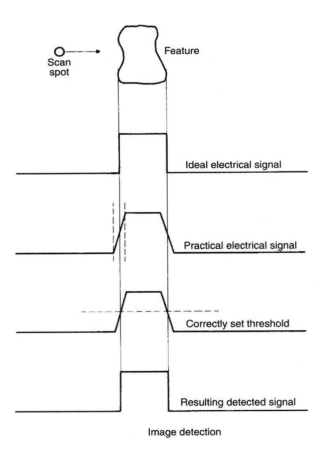

**Figure 13**  Thresholding to obtain particle "size." *Source*: After Ref. 38.

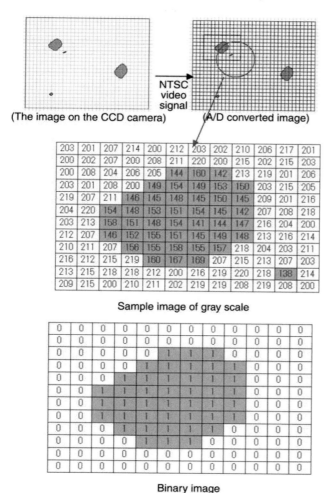

Sample image of gray scale

Binary image

**Figure 14** Oversimplified (hence incorrect) digitization. But the principle is crudely the same if a few fast Fourier transforms and Laplacian filtration is included.

in image analysis. Only in the last 5 to 10 years has sufficient computer memory become affordable for home use. We have to recall that in the 1970s, 1 MB of memory equated to around US $1 million of cost!

So let us break down the process even further. Once the image has been acquired in some sort of grey scale form, it will need to be digitized (i.e., changed to black and white only: 1's and 0's) in order that particles can be distinguished from the background. Even at this stage, there is discrimination to be had and the threshold setting here will determine what is an edge of a particle (Fig. 13).

| 0 | 0 | 0 | 0 | 0 | 0 | 0 | 0 | 0 | 0 | 0 | 0 |
|---|---|---|---|---|---|---|---|---|---|---|---|
| 0 | 0 | 0 | 0 | 0 | 0 | 0 | 0 | 0 | 0 | 0 | 0 |
| 0 | 0 | 0 | 0 | 0 | 1 | 1 | 1 | 0 | 0 | 0 | 0 |
| 0 | 0 | 0 | 0 | 1 | 0 | 0 | 0 | 1 | 0 | 0 | 0 |
| 0 | 0 | 0 | 1 | 0 | 0 | 0 | 0 | 1 | 0 | 0 | 0 |
| 0 | 0 | 1 | 0 | 0 | 0 | 0 | 0 | 1 | 0 | 0 | 0 |
| 0 | 0 | 1 | 0 | 0 | 0 | 0 | 0 | 1 | 0 | 0 | 0 |
| 0 | 0 | 1 | 0 | 0 | 0 | 0 | 0 | 1 | 0 | 0 | 0 |
| 0 | 0 | 0 | 1 | 0 | 0 | 0 | 1 | 0 | 0 | 0 | 0 |
| 0 | 0 | 0 | 0 | 1 | 1 | 1 | 0 | 0 | 0 | 0 | 0 |
| 0 | 0 | 0 | 0 | 0 | 0 | 0 | 0 | 0 | 0 | 0 | 0 |
| 0 | 0 | 0 | 0 | 0 | 0 | 0 | 0 | 0 | 0 | 0 | 0 |

**Figure 15**   Edge isolation by considering the pixel in relation to its neighbors.

Thus for small particles where diffraction limitation is an issue we still have plenty of room to play! We also need to remember that the acquired image may only be a few pixels in size at the so-called lower range of the device we are using. Obviously we must be aware that shape analysis on something six pixels in total size is meaningless. The light that we are illuminating the particle with then plays an important role and it will need to be kept constant—lamps warming up will alter the point around the particle at which the thresholding takes effect. If there is too little light then the particle could appear larger. With too much light, a smaller particle could be synthesized.

We will quickly obtain a binary image. This is where many choices can now be made:

- "Holes" in binary images of particles can be filled. A good example of applying this is with glass beads, which can act as a miniature lens and

Class 2 (Detection count : 1438)

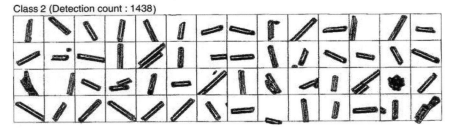

**Figure 16**   Wet images – Glass fiber + Latex. *Source*: From FPIA, Sysmex Corporation, Kobe-Osaka, Japan.

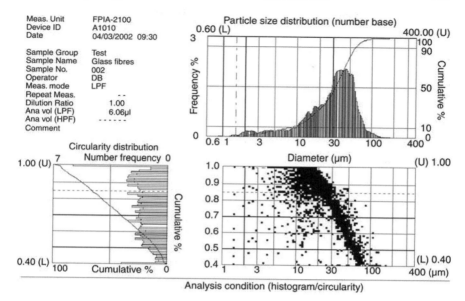

**Figure 17** Wet measurement – Glass fiber + Latex. Calculated data and graphs.

focus light to a bright spot behind. They are not actually donuts but could appear as so if this hole filling routine is not practiced. Now what would be the situation if this were a genuine donut? This is a

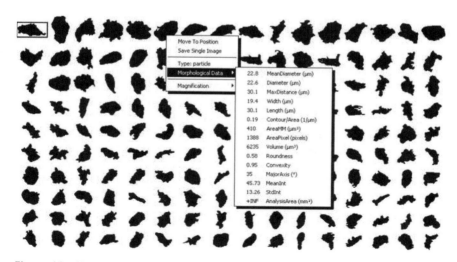

**Figure 18** Dry measurement indicating the wide variety of possible derived data. *Source*: From Pharmavision Systems, Lund, Sweden.

philosophical question again, as we would have to consider internal and external radii of the "particle."

■ Segmentation. Particles that are touching need to be separated. Ideally we would want to see only single particles, but in practice this never likely or possible. The technique of erosion and dilation developed by Jean Serra and coworkers at the London Academic Press (41) in the mid-1970s is still the main route to achieve this.

We then end up with the "particles" as binary images on a background. This is when the mathematical entertainment starts and all sorts of numbers to many decimal places can be calculated and displayed in the true spirit of "garbage in = garbage out" and in a fashion that the computer is well equipped to generate.

Different definitions of circularity and convexity, etc., are to be found in propriety software so the wise user will determine how these were derived. ISO 9276–6 (in progress) is attempting to standardize these definitions.

So what is the type of output analysis that we can obtain? As an example we will look at two materials dispersed both dry and wet and measured on two techniques (wet: FPIA, Sysmex Corporation, Kobe-Osaka, Japan; dry: Pharma Vision Systems AB, Lund, Sweden):

■ wet images: glass fiber + latex (Fig. 14),
■ wet measurement: glass fiber + latex. Calculated data and graphs. Note the circularity diagram illustrating how, as a rod is shortened, it becomes more "spherical" (Fig. 15), and
■ dry measurement.

## CONCLUSIONS

So after this journey where have we got to? Indeed have we even begun the journey? The measurement and characterization of our particulate system is so vital that it must be tackled in a systematic and logical fashion and there is no substitute for building a firm foundation on the basic principles outlined in this chapter. Careful and systematic experimental work and observation is of considerably more value than any number of Greek symbols in a text. Indeed the latter are probably a crutch for lack of fundamental understanding or "feel" for the system. If this text has gone even a footstep on the never-ending journey of equipping the reader for a lifetime's improvement (3), then it will have fulfilled its purpose.

## REFERENCES

1. Heywood H. Proceedings of the First Particle Size Anal. Conf. Heffer, Loughborough, U.K., September 1966:355–9.

2. Noyes AA, Whitney WR. The rate of solution of solid substances in their own solutions. J Am Chem Soc 1897; 19:930.

3. Nelligan T. Chris Leslie: wood, wire and wit. Dirty Linen June/July 2000; 88: 47–50 (The quotation appears on page 49).

4. Rawle AF. The Basic Principles of Particle Size Analysis. Technical Paper. Malvern Instruments, UK, 1993. Downloadable from http://www.malvern.co.uk.

5. USP General Test <776>, USP XXXIV. Rockville, MD: The United States Pharmacopoeial Convention, 2000:1965–7.

6. Scarlett B. Measurement of particle size and shape, some reflections on the BCR reference material programme. Part Charact 1985; 2:1–6.

7. Muegle RA, Evans HD. Droplet size distributions in sprays. Ind Eng Chem 1953; 43(6):1317–24.

8. Allen T. Particle Size Measurement, Vol. 1, 5th ed. Chapman and Hall, 1997.

9. ISO9276-2. Representation of results of particle size analysis. Part 2. Calculation of average particle sizes/diameters and moments from particle size distributions.

10. Hatch T, Choate SP. Statistical description of the size properties of non-uniform particulate substances. J Franklin Inst 1929; 207:369–87.

11. http://pharmlabs.unc.edu/parenterals/equipment/ch16.htm.

12. Gregg SJ, Sing KSW. Adsorption Surface Area and Porosity. London: Academic Press, 1967.

13. Cadle RC. Particle Size: Theory and Industrial Applications, 1st ed. New York: Reinhold Pub Corp, 1965.

14. Wills BA. Mineral Processing Technology. 4th ed. Oxford: Pergamon Press, 1988. ISBN 0-08-034936-6.

15. Heywood H. The origins and development of particle size analysis (Plenary Lecture). In: Groves MJ, Wyatt JL, eds. Proceedings of Particle Size Analysis 1970 Conference held at the University of Bradford, 9–11 September 1970. The Society for Analytical Chemistry. Cambridge: W Heffer, 1972:1–18. The descriptions of sieving are to be found on pages 4–8 of this article.

16. Kaye BH. New perspectives in pharmaceutical technology. In: Proceedings of the Hosokawa Powder Systems' Pharmaceutical Technical Seminar Summit, New Jersey, U.S.A.: Hosokawa Micron Systems, 19–20 May 1998.

17. Bleininger AV. The manufacture of hydraulic cements. Geological Survey of Ohio. Fourth Series, Bulletin No. 3, Columbus, Ohio, December 1904.

18. Leschonski K. Proceedings of Particle Size Anal. Conf. Bradford, Heyden: Bradford Anal. Div. Chem. Soc. 1977:186.

19. Rose HE. The Measurement of Particle Size in Very Fine Powders. New York: Chemical Publishing, 1954.

20. Davies CN, ed. Aerosol Science. London and New York: Academic Press, 1966.

21. ISO13320. Particle Size Analysis—Laser Diffraction Methods. Part 1: General Principles ISO Standards Authority, 1999. Can be downloaded from http://www.iso.ch on payment with credit card.

22. Rawle AF. Attrition, dispersion and sampling effects in dry and wet particle size analysis using laser diffraction. Paper 0208. Proceedings of the 14th International Congress of Chemical and Process Engineering, CHISA. 27–31 August 2000, Praha, Czech Republic.

23. Nichols G, Byard S, Bloxham MJ, et al. A review of the terms agglomerate and aggregate with a recommendation for nomenclature used in powder and particle characterization. J Pharm Sci 2002; 91(10):2103–9.
24. Irani RR, Callis CF. Particle Size: Measurement, Interpretation and Application. New York: John Wiley, 1963.
25. Brittain HG. Particle size distribution. Part 1. Representations of particle shape, size and distribution. Pharm Technol December 2001:38–45.
26. Wadell H. Volume, shape, and roundness of rock-particles. J Geol 1932; 40: 443–51.
27. Wentworth CK. A laboratory and field study of cobble abrasion. J Geol 1919; 27:507–21.
28. Powers MC. A new roundness scale for sedimentary particles. J Sedimentary Petrol 1953; 23:117–9.
29. Folk RL. Student operator error in determination of roundness, sphericity and grain size. J. Sedimentary Petrol 1955; 25:297–301.
30. David Wells. The Penguin Dictionary of Curious and Interesting Numbers. London: Penguin Books, 1986.
31. Dragoo AL, Hsu SM, and Robbins CR, Critical assessment of requirements for ceramic powder characterization. In Ceramic Powder Science II, Messing GL et al., eds., Westerville, Ohio: American Ceramic Society, 1987.
32. Lang HR, ed. Proceedings of the Physics of Particle Size Analysis Conference arranged by The Institute of Physics and held in the University of Nottingham. The Institute of Physics, London. Br J Appl Phys 1954; Supplement No. 3.
33. Rawle AF. Sampling of powders for particle size characterization. Invited Lecture (AME.2-A-02-2002). Session E2 Practical Issues in Ceramic Powder Size Characterization. Proceedings of the 104th American Ceramic Society Meeting. St. Louis, 29 April 2002.
34. Masuda H, Gotoh K. Study on the sample size required for the estimation of mean particle diameter. Adv Powder Technol 1999; 10(2):159–73.
35. Wedd MW. Procedure for predicting a minimum volume or mass of sample to provide a given size parameter precision. Part Part Syst Charact 2001; 18: 109–13.
36. Mandelbrot BB. The Fractal Geometry of Nature. New York: WH Freeman, 1983.
37. Kaye BH. Chaos and Complexity; Discovering the Surprising Patterns of Science and Technology. Weinheim: VCH, 1993.
38. Yamate G, Stockham JD. Sizing particles using the microscope. In: Stockham JD, Fochtman EG, eds. Particle Size Analysis. Ann Arbor: Ann Arbor Science Publishers, 1977. ISBN: 0-250-40189-4.
39. Washington C. Particle Size Analysis in Pharmaceutics and Other Industries. West Sussex, U.K.: Ellis Horwood, 1992:215–235.
40. Russ JC Computer-Assisted Microscopy: The Measurement and Analysis of Images. New York: Plenum Press, 1992.
41. Serra J. Image Analysis and Mathematical Morphology, Vol. 1, 4th ed. London: Academic Press, 1993.
42. Joyce Loebl. Image Analysis: Principles and Practice. Marquisway, Team Valley, Gateshead: Tyne and Wear, 1985.

# Preparation and Identification of Polymorphs and Solvatomorphs

**Harry G. Brittain**

*Center for Pharmaceutical Physics, Milford, New Jersey, U.S.A.*

## INTRODUCTION

It is now very well known that the majority of organic compounds are capable of being crystallized into more than one structural form (1–11). Polymorphism is defined as the situation where the different crystal forms of a compound are found to be identical in their elemental composition, while solvatomorphism is defined as the situation where the various crystal forms of a compound differ in their solvation or hydration state. The development of a full understanding of the stability relationships between polymorphs and solvatomorphs is vitally important to a preformulation program, as the selection of the proper form is crucial even at the earliest stages of development.

The preparation and identification of polymorphs and solvatomorphs have become extremely important, since the nature of the crystal structure adopted by a given compound upon crystallization exerts a profound effect on the solid-state properties of that system. It is now well established that different crystal forms can have different solubility characteristics, as well as different intrinsic dissolution rates (IDRs) and possibly even different bioavailabilities. In addition, different forms may have different degrees of stability with respect to humidity, temperature, light, and formulation excipients. The manufacturing process may be affected if the different forms exhibit differences in flow characteristics, crystal habit, or thermal stability.

Since these structural variations can translate into significant differences in properties of pharmaceutical importance, it is extremely important that a search for all accessible crystal forms should be carried out as part of the preformulation program. The results of this work are ordinarily included in the Chemistry, Manufacturing, and Control section of a New Drug Application, since such knowledge is considered vital to demonstrating an understanding of the drug substance manufacturing process.

## OVERVIEW OF POLYMORPHISM AND SOLVATOMORPHISM

An ideal crystal is constructed by the infinite regular repetition in space of identical fundamental structural units, with each unit containing one or more molecules. One may describe the structure of all crystals in terms of a single periodic lattice, which represents the translational repetition of the fundamental structural unit. For organic molecules, a group of atoms is often attached to a lattice point or is situated in an elementary parallelepiped.

A lattice is defined as a regular periodic arrangement of points in space, and is by definition a purely mathematical abstraction. The nomenclature is in allusion to the fact that a three-dimensional grid of lines can be used to connect the lattice points. It is important to note that the points in a lattice may be connected in various ways to form an infinite number of different lattice structures. The crystal structure is formed only when a fundamental unit is attached identically to each lattice point and extended along each crystal axis through translational repetition. The points on a lattice are defined by three fundamental translation vectors, a, b, and c, such that the atomic arrangement looks the same in every respect when viewed from any point r as it does when viewed at point r':

$$r' = r + n_1 a + n_2 b + n_3 c \qquad (1)$$

where $n_1$, $n_2$, and $n_3$ are arbitrary integers.

It is common practice to use the primitive translation vectors to define the axes of the crystal, although other nonprimitive crystal axes can be used for the sake of convenience. A lattice translation operation is defined as the displacement within the lattice, with the vector describing the operation given by

$$T = n_1 a + n_2 b + n_3 c \qquad (2)$$

The crystal axes a, b, and c form three adjacent edges of a parallelepiped. The smallest parallelepiped built upon the three unit translations is known as the unit cell. Although the unit cell is an imaginary construct, it has an actual shape and definite volume. The entire crystal structure is generated through the periodic repetition, by the three unit translations, of matter contained within the volume of the unit cell. A unit cell does not necessarily have a definite absolute origin or position, but does have the definite orientation and shape defined by the translation vectors. A cell will fill all space under the action of suitable crystal translation operations and will occupy the minimum volume permissible.

The unit cell is defined by the lengths ($a$, $b$, and $c$) of the crystal axes, and by the angles ($\alpha$, $\beta$, and $\gamma$) between these. The convention is that $\alpha$ defines the angle between the $b$ and $c$ axes, $\beta$ defines the angle between the $a$ and $c$ axes, and $\gamma$ defines the angle between the $a$ and $b$ axes. There are seven fundamental types of primitive unit cell, which define the seven crystal classes. As stated earlier, each unit cell will occupy one lattice point in the structure.

Polymorphs and solvatomorphs must necessarily be different in the details of their unit cells, and therefore will exhibit differing degrees of stability. At a given temperature and pressure, one particular form must be more stable than all others, enabling a differentiation between the stable form of a drug substance and its metastable forms. Most often, one will seek to develop the stable form of a drug candidate unless overwhelming arguments exist for the development of a metastable form. Polymorphic or solvatomorphic systems will either exhibit enantiotropy (for each possible form, a defined and accessible temperature/pressure region exists where it is the most stable form) or monotropy (only one form is the most stable at all accessible temperatures and pressures).

Generally speaking, the concepts of monotropy and enantiotropy in phase theory appear to coincide with the structural concepts of unrelated and related lattices. Nevertheless, one must avoid equating the two, for it is certainly possible that one of two related lattices of the same substance is less stable than is the other under all conditions of temperature and pressure. This would indicate the existence of monotropy in spite of the existence of related lattices. This situation becomes especially important for polymorphic organic compounds, which form molecular lattices.

For substances that form molecular lattices, structural modifications can arise in two main distinguishable ways. Should the molecule exist as a rigid group of atoms with definite symmetry, these can be stacked differently to occupy the points of different lattices. This type of behavior is known as packing polymorphism, and can be described in terms of packing equivalent or nonequivalent spheres (or ellipsoids). On the other hand, if the molecule is not rigidly constructed and can exist in multiple conformational states, then it can form structural variations through conformational polymorphism.

## PREPARATION OF POLYMORPHS AND SOLVATOMORPHS

As part of the preformulation development program, one ordinarily establishes a protocol that serves to define the experiments needed to identify the possible crystalline states of a drug substance. The protocol should also describe the analytical techniques to be used in the detection and characterization of new crystalline forms. Ultimately, the goal of this work is to ensure that the most appropriate crystalline form for development is determined, and that its stability and transformation relationships with all other forms be understood.

As part of the preliminary preformulation work, a substantial amount of information regarding the substance under study must be known. Prior to the implementation of the polymorphism study, the chemical form of the drug entity has been defined, and the decision as to whether to develop a salt form of the substance has already been made (12). The scientists conducting the work will therefore know the systematic chemical name, empirical formula, molecular weight, and structural formula, and will have a good idea as to the magnitudes of all accessible ionization constants.

It is worth pointing out that in order to minimize artifacts due to impurities, a highly purified drug substance should be used for this phase of study. Once the system becomes defined, one can then consider the effect of impurities on the accessible crystal forms. One must always remember that in addition to identifying all crystal forms, a second objective is to choose a crystallization process for the final crystallization of the drug substance.

## Solvent-Mediated Studies

In practically every protocol for the study of polymorphs and solvato-morphs, the first sequence of study entails crystallization of the substance out of a variety of solvents and under a variety of conditions. Since it has been found that the crystal form of a substance often depends on the nature and identity of the crystallization solvent, it is necessary to precipitate the drug substance from a wide range of solvent types and under a variety of crystallization rates (13). The essence of this work is to use differences in solvent properties and isolation modes to induce the nucleation and subsequent growth of all possible crystal types.

It is obvious that crystal growth cannot proceed out of either an unsaturated or even a saturated solution, and that only through the establishment of a supersaturation condition can such growth be achieved. It has been recognized since the earliest studies of Ostwald (14) that the phase diagram for solubility is more complicated than is most commonly envisioned. A supersaturated solution will not spontaneously adjust to the equilibrium condition required by the phase rule (i.e., the equilibrium solubility) unless the degree of supersaturation exceeds a certain value. The concentration region where supersaturation can be obtained without the spontaneous formation of crystal nuclei is termed the metastable zone, while the concentration region where the formation of crystal nuclei cannot be stopped is termed the labile zone. This behavior has been illustrated in Figure 1.

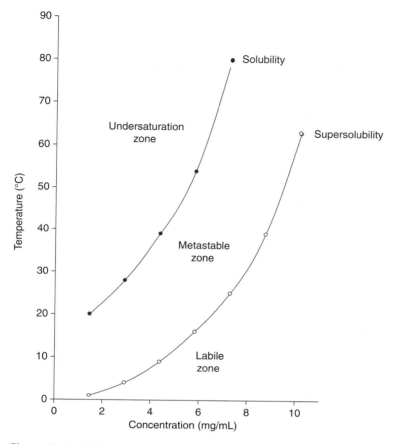

**Figure 1** Solubility (●) and supersolubility (○) curves of a new chemical entity, illustrating the various concentration zones for this compound.

When attempting to obtain as many polymorphs or solvatomorphs as can exist for a given compound, one ordinarily seeks to either rapidly or slowly place the system into the labile zone, and to then identify the various crystal forms that are obtained. The usual practice is to make up a saturated solution near the boiling point of the solvent, and then create the super-saturation by either rapidly or slowly cooling the solution. One often finds the formation of the more metastable phases through the rapid discharge of supersaturation. Rapid crystallization can also be achieved by the addition of a miscible solvent in which the substance exhibits little solubility (an antisolvent), or by a rapid change in acidity or basicity for substances having a strong pH dependence of solubility. The more stable phases are usually obtained through the slow alleviation of supersaturation. An alternative to slow cooling is crystallization by evaporation.

Ostwald recognized that when a system was capable of existing in multiple crystal forms, these could interconvert during the time they were suspended in solution. As he stated: "When a given chemical system is left in an unstable state, it tends to change not into the most stable form, but into the form the stability of which most nearly resembles its own; that is, into that transient stable modification whose formation from the original state is accomplished by the smallest loss of free energy" (14). The practical implication of the Rule of Stages is that when rapidly discharging supersaturation, investigators must quickly isolate the precipitated solids before they have a change to transform into a new form.

When the direct crystallization methods produce only metastable forms, one can use Ostwald ripening experiments to obtain new polymorphic or solvatomorphic crystal forms, if these are more stable than the starting crystal forms. These studies are executed by suspending an excess of solid material in its saturated solution for an extended period of time. Often, it is worthwhile to maintain the suspension at both low and elevated temperatures if there is an indication that the crystal forms might be enantiotropic in nature. After a period of standing, the metastable forms will convert to a more stable form if the energetics of the system so permit.

It is quite clear that the temperature-concentration zones of Figure 1 will be highly dependent on the solvent system employed, and hence solvent-mediated studies are performed using a variety of crystallization solvents. Owing to their differing chemical and physical properties, crystallizing solvents can often exert a strong influence on the nature of packing or conformation polymorphism associated with a given compound (15). Solvents have been classified on the basis of their proton-donating, proton-accepting, and dipole-interaction abilities (16), and divided according to high performance liquid chromatography–related properties (17). Workers needing more information about solvent classifications and properties of individual solvents can find this information in the extraordinary compilation of Riddick and Bunger (18). A more limited, but still useful, solvent classification scheme and suggestions for the nomenclature of appropriate solvent systems are shown in Table 1.

Out of the hundreds of potential crystallization solvents, Mullin has listed the useful ones as belonging to seven groups: water, acetic acid and its esters, lower alcohols and ketones, ethers, chlorinated hydrocarbons, aromatic hydrocarbons, and light petroleum fractions (19). He has also suggested the use of mixed solvent systems, specifically citing alcohol–water, alcohol–ketone, alcohol–ether, alcohol–chloroform, and alcohol–toluene, as well as others that would not be applicable in a pharmaceutical setting.

The goal in solvent-mediated studies is to set up as many different experimental conditions as possible so as to cause self-nucleation of all possible polymorphs or solvatomorphs. The nucleation process can be facilitated through the inclusion of epitaxial surfaces in the supersaturated

**Table 1** Classification of Crystallization Solvent Types

| Solvent system type | Preferred solvents | Alternative solvents |
|---|---|---|
| Dipolar aprotic | Acetonitrile | Dimethyl formamide, dimethyl sulfoxide, N-methyl-pyrrolidone |
| Protic | Water (pH 3, 7, 10), methanol | Acetic acid, ethanol, i-propanol, n-butanol |
| Lewis acidic | Dichloromethane | Chloroform |
| Lewis basic | Acetone, ethyl acetate | Tetrahydrofuran, methyl ethyl ketone, methyl butyl ether, butyl acetate |
| Aromatic | Toluene | Xylene, pyridine, anisole, ethylbenzene |
| Nonpolar | Hexane | Heptane, cyclohexane |

crystallization solution (20,21). This process has been used for years in the form of scratching the sides of a vessel, but more recently through the deliberate inclusion of solid materials whose surfaces present a wide variety of nucleation conditions. The epitaxial agents can be crystalline organic substances, fractured polymeric solids, or any insoluble material presenting a variety of crystal planes to the crystallizing medium.

It necessarily follows that the polymorphic or solvatomorphic form of each and every solid material isolated after a solvent-meditated study must be determined. This work is usually performed using X-ray powder diffraction (XRPD) in conjunction with at least one other technique, such as differential scanning calorimetry (DSC), vibrational spectroscopy (either infrared absorption or Raman spectroscopy), or solid-state nuclear magnetic resonance (NMR) (usually [13]C-NMR). A unique crystal form is indicated by a distinct and characteristic XRPD powder pattern, confirmed by the ancillary technique. One should not be surprised to observe the formation of solvatomorphs as well as polymorphs, as the existence of these crystal forms are widely known for organic compounds (22).

It is also appropriate to conduct solubility studies for each unique form isolated after a solvent-meditated study. This work will include the aqueous solubility characteristics (pH dependence of solubility and partition coefficient, IDRs) as well as the nonaqueous solubility characteristics (the saturated solutions remaining after crystallization studies are used to obtain the solubilities in these systems).

## Solid-State Transformation Studies

Very often, several polymorphs and solvatomorphs are identified upon completion of the solvent-mediated studies. Each of these forms should then be subjected to a series of "substance abuse" experiments (i.e., intentionally imposed solid-state stress conditions) that are designed to learn if other crystalline forms are attainable by these means. These studies can provide information useful in determining milling, drying, and tableting conditions.

One of the most important studies in this part of the protocol entails measurements of water vapor adsorption. Each unique form identified after the solvent-mediated studies can, in principle, interact differently with water vapor. Additional experimentation can be performed using dynamic vapor sorption instrumentation, if appropriate. In the typical procedure, one exposes the various unique forms to selected equilibrium relative humidity (RH) conditions, usually established through the use of saturated salt solutions. The storage chambers should have RH values of 0% and 100%, and at least five intermediate humidity conditions. After the complete equilibration of the sample with the environment, one measures the water content and plots the total water content as a function of RH.

When a compound does not form a hydrate, a plot of water content against RH will usually consist of a simple concave-up type of plot. However, when a substance can form a stoichiometric hydrate, the hydrate should exhibit stability over a range of RH values (23,24). This type of behavior has been illustrated in Figure 2, where the existence of a definite

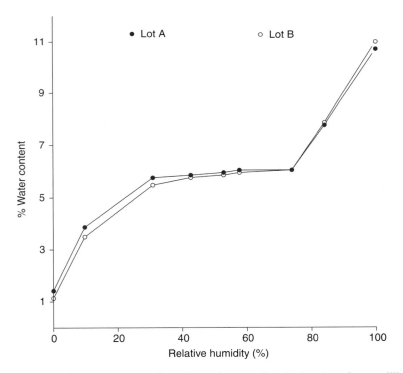

**Figure 2**  Water content of two lots of a new chemical entity after equilibration at various relativity conditions.

state of hydration is indicated by a plateau over the range of 30% to 75% RH in the plot of water composition against RH. One can then use the measured water content to calculate the stoichiometry of the hydrate through simple calculations.

Since new crystal forms can often be obtained through thermal processing, an important aspect of the screening program consists of isothermal heating of the unique forms obtained from the solvent-mediated and moisture-uptake experiments. One can identify appropriate isothermal heating regions of interest by studying the DSC thermograms of each unique form. Typically, one heats bulk samples at temperatures close to or at the onset of desolvation, phase transformation, or melting. The heated samples are then thermally quenched by either slow or rapid cooling.

A second approach to generating new crystal forms by means of thermal processing can be executed through the use of temperature cycling. One heats all identified unique forms from the preceding studies above each thermal event noted in its DSC thermogram, cools the sample to ambient temperature, and then reruns the full DSC thermogram. The thermal events noted during the DSC studies of each unique form should be studied using hot stage microscopy. Of particular interest will be changes in birefringence and thermally induced visual phenomena.

An additional method to find new crystal forms entails the use of sublimation. Since each unique crystal form must be characterized by a unique lattice energy, the various substances can exhibit different sublimation behaviors. In addition, the sublimed form of the compound may itself represent a new crystal form. The experiment is best conducted by setting the temperature of each sample in the sublimation system, and continuously lowering the system pressure until the substance is observed to sublime. Polymorphs can be differentiated on the basis of their differing sublimation pressures.

The investigation of potential solid-state phase transformations cannot be considered as being complete until a sequence of grinding and compression experiments are conducted. One may study the effect of particle size reduction and milling by simply manually grinding portions of each of the unique polymorphic and solvatomorphic forms in an agate mortar for a few minutes, and then using the usual characterization methodology to determine if any phase change had taken place. To study the effect of compaction, one would compress each unique form in a press and then study the resulting compact with as little mechanical disruption as possible.

It is worth reiterating at this point that full characterization should be performed on each and every solid material isolated after a solid-state study. At the minimum, this work will feature XRPD, but this should be supplemented with polarizing light microscopy, thermal analysis, vibrational spectroscopy, and solid-state NMR. For any new crystal forms discovered during this part of the program, it is also important to record the solubility characteristics (pH dependence of solubility and partition coefficient, IDRs, and solubilities in nonaqueous systems).

## IDENTIFICATION OF POLYMORPHS AND SOLVATOMORPHS

Every time a chemical entity is processed using any of the methodologies outlined in the previous section, its appropriate properties must be catalogued so that one may know whether a new crystal form has been obtained or not. For identification purposes, it is appropriate to identify the crystal form of an isolated solid using a combination of XRPD and one other supporting technique (8). The ancillary technique will usually be one or more of the following: polarizing light microscopy (i.e., optical crystallography), thermal methods of analysis [usually a combination of DSC and thermogravimetry (TG)], solid-state vibrational spectroscopy (either infrared absorption or Raman spectroscopy), and solid-state NMR spectrometry (usually $^{13}$C-NMR).

Since other chapters in this book will discuss these techniques in great detail, the discussion of characterization methodology will be sufficiently brief to enable an understanding of the forthcoming case histories. Illustrations of the applicability of each method to studies of polymorphism and solvatomorphism will be made in a subsequent section.

### X-Ray Powder Diffraction

Since polymorphism and solvatomorphism are crystallographic phenomena, it follows that a crystallographic technique would be most appropriate for the identification of new crystal forms. XRPD has become exceedingly important to pharmaceutics because it represents the primary method whereby one can obtain fundamental structural information on the structure of a crystalline substance (25). The technique is ideally suited for the study of large numbers of polycrystalline samples and has found widespread use in the evaluation of crystal structures, comparison of polymorphism and solvate structures, evaluation of degrees of crystallinity, and the study of phase transitions (26). The applicability of the methodology for qualitative (27) and quantitative (28) analysis has been demonstrated.

Bragg and Bragg (29) explained the diffraction of X-rays by crystals using a model where the atoms of a crystal are regularly arranged in space so that they can be regarded as lying in parallel sheets separated by a definite and defined distance. Then they showed that scattering centers arranged in a plane act like a mirror to X-rays incident on them, so that constructive interference would occur for the direction of specular reflection. Within a given family of planes, defined by a Miller index of ($h$ $k$ $l$) and each plane being separated by the distance $d$, each plane produces a specular reflectance of the incident beam. If the incident X-rays are monochromatic (having wavelength equal to $\lambda$), then for an arbitrary glancing angle of $\theta$, the reflections from successive planes are out of phase with one another. This yields destructive interference in the scattered beams. However, by varying $\theta$, a set of values for $\theta$ can be found so that the path difference between X-rays reflected by successive planes will be an integral number ($n$) of wavelengths, and constructive interference will occur. One ultimately obtains the expression known as Bragg's law that explains the phenomenon:

$$2d\sin\ \theta = n\lambda \tag{3}$$

Unlike the case of diffraction of light by a ruled grating, the diffraction of X-rays by a crystalline solid leads to observation of constructive interference (i.e., reflection) occurs only the critical Bragg angles. When reflection does occur, it is stated that the plane in question is reflecting in the $n$th order, or that one observes $n$th order diffraction for that particular crystal plane. Therefore, one will observe an X-ray scattering response for every plane defined by a unique Miller index of ($h\ k\ l$).

Since the microcrystals of a randomly oriented powdered sample will present all possible crystal faces at a given interface, the diffraction off this powdered surface will therefore provide information on all possible atomic spacings (i.e., defining the crystal lattice). The powder pattern will therefore consist of a series of peaks, having varying relative intensities, which are detected at various scattering angles. These angles, and their relative intensities, are correlated with computed $d$-spacings to provide a full crystallographic characterization of the powdered sample. After indexing all the scattered bands, it is possible to derive unit cell dimensions and other crystallographic information from a high-resolution powder pattern of a substance (30).

To measure a powder pattern, a randomly oriented powdered sample is so prepared as to expose all its planes. The scattering angle is determined by slowly rotating the sample and measuring the angle of diffracted X-rays (typically using a scintillation detector) with respect to the angle of the incident beam. Alternatively, the angle between sample and source can be kept fixed, while moving the detector to determine the angles of the scattered radiation. By knowing the wavelength of the incident beam, the spacing between the planes (identified as the $d$-spacings) is calculated using Bragg's law.

As an example of how XRPD can be used to identify polymorphs of a new chemical entity, two powder patterns of a compound under development are shown in Figure 3. The two forms are readily distinguishable, and one could continue the analysis through a listing of the characteristic scattering angles, computed $d$-spacings, and relative intensities.

A very useful complement to ordinary powder X-ray diffraction is variable temperature X-ray diffraction. In this method, the sample is

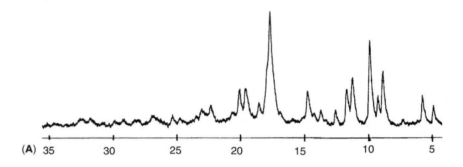

(A) 35  30  25  20  15  10  5

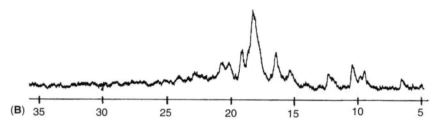

(B) 35  30  25  20  15  10  5

**Figure 3** X-ray powder diffraction patterns of the two polymorphs of a new chemical entity.

contained on a stage that can be heated to any desired temperature. The method is extremely useful in the study of thermally induced phenomena (31,32) and is especially useful in the study of thermally induced desolvation of solvatomorphs (33).

## Microscopy and Optical Crystallography

Evaluation of the morphology of a pharmaceutical solid is of extreme importance, since this property exerts a significant influence over the micromeritic and bulk powder properties of the material (34,35). The value of a preformulation program is that one can deduce crystallographic information that is comparable in its utility to that obtainable by means of XRPD. When employed in conjunction with polarizing optics, simple optical microscopy becomes optical crystallography, and becomes far more suitable for the identification of polymorphs and solvatomorphs (36).

The polarizing microscope is a light microscope equipped with a linear polarizer located below the condenser, and an additional polarizer mounted on top of the eyepiece. A rotating stage is also found to be very useful, as is the ability to add other optical accessories (such as phase contrast).

Polarization optical analysis is based on the action of the analyte crystal on the properties of the transmitted light. This method can yield several directly measured parameters, such as the sign and magnitude of any observed birefringence, the refractive indices associated with each crystal direction, the axis angles, and the relations between the optical axes.

The refractive index of light passing through an isotropic crystal will be identical along each of the crystal axes, and such crystals therefore possess single refraction. Anisotropic substances will exhibit different refractive indices for light polarized with respect to the crystal axes, thus exhibiting double refraction. Crystals within the hexagonal and tetragonal systems possess one isotropic direction, and are termed uniaxial. Anisotropic crystals possessing two isotropic axes are termed biaxial, and include all crystals belonging to the orthorhombic, monoclinic, and triclinic systems. Biaxial crystals will exhibit different indices of refraction along each of the crystal axes.

Isotropic samples are characterized by the existence of equivalent crystal axes; they therefore exhibit isotropic extinction and have no effect on the polarized light no matter how the crystal is oriented. When a sample is capable of exhibiting double refraction, the specimen will appear bright against a dark background. For example, when a uniaxial crystal is placed with the unique $c$ axis horizontal on the stage, it will be alternately dark and bright as the stage is rotated. Furthermore, the crystal will be completely dark when the $c$ axis is parallel to the transmission plane of the polarizer or analyzer. If the crystal has edges or faces parallel to the $c$ axis, then it will be extinguished when such an edge or face is parallel to one of the polarizer directions, a condition known as parallel extinction. At all intermediate positions, the crystal will appear light and usually colored. A rhombohedral or pyramidal crystal will be extinguished when the bisector of a silhouette angle is parallel to a polarization direction, and this type of extinction is termed symmetrical extinction. For biaxial crystals, similar results are obtained as with uniaxial crystals. The exception to this rule is that in monoclinic and triclinic systems, the polarization directions need not be parallel to the faces or to the bisectors of face angles. If the prominent faces or edges of an extinguished crystal are not parallel to the axes of the initial polarizer, the extinction is said to be oblique. Knowledge of the type of extinction therefore permits one to make a determination of the system to which a given crystal belongs.

Different polymorphs ordinarily exhibit morphologies, as well as differing optical crystallographic parameters. Figure 4 shows the crystals corresponding to the two forms of the new chemical entity being charted in this article.

The ability to observe the optical properties of crystals during heating and cooling processes is termed "thermal microscopy," and this can be a profoundly useful technique in the study of polymorphs and solvatomorphs

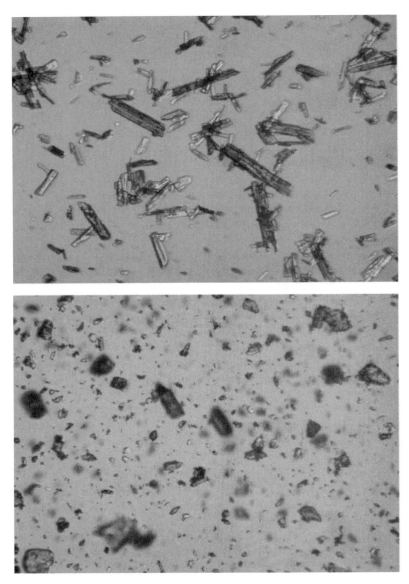

**Figure 4** Photomicrographs obtained using optical microscopy of the two polymorphs of a new chemical entity.

(37,38). Crystal polymorphs ordinarily exhibit different melting points, with the order of melting points being indicative of the order of stability at the elevated temperature condition. The interconversion of such crystal forms is classified as being either enantiotropic or monotropic, according to whether the transformation of one modification into the other is reversible or not. Enantiotropic modifications interchange reversibly at the ordinary transition point, and each form is characterized by having its own stability range of temperature. Monotropic substances are characterized by the existence of a purely hypothetical transition point, since this point is predicted to be higher in temperature than the melting point of one of the polymorphic forms. Monotropic polymorphs are characterized by the fact that one form is stable at all temperatures below its melting point, while the second form is metastable at all temperatures (35).

## Thermal Methods of Analysis

Thermal analysis methods are defined as those techniques in which a property of the analyte is determined as a function of an externally applied temperature (39). In practice, the sample temperature is increased in a linear fashion, while the property in question is evaluated on a continuous basis. The technology is used to characterize compound purity, polymorphism, solvation, degradation, and excipient compatibility (40). Thermal analysis methods are normally used to monitor endothermic processes (melting, boiling, sublimation, vaporization, desolvation, solid–solid phase transitions, and chemical degradation) as well as exothermic processes (crystallization and oxidative decomposition) (41).

Significant insight into the principles of thermal analysis can be obtained from an evaluation of the determination of ordinary melting points by means of fusion curves. In this experiment, one places the sample within a suitable container, immerses it in a bath whose temperature is increased at a fixed rate, and monitors the temperature of the sample. As long as the substance is a solid, it has a fixed and finite heat capacity; so its temperature linearly increases at a rate governed by the rate of heat flow. Once the substance begins to melt, the heat capacity of the system becomes effectively infinite, since all of the absorbed heat is used to transform the solid phase into the liquid phase. The temperature of the sample cannot change during this process owing to the infinite value of the heat capacity, and the fact that any heat entering the system acts only to redistribute the relative amounts of the two phases. Once the entire sample has melted, however, the heat capacity again becomes fixed and finite since the substance is now a simple liquid. Further heating results in a linear rate of temperature increase up to the next phase transition.

Differential thermal analysis (DTA) represents an improvement to the melting point determination in that one monitors the difference in temperature between the sample and a reference as a function of temperature (42). As long as no thermal transitions take place, the temperature of the sample and reference will be the same since the heat capacities of the two will be roughly equivalent. However, differences in temperature between the sample and reference will be manifest when changes occur that require a finite heat of reaction. If $\Delta H$ for the transition is positive (endothermic reaction), the temperature of the sample will lag behind (since more heat will be absorbed by the sample than by the reference), and this event will be recorded as a negative-going peak in the thermogram. If the $\Delta H$ of the transition is negative (exothermic reaction), the temperature of the sample will exceed that of the reference (since the sample itself will be a source of additional heat), and the event will be recorded as a positive-going peak in the thermogram.

DSC represents a significant improvement to DTA analysis and has become the most widely used method of thermal analysis (41). In the DSC method, the sample and reference are kept at the same temperature, and the heat flow required to maintain the equality in temperature between the two is measured (43). This can be achieved by placing separate heating elements in the sample and reference cells, with the rate of heating by these elements being controlled and measured. This method of measurement is termed power-compensation DSC, and it yields positive-going peaks for endothermic transitions and negative-going peaks for exothermic transitions. Another methodology is heat-flux DSC, where the sample and reference cells are heated by the same element, and one monitors the direction and magnitude of the heat being transferred between the two. Heat-flux DSC is probably a preferable method in that it yields superior baselines compared to power-compensation DSC. In addition, one obtains negative-going peaks for endothermic transitions and positive-going peaks for exothermic transitions (the same as for DTA analysis) that are in harmony with the IUPAC guidelines.

DSC plots are obtained as the differential rate of heating (in units of W/sec, cal/sec, or J/sec) against temperature and thus represent direct measures of the heat capacity of the sample. The area under a DSC peak is directly proportional to the heat absorbed or evolved by the thermal event, and integration of these peak areas yields the heat of reaction (in units of cal/sec g or J/sec g). Owing to its ability to facilitate quantitative data interpretation, DSC analysis has virtually supplanted DTA analysis.

Figure 5 shows the DSC thermograms corresponding to the two forms of the new chemical entity being charted in this article. Form A is clearly the most stable form near the melting point, exhibiting a single melting endotherm having a maximum at 148°C. Form B is found to exhibit a maximum in its melting endotherm at 131°C, followed by a recrystallization exotherm and subsequent melting endotherm of form A (endothermic maximum at 147°C).

One other commonly used thermoanalytical technique is TG, where one measures the thermally induced weight loss of a material as a function of the applied temperature (44). TG analysis is restricted to studies that involve either a mass gain or loss (usually loss) and is most commonly used to study desolvation processes and compound decomposition. The major

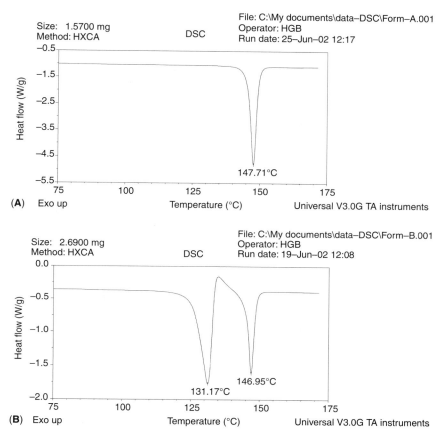

**Figure 5** Differential scanning calorimetry thermograms of the two polymorphs of a new chemical entity.

utility of TG analysis in the identification of polymorphs and solvates is that it enables one to demonstrate that a given substance is nonsolvated or to calculate the compound-to-solvent stoichiometry in a solvatomorph.

## Solid-State Vibrational Spectroscopy

The energies associated with the fundamental vibrational modes of a chemical compound lie within the range of 400 to 4000 $cm^{-1}$, and the electromagnetic radiation having the proper energies to promote transitions between these modes corresponds to the mid-infrared region (45). Transitions between vibrational energy levels can be observed directly through their absorbance in the infrared region of the spectrum, with Fourier-transform infrared spectroscopy (FTIR) now being the method of choice. In addition, these transitions can also be observed using Raman spectroscopy, where the inelastic scattering of incident energy is used to obtain vibrational spectra. Overtones and combination bands of the fundamental vibrational modes are observed in the near-infrared region of the spectrum (4000 to 13,350 cm$^{-1}$) (46).

Infrared absorption spectroscopy, especially when measured by means of the Fourier transform method (FTIR), is a powerful technique for the physical characterization of pharmaceutical solids (47). When the structural details associated with polymorphism or solvatomorphism perturb the pattern of vibrational motion for a given molecule, one can use the differences in vibrational frequencies between crystal forms as a means to study the solid-state chemistry (48). In addition, solid-state vibrational spectra can be very useful in studies of the solvation phenomena associated with a solvatomorphic system. Solid-state infrared absorption spectra are most appropriately obtained on powdered solids through the combined use of FTIR and a nonperturbing sampling system (diffuse reflectance or attenuated total reflectance detection), and interpreted through the conventional group frequency compilations (49).

Figure 6 shows the infrared absorption spectra, obtained using the attenuated total reflectance detection mode, of the two forms of the new chemical entity being charted in this article. The two forms are readily distinguishable, and a number of infrared absorption peaks serve to differentiate the two forms. At the same time, some of the infrared absorption bands are the same in the two forms, indicating that those particular vibrational modes were not affected by the differences in crystal structure between the two forms.

Another technique of vibrational spectroscopy that is ideally suited for the characterization of polymorphism or solvatomorphism in solids is Raman spectroscopy. In this methodology, the sample is irradiated with monochromatic laser radiation, and the inelastic scattering of the source energy is used to obtain a vibrational spectrum of the analyte (50). Since most compounds of pharmaceutical interest are of low symmetry, the Raman spectrum will contain spectra features at the same energies as those obtained using the FTIR method. However, owing to the fundamentally different selection rules associated with the phenomenon, differences in peak intensity are often observed. In general, symmetric vibrations and nonpolar groups yield the most intense Raman scattering bands, while antisymmetric vibrations and polar groups yield the most intense infrared absorption bands. These differences can, at times, be quite profound and can therefore be successfully exploited in the characterization of solid materials.

## Solid-State NMR Spectrometry

An extremely detailed characterization of a pharmaceutical material can be performed at the level of the individual chemical environments of each atom

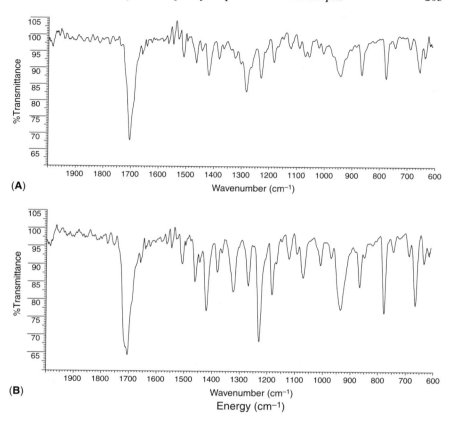

**Figure 6** Infrared absorption spectra of the two polymorphs of a new chemical entity, obtained in the attenuated total reflectance mode.

in the solid compound, and this information is obtained using NMR spectroscopy. With recent advances in instrumentation and computer pulse sequences, these studies can now be routinely carried out in the solid state (51). Although any nucleus that can be studied in the solution phase can also be studied in the solid state, most of the work has focused on $^{13}$C studies. $^{1}$H-NMR remains an extremely difficult measurement in the solid state, and the data obtained from such work are only obtained at medium resolution. The main problem is that $^{1}$H-NMR has one of the smallest isotropic chemical shift ranges (12 ppm), but with peak broadening effects that can span several ppm in magnitude.

The local magnetic field ($B_{loc}$) at a $^{13}$C nucleus in an organic solid is given by

$$B_{loc} = \pm \{h\gamma_H/4\pi\}\{(3 \ \cos^2 \theta - 1/r^3)\} \tag{4}$$

where $\gamma_H$ is the magnetogyric ratio of the proton, $r$ is the internuclear C–H distance to the bonded proton, and $\theta$ is the angle between the C–H bond and the external applied field ($B_o$). The $\pm$ sign results from the fact that the local field may add to or subtract from the applied field, depending on whether the neighboring proton dipole is aligned with or against the direction of $B_o$. In a microcrystalline organic solid, there is a summation over many values of $\theta$ and $r$, resulting in a proton dipolar broadening of many kilohertz. A rapid reorientation of the C–H internuclear vectors (such as those associated with the random molecular motions that take place in the liquid phase) would result in a reduction of the dipolar broadening. In solids, such rapid isotropic tumbling is not possible, but since the term $(3 \cos^2\theta - 1)$ equals zero if $\theta$ equals $\cos^{-1} 3^{-1/2}$ (approximately 54°44'), spinning the sample at the so-called "magic angle" of 54°44' with respect to the direction of the applied magnetic field results in an averaging of the chemical shift anisotropy. In a solid sample, the anisotropy reflects the chemical shift dependence of chemically identical nuclei on their spatial arrangement with respect to the applied field. Since it is this anisotropy that is primarily responsible for the spectral broadening associated with $^{13}$C samples, spinning at the magic angle makes it possible to obtain high-resolution $^{13}$C-NMR spectra of solid materials.

An additional method for the removal of $^{13}$C–$^1$H dipolar broadening is to use a high-power proton decoupling field, often referred to as dipolar decoupling. One irradiates the sample using high power at an appropriate frequency, which results in the complete collapse of all $^{13}$C–$^1$H couplings. With proton dipolar coupling alone, the resonances in a typical solid-state $^{13}$C spectrum will remain very broad (on the order of 10–200 ppm). This broadening arises from the fact that the chemical shift of a particular carbon is directional, depending on the orientation of the molecule with respect to the magnetic field.

Even though high-resolution spectra can be obtained on solids using the magic angle spinning (MAS) technique, the data acquisition time is lengthy due to the low sensitivity of the nuclei and the long relaxation times exhibited by the nuclei. This problem is circumvented by using cross polarization (CP), where spin polarization is transferred from the high-abundance, high-frequency nucleus ($^1$H) to the rare, low-frequency nucleus ($^{13}$C). This process results in up to a fourfold enhancement of the normal $^{13}$C magnetization and permits a shortening of the waiting periods between pulses. The CP experiment also allows the measurement of several relaxation parameters that can be used to study the dynamic properties of the solid under investigation.

When the crystallography of compounds related by polymorphism is such that nuclei in the two structures are magnetically nonequivalent, it follows that the resonances of these nuclei will not be equivalent. Since it is normally not difficult to assign organic functional groups to observed resonances, solid-state NMR spectra can be used to deduce the nature of polymorphic variations, especially when the polymorphism is conformational in nature (52). Such information has proven to be extremely valuable during various stages in the development of numerous pharmaceutical substances (53).

Figure 7 shows the solid-state $^{13}$C-NMR spectra of the two forms of the new chemical entity being charted in this article. For this polymorphic pair, the SS-NMR spectra would not represent the optimal methodology for the differentiation of the two forms, since the spectra happen to be rather similar. This finding simply means that most of the chemical environments of the nuclei of the two forms are effectively equivalent. For this compound, one would not use SS-NMR as the supporting technique to bolster the XRPD identifications, and often knowing this type of information is equal in importance to determining what technique would be a good supporting technique.

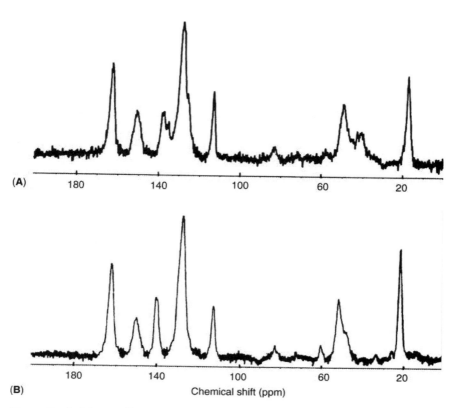

**Figure 7**  Solid-state $^{13}$C-NMR spectra of the two polymorphs of a new chemical entity.

## CASE STUDIES OF PREFORMULATION STUDIES OF POLYMORPHISM AND SOLVATOMORPHISM

The number of preformulation studies reported in the literature that relate to the identification of polymorphs and solvatomorphs is simply astounding, and the field cannot be reviewed in any comprehensive manner. However, it is useful to see how the current practice is being executed through the examination of a number of recent investigations and to learn from the examples.

### Production of Polymorphs and Solvatomorphs Through Direct Crystallization

Two polymorphs of TKS-159

have been prepared by direct crystallization (54). One form was obtained by crystallization from 1:1 water/ethanol, water, ethyl acetate, or methyl ethyl ketone, and the other form was obtained by crystallization out of acetone. The compounds were identified on the basis of their characteristic XRPD, DSC, SS-infrared, and SS-NMR features. Interestingly, the solid-state $^{13}$C-NMR spectrum of the metastable $\beta$-form tended to resemble the solution phase spectrum of TKS-159 more than did the spectrum of the more stable $\alpha$-form.

Three different crystal forms of CHF-1035

were obtained by recrystallization out of ordinary solvent systems (55). The procedure followed was to saturate 10 mL of solvent with the product near the boiling point, and rapidly cool this to either ambient or ice–water temperature. Form I was obtained under both crystallization conditions from both methanol and ethanol, while form II was obtained under both crystallization conditions from methyl ethyl ketone. Cooling of acetone solutions to room temperature yielded form I, while cooling of acetone solutions to 0°C yielded form III.

The $\alpha, \beta$, and $\delta$ polymorphs of TA-270

were obtained by recrystallization from acetonitrile, ethanol, and acetone, respectively, and an amorphous form obtained by milling the $\beta$-form (56). The $\beta$ and $\delta$ polymorphs could be transformed into the $\alpha$-form by heating. The intrinsic dissolution of the most stable $\alpha$-form was found to be significantly slower than any of the other forms, which all exhibited somewhat comparable IDRs. In accompanying biostudies, it was found that the rat plasma concentration of the $\alpha$-form of TA-270 exhibited a time dependence different from that of the other forms.

Two polymorphs of the antispastic chemical entity E2101

were prepared by direct crystallization methods (57). Form I was the usual product resulting from crystallization out of most solvent systems (isopropyl acetate, ethyl acetate, ethanol, and aqueous ethanol), but interesting behavior was noted in the mixed ethyl acetate/alkane system. Form I was obtained by crystallization out of 75:25 v/v ethyl acetate/n-heptane, while form II was obtained by crystallization out of 25:75 v/v ethyl acetate/ *n*-hexane. This observation demonstrates the requirement to investigate mixed solvent systems in order to ensure production of all crystal forms during a polymorphic screening study.

Turning to named compounds, the new form II of chlordiazepoxide

was prepared by crystallization of the compound out of methanol (58). Form I had been obtained from other alcoholic solvents (i.e., ethanol, propanol, and butanol), illustrating that one can sometimes obtain different crystal forms even when crystallizing out of systems of the same solvent type. Studies of the single-crystal structures of the two forms indicated the existence of similar molecular conformations, but with different modes of crystal packing. The enantiotropic transition between the forms was attributed to a molecular rearrangement of dimeric units in the two structures.

Two polymorphs and three solvates of fluconazole

were obtained by crystallization out of different solvents at different cooling rates (59). Anhydrate form I was obtained by room temperature crystallization out of *iso*-propanol, while anhydrate form II was crystallized from dichloromethane at room temperature. An acetone 1/4-solvatomorph was obtained by cooling a hot solution to room temperature, while a benzene 1/7-solvatomorph was obtained by cooling the hot solution to 4 °C. Finally, a monohydrate form was obtained by cooling aqueous solutions to room temperature. The IDRs of the various forms were all found to be significantly different to within a 95% confidence interval, as were most of their other characterization properties.

Three polymorphs of glisentide

have been prepared by crystallization from different solvents (60). Form I was obtained from the room temperature crystallization from ethanol, methanol, acetone, acetonitrile, and *N*, *N*-dimethyl formamide. Form II was obtained by dissolving the drug substance in a small amount of hot acetone and then slowly precipitating by the addition of an antisolvent (ethyl acetate) in conjunction with a slowly programmed cooling rate. Form III was obtained by the rapid cooling of a hot dioxane solution to 4°C. One other anhydrous form was obtained by heating form III at 100°C.

Two crystalline polymorphs forms of glybuzole

were ultimately discerned after a screening study involving 11 solvents and six kinds of preparation methods (111). Cooling hot saturated solutions of the substance to room temperature yielded form I (out of ethanol, *n*-propanol, *iso*-butanol, chloroform, or acetone), form II (out of methanol or benzene), or a mixture of forms I and II (out of toluene). When the hot saturated solutions of the substance were rapidly cooled to 5°C, Form I was obtained out of methanol and toluene, while form II was obtained out of ethanol, *n*-propanol, *iso*-butanol, chloroform, or acetone. Dropping saturated solutions of the substance into water (i.e., antisolvent precipitation) yielded only form I (methanol, ethanol, *n*-propanol, *n*-butanol, *iso*-butanol, or acetone). Lyophilization of a benzene solution yielded form I, while freeze-drying a dioxane solution was found to yield form II.

Three polymorphic forms of lifibrol

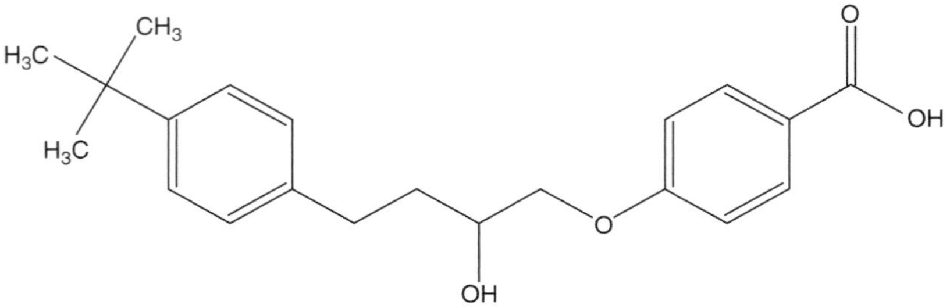

were produced by typical solvent-mediated studies (61). Form I was obtained by crystallization from acetone, chloroform, carbon tetra-chloride, xylene, or ethyl acetate. It could also be obtained through pH modification (addition of acid to alkaline solutions) or through addition of an antisolvent (addition of petroleum ether to a benzene solution). The more stable form II was obtained by crystallization from methanol or ethanol or by the slow addition of an antisolvent (specifically water) to alcoholic solutions. The metastable form III was produced by heating a solidified glassy melt up to 50°C to 60°C on the hot stage microscope.

The use of solvent-mediated polymorphic transformations as a means to discover the most stable crystal form has been investigated for sulfa-merazine (62):

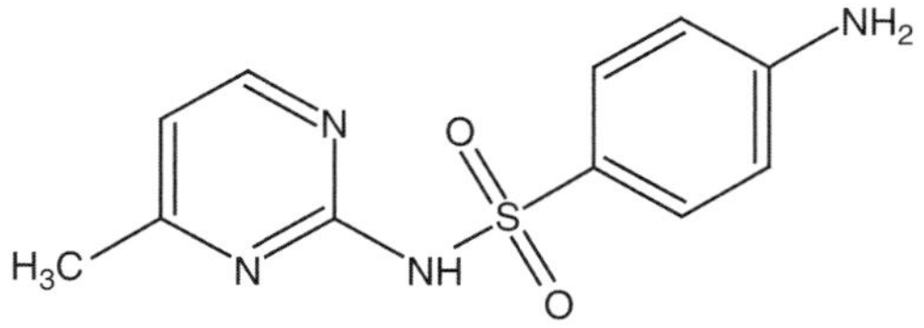

Form I was prepared from the commercial product by recrystallization from *iso*-propanol, while form II was obtained by the suspension of form I in acetonitrile for 20 days. The transition from form I to form II was studied at different temperatures by preparing suspensions of the two forms and allowing these to equilibrate over time. The kinetics of the process was followed by filtering portions of the suspensions and subjecting these to XRPD analysis.

Four anhydrous polymorphs and six solvatomorphs of tenoxicam

were prepared by direct crystallization methods (63). In each preparative method, a relatively concentrated solution of the substance was prepared at 60°C and then cooled to precipitate the product. Form I was obtained by cooling a chloroform solution to 4°C, while form II was obtained out of either ethanol or *n*-butanol. Form III was obtained by cooling either tetrahydrofuran or *iso*-propanol solutions to 4°C, while form IV was obtained by allowing methanol or *N,N*-dimethyl acetamide solutions to remain at room temperature. The dioxane, *N,N*-dimethyl formamide, ethyl acetate, acetone, and *iso*-propanol solvatomorphs were obtained by allowing cooled solutions to remain for extended time periods. It was found that desolvation of the acetonitrile or dioxane solvatomorphs yielded form I, while desolvation of the *N,N*-dimethyl formamide solvatomorph yielded form III.

Crystallization studies performed on torasemide

yielded two polymorphs and a pseudopolymorphic channel inclusion compound (64). Form I crystallizes from hot saturated solutions of methanol, ethanol, *n*-propanol, or *iso*-propanol by slowing cooling down to 20°C. Form II is prepared through a pH adjustment method, where an alkaline solution is treated with acetic acid at 20°C to precipitate the substance. The channel inclusion form is obtained by rapidly cooling a hot saturated aqueous alkanol solution (either 2:2 v/v methanol/water or ethanol/water) to 7°C. This latter form cannot be obtained from pure alcohol or water, but in the presence of small quantities of water crystal of the channel form are obtained if the hot solution is rapidly cooled down to 7°C.

A thorough examination of the polymorphism of 2,4,6-trinitrotoluene (TNT)

as crystallized from solution has provided considerable insight into some of the mechanisms of solvent-mediated solvent methods (65). The two polymorphs are well known and can be prepared by a variety of cooling and antisolvent precipitation mechanisms. In this work, it was shown that even though the identity of the isolated polymorph was strongly affected by the mode of its isolation, this dependence could not be linked to any stereospecific direction that was induced by solvent–solute interactions. Rather, the polymorphic form was simply the result of the initial precipitation of the metastable orthorhombic form, followed by its conversion to the more stable monoclinic form, as would be predicted on the basis of Ostwald's Rule of Stages. Systems favoring the ultimate isolation of the metastable orthorhombic form were those where the solubility was very low, not favoring an Ostwald ripening process that could eventually lead to a phase conversion. Where the compound solubility in the crystallization medium was high, phase conversion took place easily, and one isolated only the more stable monoclinic form. These observations are very important when one attempts to interpret trends in solvent crystallization phenomena, as anomalous behavior may arise owing to the existence of secondary reactions.

## Production of Polymorphs and Solvatomorphs Through Solid-State Transformation Studies

The crystal structures of two enantiotropic polymorphs of finasteride

were determined, and related to their spectroscopic characteristics (66). Form I is produced by direct crystallization out of dry ethyl or isopropyl acetate, while form II can be produced by heating form I through its solid–solid phase transition. The true thermodynamic transition temperature was determined to be 129°C by means of solubility studies performed in cyclohexane. In order to obtain a crystal of form II suitable for single-crystal structural analysis, these workers seeded a molten sample of the drug with a form II crystal, and over a period of several hours, the sample crystallized to yield a suitable crystal.

Upon completion of a conventional crystallization study, two polymorphic forms (identified as forms A and B) of the central nervous system–active drug compound Org 13011 were obtained (67):

When the two low temperature forms were heated at temperatures exceeding 70°C, two additional polymorphs of this compound were discovered. In particular, form A converted to the new form C, while form B converted to the new form D. Both phase transitions took place rapidly and were completely reversible. Upon cooling back to room temperature, forms C and D transformed back into forms A and B, respectively.

When originally prepared, cilostazol

was thought to exist in only a single-crystal form (68). However, it was found that when the substance was melted at 159°C and cooled down to room temperature, the resulting glass could crystallize into two new forms characterized by melting points of 136°C and 146°C. The two thermally derived forms exhibited a monotropic relationship to the stable phase, and each underwent rapid solution-mediated transformations back to the stable phase.

The hydrochloride salt of an NK1 receptor antagonist

has been found to be able to exist in two polymorphic forms at room temperature, and in two different forms at elevated temperatures (69). The system is interesting in that two pairs of low/high temperature forms each bear an enantiotropic relationship, but that conversion to members of the other related pair is much more difficult.

The phase stability and interphase conversion of caffeine and its monohydrate phase relate to the strength of the available hydrogen bonds (70). The hydrogen-bonded branched spine of water molecules present in caffeine monohydrate, which defines its characteristic structure, can be dehydrated to yield the β-anhydrate form. This β-anhydrate form can be heated at 155°C to obtain the trigonal α-anhydrous phase.

The effect of temperature and humidity on the kinetics of dehydration of diclofenac N-(2-hydroxyethyl)pyrollidine dihydrate have been studied (71). In the temperature range of 34°C to 40°C, a diffusion model yielded the best fit to the data. In the temperature range of 42°C to 48°C, the best fit to the data was provided by a phase boundary model. Interestingly, the choice of dehydration model did not significantly affect the calculated activation energy values.

The commercially available hemihydrate form of aspartame

was found to differ from the form whose crystal structure had been reported (72). Although both hemihydrate polymorphs could be heated to form a crystalline anhydrate, they did so at different temperatures. At higher temperatures, the anhydrate phase derived from both hemihydrates formed a dioxopiperazine through a cyclization reaction. In addition, when both hemihydrate forms were contacted with liquid water one obtained a 2.5-hydrate phase.

## CASE STUDY: THE NEDOCROMIL SYSTEM

Nedocromil has been used in various salt forms for the treatment of reversible obstructive airway diseases, and the salt forms have been the subject of extensive study. The sodium salt has been found to exist as a heptahemihydrate, a trihydrate, and a monohydrate (73). For crystalline hydrate phases maintained at 22°C and at varying degrees of RH, a number of stability ranges were determined. The monohydrate was found to be stable from 0% to 6.4% RH, the trihydrate stable from 6.4% to 79.5% RH, and the heptahemihydrate stable above 80% RH. The IDRs of the hydrates decreased in the order of monohydrate > trihydrate > heptahemihydrate, which corresponded with the ordering of free energy with respect to the aqueous solution.

The various crystal forms of nedocromil sodium were characterized using solid-state infrared spectroscopy and NMR (74). It was found that the $^{13}$C-NMR spectrum provided information related to the conformation of the nedocromil anion, while the infrared spectrum was sensitive to the interactions of water molecules in the solid state.

The trihydrate phase of nedocromil sodium was fully dehydrated in vacuum, and the water vapor adsorption characteristics studied at different water vapor pressures over the temperature range of 20°C to 40°C (75). Arrhenius-type plots were interpreted as showing that control of the process is dependent on the ability of the surface to hold water molecules. In a subsequent work, this group used a six-stage model to describe the overall process of sorption of water vapor on and into anhydrous nedocromil sodium (76). It was concluded that up to 27°C, the hydration was controlled by a nucleation and growth mechanism. Between 27°C and 31°C, the hydration process was dominated by diffusion of water molecules into the crystal. At temperatures higher than 31°C, the nature of the process was not defined.

Two independent nonthermal methods were used to determine the activation energies associated with the dehydration of nedocromil sodium hydrate forms (77). For the dehydration of the monohydrate to the anhydrate, it was concluded that the pathway entailed a three-dimensional nucleation mechanism in the bulk of the crystal with subsequent three-dimensional growth of the anhydrate phase.

A number of hydrate phases derived from the bivalent metal salts of nedocromil have also been reported. Three hydrates of the magnesium salt have been reported (78), while the zinc salt of nedocromil was found to form an octahydrate, a heptahydrate, and a pentahydrate (79). The pentahydrate phase was found to be capable of existing in two different crystal structures, differing in their long-range order but being similar in their short-range order. The calcium salt of nedocromil was found to be able to crystallize as a crystalline pentahydrate and a crystalline 8/3-hydrate (80), while the nickel salt was found to form an octahydrate phase (81).

## THE ROLE OF SOLUBILITY STUDIES IN A PREFORMULATION PROGRAM

Once the accessible polymorphs and solvatomorphs of a system have been identified, it is appropriate and necessary in a preformulation program to determine the relative order of stability of these. Ordinarily, one would seek to develop the most stable crystal form into the final drug product, so it is necessary to develop methods that enable this determination. At the same time, it is equally important during dosage form development to determine the relative solubilities of the various crystal forms. Fortunately these two questions can be answered through properly designed solubility studies.

If the pressure of the system is fixed, then the Gibbs free energy difference between the two phases is determined by their relative fugacities:

$$\Delta G = RT \ln(f_2/f_1) \tag{5}$$

The fugacity of each phase can be approximated by its vapor pressure:

$$\Delta G \approx RT(p_2/p_1) \tag{6}$$

In a condensed phase, the fugacity is proportional to the activity, so the Gibbs free energy difference between the two phases is determined by their relative activities:

$$\Delta G \approx RT(a_2/a_1) \tag{7}$$

The activity of each phase can be approximated by its solubility, and so

$$\Delta G \approx RT(S_2/S_1) \tag{8}$$

Since the most stable polymorph under defined conditions of temperature and pressure must have the lowest Gibbs free energy, it must also have the lowest fugacity, vapor pressure, thermodynamic activity, solubility in any given solvent, and IDR.

Of the various parameters, the measurements of solubility and IDR are often the most accessible. Since the choice of crystal form to be developed often depends on solubility characteristics, every preformulation program should contain solubility studies. Not only will such work facilitate the choice of the final crystal form, but it will also yield the relative order of stability and valuable information regarding the thermodynamics of the system.

Methods for the determination of solubility have been reviewed (82–84), especially with respect to the characterization of pharmaceutical solids (85) and polymorphic substances (86). For most solids, solubility is highly dependent on temperature, and therefore in addition to the composition of the system, one must also record the temperature for each solubility measurement. Plots of solubility against temperature are commonly used for characterizing pharmaceutical solids and have been extensively discussed (82,87).

It is highly useful to determine the solubility values as a function of temperature and to reduce the data to the linear relationship associated with the van't Hoff equation,

$$\ln X_2^{sat} = (-a/RT) + c' \tag{9}$$

or by the Hildebrand equation,

$$\ln X_2^{sat} = (b/R) \ln T + c'' \tag{10}$$

In Equations 7 and 8, $X_2^{sat}$ is the mole fraction solubility of the solid solute at an absolute temperature $T$, $a$ is the apparent molar enthalpy of solution, $b$ is the apparent molar entropy of solution, and $c'$ and $c''$ are constants.

The hydrochloride salt of gepirone

has been found to exist in at least three polymorphic forms whose melting points were reported to be 180°C (form I), 212°C (form II), and 200°C (form III) (88). Forms I and II, and forms I and III were determined to bear an enantiotropic relationship, while form III was found to be monotropic with respect to form II. The solubility data illustrated in Figure 8 were used to estimate a transition temperature of 74°C for the enantiotropic forms I and II, while the reported enthalpy difference was 4.5 kcal/mot at 74°C and 2.54 kcal/mot at 25°C. The most stable polymorph below 74°C was form I, whereas form II was the most stable above 74°C.

The effect of solvent composition on the solubility of polymorphs was investigated with cimetidine (89).

Both forms exhibited almost identical melting points, but form B was found to be less soluble than form A, identifying it as the most stable polymorph

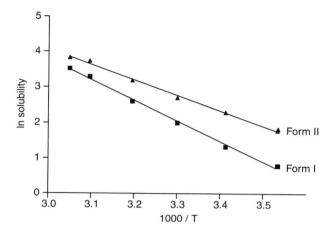

**Figure 8** Temperature dependence of the equilibrium solubilities of two poly-morphic forms of gepirone hydrochloride, plotted according to the van't Hoff equation. *Source*: Adapted from Ref. 88.

at room temperature. The two forms were more soluble in mixed water–isopropanol solvents than in either of the pure solvents, reflecting the balance between the solvation of the molecules by water and isopropanol in determining the activity coefficient of the solute and hence the solubility. At constant temperature, the difference in the Gibbs free energy and the solubility ratio was constant, independent of the solvent system.

The hydrochloride salt of amiloride

can be obtained in two polymorphic dihydrate forms, A and B (90). However, each solvate dehydrates around 115°C to 120°C, and the resulting anhydrous solids melt at the same temperature. However, form B was found to be slightly less soluble than form A between 5°C and 45°C, indicating that it is the thermodynamically stable form at room temperature. The temperature dependencies of the solubility data were processed by the van't Hoff equation to yield the apparent enthalpies of solution of the two polymorphic dihydrates.

Because only one member of a family of polymorphs or solvates can be the most thermodynamically stable form under a given set of environmental conditions defined by the phase rule, one frequently finds that one form spontaneously converts to another form during the time required to establish an equilibrium solubility. The existence of an unexpected metastable solubility can lead to important (and possibly undesirable) consequences. Any metastable phase will have a higher free energy than would a thermodynamically more stable phase, and it will undergo a phase transformation to the more stable phase once the activation energy barrier is overcome. Often the barrier to phase transformation is merely the improbability of a suitable nucleation step. Hence, only fortuitously unfavorable kinetics permitted a determination of the equilibrium solubility of the various higher-energy phases discussed in the preceding section.

Conversions of a metastable phase into a more stable phase may include the transformation of one polymorphic phase into another, the solvation of an anhydrous phase, the desolvation of a solvate phase, the transformation of an amorphous phase into a crystalline anhydrate or solvate phase, the degradation of a crystalline anhydrate or solvate phase to an amorphous phase, or in the case of digoxin, the conversion of imperfect (less crystalline, more amorphous) crystals with a high density of defects into more perfect (more crystalline) crystals with a lower density of defects. While it is straightforward to determine the equilibrium solubility of a phase that is stable with respect to conversion, the measurement of solubilities of metastable phases that are susceptible to conversion is not a trivial matter.

Because determinations of the solubility of solid materials are often made by suspending an excess of the compound in question in the chosen solvent or other dissolution medium, the application of this equilibrium method to a metastable phase will result in a determination of the solubility of the stable phase. One of the attempts to measure the solubility of a metastable polymorph was made by Milosovich, who developed a method based on the measurement of the IDRs and used it to deduce the relative solubilities of sulfathiazole forms I and II (91). This method assumes that the IDR is proportional to the solubility, the proportionality constant being the transport rate constant, which is constant under constant hydrodynamic conditions in a transport-controlled dissolution process.

Carbamazepine

is known to exist in both an anhydrate and a dihydrate form, with the anhydrate spontaneously transforming to the dihydrate upon contact with bulk liquid water (92). The anhydrous phase is reported to be practically insoluble in water, but this observation is difficult to confirm owing to its rapid transition to the dihydrate phase. The rates associated with the phase transformation process have been studied and appear to follow first-order kinetics (93). Interestingly, the only difference in pharmacokinetics between the two forms was a slightly higher absorption rate for the dihydrate (94). The slower absorption of anhydrous carbamazepine was attributed to the rapid transformation to the dihydrate, accompanied by a fast growth in particle size. Comparison of the bioavailabilities of different polymorphs of a given drug suggest that significant differences are found only when the polymorphs differ significantly in the Gibbs free energy deduced from the ratio of solubilities or IDRs.

Recognizing that the hydration state of a hydrate depends on the water activity, in the crystallization medium, Zhu and Grant investigated the influence of solution media on the physical stability of the anhydrate, tri-hydrate, and amorphous forms of ampicillin (95).

The crystalline anhydrate was found to be kinetically stable in the sense that no change was detected by powder X-ray diffraction for at least five days in methanol/water solutions over the whole range of water activity ($a_v = 0$ for pure methanol to $a_v = 1$ for pure liquid water). However, addition of trihydrate seeds to ampicillin anhydrate suspended in methanol/water solutions at $a_v \geq 0.381$ resulted in the conversion of the anhydrate to the thermodynamically stable trihydrate. The trihydrate converted to the amorphous form at $a_w \leq 0.338$ in the absence of anhydrate seeds, but converted to the anhydrate phase at $a_w \leq 0.338$ when the suspension was seeded with the anhydrate. The metastable amorphous form took up water progressively with increasing $a_w$ from 0.000 to 0.338 in the methanol/water mixtures. It was concluded that water activity was the major thermodynamic factor deter-mining the nature of the solid phase of ampicillin that crystallized from methanol/water mixtures.

Evaluation of the dissolution rates of polymorphic or solvatomorphic drug substances is especially important in the preformulation program since possible bioavailability differences may arise from differences in dissolution rate, which are themselves due to differences in solubility (8). The wide variety of methods for determining the dissolution rates of solids may be categorized either as batch methods or as continuous-flow methods, for which detailed experimental protocols have been provided (96).

Batch-type dissolution rate studies of loose powders and compressed disks have played a major role in the characterization of essentially every polymorphic or solid-state solvated system (97–99). Stagner and Guillory used these two methods of dissolution to study the two polymorphs and the amorphous phase of iopanoic acid (100).

The two polymorphs were found to be stable with respect to phase conversion, but the amorphous form rapidly converted to form I under the dissolution conditions. In the powder dissolution studies, the initial solubilities of the different forms followed the same rank order as did their respective IDRs, but the subsequent phase conversion of the amorphous form to the stable form I appeared to change the order. The amorphous form demonstrated a 10-fold greater IDR relative to form I, while the IDR of form II was 1.5 times greater than that of form I.

It has been generally noted that, for many substances, the dissolution rate of an anhydrous phase usually exceeds that of any corresponding hydrate phase. These observations have a thermodynamic base, where it is reasoned that the hydrates possessed less activity and would be in a more stable state relative to their anhydrous forms (101). This general rule was found to hold for the anhydrate/hydrate phases of theophylline (102–104), ampicillin (95), metronidazole benzoate (105), carbamazepine (92,94), glutethimide (24), and oxyphenbutazone (106), as well as for many other systems not mentioned here. In addition, among the hydrates of urapidil, the solubility decreases with increasing crystal hydration (107). It should be recognized, however, that there exist exceptions to this general rule.

It is recognized that the final concentration measured using the loose powder dissolution method is the equilibrium solubility, and that the initial stages of this dissolution are strongly affected by the particle size and surface area of the dissolving solids. For this reaction, many workers have chosen to study the dissolution of compacted materials, where the particle size and surface area are regulated by the process of forming the compact.

In the disk method for conducting intrinsic dissolution studies, the powder is compressed in a die to produce a compact. One face of the disk is exposed to the dissolution medium and rotated at a constant speed without wobble. The dissolution rate is determined as for a batch method, while the wetted surface area is simply the area of the disk exposed to the dissolution medium. It is good practice to compare the powder X-ray diffraction patterns of the compacted solid and of the residual solid after the dissolution experiment with that of the original powder sample. In this manner, one may test for possible phase changes during compaction or dissolution.

The dissolution rate of a solid from a rotating disc is governed by the controlled hydrodynamics of the system, which has been treated theoretically by Levich (108). In this system, the IDR ($J$) may be calculated using either of the following relations:

$$J = 0.620D^{2/3}v^{-1/6}(c_s - c_b)\omega^{1/2} \tag{11}$$

or

$$J = 1.555D^{2/3}v^{-1/6}(c_s - c_b)W^{1/2} \tag{12}$$

where $D$ is the diffusivity of the dissolved solute, $\omega$ is the angular velocity of the disc in radians per second, $v$ is the kinematic viscosity of the fluid, $c_b$ is the concentration of solute at time $t$ during the dissolution study, and $c_s$ is the equilibrium solubility of the solute.

Under constant hydrodynamic conditions, the IDR is usually proportional to the solubility of the dissolving solid. Consequently, in a polymorphic system, the most stable form will ordinarily exhibit the slowest IDR.

IDR studies proved useful during the characterization of the two anhydrous polymorphs and one hydrate modification of alprazolam (109).

The equilibrium solubility of the hydrate phase was invariably less than that of either anhydrate phase, although the actual values obtained were found to be strongly affected by pH. Interestingly, the IDR of the hydrate phase was higher than that of either anhydrate phase, with the anhydrous phases

**Table 2**  IDRs for the Various Polymorphs of Alprazolam at Different
Spindle Speeds

| Crystalline form | IDR, 50 rpm ($\mu$g/min/cm$^2$) | IDR, 75 rpm ($\mu$g/min/cm$^2$) |
|---|---|---|
| Form I | 15.8 | 21.8 |
| Form II | 18.4 | 21.9 |
| Form V | 20.7 | 27.3 |

*Abbreviation*: IDR, intrinsic dissolution rates.
*Source*: From Ref. 109.

exhibiting equivalent dissolution rates. The IDR data of Table 2 reveal an
interesting phenomenon, where discrimination between some polymorphs
was noted at slower spindle speeds, but not at higher rates. Thus, if one is to
use IDR rates as a means to determine the relative rates of solubilization of
different rates, the effect of stirring speed must be investigated before the
conclusions can be judged genuine.

One area of concern associated with intrinsic dissolution measurements involves the preparation of the solid disc by compaction of the drug
particles. If a phase transformation is induced by compression, one might
unintentionally measure the dissolution rate of a polymorph different from
the intended one. This situation was encountered with phenylbutazone,
where form III was transformed to the most stable modification (form IV)
during the initial compression step (110).

## SUMMARY

Through the performance of an appropriately designed series of solvent-
mediated and solid-state transformations, one can be reasonably assured of
finding all of the accessible polymorphs and solvatomorphs of a given drug
substance. With the performance of this work comes an evaluation of the
relative stabilities of the polymorphs and solvatomorphs, studies of the
absolute stabilities of each form, and recommendation of the physical form
that should receive continued development.

## REFERENCES

1. Brittain HG. Polymorphism in Pharmaceutical Solids. New York: Marcel
   Dekker, 1999.
2. Byrn SR, Pfeiffer RR, Stowell JG. Solid State Chemistry of Drugs, 2nd edn.
   West Lafayette, IN: SSCI Inc., 1999.
3. WC McCrone. Polymorphism (chap. 8). In: Fox D, Labes MM, Weissberger
   A, eds. Physics and Chemistry of the Organic Solid State, Vol. II. New York:
   Interscience Publishers, 1965, pp. 725–67.
4. Haleblian JK, McCrone WC. Pharmaceutical applications of polymorphism.
   J Pharm Sci 1969; 58:911–29.

5. Haleblian JK. Characterization of habits and crystalline modification of solids and their pharmaceutical applications. J Pharm Sci 1975; 64:1269–88.
6. Borka L. Review on crystal polymorphism of substances in the European Pharmacopeia. Pharm Acta Helv 1991; 66:16–22.
7. Byrn SR, Pfeiffer RR, Stephenson G, Grant DJW, Gleason WB. Solid-state pharmaceutical chemistry. Chem Mater 1994; 6:1148–58.
8. Byrn SR, Pfeiffer RR, Ganey M, Hoiberg C, Poochikian G. Pharmaceutical solids: a strategic approach to regulatory considerations. Pharm Res 1995; 12: 945–54.
9. Brittain HG. The impact of polymorphism on drug development: a regulatory viewpoint. Am Pharm Rev 2000; 3:67–70.
10. Vippagunta SR, Brittain HG, Grant DJW. Crystalline solids. Adv Drug Dev Rev 2001; 48:3–26.
11. Brittain HG. Polymorphism: pharmaceutical aspects. In: Swarbrick J, Boylan JC, eds. Encyclopedia of Pharmaceutical Technology. New York: Marcel Dekker, 2002, pp. 2239–49.
12. Newman AW, Stahly GP. Form selection of pharmaceutical compounds (chap. 1). In: Ohannesian L, Streeter AJ, eds. Handbook of Pharmaceutical Analysis. New York: Marcel Dekker, 2001, pp. 1–57.
13. Threlfall T, Org Proc Res Dev 2000; 4:384–90.
14. Ostwald W. Lehrbuch, Vol. 2. Leipzig: Engelmann Press, 1897.
15. Guillory JK. Generation of polymorphs, hydrates, solvates, and amorphous solids (chap. 5). In: Brittain HG, ed. Polymorphism in Pharmaceutical Solids. New York: Marcel Dekker, 1999, pp. 183–226.
16. Snyder LR. J Chrom Sci 1978; 16:223.
17. Sadek PC. The HPLC Solvent Guide. New York: John Wiley & Sons, 1996.
18. Riddick JA, Bunger WB. Organic Solvents, 3rd edn. New York: Wiley-Interscience, 1970.
19. Mullin JW. Crystallization, 2nd edn. Cleveland, OH: CRC Press, 1972, pp. 52–3.
20. Bonafede SJ, Ward MD. J Am Chem Soc 1995; 117:7853–61.
21. Mitchell CA, Yu L, Ward MD. J Am Chem Soc 2001; 123:10830–9.
22. Gorbitz CH, Hersleth H-P. Acta Cryst B 2000; 56:526–34.
23. Morris KR, Rodriguez-Hornedo N. Encyclopedia of Pharmaceutical Technology, vol. 7. New York: Marcel Dekker, 1993, pp. 393–440.
24. Khankari RK, Grant DJW. Thermochim Acta 1995; 248:61–79.
25. Suryanarayanan R. X-ray powder diffractometry (chap. 7). In: Brittain HG, ed. Physical Characterization of Pharmaceutical Solids. New York: Marcel Dekker, 1995, pp. 187–221.
26. Klug HP, Alexander LE. X-ray diffraction procedures for polycrystalline and amorphous materials, 2nd edn. New York: Wiley-Interscience, 1974.
27. Phadnis NV, Cavatus RK, Suryanarayanan R. J Pharm Biomed Anal. 1997; 15:929–43.
28. Pirttmaki J, Lehto V-P, Laine E. Drug Dev Ind Pharm 1993; 19:2561–77.
29. Bragg WH, Bragg WL. X-Rays and Crystal Structure. London: G. Bell & Sons, 1918.

30. Rousseau JJ. Basic Crystallography. Chichester: John Wiley & Sons, 1998, pp. 188–91.
31. Epple M, Cammenga HK. Ber Bunsenges Phys Chem 1992; 96:1774–8.
32. Conflant P, Guyot-Hermann A-M. Eur J Pharm Biopharm 1994; 40:388–92.
33. Rastogi S, Zakrzewski M, Suryanarayanan R. Pharm Res 2001; 18:267–73; ibid., 2002; 18:1265–73.
34. McCrone WC, McCrone LB, Delly JG. Polarized Light Microscopy., Ann Arbor, MI: Ann Arbor Science Publishers, 1978.
35. Rochow TG, Rochow EG. An Introduction to Microscopy by Means of Light, Electrons, X-Rays, or Ultrasound. New York: Plenum Press, 1978.
36. Newman AW, Brittain HG. Particle morphology: optical and electron microscopies (chap. 5). In: HG Brittain, ed. Physical Characterization of Pharmaceutical Solids. Marcel Dekker, New York, 1995, pp. 127–56.
37. McCrone WC. Fusion Methods in Chemical Microscopy. New York: Interscience Publishers, 1957.
38. Kuhnert-Brandstätter M. Thermomicroscopy in the Analysis of Pharmaceuticals. Oxford: Pergamon Press, 1971.
39. Wendlandt WW. Thermal Analysis, 3rd edn. New York: John Wiley & Sons, 1986.
40. Ford JL, Timmins P. Pharmaceutical Thermal Analysis. Chichester: Ellis Horwood Ltd., 1989.
41. McCauley JA, Brittain HG. Thermal methods of analysis (chap. 8). In: HG Brittain, ed. Physical Characterization of Pharmaceutical Solids. New York: Marcel Dekker, 1995, pp. 223–51.
42. Pope MI, Judd MD. Introduction to Differential Thermal Analysis. London: Heyden, 1977.
43. Dollimore D. Thermoanalytical instrumentation. In: Ewing GW, ed. Analytical Instrumentation Handbook. New York: Marcel Dekker, 1990, pp. 905–60.
44. Keattch CJ, Dollimore D. Introduction to Thermogravimetry, 2nd edn. London: Heyden, 1975.
45. Wilson EB, Decius JC, Cross PC. Molecular Vibrations. New York: McGraw Hill, 1955.
46. Ciurczak EW, Drennen JK. Pharmaceutical and Medical Applications of Near-Infrared Spectroscopy. New York: Marcel Dekker, 2002.
47. Bugay DE, Williams AC. Vibrational spectroscopy (chap. 3). In: Brittain HG, ed. Physical Characterization of Pharmaceutical Solids. New York: Marcel Dekker, 1995, pp. 59–91.
48. Brittain HG. J Pharm Sci 1997; 86:405–12.
49. Conley RT. Infrared Spectroscopy. Boston: Allyn and Bacon, 1966.
50. Lewis IR, Edwards HGM. Handbook of Raman Spectroscopy. New York: Marcel Dekker, 2001.
51. Fyfe CA. Solid State NMR for Chemists. Guelph: CFC Press, 1983.
52. Bugay DE. Magnetic resonance spectrometry (chap. 4). In: Brittain HG, ed. Physical Characterization of Pharmaceutical Solids. New York: Marcel Dekker, 1995, pp. 93–125.
53. Bugay DE. Pharm Res 1993; 10:317–27.

54. Yanagi T, Mizoguchi J-I, Adachi T, et al. Chem Pharm Bull 2000; 48:366–9.
55. Giordano F, Rossi A, Moyano JM, et al. J Pharm Sci 2001; 90:1154–63.
56. Kimura N, Fukui H, Takagaki H, Yonemochi E, Terada K. Chem Pharm Bull 2001; 49:1321–5.
57. Kushida I, Ashizawa K. J Pharm Sci 2002; 91:2193–202.
58. Singh D, Marshall PV, Shields L, York P. J Pharm Sci 1998; 87:655–62.
59. Alkhamis KA, Obaidat AA, Nuseirat AF. Pharm Dev Tech 2002; 7:491–503.
60. Zornoza A, de No C, Martin C, Goni MM, Martinez-Oharriz MC, Valaz I. Int J Pharm 1999; 186:199–204.
61. Burger A, Lettenbichler A. Eur J Pharm Biopharm 2000; 49:65–72.
62. Gu C-H, Young V, Grant DJW. J Pharm Sci 2001; 90:1878–90.
63. Canterau RG, Leza MG, Bachiller CM. J Pharm Sci 2002; 91:2240–51.
64. Vrcelj RM, Gallagher HG, Sherwood JN. J Am Chem Soc 2001; 123:2291–5.
65. Rollinger JM, Gstrein EM, Burger A. Eur J Pharm Biopharm 2002; 53:75–86.
66. Wenslow RM, Baum MW, Ball RG, McCauley JA, Varsolona RJ. J Pharm Sci 2000; 89:1271–85.
67. van Hoof P, Lammers R, Puijenbroek R, Schans M, Carlier P, Kellenback E. Int J Pharm 2002; 238:215–28.
68. Stowell GW, Behmne RJ, Denton SM, et al. J Pharm Sci 2002; 91:2481–8.
69. Yang Y, Wenslow RM, McCauley JA, Crocker LS. Int J Pharm 2002; 243: 147–59.
70. Edwards HGM, Lawson E, de Matas M, Shields L, York P. J Chem Soc Perkin Trans 1997; 2:1985–90.
71. Ledwidge MT, Corrigan OI. Int J Pharm 1997; 147:41–9.
72. Leung SS, Padden BE, Munson EJ, Grant DJW. J Pharm Sci 1998; 87:501–7; ibid., 1998; 87:508–13.
73. Khankari R, Chen L, Grant DJW. J Pharm Sci 1998; 87:1052–61.
74. Chen LR, Padden BE, Vippagunta SR, Munson EJ, Grant DJW. Pharm Res 1999; 17:619–24.
75. Richards AC, McColm IJ, Harness JB. J Pharm Sci 1999; 88:780–5.
76. Richards AC, Harness JB, McColm IJ. J Pharm Sci 2000; 89:1187–95.
77. Richards AC, McColm IJ, Harness JB. J Pharm Sci 2002; 91:1101–16.
78. Zhu H, Khankari RK, Padden BE, Munson EJ, Gleason WB, Grant DJW. J Pharm Sci 1996; 85:1026–34.
79. Zhu H, Halfen JA, Young VG, et al. J Pharm Sci 1997; 86:1439–47.
80. Zhu H, Padden BE, Munson EJ, Grant DJW. J Pharm Sci 1996; 86:418–29.
81. Zhu H, Young VG, Grant DJW. Int J Pharm 2002; 232:23–33.
82. Grant DJW, Higuchi T. Solubility Behavior of Organic Compounds., New York: John Wiley & Sons, 1990.
83. Mader WJ, Vold RD, Vold MJ. In: Weissberger A, ed. Physical Methods of Organic Chemistry, 3rd edn. Vol. 1, part I. New York: Interscience Publishers, 1959, pp. 655–88.
84. Yalkowsky SH, Banerjee S. Aqueous Solubility Methods of Estimation for Organic Compounds. New York: Marcel Dekker, 1992, pp. 149–54.
85. Grant DJW, Brittain HG. Solubility of pharmaceutical solids (chap. 11). In: Brittain HG, ed. Physical Characterization of Pharmaceutical Solids. New York: Marcel Dekker, 1995, pp. 321–86.

86. Brittain HG, Grant DJW. Effects of polymorphism and solid-state solvation on solubility and dissolution rate (chap. 7). In: Brittain HG, ed. Polymorphism in Pharmaceutical Solids. New York: Marcel Dekker, 1999, pp. 279–330.
87. Grant DJW, Mehdizadeh M, Chow AH-L, Fairbrother JE. Int J Pharm 1984; 18:25.
88. Behme RJ, Brooke D, Farney RF, Kensler TT. J Pharm Sci 1985; 74:1041.
89. Sudo S, Sato K, Harano Y. J Chem Eng Japan 1991; 24:237.
90. Jozwiakowski MJ, Williams SO, Hathaway RD. Int J Pharm 1993; 91:195.
91. Milosovich G. J Pharm Sci 1964; 53:781.
92. Laine E, Tuominen V, Ilvessalo P, Kahela P. Int J Pharm 1984; 20:307.
93. Young WWL, Suryanarayanan R. J Pharm Sci 1991; 80:496.
94. Kahela P, Aaltonen R, Lewing E, Anttila M, Kristoffersson E. Int J Pharm 1983; 14:103.
95. Zhu H, Grant DJW. Int J Pharm 1996; 139:33.
96. United States Pharmacopoeia 26. United States Pharmacopoeial Convention, Inc., Rockville MD, 2003, pp. 2155–6.
97. Higuchi WI, Lau PK, Higuchi T, Shell JW. J Pharm Sci 1963; 52:150.
98. Poole JW, Bahal CK. J Pharm Sci 1968; 57:1945.
99. Shefter E, Higuchi T. J Pharm Sci 1963; 52:781.
100. Stagner WC, Guillory JK. J Pharm Sci 1979; 68:1005.
101. Yalkowsky SH. Techniques of Solubilization of Drugs. New York: Marcel Dekker, 1981, pp. 160–80.
102. Fokkens JG, van Amelsfoort JGM, de Blaey CJ, de Kruif CC, Wilting J. Int J Pharm 1983; 14:79.
103. de Smidt JH, Fokkens JG, Grijseels H, Crommelin DJA. J Pharm Sci 1986; 75:497.
104. Zhu H, Yuen C, Grant DJW. Int J Pharm 1996; 135:151.
105. Hoelgaard A, Moller N. Int J Pharm 1983; 15:213.
106. Stoltz M, Caira MR, Lötter AP, van der Watt JG. J Pharm Sci 1989; 78:758.
107. Botha SA, Caira MR, Guillory JK, Lötter AP. J Pharm Sci 1988; 77:444.
108. Levich VG. Physicochemical Hydrodynamics. Englewood Cliffs, NJ: Prentice-Hall, 1962.
109. Laihanen N, Muttonen E, Laaksonen M. Pharm Dev Tech 1996; 1:373.
110. Ibrahim HG, Pisano F, Bruno A. J Pharm Sci 1977; 66:669.
111. Otsuka M, Ofusa T, Matsuda Y. Drug Dev Indust Pharm 1999; 25:197–203.

# 3.4

# X-Ray Diffraction Methods for the Characterization of Solid Pharmaceutical Materials

## J. R. Blachére

*Department of Materials Science and Engineering, University of Pittsburgh, Pittsburgh, Pennsylvania, U.S.A.*

## Harry G. Brittain

*Center for Pharmaceutical Physics, Milford, New Jersey, U.S.A.*

## INTRODUCTION

All properly designed investigations into the solid state of a pharmaceutical compound or its formulation begin with an understanding of the structural aspects involved, and it is generally accepted that the primary tool for the study of solid-state crystallography is that of X-ray diffraction (XRD). The history associated with the preparation of materials of various types determines their structure, which in turn determines their properties beyond the role of mere chemistry. The interrelationship between structure, properties, and processing is very important in pharmaceutics, as well as in materials science. Therefore, it is critical to characterize the structures of a drug and its nonactive components in a given formulation, to relate these to desired properties, and to use this information to understand the consequences of preparation procedures.

The structure of materials entails descriptions of the arrangement of atoms in a solid, and crystallography is the science concerned with the structure of crystals. This matter has been treated previously in this volume (1), as well as in many books (2–6), some of which have been specifically devoted to the crystallography of organic molecules (7,8). Many products consist of agglomerations of many small crystals (sometimes called crystallites) into the larger grains of an agglomerated powder, which may be bonded further into pellets upon compression. The structure of the grains and pellets also plays an important role in the performance of solid pharmaceutical products. In solid pharmaceutical substances and preparations, it is important to determine the overall structure as well as any micro-structural features.

XRD is used extensively to characterize the solid components of pharmaceutical products, any changes resulting from preparation methods or secondary processing, and exposures to various conditions. After a short introduction to X-rays and diffraction phenomena, with emphasis on the powder method, the uses of this methodology for phase analysis (qualitative and quantitative), the measurement of crystallite size and crystallinity, and structure determination will be presented. More extensive treatments of XRD can be found in several excellent books (9–12).

## X-RAYS, XRD, AND THE BRAGG LAW

### Historical Background

X-ray crystallography has its origins in studies performed to discover the nature of the radiation emitted by cathode ray tubes, known at the time as "Roentgen rays" or "x-radiation." It was not clear at the end of the 19th century whether these rays were corpuscular or electromagnetic in nature. Since it was known that they moved in straight lines, cast sharp shadows, were capable of crossing a vacuum, acted on a photographic plate, excited substance to fluoresce, and could ionize gases, it appeared that they had the characteristics of light. But at the same time, the mirrors, prisms, and lenses that operated on ordinary light had no effect on these rays, they could not be diffracted by ordinary gratings, and neither birefringence nor polarization could be induced in such beams by passage through biaxial crystals, suggesting a corpuscular nature.

The nature of "x-radiation" ultimately became understood through studies of their diffraction, although the experimental techniques differed from those of classical diffraction studies. The existence of optical diffraction effects had been known since the 17th century, when it was shown that shadows of objects are larger than they ought to be if light traveled past the bodies in straight lines undetected by the bodies themselves. During the 19th century, the complete theory of the diffraction grating was worked out, where it was established that in order to produce diffraction spectra from an ordinary grating, the spacings of the lines on the grating had to be of the same size magnitude as the wavelength of the incident light. Laue argued that if X-rays consisted of electromagnetic radiation having a very short wavelength, it should be possible to diffract the rays once a grating having sufficiently small spacings could be found.

The theory of crystals developed by Bravais suggested that the atoms in a solid were in regular array, and estimates of atomic size showed that the distances between the sheets of atoms were probably about the same as the existing estimates for the wavelengths of the x-radiation. Lane suggested the experiment of passing an X-ray beam through a thin slice of crystalline zinc blende, since this material had an understood structure. Friedrich and Knipping tried the experiment and found a pattern of regularly placed diffracted spots arranged round the central undeflected X-ray beam, thus showing that the rays were diffracted in a regular manner by the atoms of the crystal. In 1913, Bragg reported the first XRD determination of a crystal structure, deducing the structures of KCl, NaCl, KBr, and KI.

Bragg established that the diffraction angles were governed by the spacings between atomic planes within a crystal. He also reported that the intensities of diffracted rays were determined by the types of atoms present in the solid, and their arrangement within a crystalline material. Atoms with higher atomic numbers contain larger numbers of electrons and, consequently, scatter X-rays more strongly than atoms characterized by lower atomic numbers. This difference in scattering power leads to marked differences in the intensities of diffracted rays, and such data provide information on the distribution of atoms within the crystalline solid.

## The Nature of X-Rays

The characterization of materials by XRD requires a probing of the structure on the atomic scale, and therefore the probe to be used must be of the order of atomic dimensions or smaller. X-rays, which are one type of electromagnetic radiation, are characterized by wavelengths in the range 0.05 to 0.25 nm and are ideal for this task. X-rays are generated by the bombardment of metallic targets, such as Cu or Mo, by an electron beam. The beam is decelerated by its interaction with the electrons of the target, and this generates heat and a broad X-ray spectrum that is termed the continuous spectrum. The continuous spectrum is used for some diffraction experiments on single crystals.

Characteristic X-rays are also generated (Fig. 1) when an electron beam has sufficient energy to promote the excitation of core electrons in the target atoms to higher energy states, and the system relaxes back to the ground state. For example, $K_\alpha$ radiation is generated by the transition from of L shell electrons to the K shell. This process can yield sources that are rendered fairly monochromatic through the use of appropriate filters or through the use of a monochromator to remove lower intensity radiation also emitted along with the $K_\alpha$ (e.g., $K_\beta$ radiation resulting from the M shell to the K shell transition). $K_\alpha$ radiation actually consists of a doublet, referred to as $K_{\alpha 1}$ and $K_{\alpha 2}$. This doublet is not always resolved in diffraction experiments, although it can be deconvoluted during processing of the data.

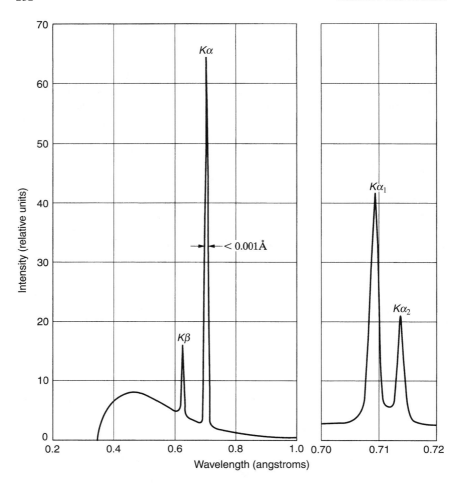

**Figure 1**   Spectrum of Mo at 35 kV (*schematic*); line width not to scale. *Source*: From
Ref. 10.

These characteristic X-rays are often used in diffraction studies and have
found particular use in the study of powdered solids.

## The Nature of Crystalline Solids

To understand the phenomenon of XRD by crystalline materials, it is first
necessary to understand the nature of crystalline solids. An ideal crystal is
constructed by an infinite regular spatial repetition of identical structural
units. For the organic molecules of pharmaceutical interest, the simplest
structural unit will contain one or more molecules. The structure of crystals

is ordinarily explained in terms of a periodic lattice, or a three-dimensional grid of lines connecting points in a given structure. For organic molecules, a group of atoms is attached to a lattice point. It is important to note that the points in a lattice may be connected in various ways to form an infinite number of different lattice structures. The crystal structure is formed only when a fundamental unit is attached identically to each lattice point and extended along each crystal axis through translational repetition.

The points of a crystal lattice can be considered as lying in various sets of parallel planes. These, of course, are not limited to lying along a single Cartesian direction, but can instead be situated along any combination of axis directions permitted by the structure of the lattice. Consider a given set of parallel planes, which cuts across the $a$-, $b$-, and $c$-axes at different points along each axis. If the $a$-axis is divided into $h$ units, the $b$-axis into $k$ units, and $c$-axis into $l$ units, then $(h\ k\ l)$ are the Miller indices of that set of planes, and the set of planes is identified by its Miller indices as $(h\ k\ l)$. If a set of planes happens to be parallel to one axis, then its corresponding Miller index is zero. For instance, a plane that lies completely in the $ab$-plane is denoted as the $(0\ 0\ 1)$ plane, a plane that lies completely in the $ac$-plane is denoted as the $(0\ 1\ 0)$ plane, a plane that lies completely in the $bc$-plane is denoted as the $(1\ 0\ 0)$ plane, and the plane that equally intersects the $a$-, $b$-, and $c$-axes is denoted as the $(1\ 1\ 1)$ plane. The values of $h$, $k$, and $l$ are independent quantities and are defined by their spatial arrangements within the unit cell.

Bragg provided the simplest treatment of X-ray scattering phenomena by crystalline solids. He assumed that the atoms of a crystal are regularly arranged in space and that they can be regarded as lying in parallel sheets separated by a definite and defined distance. Then he showed that scattering centers arranged in a plane act like a mirror to X-rays incident on them, so that constructive interference would occur for the direction of specular reflection. Thus, one can draw an infinite number of sets of parallel planes passing through the points of a space-lattice. If one considers a set of planes, defined by a Miller index of $(h\ k\ l)$, each plane of this set produces a specular reflectance of the incident beam. If the incident X-rays are monochromatic, then for an arbitrary glancing angle, the reflections from successive planes are out of phase with one another (i.e., destructive interference in the scattered beams). However, by varying the glancing angle, a set of angles can be found so that the path difference between X-rays reflected by successive planes will be an integral number of wavelengths, and then constructive interference occurs. This results in the observation of a scattered X-ray beam from the solid.

## The Phenomenon of X-Ray Scattering

The major source of X-rays scattering in solid materials is the electrons, which will scatter the X-rays in all directions. The coherently scattered waves have the same wavelength (that of the incident beam) and tend to add in either a constructive or destructive manner depending on their phase. In order to detect a scattered (diffracted) beam outside the sample, a net addition of the waves scattered in the direction of the X-ray detector must occur. It is convenient to process this sum in three conceptual stages. The first is to sum the waves scattered by the electrons of individual atoms. This results in the atomic scattering factor, $f$. The second step is to sum the contributions of the atoms in the unit cell of the crystal, which yields the structure factor, $F$:

$$F_{hkl} = \sum_n f_n e^{2\pi i(hu_n + kv_n + lw_n)} \tag{1}$$

where $u_n$, $v_n$, and $w_n$ are the coordinates of the $n$th atom in the unit cell. In general, $F$ sums the contributions of all atoms, ions, and molecules to the scattering in terms of their location in the unit cell. It is the sum of the contributions of the structural units associated with the equipoints of the structure. The third step is to sum the contributions of all the unit cells of the sample in the X-ray beam.

The scattered intensity is proportional to the square of the amplitude of the scattered wave and to the volume irradiated. The integrated intensity of the beam takes the form

$$I_{hkl} \propto \frac{I_c(h\ k\ l)F_{hkl}^2 V_s}{V_{uc}^2 \sin^2 \theta} \tag{2}$$

where $V_s$ is the irradiated sample volume, $V_{uc}$ the volume of the unit cell, and $I_e(h\ k\ l)$ the intensity scattered by an electron. While Equation 1 is used extensively, $F_{hkl}$ is in general a complex number, and $F2_{hkl}$ is really $F_{hkl}F^*_{hkl}$.

Bragg simplified this treatment by considering that the atoms of a crystal are located on atomic planes, and assuming that these planes behave as partially transparent mirrors (Fig. 2). For one set of parallel atomic planes $(h\ k\ l)$ to give a diffracted beam in a given direction, the beams reflected by the individual planes must add, that is, they must be in phase. Therefore the path difference, ABC, for beams reflected by neighboring planes must be a multiple of the wavelength. This relation is expressed as the Bragg law:

$$2d\sin\theta = n\lambda \tag{3}$$

where $n$ is an integer, $\lambda$ the wavelength of the X-rays used, $d$ the spacing between the diffracting planes, and $\theta$ the angle of incidence and reflection of the X-rays from the diffracting planes.

In the practical implementation of Bragg's law, two of the three variables are usually varied in tandem while the third is held constant. For example, in the XRD powder method, by running the experiment at

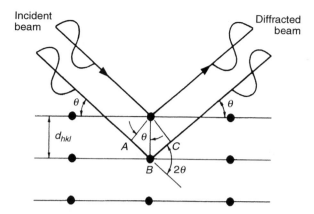

**Figure 2** Derivation of Bragg's law, considering the atomic planes as diffraction planes.

constant $\lambda$ (i.e., monochromatic radiation), one varies $\theta$ and obtains the $d$-spacings of the families of $(h\,k\,l)$ planes for which the Bragg law is obeyed. On the other hand, if one fixes $\theta$ and instead uses a broad range of $\lambda$ (i.e., a continuous spectrum), the Bragg law will be obeyed for a set of $d$-spacings and their corresponding wavelengths. This latter approach is used in the study of single crystals.

## POWDER X-RAY DIFFRACTOMETRY

Although single-crystal XRD undoubtedly represents the most powerful method for the characterization of crystalline materials, it does suffer from the drawback of requiring the existence of a suitable single crystal. Very early in the history of XRD studies, it was recognized that the scattering of X-ray radiation by powdered crystalline solids could be used to obtain structural information, leading to the practice of powder X-ray diffraction (PXRD).

The PXRD technique has become exceedingly important to pharmaceutical scientists, since it represents the easiest and fastest method to obtain fundamental information on the structure of a crystalline substance in its ordinarily obtained form. Since the majority of drug substances are obtained as crystalline powders, the powder pattern of these substances is often used as a readily obtainable fingerprint for determination of its structural type.

The powder method was developed using cameras and photographic film to record observed patterns, but the technique is now practiced through the use of counter diffractometers. The sample is scanned in a diffractometer by a beam of monochromatic radiation (typically the $K_\alpha$ line of copper), while maintaining the reflection geometry between the incident and reflected beams with the surface of the sample as the mirror (Fig. 3). The

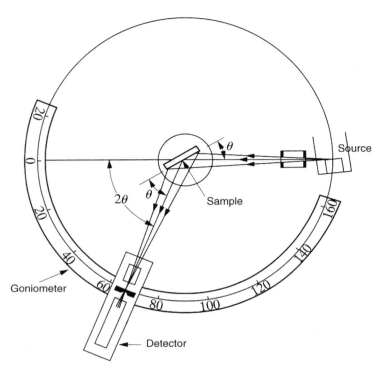

**Figure 3**   Schematic of X-ray diffractometer. *Source*: From Ref. 10.

configuration in Figure 3 shows the usual parafocusing (Bragg-Brentano) geometry. The goniometers may be horizontal or vertical. In some systems the source is fixed, and the sample is rotated at $\theta$ degrees/sec while the detector rotates at $2\theta$ degrees/sec. In other systems, the sample is fixed and the source and the detector each rotate at $\theta$ degrees/sec in opposite directions. The axis of rotation in all cases is in the plane of the surface of the sample.

Unlike the case of diffraction of light by a ruled grating, the diffraction of X-rays by a crystalline solid leads to an observation that constructive interference (i.e., reflection) occurs only for the critical Bragg angles. When reflection does occur, it is stated that the plane in question is reflecting in the *n*th order, or that one observes *n*th order diffraction for that particular crystal plane. Therefore, one will observe an X-ray scattering response for every plane defined by a unique Miller index of (*h k l*).

To measure a powder pattern, a randomly oriented powdered sample is prepared so as to expose all possible planes of a crystalline powder. The scattering angle, $\theta$, is measured for each family of crystal planes by slowly rotating the sample and measuring the angle of diffracted X-rays with respect to the angle of the incident beam. Alternatively, the angle between sample and source can be kept fixed, while moving the detector to determine the angles of the scattered radiation. Knowing the wavelength of the incident beam, the spacing between the planes (identified as the *d*-spacings) is calculated from the scattering angle using Bragg's law.

As a typical diffraction pattern, the PXRD pattern of ibuprofen is shown in Figure 4 (13). This figure illustrates the usual mode of presentation where the X-ray intensity is plotted as a function of the scattering angle (in units of degrees $2\theta$) between the incident and the reflected beams during the scan. Each peak in the powder pattern is due to the constructive interference of the beams reflected by one set of parallel atomic planes when the Bragg law is obeyed. In this symmetric geometry, the only planes that can contribute to the reflections must be parallel to the surface of the sample.

In order to obtain all reflections from all of the various ($h$ $k$ $l$) planes with reproducible intensities, the sample must contain a large number of grains with a random orientation. The usual practice to achieve this end is to pack the powdered sample in a holder, or to smear it onto tape held on a glass slide. The sample can also be a solid polycrystalline material, possibly obtained through the compaction of powders. Ideal grain sizes are of the order of 1 μm, but one can work with powders of grain size less than 20 μm with less than about 10% error in the pattern intensities. When the grains are too small (i.e., less than 0.1 μm), the pattern deteriorates and one observes considerable peak broadening.

In powder diffraction patterns, such as that in Figure 4, the location of the peaks (in units of degrees $2\theta$) is determined by the size and shape of the unit cell. The *d*-spacing associated with the set of ($h$ $k$ $l$) planes giving a reflection at a characteristic angle is governed by the Bragg equation. The intensities of the peaks depend on the content of the unit cell, namely the

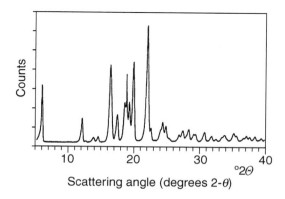

**Figure 4** XRD powder pattern of ibuprofen. *Abbreviation*: XRD, X-ray diffraction. *Source*: From Ref. 13.

atoms and their location in the unit cell. This is introduced by the structure factor $F$ (Eq. 1), which takes into account the phase difference between beams scattered by atoms at different locations in the unit cell. From Equation 2, the intensity of a line will equal 0 when $F$ equals 0, thus resulting in absences of lines even when Bragg's law is obeyed. The intensities of the peaks are further modified by the polarization, multiplicity, Lorentz, absorption, and temperature factors (5,6).

Indexing is the assignment of the observed peaks in an XRD pattern to the $(h\ k\ l)$ planes that are responsible for each reflection. Based on the properties of a diffraction pattern, it is clear that the shape and size of the unit cell can be obtained from the location of the lines of an XRD pattern. One can assume a crystal system and compare the expected lines with the measured ones. This is quite easy for cubic structures, but it becomes more difficult as the symmetry of the structure decreases. For low symmetry structures such as those typified by organic molecules, the accuracy of the pattern becomes critical. Indexing can be performed through the use of simple calculations for high symmetry structures and with a variety of computer programs (9–12).

## APPLICATIONS OF XRD IN PHARMACEUTICS AND PREFORMULATION

Crystals of the same chemical composition may have different structures and therefore different properties. Once the structures of crystals have been established, they are ordinarily recorded into reference files, termed "powder diffraction files" (14), which are then used in the XRD identification of unknown products. This phase identification is a major part of the XRD characterization of materials and is an analysis based solely on the crystal structure of the substances. As such, it differs from ordinary chemical analysis, although it may indirectly yield the chemical composition of the phase.

Besides the identification methods, other applications of X-ray powder diffraction methodology include the evaluation of polymorphism and solvatomorphism, the study of phase transitions, and evaluation of degrees of crystallinity. More recently, advances have been made in the use of powder diffraction as a means to obtain solved crystal structures. A very useful complement to ordinary PXRD is variable temperature XRD. In this method, the sample is contained on a stage that can be heated to any desired temperature. The method is extremely useful for the study of thermally induced phenomena and can be a vital complement to thermal methods of analysis.

Detailed reviews of the utility of XRD in pharmaceutics are available in Refs. 15–17.

### Determination of Crystal Structure Using Powder Diffraction

Very often during the conduct of preformulation studies, the quantity of substance present is so limited that the only plausible XRD work is conducted via the powder method. When new substances are studied, and their powder patterns observed for the first time, the deduction of structural information from a powder pattern (when possible) can be of great value (18,19).

As seen earlier, the intensity ($I_{hkl}$) of a peak in an X-ray pattern can be calculated from the structure factor of Equation 1, as shown in Equation 2. $F$ is calculated from the position of the atoms in the unit cell and their atomic scattering factor, $f$. The task of crystal structure determination is to reverse this procedure by accurately measuring the intensities of the XRD pattern in order to calculate the structure factor and determine from it the location of the atoms in the unit cell. However, the structure factor is a complex number and the phase information is lost, since the product $F_{hkl}F^{*}_{hkl}$ is only obtained from the line intensity. In addition, the observed X-ray powder pattern will usually contain many overlapping and incompletely resolved peaks. Both of those complications make the structural interpretation difficult (3–5,11,20).

Nevertheless, when powder diffraction data of sufficient quality are available (such as those obtained when using synchrotron radiation as a source), structural information can be deduced from powder data. A traditional path for structural determinations of this type can be envisioned as being composed of three steps.

The first step entails an indexing and symmetry determination of the powder pattern. As stated earlier, indexing defines the unit cell from the XRD powder pattern and is accomplished by assigning each of the observed diffraction peaks to a particular ($h$ $k$ $l$) diffraction plane. The symmetry determination (space group assignment) is made from the intensity of the lines of the PXRD pattern. The number of atoms per unit cell is calculated from the size of the unit cell, the chemical composition, and the density of the specimens.

The second step entails proposal of a structure solution. Based on the results of the first step, a structure is assumed and tested by calculation of the PXRD pattern expected for this structure. Different possible structures are thus evaluated, and this leads to an initial approximate structure model. The third step is a structure refinement, where the most promising structure identified during performance of the second step is processed, usually by the Rietveld profile refinement technique (21).

Another approach for structural determination is to generate a trial crystal structure independently from the X-ray pattern and to calculate the expected powder pattern. The predicted and experimental patterns are then compared and the agreement evaluated for various possible structures.

## Qualitative Analysis and Phase Identification

The set of lines, their location, and relative intensity, obtained for an XRD powder pattern of a crystalline phase, is characteristic for that phase and represents a kind of fingerprint. All published XRD patterns of crystalline phases are recorded in the powder diffraction files (14), which can be searched to identify the phases present in preparations. These searches are ordinarily accomplished using computer search engines, and various search methods are discussed in detail in many publications (10,11).

The United States *Pharmacopeia* contains a general chapter on XRD (22), which sets out the criterion that identity is established if the scattering angles in the powder patterns of the sample and reference standard agree to within the calibrated precision of the diffractometer. It is noted that it is generally sufficient that the scattering angles of the 10 strongest reflections obtained for an analyte agree to within either $\pm 0.10$ or $\pm 0.20$ degrees $2\theta$, whichever is more appropriate for the diffractometer used. It is usually convenient to identify the angles of the 10 most intense scattering peaks in a powder pattern and to then list the accepted tolerance ranges of these based on the diffractometer used for the determinations.

PXRD can be used to differentiate between the members of a polymorphic system, a solvatomorphic system, or a system composed of both polymorphs and solvatomorphs. For instance, the powder patterns obtained for the anhydrate and monohydrate phases of lactose are shown in Figure 5 (Brittain HG, unpublished results). The existence of structural similarities in the two forms is suggested since the main scattering peaks of each form are clustered near 20 degrees $2\theta$, but the two phases are easily differentiated from an inspection of the patterns.

Although it is well known that PXRD is a very powerful phase identification technique, its use becomes more difficult for mixtures of phases. This difficulty is most evident when the phases to be identified are not well crystallized or characterized. In a mixture of crystalline phases, each phase contributes its ensemble of scattering peaks to the measured PXRD pattern, which can then become very complex, making phase identification difficult. The intensities of the PXRD scattering peaks associated with a particular phase in a mixture are directly related to the phase content. As a result, with increasing dilution of a phase in a mixture, the PXRD peaks of a phase become unobservable in a well-sequenced order: the weaker peaks will disappear first, followed eventually by the stronger lines. For a positive identification of a phase in a mixture, at least five of the strongest lines detected in its reference pattern must be present in the pattern of the mixture, and their intensity ratios must be approximately the same as in the reference pattern.

Although exact value for the limit of detection for the presence of a given phase in a complex mixture will vary depending on the exact degree of overlap associated with the various peaks, a rule of thumb is that the detection limit would be on the order of 1% to 2% for a well-crystallized phase. With very long data acquisition times and signal averaging, theoretical detection limits as low as 10 ppm have been reported (11). For

Anhydrate phase

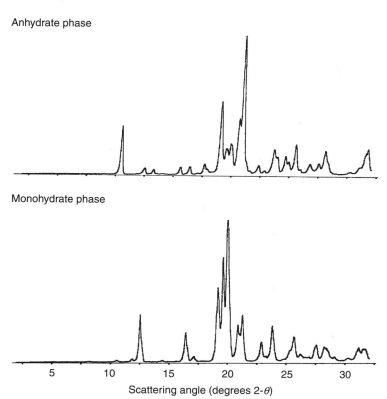

Monohydrate phase

Scattering angle (degrees 2-θ)

**Figure 5** X-ray powder diffraction patterns of the anhydrate and monohydrate phases of lactose. *Source*: From Brittain HG, unpublished results.

qualitative analysis of complex mixtures, investigators routinely make use of other methodologies, such as chemical analysis, differential scanning calorimetry (DSC), infrared and Raman spectroscopies, and X-ray microanalysis. Such multidisciplinary approaches to phase analysis have been widely employed in the pharmaceutical field and have indeed become the norm (15–17).

## Thermodiffractometry

The performance of PXRD on a hot stage enables one to obtain powder patterns at elevated temperatures and permits one to deduce structural assignments for thermally induced phase transitions (23,24). Determination of the origin of thermal events taking place during the conduct of differential thermal analysis or DSC is not always straight forward, and the use of supplementary PXRD technology can be extremely valuable to elucidate the

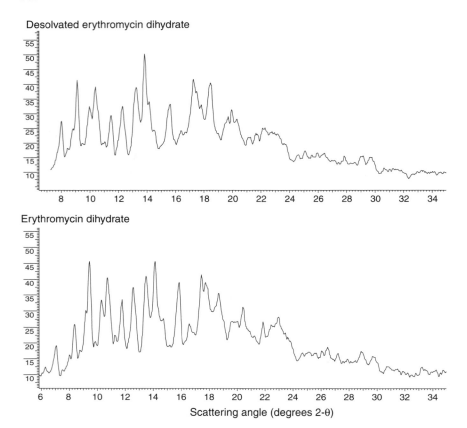

**Figure 6** X-ray powder diffraction patterns of erythromycin dihydrate (*lower trace*), and the anhydrate phase obtained by thermal dehydration of the dihydrate phase (*upper trace*). *Source*: From Brittain HG, unpublished results.

structural course of thermally induced reactions. By conducting PXRD studies on a hot stage, one can bring the system to positions where a DSC thermogram indicates the existence of an interesting point of thermal equilibrium.

One of the uses for thermodiffractometry that immediately comes to mind concerns the desolvation of solvatomorphs. For instance, after the dehydration of a hydrate phase, one may obtain either a crystalline anhydrate phase or an amorphous phase. The PXRD pattern of a dehydrated hydrate will clearly indicate the difference. In addition, should one encounter an equivalence in powder patterns between the hydrate phase and its dehydrated form, this would indicate the existence of channel-type water (as opposed to genuine lattice water) (25). For instance, as shown in Figure 6 for the desolvation of erythromycin dihydrate, the removal of the two waters of hydration does not alter the PXRD pattern (Brittain HG, unpublished results).

A PXRD system equipped with a heatable sample holder has been described, which permitted highly defined heating up to 250°C (23). The system was used to study the phase transformation of phenanthrene and the dehydration of caffeine hydrate. An analysis scheme was developed for the data that permitted one to extract activation parameters for these solid-state reactions from a single nonisothermal study run at a constant heating rate.

In another study, thermodiffractometry was used to study phase transformations in mannitol and paracetamol, as well as the desolvation of lactose monohydrate and the dioxane solvatomorph of paracetamol (24). The authors noted that in order to obtain the best data, the heating cycle must be sufficiently slow to permit the thermally induced reactions to reach completion. At the same time, the use of overly long cycle times can yield sample decomposition. In addition, the sample conditions are bound to differ relative to the conditions used for a DSC analysis, so one should expect some differences in thermal profiles when comparing data from analogous studies.

The commercially available form of Aspartame is hemihydrate form II, which transforms into hemihydrate form I when milled, and a 2.5-hydrate species is also known (26,27). PXRD has been used to study the desolvation and ultimate decomposition of the various hydrates. When heated to 150°C, both hemihydrate forms dehydrate into the same anhydrous phase, which then cyclizes to 3-(carboxymethyl)-6-benzyl-2,5-dioxopiperazine if heated to 200°C. The 2.5-hydrate was shown to dehydrate to hemihydrate form II when heated to 70°C, and this product was then shown to undergo the same decomposition sequence as directly crystallized hemihydrate form II.

## Quantitative Phase Analysis

Once the characteristic PXRD patterns of one or more analytes have been established, it is usually possible to develop quantitative methods of analysis. The methodology is based on the premise that each component will contribute to the overall scattering by an amount that is proportional to its weight fraction in a mixture, and that the powder pattern of each analyte contains one or more peaks whose scattering angle is unique to that analyte. As will be discussed below, quantitative analysis requires the use of reference standards that contribute known scattering peaks at appropriate scattering intensities.

Although simple intensity correction techniques can be used to develop very adequate PXRD methods of quantitative analysis, the introduction of more sophisticated data acquisition and handling techniques can greatly improve the quality of the developed method. For instance, improvement of the powder pattern quality through the Rietveld method has been used to evaluate mixtures of two anhydrous polymorphs of carbamazepine and the dihydrate solvatomorph (28). The method of whole pattern analysis developed by Rietveld (21) has found widespread use in crystal structure refinement and in the quantitative analysis of complex mixtures. Using this approach, the detection of analyte species was possible even when their concentration was less than 1% in the sample matrix. It was reported that good quantitation of analytes could be obtained in complex mixtures even without the requirement of calibration curves.

The effects of preferred orientation in quantitative PXRD analysis can be highly significant and are most often encountered when working with systems whose polymorphs or solvatomorphs are characterized by differing crystal morphologies. A viable PXRD sample is one that presents equal numbers of all scattering planes to the incident X-ray beam. Any orientation effect that minimizes the degree of scattering from certain crystal planes will strongly affect the observed intensities, and this will in turn strongly affect the quantitation. For instance, the three polymorphs of mannitol are obtained as needles, and represent a good system for evaluating the effect of preferential orientation on quantitative PXRD (29). Through the use of small particle sizes and sample rotation, the preferential orientation effects were held to a minimum, and the investigators obtained discrimination of the polymorphs at around the 1% level.

The complications associated with preferential orientation effects were addressed in detail during studies of a benzoic acid/benzyl system (30). The use of various sample packing methods was considered (vacuum free-fall, front-faced packing vs. rear-faced packing, etc.), but the best reduction in the effect was achieved by using materials having small particle sizes that were produced by milling. Through the use of sieving and milling, excellent linearity in diffraction peak area as a function of analyte concentration was attained. The authors deduced a protocol for development of a quantitative PXRD method that consisted of six main steps:

1.  calculation of the mass absorption coefficient of the drug substance,
2.  selection of appropriate diffraction peaks for quantification,
3.  evaluation of the loading technique for adequate sample size,
4.  determining that whether preferred orientation effects can be eliminated through control of the sample particle size,
5.  determination of appropriate milling conditions to obtain reproducibility in peak areas, and
6.  generation of calibration curves from physical mixtures.

After completion of these steps, one then should have a quantitative PXRD method that is suitable for analysis of real samples.

In a multiphase system, the intensity of the peaks in the diffraction pattern of the α-phase is proportional to the volume fraction, $c_\alpha$, of that phase in the mixture. However, the intensity of an X-ray line, $I_\alpha$, is also dependent on the X-ray absorption of the mixture. This means that the relationship between the line intensity for one phase and the concentration of that phase is usually not linear. The relationship is described by

$$I_\alpha = \frac{Kc_\alpha}{\mu_m} \tag{4}$$

where $I_\alpha$ is the integrated intensity for the XRD line, and $\mu_m$ is the linear absorption coefficient for the mixture. $K$ is an unknown proportionality constant, which will cancel out when the intensity is divided by that of a standard reference peak. Therefore, quantitative analysis is a measurement of this ratio.

The three main methods of quantitative analysis differ in the approach used for measurement of the reference. The first of these is the external standard method, where the separately measured peaks of a reference standard of the same material are used. In this method, a particular peak in the PXRD pattern of the reference is chosen as the standard, and the intensity of the corresponding peak in the sample is also measured. As long as the two diffraction patterns are obtained under the same set of conditions, one may use the intensity ratio of the two peaks to calculate the amount of substance present in the analyzed mixture.

Another approach for quantitative analysis is known as the internal standard method. Here, a known weight fraction of the standard is mixed with the powdered sample that is to be analyzed. The diffraction results are calibrated by measurements of the intensity of the selected PXRD line(s) for the analyte in the mixture, and the intensity of the scattering peak of standard. The ratio of these can be used to develop a calibration curve, which is developed in the usual manner by the method of standard additions. Most workers have found that elemental silicon or powdered lithium fluoride is most suitable as internal standards. Yet another technique for quantitative PXRD analysis is the direct comparison method. Here, the reference is a peak from another phase present in the multiphase mixture.

The Rietveld method is totally different, being a profile refinement method applied to the entire diffraction pattern. This method generates weighing factors for the phases in the sample that are related to the phase contents (9).

The phase analysis of prazosin hydrochloride represents an example of a well-designed method for the quantitative PXRD determination of polymorphs (31). The utility of this methodology for the determination of solvatomorphs was demonstrated for the quantitation of cefepime dihydrochloride dihydrate in bulk samples of cefepime dihydrochloride monohydrate (32). Here, a limit of detection of 0.75% w/w and a limit of quantitation of 2.5% w/w were associated with a working range of 2.5% to 15% w/w.

Quantitative PXRD methods have also been developed for the determination of drug substances in excipient matrices. For instance, it was found that approximately 2% of selegilin hydrochloride can be observed reliably in the presence of crystalline mannitol or amorphous modified starch (33). The effects of temperature on the polymorphic transformation of chlorpropamide forms A and C during tableting were investigated using PXRD (34). Even though form A was the stable phase and form C was metastable, the results suggested that the two forms were mutually transformed. It was found that the crystalline forms were converted to a noncrystalline solid by the mechanical energy, and that resulting noncrystalline form transformed into either form A or form C depending on the nature of the compression process.

## Degree of Crystallinity

During the conduct of preformulation work, it is important to determine the degree of crystallinity for a given substance. When reference samples of the pure amorphous and pure crystalline phases of a substance are available, calibration samples of known degrees of crystallinity can be prepared by the mixing of these. Establishment of a calibration curve (PXRD response vs. degree of crystallinity) permits the evaluation of unknown samples to be performed. Since this type of work represents a specific aspect of quantitative PXRD analysis, all of features of the previous discussion are obviously incorporated into this section. However, this discussion must be preceded by a preliminary discussion of peak broadening. Extensive treatments on crystallinity are available in Refs. (35,36).

After correction for background, the peak shape of a PXRD peak can be described by Gaussian or Lorentzian functions, or by a combination of these. The peaks may be defined by their height and width at half height (FWHM). The width of powder XRD peaks is affected by instrumental factors (instrumental broadening) and by the characteristic features of the sample. The sample characteristics provide two major sources of peak broadening. In the first case, the microstructural units generating the pattern are too small to give sharp lines because there are too few planes generating the Bragg reflection in each unit. This happens for powders or solid materials with very fine crystals (crystallites or grain size), and with the mosaic structure of single crystals. The other sources of peak broadening are associated with deformation and strain and compositional heterogeneity, which result in a range of *d*-spacings for individual PXRD peaks.

The influence of crystallite size is usually represented by the Scherrer equation:

$$W_{\text{FWHM}} = \frac{K\lambda}{D\cos\theta} \tag{5}$$

in which $W_{\text{FWHM}}$ is in radians, $D$ the crystal size, $\lambda$ the wavelength of the X-rays, and $K$ a constant of about 0.9. For Gaussian shaped peaks, the widths are corrected for instrumental broadening according to

$$W^2_{\text{FWHM}} = W^2_{o} - W^2_{i} \tag{6}$$

In Equation 6, $W_o$ is the FWHM measured for the PXRD line of the sample, and $W_i$ is the FWHM measured for the same line in a well-crystallized reference material having crystallites or grains larger than 1 µm. The Scherrer equation may be used to estimate grain (crystallite) sizes smaller than about 0.1 µm, assuming no broadening due to variations in $d$-spacing. More sophisticated procedures take into account the shape of the peaks (11) and separate the two major types of sample contributions to the broadening (for instance using Williamson-Hall plots) (10–12).

The degree of crystallinity is of great importance to pharmaceutics since it is related to the stability, solubility, and other important properties of pharmaceutical compounds. Often, this quantity involves a qualitative comparison of the intensity of powder patterns for the same compositions (13). A sample of high crystallinity will yield strong diffraction pattern characterized by intense and narrow scattering peaks. The other extreme is associated with noncrystalline, glassy, or amorphous substances. Glasses exhibit very broad diffraction patterns, characterized by one broad scattering feature of very low amplitude, often termed the "amorphous halo." Figure 7 shows the amorphous halo measured for amorphous polyethylene (37).

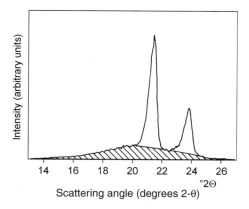

**Figure 7** XRD pattern for a medium density polyethylene; the amorphous halo is shaded. *Abbreviation*: XRD, X-ray diffraction. *Source*: From Ref. 37.

Many substances can exist in noncrystalline (glassy or amorphous) or crystalline forms. The same substances may also be partially crystallized, and XRD is a powerful tool for estimation of the degree of crystallinity. This procedure could be performed on the data of Figure 7 by separating the crystalline and amorphous contributions to the pattern (as shown schematically in the figure), and then evaluating their relative areas. This pattern may be compared with that of completely amorphous polyethylene, or a sample containing a known mass fraction of crystalline phase, and the composition may be calculated from the ratio

$$X_c = \frac{A_c}{A_a + A_c} \tag{7}$$

where $A_c$ is the crystalline peak area, and $A_a$ is the amorphous "peak" area. A number of corrections may be performed in addition to correcting for background (37). For instance, Crocker and McCauley used the "backgrounds" of crystalline and amorphous phases to measure degrees of crystallinity (38).

In one study that illustrates the principles of the method, a PXRD procedure was described for estimation of the degree of crystallinity in digoxin samples (39). Crystalline product was obtained commercially, and the amorphous phase was obtained through ball-milling of this substance. Calibration mixtures were prepared as a variety of blends prepared from the 100% crystalline and 0% crystalline materials, and acceptable linearity and precision were obtained in the calibration curve of PXRD intensity versus actual crystallinity. Other studies have used quantitative PXRD to evaluate the degree of crystallinity in bulk drug substances, such as calcium gluceptate (40) and cefditoren pivoxil (41).

When the excipient matrix in a formulation is largely amorphous, similar PXRD methods can be used to determine the amount of crystalline drug substance present in a drug product. The principles were established in a study that included a number of solid dose forms (42) and also in another study involving a determination of the amount of crystalline acetaminophen in some solid dispersions (43). The same principles have been used to characterize the crystalline content within lyophilized solids (44), where the matrix is again an amorphous material.

## PXRD as a Stability-Indicating Method

A crucial aspect of preformulation work concerns the stability of the bulk drug substance over time, whether in its pure form or in its formulated state. When the phase identity, or degree of crystallinity, of a drug substance is important to its performance in a drug product, PXRD can serve as a vital stability-indicating method. There is no doubt that PXRD can be validated to the status of any other stability-indicating assay, and that one can use the usual criteria of method validation to establish the performance parameters of the method. This aspect would be especially important when either a metastable or an amorphous form of the drug substance has been chosen for development. One may conduct such work either on samples that have been stored at various conditions and pulled at designated time points, or on substances that are maintained isothermally and the PXRD periodically measured.

For example, amorphous clarithromycin was prepared by grinding and spray-drying processes, and PXRD was used to follow changes in crystallinity upon exposure to elevated temperature and relative humidity (45). Exposure of either substance to a 40°C/82% RH environment for seven days led to the formation of the crystalline form, but the spray-dried material yielded more crystalline product than did the ground material. This finding, when supported with thermal analysis studies, led to the conclusion that the amorphous substances produced by the different processing methods were not equivalent.

## SUMMARY

XRD has now become a commonly applied tool for the structural characterization of single crystals and polycrystalline powders. Owing to the presence of the functional groups in drug substance molecules that promote their efficacious action, the crystallization possibilities for such materials can be wide-ranging, leading to multitudes of interaction possibilities that represent the center of preformulation research.

X-ray powder diffraction represents the methodology of choice for the crystallographic characterization of drug substances produced on a routine, batch-type basis. Properly prepared samples yield powder patterns that contain a scattering peak for each set of crystal plane/face, and therefore constitute an identification test for a given crystalline phase. When the data are of suitable quality, PXRD can be used to deduce details of the unit cell and the crystal structure. With the generation of appropriate calibration data, PXRD can be used as a means to deduce the degree of crystallinity in a given sample, of the composition of a physically heterogeneous mixture. Since polymorphism and solvatomorphism are crystallographic occurrences, PXRD will always be the primary determinant of the existence of such phenomena. Variable temperature PXRD is a valuable tool to understand thermally induced reactions and to characterize materials during the conduct of stability studies.

## REFERENCES

1. Spanton S. Prediction of crystallographic characteristics. In: Adeyeye C, Brittain HG, eds. Preformulation. New York: Informa, 2008.
2. Burger MJ. X-ray Crystallography. New York: Wiley, 1942.

3.  Bunn CW. Chemical Crystallography. Oxford: Clarendon Press, 1945.
4.  Bijvoet JM, Kolkmeyer NH, MacGillavry CH. X-ray Analysis of Crystals. London: Butterworths, 1951.
5.  Woolfson MM. An Introduction to X-ray Crystallography. Cambridge: Cambridge University Press, 1970.
6.  Rousseau J-J. Basic Crystallography. Chichester: Wiley, 1999.
7.  Robertson JM. Organic Crystals and Molecules. Ithaca: Cornell University Press, 1953.
8.  Kitaigorodskii AI. Organic Chemical Crystallography. New York: Consultants Bureau, 1957.
9.  Krawitz AD. Introduction to Diffraction in Materials Science and Engineering. New York: Wiley, 2001.
10. Cullity BD, Stock SR. Elements of X-ray Diffraction, 3rd ed. New York: Prentice-Hall, 2001.
11. Snyder RL. X-ray diffraction. In: Lifshin E, ed. X-ray Characterization of Materials. New York: Wiley, 1999:1–103.
12. Klug HP, Alexander LE. X-ray Diffraction Procedures. New York: Wiley, 1974.
13. Janjikhel RV, Adeyeye CM. Dissolution of ibuprofen enantiomers from coprecipitates and suspensions containing chiral excipients. Pharm Dev Tech 1999; 4:9–17.
14. Powder Diffraction Files. Newton Square, PA: International Centre for Diffraction Data (ICDD).
15. DeRanter CJ. Applications of X-ray diffractometric techniques in the analysis of drugs. J Pharm Biomed Anal 1986; 4:747–54.
16. Suryanarayanan R. X-ray powder diffractometry. In: Brittain HG, ed. Physical Characterization of Pharmaceutical Solids. New York: Marcel Dekker, 1995: 187–221.
17. Brittain HG. X-ray diffraction of pharmaceutical materials. In: Brittain HG, ed. Profiles of Drug Substances, Excipients, and Related Methodology. Amsterdam: Elsevier Academic Press, 2003:273–319.
18. Poojary DM, Clearfield A. Applications of X-ray powder diffraction techniques to the solution of unknown crystal structures. Acc Chem Res 1997; 30:414–22.
19. Stephenson GA. Structure determination from conventional powder diffraction data: application to hydrates, hydrochloride salts, and metastable polymorphs. J Pharm Sci 2000; 89:958–66.
20. Harris KDM, Tremayne M, Kariuki BM. Contemporary advances in the use of powder X-ray diffraction for structure determination. Angew Chem Int Ed 2001; 40:1626–51.
21. Rietveld HM. A profile refinement method for nuclear and magnetic structures. J Appl Crystallogr 1969; 2:65–71.
22. X-ray diffraction. General test <941>. United States Pharmacopoeia 26. Rockville, MD: The United States Pharmacopoeial Convention, 2003:2233–34.
23. Epple M, Cammenga HK. Investigation of solid state reactions and solid-solid phase transformations with time- and temperature-resolved X-ray powder diffractometry. Ber Bunsenges Phys Chem 1992; 96:1774–8.

24. Conflant P, Guyot-Hermann A-M. Contribution of X-ray powder diffraction versus temperature to the solid state study of pharmaceutical raw materials. Eur J Pharm Biopharm 1994; 40:388–92.

25. Stephenson GA, Groleau EG, Kleemann RL, Xu W, Rigsbee DR. Formation of isomorphic desolvates: creating a molecular vacuum. J Pharm Sci 1998; 87: 536–42.

26. Leung SS, Grant DJW. Solid state stability of model dipeptides: aspartame and aspartylphenylalanine. J Pharm Sci 1997; 86:64–71.

27. Rastogi S, Zakrzewski M, Suryanarayanan R. Investigation of solid-state reactions using variable temperature X-ray powder diffractometry. I. Aspartame hemihydrate. Pharm Res 2001; 18:267–73.

28. Suryanarayanan R. Determination of the relative amounts of anhydrous carbamazepine and carbamazepine dihydrate in a mixture by powder X-ray diffractometry. Pharm Res 1989; 6:1017–24.

29. Campell Roberts SN, Williams AC, Grimsey IM, Booth SW. Quantitative analysis of mannitol polymorphs: X-ray powder diffractometry exploring preferred orientation effects. J Pharm Biomed Anal 2002; 28:1149–59.

30. Kidd WC, Varlashkin P, Li CY. The applicability of powder X-ray diffraction to the quantification of drug substance polymorphs using a model organic system. Powder Diffraction 1993; 8:180–7.

31. Tanninen VP, Yliruusi J. X-ray powder diffraction profile fitting in quantitative determination of two polymorphs from their powder mixture. Int J Pharm 1992; 81:169–77.

32. Bugay DE, Newman AW, Findlay WP. Quantitation of cefepime dihy-drochloride dihydrate in cefepime dihydrochloride monohydrate by diffuse reflectance IR and powder X-ray diffraction techniques. J Pharm Biomed Anal 1996; 15:49–61.

33. Pirttimaki J, Lehto V-P, Laine E. The determination of relative amounts of phases in binary mixtures with quantitative X-ray diffraction. Drug Dev Indust Pharm 1993; 19:2561–77.

34. Otsuka M, Matsuda Y. Effects of environmental temperature and compression energy on polymorphic transformation during tabletting. Drug Dev Indust Pharm 1993; 19:2241–69.

35. Alexander LE. X-ray Diffraction Methods in Polymer Science. Miami: R.E. Krieger, 1979.

36. Balta-Calleja FJ, Wonk CG. X-ray Scattering of Synthetic Polymers. Amsterdam: Elsevier, 1989.

37. Young RI, Lowell PA. Introduction to Polymers (Chapter 4). Chapman and Hall, 1991.

38. Crocker LS, McCauley JA. Comparison of the crystallinity of imipenen samples by X-ray diffraction of amorphous materials. J Pharm Sci 1995; 84: 226–7.

39. Black DB, Lovering EG. Estimation of the degree of crystallinity in digoxin by X-ray and infrared methods. J Pharm Pharmacol 1977; 29:684–7.

40. Suryanarayanan R, Mitchell AG. Evaluation of two concepts of crystallinity using calcium gluceptate as a model compound. Int J Pharm 1985; 24:1–17.

41. Ohta M, Tozuka Y, Oguchi T, Yamamoto K. Comparison of crystallinity of cefditoren pivoxil determined by X-ray, differential scanning calorimetry and microcalorimetry. Chem Pharm Bull 1999; 47:1638–40.

42. Phadnis NV, Cavatur RK, Suryanarayanan R. Identification of drugs in pharmaceutical dosage forms by X-ray powder diffractometry. J Pharm Biomed Anal 1997; 15:929–43.

43. de Villiers MM, Wurster DE, Van der Watt JG, Ketkar A. X-ray powder diffraction determination of the relative amount of crystalline acetaminophen in solid dispersions with polyvinylpyrrolidone. Int J Pharm 1998; 163:219–24.

44. Clas S-D, Faizer R, O'Connor RE, Vadas EB. Quantification of crystallinity in blends of lyophilized and crystalline MK-0591 using X-ray powder diffraction. Int J Pharm 1995; 121:73–9.

45. Yonemochi E, Kitahara S, Maeda S, Yamamura S, Oguchi T, Yamamoto K. Physiochemical properties of amorphous clarithromycin obtained by grinding and spray drying. Eur J Pharm Sci 1999; 7:331–8.

# 3.5

# Spectroscopic Methods for the Characterization of Drug Substances

**Harry G. Brittain**

*Center for Pharmaceutical Physics, Milford, New Jersey, U.S.A.*

## INTRODUCTION

A great number of characterization methodologies can be employed during the preformulation stage of drug development, and each has its associated utility and function for the physical characterization of a drug substance. However, when a large amount of information is to be gleaned from a small amount of sample, spectroscopic methods of analysis can be of the greatest use. Most of the methods are nondestructive in nature, and the analyzed material can be recycled for additional study once the measurements are complete. Of particular importance during the preformulation program is the study of crystal forms of the drug substance, and spectroscopic techniques can prove to be valuable adjuncts to the standard range of crystallographic procedures.

The fact that elements and chemical compounds can be obtained in more than one crystal form has been known for a very long time, and the properties of these solids have been studied using the appropriate characterization tools (1). Significant advances were made using optical and structural crystallographies, particle morphology, and phase transition phenomena. The term "polymorphism" is used to denote crystal systems where a substance can exist in different crystal packing arrangements, all of which have the same elemental composition (2). The term "solvatomorphism" is finding use as a descriptor for those crystal systems where the structural variations are caused by the inclusion of solvent in the crystal, thus causing the different crystal forms to have different elemental compositions (3). These phenomena have been discussed in much more detail in monographs on the subject (4–6).

The deduction of all possible crystal forms that can be obtained for a given drug substance is routinely required by regulatory authorities. However, during the preformulation stage of drug development, the rationale for developing knowledge regarding the polymorphic and solvatomorphic tendencies of a substance is primarily associated with the requirement of obtaining a sufficient quantity of information so as to enable the substance to be formulated. This is because the nature of the structure adopted by a given compound upon crystallization exerts a strong influence on the solid-state properties of that system. For instance, the heat capacity, conductivity, volume, density, viscosity, surface tension, diffusivity, crystal hardness, crystal shape and color, refractive index, electrolytic conductivity, melting or sublimation properties, latent heat of fusion, heat of solution, solubility, dissolution rate, enthalpy of transitions, phase diagrams, stability, hygroscopicity, and rates of reactions, can all be affected by the nature of the crystal structure.

Since it is usually the goal in pharmaceutical manufacturing to produce a drug substance that is phase pure and remains in that state as long as the bulk material is stored, knowledge of crystal forms and their tendency to interconvert is essential. It is equally vital to formulate the drug substance in a manner so that it remains in the same phase pure state during the manufacture of the drug product, and during any subsequent storage. These requirements demonstrate the need for development and validation of assay methodology for the determination of phase composition. The use of suitable techniques for the physical characterization of polymorphic and solvatomorphic solids has been discussed before (7–10), and a significant amount of appropriate methodology utilizes spectroscopy.

For the purposes of this chapter, it will be assumed that the crystallography of any given system will have been investigated using the structural methods of single crystal of powder X-ray diffraction. Once the polymorphic and solvatomorphic forms of the substance under investigation have been established after performance of a screening study, and the forms identified using crystallography, then spectroscopic methods can play an extremely important role in the preformulation characterization of the substance. Vibrational spectroscopy [infrared (IR) absorption or Raman scattering, or a combination of both] will yield information about the group motion of functional groups in the solid, and if the molecular vibrations are affected by the structural differences that characterize different crystal forms, then studies of these will be useful for an evaluation as to the origin of the effect. Similarly, nuclear magnetic resonance can be used to probe the environments of atoms in the solid state, and structurally nonequivalent nuclei in different crystal forms would resonate at observably different frequencies. It goes without saying that either approach could be used to study the structural variations that exist in solvatomorphic forms.

In this chapter, the basic principles underlying each spectroscopic method will be briefly outlined, and then the use of such methodology will be illustrated through the use of representative examples.

## SOLID-STATE VIBRATIONAL SPECTROSCOPY

The energies associated with the vibrational modes of a chemical compound are typically taken to be within the range of 400 to 4000 cm$^{-1}$, although with Raman spectroscopy one can typically observe lattice modes at even lower energies. The vibrational modes can be observed directly through their absorbance in the infrared region of the spectrum, or through the observation of the low-energy scattered bands that accompany the passage of an intense beam of light through the sample (the Raman effect). In either case, the use of Fourier-transform methodology has vastly improved the quality of the data that can be thusly obtained (11). It is now widely recognized that the vibrational spectra of solid materials often reflect details of the crystal structure, and hence these methods can be used in the spectroscopic investigation of polymorphs and solvatomorphs (12–14).

In studies of polymorphic or solvatomorphic systems, the purpose of the vibrational spectroscopic investigation is to gather information from the observed pattern of vibrational frequencies and to use this data to obtain a deeper understanding of the structural and crystallographic differences that characterize the various crystal forms. The first step in this analysis is to determine which spectral features are most appropriate for the discrimination of one crystal form over another. In the most limited application, the vibrational spectra of various polymorphs and/or solvatomorphs can simply be used as a method for identity testing, but in more advanced applications, features in the vibrational spectra can be exploited for the development of rugged and robust methods for the quantitative analysis of one polymorph or solvatomorph in the presence of the other. The latter application becomes very important when isolation procedures yield mixtures of crystal forms, and assay methodology must be developed for the quantitative analysis of such mixtures.

## Infrared Absorption Spectroscopy

### Principles

The acquisition of high-quality infrared absorption spectra appropriate for the characterization of polymorphs and solvates is most appropriately performed using Fourier transform technology (the FTIR method), since this approach minimizes transmission and beam attenuation problems.

Essentially all FTIR spectrometers use a Michelson interferometer, where radiation entering the interferometer is split into two beams by means of a beam splitter. One beam follows a path of fixed distance before being reflected back into the beam splitter, while the other beam travels a variable distance before being recombined with the first beam. The recombination of these two beams yields an interference pattern, where the time-dependent constructive and destructive interferences have the effect of forming a cosine signal.

Each component wavelength of the source will yield a unique cosine wave, having a maximum at the zero path length difference (ZPD) and which decays with increasing distance from the ZPD. The detector is placed so that radiation in the central image of the interference pattern will be incident upon it, and therefore intensity variations in the recombined beam are manifest as phase differences. The observed signal at the detector is a summation of all the cosine waves, having a maximum at the ZPD, and which decays rapidly with increasing distance from the ZPD. If the component cosine waves can be resolved, then the contribution from individual wavelengths can be observed. The frequency domain spectrum is obtained from the interferogram by performing the Fourier transformation mathematical operation. More detailed descriptions of FTIR instrumentation and its methodology are available in Ref. (15).

Acquisition of solid-state FTIR spectra suitable for use in the characterization of different crystal forms can be performed using Nujol mull, diffuse reflectance, or (most preferably) attenuated total reflectance (ATR) techniques. Any use of pelleting techniques is to be strictly avoided, since too many complications and spurious effects can arise with compaction of the KBr pellet, and these can limit the utility of the spectroscopic method. The main drawback to the mull technique is that regions in the IR spectrum overlapping with carbon–hydrogen vibrational modes will be obliterated owing to absorbance from the oil.

The measurement of diffuse reflectance effectively involves focusing the infrared source beam onto the surface of a powder sample and using an integrating sphere to collect the scattered infrared radiation (16). The technique requires careful attention to sample preparation, and often one must dilute the analyte with KBr powder to reduce the occurrence of anomalous effects (17). In practice, one obtains the spectrum of the finely ground KBr dispersant and then ratios this to the spectrum of KBr containing the analyte. The relative reflectance spectrum is converted into Kubelka-Munk units using standard equations (18), thus obtaining a diffuse reflectance spectrum that resembles a conventional IR absorption spectrum. The main drawback to the diffuse reflectance infrared Fourier transform (DRIFT) technique is that one needs to dilute the sample with KBr to order to obtain good-quality spectra, and the ratio of KBr to analyte is crucial to the outcome.

The ATR method of detection is emerging as a highly useful approach to obtaining IR absorption spectra with minimal sample preparation (19). If an IR-transparent crystal is sandwiched by the sample, and if the refractive index of the crystal exceeds that of the sample, at certain orientations an infrared beam entering the crystal will undergo multiple internal reflections. At each reflection, some of the incident energy is absorbed by the vibrational modes of the sample, and the degree of this absorption builds with the number of internal reflections. When the beam finally emerges from the crystal, it can be processed in the usual way to obtain a pattern of the IR absorption bands of the sample in contact with the crystal.

With the advent of high-efficiency ATR accessories, this particular technique undoubtedly represents the simplest approach to the necessary step of sample handling. One merely needs to place a few milligrams of powder on the ATR crystal and then use a clamping device to press the powder against the crystal to obtain high-quality spectra. Hence, for ease of routine use, the ATR method of sampling is difficult to surpass.

Representative Applications

When coupled with a nonperturbing sampling mode such as diffuse reflectance or ATR, infrared spectroscopy can also be used to establish the phase identity of a potentially polymorphic substance. For example, as shown in Figure 1, the polymorphic identity of famotidine can be readily established using FTIR-ATR spectroscopy, since the spectra are sufficiently different in the fingerprint region to enable such a distinction to be made (20). It should be noted, however, that the magnitude of peak shifting between two forms can often be as little as $10 \, \text{cm}^{-1}$, so careful attention needs to be paid to sample handling and peak measurement.

A combination of theory and experiment was used to obtain more information on the three polymorphs of octahydro-1,3,5,7-tetranitro-1,3,5,7-tetrazocine than was available from X-ray powder diffraction (21). Density functional theory and scaled force-field methods were used to calculate the gas phase vibrational spectroscopy for the molecule in different conformations and molecular symmetries, and the authors compared these calculated spectra with experimentally observed data to interpret the various crystal spectra. It was concluded that the molecule existed in different conformations in each of the three polymorphs, with the molecule in the β-phase exhibiting $C_i$ symmetry, and the molecules in the α- and δ-phases being characterized by $C_{2v}$ symmetry.

The infrared spectra obtained on the polymorphs of acetohexamide and several of its derivatives have been used to study the tautomerism associated with the drug substance in its various solid-state forms (22). It was concluded that Form A existed in the enol form, being stabilized by the intramolecular bonding between the O–H and S=O groups that produced a six-membered ring. Form B was characterized by the existence of

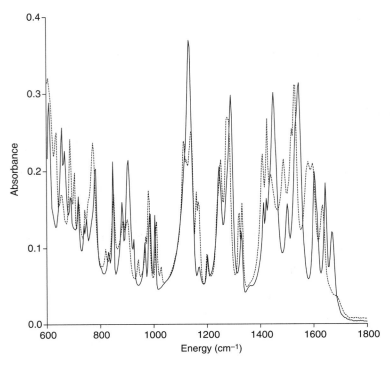

**Figure 1** FTIR-ATR spectra in the fingerprint region of famotidine form A (*solid trace*) and form B (*dashed trace*) (20). *Abbreviations*: FTIR, Fourier transform technology; ATR, attenuated total reflectance.

the keto form, where the urea carbonyl group was bound intermolecular to the sulfonamide N–H functional group. This behavior is quite different from that associated with spironolactone, where no evidence was found for the existence of enoic tautomers in any of the four polymorphs (23).

Infrared absorption spectroscopy has been found to be an extremely powerful tool for the identification and study of solvatomorphic systems. For example, the characteristic absorption bands of lactose anhydrate and lactose monohydrate shown in Figure 2 demonstrate the facile differentiation of the two forms from each other (20). The presence of a strong absorption band at an energy of 1068 cm$^{-1}$ in the fingerprint region readily identifies a lactose sample as consisting of the monohydrate phase, and the presence of crystalline water in the monohydrate phase is further demonstrated in the high frequency region by the well-defined absorbance band observed at 3522 cm$^{-1}$.

Fourier transform infrared spectroscopy was used to examine the structural changes of norfloxacin that were associated with the hydration/

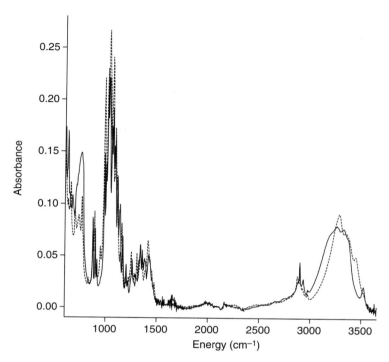

**Figure 2** FTIR-ATR spectra of lactose monohydrate (*solid trace*) and lactose anhydrate (*dashed trace*) (20). *Abbreviations*: FTIR, Fourier transform technology; ATR, attenuated total reflectance.

dehydration processes that took place at different relative humidities (24). It was found that when norfloxacin anhydrate was converted to its hydrate, the intensities of the absorption bands at 1732 and 1253 cm$^{-1}$ (assigned to the C=O and C–O moieties of the carboxylic acid group) decreased gradually with increasing water content. On the other hand, the intensities of the absorption bands at 1584 and 1339 cm$^{-1}$ (corresponding to asymmetric and symmetric carboxylate modes) increased with the water content. In addition, the peak at 2553 cm$^{-1}$ (assigned to the NH$_2^+$ group) shifted from 2558 cm$^{-1}$ as the water content increased. These spectral changes correlated with transformations of COOH to COO$^-$ and from NH to NH$_2^+$, attributable to a proton transfer from carboxylic acid group, and suggestive that hydration could induce proton transfer processes in the solid state.

Fluconazole has been isolated in a number of solvated and non-solvated forms, and infrared spectroscopy has proven to be an important tool in their characterization. In one study involving two nonsolvated polymorphs (forms I and II) and several solvatomorphs (the ¼-acetone solvate, a 1/7-benzene solvate, and a monohydrate), the infrared spectra of the different forms showed differentiation in bands associated with the triazole and 2,4-difluorobenzyl groups, and in the propane backbone (25). In another study, the diagnostic infrared spectral properties of nonsolvated form III and two solvatomorphs (the ¼-ethyl acetate solvate and a monohydrate) were used to demonstrate the novelty of the new forms relative to those in the literature (26).

The power of infrared absorption spectroscopy to characterize new crystal forms is illustrated in Figure 3, which shows the FTIR-ATR spectra obtained for the hydrochloride and sulfate salts of (RS)-α-methylphenethylamine (dashed trace) (20). The two salts are easily differentiated from each other since the spectrum of the sulfate salt is dominated by the absorbance of the anion at $1053 \, cm^{-1}$, which is necessarily absent in the spectrum of the hydrochloride salt. In addition, bands in the –OH portion of the high-frequency region (3371 and $3404 \, cm^{-1}$) demonstrate the sulfate salt

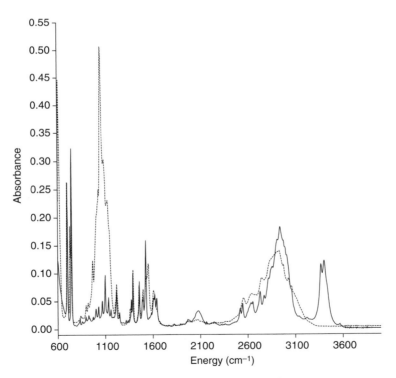

**Figure 3**   FTIR-ATR spectra of (RS)-α-methylphenethylamine hydrochloride (*solid trace*) and (RS)-α-methylphenethylamine sulfate (*dashed trace*) (20). *Abbreviations*: ATR, attenuated total reflectance; FTIR, Fourier transform technology.

to be an anhydrate crystal form and the hydrochloride salt to be a hydrate species.

In a study of the amorphous salt obtained through the coprecipitation of cimetidine and diflunisal, solid-state infrared absorption spectroscopy was used to prove the existence of the salt species (27). The prominent carbonyl absorption band observed at 1650 cm$^{-1}$ in crystalline diflunisal was not observed in the spectrum of the amorphous salt, but a new peak was noted at 1580 cm$^{-1}$ that was assigned to an asymmetric stretching mode of a carboxylate group. The shift of the carbonyl stretching frequency from high to low frequency is invariably observed when a salt form of an acid has been formed. These findings were taken to indicate that the amorphous character of precipitates formed by cimetidine and other nonsteroidal anti-inflammatory agents was due to salt formation and not because of the existence of nonbonding intermolecular interactions.

Given its ability to report on the chemical composition of a mixture, it is no surprise that infrared absorption spectroscopy can play a key role in preformulation studies. For example, it is well known that omeprazole is unstable when exposed to acid and moisture, and, as a result, the substance undergoes rapid decomposition when exposed to acidic and humid conditions (28). To illustrate how one would use FTIR to study the reaction, a 50% w/w blend of omeprazole and salicylic acid was prepared. As shown in Figure 4, the infrared spectrum of the initial blend consisted of the super-imposition of the individual spectral components, but after this blend was exposed to an environment of 40 °C and 75% relative humidity for 14 days, the infrared spectrum consisted almost entirely of that of salicylic acid (20). This study demonstrates the incompatibility of the two substances, since the omeprazole was effectively completely decomposed during the accelerated stability study.

The interaction of dextro-amphetamine sulfate with lactose has been studied in detail, with the degree of Maillard reaction being more pronounced with spray-dried lactose owing to the higher amounts of 5-hydroxymethylfurfural present in the processed excipient (29). The presence of a C$=$N vibrational band in the infrared absorption spectrum of the decomposition product, which was not observed in the initial mixtures of materials, was used to assist in an identification of the brown product as being the amphetamine-hydroxymethylfurfural Schiff base reaction product.

Differential scanning calorimetry (DSC) and diffuse reflectance infrared spectroscopy have been used to study the yellow or brown color that develops when aminophylline is mixed with lactose (30). The DSC thermogram of the aminophylline/lactose mixture was not found to be a simple superposition of the individual components, therefore indicating the existence of incompatibility between the substances. After a complete analysis of the infrared spectra of the individual components, physical mixtures

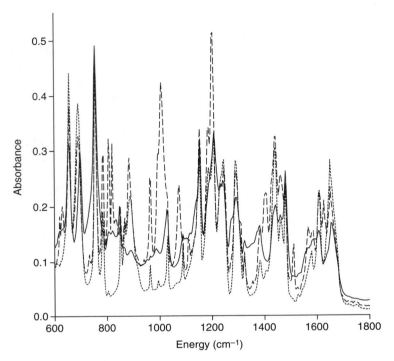

**Figure 4** Fingerprint region FTIR-ATR spectra in the of a 50% w/w blend of omeprazole with salicylic acid (*dashed trace*), and the same sample after being exposed to the 40°C and 75% relative humidity storage condition for 14 days (*solid trace*). Also shown for comparison purposes is the reference spectrum of salicylic acid (*dotted trace*) (20). *Abbreviations*: ATR, attenuated total reflectance; FTIR, Fourier transform technology.

of these, and various blended samples subjected to stress conditions (60°C for three weeks), it was concluded that ethylenediamine was being liberated from the aminophylline complex, and this reacted with lactose through the usual Schiff base intermediate. This reaction results in the observed brown discoloration of the sample.

## Raman Spectroscopy

### Principles

The vibrational modes of a compound may also be studied using Raman spectroscopy, where one measures the inelastic scattering of radiation by a nonabsorbing medium (31). When a beam of light is passed through a material, approximately one in every million incident photons is scattered with a loss or gain of energy. The inelastically scattered radiation can occur at lower

(Stokes lines) and higher (anti-Stokes lines) frequencies relative to that of the incident (or elastically scattered) light, and the energy displacements relative to the energy of the incident beam correspond to the vibrational transition frequencies of both the media. The actual intensities of the Stokes and anti-Stokes lines are determined by the Boltzmann factor characterizing the vibrational population. For high-frequency vibrations, the Stokes lines are relatively intense relative to the anti-Stokes lines, so conventional Raman spectroscopy makes exclusive use of the Stokes component.

The Raman effect originates from the interaction of the oscillating induced polarization or dipole moment of the medium with the electric field vector of the incident radiation. Raman spectra are measured by passing a laser beam through the sample and observing the scattered light either perpendicular to the incident beam or through back-scatter detection. The scattered light is analyzed at high resolution by a monochromator and ultimately detected by a suitable device. One key to obtaining good spectra is through the use of a notch filter, which will eliminate the exciting line, since that is required to obtain acceptable signal-to-noise ratios.

Although both infrared absorption and Raman scattering yield information on the energies of the same vibrational bands, the different selection rules governing the band intensities for each type of spectroscopy can yield useful information. For the low-symmetry situations presented by the structures of molecules of pharmaceutical interest, every vibrational band will be active to some degree in both infrared absorption and Raman scattering spectroscopies. The relative intensities of analogous bands will differ, however, when observed by either infrared absorption or Raman spectroscopy. In general, symmetric vibrations and nonpolar groups yield the most intense Raman scattering bands, while antisymmetric vibrations and polar groups yield the most intense infrared absorption bands. A discussion on a large number of practical applications of Raman spectroscopy is available in Ref. (32), and its application to pharmaceutical analysis has been discussed (12,14,33,34).

## Representative Applications

For those instances where the differing crystal structures inherent to different polymorphs or solvatomorphs cause alterations in the frequencies of the vibrational modes of functional groups, then the use of Raman spectroscopy can be very advantageous in characterization studies. Owing to its ease of measurement and nondestructive nature of sampling, Raman spectroscopy has found widespread use for the qualitative identification and study of different solid-state forms of compounds having pharmaceutical interest. For example, the two polymorphs of famotidine exhibit substantially different Raman spectra (35) in the fingerprint region (Fig. 5), and can be readily differentiated from each other on the basis of their characteristic spectra. Although it was demonstrated earlier that similar

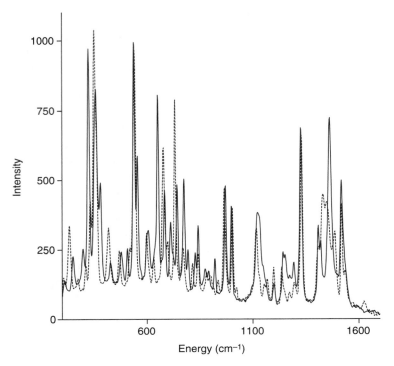

**Figure 5**   Raman spectra obtained within the fingerprint region for famotidine form A (*solid trace*) and form B (*dashed trace*) (35).

information could have been obtained through the use of infrared absorption spectroscopy, the different selection rules of the Raman effect cause different bands to be more intense in the spectrum and can often lead to a different type of selectivity.

The Raman spectra of two polymorphs of fluconazole were found to permit the ready differentiation between the crystal forms (36). Numerous differences in vibrational band energies are evident in the fingerprint and lattice regions, and even the high-frequency spectral region contains well-resolved spectral features that permit an easy characterization of the structural differences between the two systems. Thirteen samples of spironolactone, obtained from different sources, were evaluated by Raman spectroscopy, and four polymorphic forms of the drug substance were identified in these (24). When infrared absorption spectra were obtained for samples in compressed KBr pellets, no differences attributable to polymorphism could be detected, indicating interconversion during processing of the sample. However, when the samples were processed using a nondestructive method, the existence of one (or sometimes more) of the polymorphs could be readily detected.

It is frequently noted that the differences in Raman frequencies between polymorphic solids are fairly small, and a detailed analysis of such magnitudes has been reported (37). Through an evaluation of 14 systems, it was deduced that a shift exceeding $1.6\,cm^{-1}$ in the Raman spectra of the same compound isolated using different procedures was sufficient to indicate the existence of a polymorphic system. Full spectra were reduced to 10 to 17 separate peak positions, with 8 to 20 measurements being obtained for each value, and the use of standard analysis of variance methodology was critical to the quality of the analysis procedure.

The characterization of solvates and hydrates by Raman spectroscopy also requires that the differing crystal structures of the crystal forms cause a perturbation of the pattern of molecular vibrations. In many cases, the degree of crystallographic difference is large, but in other instances the solvent of crystallization only affects a small number of vibrations. For example, naproxen sodium has been shown to crystallize in an anhydrate, a monohydrate, and a dihydrate crystal form, and their physical

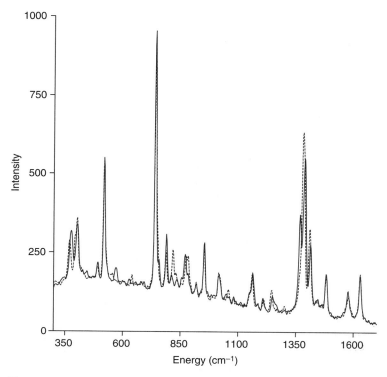

**Figure 6** Raman spectra obtained within the fingerprint region for the anhydrate form of naproxen sodium (*solid trace*) and its monohydrate phase (*dashed trace*). *Source*: From Ref. 35.

characteristics have been reported (38). As shown in Figure 6, within the fingerprint region, the anhydrate and monohydrate forms exhibit very similar Raman spectra (35). However, the two solvatomorphs can still be distinguished on the basis of their characteristic Raman peaks (such as the $1368/1388/1414\,cm^{-1}$ triplet of the anhydrate phase, compared with the $1382/1410\,cm^{-1}$ doublet of the monohydrate phase).

Three nonsolvated polymorphs of tranilast have been reported, in addition to the chloroform and methylene chloride solvatomorphs (39). The Raman spectra contained strong bands derived from the methylene stretching modes, the aromatic ring vibrations, and various low-frequency lattice modes. It was reported that the intensity of the amide band in the Raman spectrum of Form II (observed at $1643\,cm^{-1}$) was particularly strong relative to intensities of the analogous band in the other forms. Owing to the ease of its measurement, Raman spectroscopy was developed as an in-process method to evaluate any contamination by nonsolvated Forms II or III in bulk nonsolvated Form I. The pattern of lattice vibrational modes noted for nonsolvated Form I and the chloroform solvate indicated the existence of a structural similarity, and a similar conclusion was deduced for the nonsolvated Form III and the methylene chloride solvatomorph.

The Raman spectra of four hydrate forms of risedronate were found to be dominated by vibrations associated with the substituted pyridine ring (40). Both the anhydrate and the hemipentahydrate forms yielded two intense peaks derived from an in-plane pyridine ring deformation mode that was similar to that of neat pyridine. On the other hand, the monohydrate and variable hydrate forms were dominated by a single peak derived from this pyridine ring deformation. The spectroscopic differences appeared to originate from differing types of intermolecular interactions originating from hydrogen bonding between the pyridine ring and an adjacent phosphate group. Additional differences in Raman spectra between the different hydrates were observed in the high-frequency symmetric and antisymmetric methylene C–H stretching modes.

Raman spectroscopy has been used to evaluate the interactions between drug substances and polymeric excipients. The molecular structures existing in solid dispersions of indomethacin and poly(vinylpyrrolidone) (PVP) have been studied, with the carbonyl stretching mode of the drug substance being used as the spectroscopic probe (41). Addition of PVP to amorphous indomethacin increased the intensity of the non–hydrogen bonded carbonyl groups, while the carbonyl stretching band of the PVP polymer decreased to lower energies. These findings led to the conclusion that indomethacin interacted with PVP through hydrogen bonds formed between the drug hydroxyl and polymer carbonyl groups, resulting in disruption of the indomethacin dimers that existed in the bulk drug substance.

The physical state of chlorhexidine when that substance was formulated into viscoelastic, bioadhesive, semisolids has been evaluated using

Raman spectroscopy (42). The formulations were prepared by dispersing the drug substance free base into buffered polymer matrices consisting of hydroxyethylcellulose, PVP, and polycarbophil, and the Raman spectra of the drug substance were acquired within a variety of formulation conditions. The existence of an acid–base reaction between chlorhexidine and polycarbophil was demonstrated, forming the dication of the drug substance that was solubilized by the hydroxyethylcellulose component. The utility of Raman spectroscopy as a process analytical technique during formulation of topical gels and emulsions has been demonstrated, with changes in the spectral characteristics of the thickening agent carbopol and the emulsifying agent tefose being monitored after performance of major processing steps (43).

In other work, Raman spectra of promethazine, diclofenac, theophylline, and indomethacin in polymeric diluents based on polyethylene oxide, sodium alginate, and hydroxypropylmethyl cellulose were obtained (44). It was determined that the characteristic Raman spectra of each drug substance could be used to quantitate its concentration in the formulations, as well as providing information on the character of any drug–excipient interactions and incompatibilities that might exist in the formulation matrix. The latter aspect, and the ease of obtaining Raman spectral results, clearly demonstrates the utility of this technique as one of the tools in the arsenal of the preformulation scientist.

## Near-Infrared Spectroscopy

### Principles

The absorption bands found in the near-infrared (NIR) region of the spectrum (typically considered to cover 1000–2500 nm) are all due to overtones and combinations of fundamental molecular vibrational modes (45). NIR spectra are typically dominated by vibrational modes of light atoms having high bond strengths, typically hydrogen bound to nitrogen, oxygen, or carbon. The energies of the overtone bands are more affected by environmental details than are the energies of their fundamentals, so slight perturbations in the bonding can yield drastic frequency and amplitude changes in the NIR. Discussions of various pharmaceutical applications of NIR spectroscopy are available in Refs. (46,47).

Although the molar absorptivities of these bands are usually of low magnitude, the instrumental state of the art, combined with superior data deconvolution routines, has progressed to the point where their measurement has become fairly routine (48). Important requirements for the experimental aspect of NIR spectroscopy include the use of high-intensity stable light sources, sensitive detectors that do not contribute instrumental noise, and efficient methods for collecting the diffuse reflectance of the sample under study.

NIR spectroscopy became much more useful when the principle of multiple-wavelength spectroscopy was combined with the deconvolution methods of factor and principal component analysis. In typical applications, partial least squares regression is used to model the relation between composition and the NIR spectra of an appropriately chosen series of calibration samples, and an optimal model is ultimately chosen by a procedure of cross-testing. The performance of the optimal model is then evaluated using the normal analytical performance parameters of accuracy, precision, and linearity. Since its inception, NIR spectroscopy has been viewed primarily as a technique of quantitative analysis and has found major use in the determination of water in many pharmaceutical materials.

Representative Applications

A wide range of applications can be envisioned for the use of NIR spectroscopy, but the natures of the problems usually addressed by this methodology are somewhat different from those of both infrared absorption and Raman spectroscopies (46). Since NIR spectra consist of overtone transitions of fundamental vibrational modes, they are not terribly useful for identity purposes without the use of multicomponent analysis and access to spectral libraries of known materials.

Functional groups that contain unique hydrogen atoms are generally of the greatest utility to a NIR method. For example, studies of water in solids can be easily performed through systematic characterization of the characteristic –OH band, usually observed around $5170 \, cm^{-1}$. The determination of hydrate species in an anhydrous matrix can easily be performed using NIR analysis. Not surprisingly, the NIR technique has been used very successfully for moisture determination, whole tablet assay, and blending validation (49). Generally, one finds that use of the overtone and combination bands of water can yield NIR methods whose accuracy is equivalent to that associated with Karl-Fischer titration. A great advantage of NIR spectroscopy is its nondestructive nature, which represents a distinction over high-performance liquid chromatography (HPLC) methods that require destruction of the analyte materials to obtain a result.

NIR spectroscopy has been used to quantitate sulfathiazole forms I and III in binary mixtures in which one of the crystal forms was present as the dominant component (50). The spectra of each form exhibited sufficient differences so that unique wavelengths of absorbance were easily attributable to each form. Excellent linearity in graphs of calculated versus actual compositions was obtained over the concentration range of 0% to 5% for either form I in form III or form III in form I. After considering appropriate calibration models, a limit of quantitation of approximately 0.3% was ultimately deduced.

It is relatively straight forward to apply the NIR method for in situ characterization work, as was reported in the case of the EFGR tyrosine kinase inhibitor 4-(3-ethynylphenylamino)-6,7-bis(2-methoxyethoxy)quina-zolinium methanesulfonate (51). NIR spectroscopy was used to monitor the kinetics of transformation between the polymorphs and solvatomorphs and even facilitated the discovery of a new preferred form. It was determined that the in situ NIR method could be generally used in the study of practically all types of two-phase solid–liquid slurries maintained under isothermal conditions.

NIR spectroscopy has also been used to study changes in the solvatomorphic character, and the state of water, during the wet granulation of theophylline (52). The anhydrate form was wet-granulated in a planetary mixer using water as the granulation fluid, and the resulting solids subsequently characterized using a variety of methods. At a low level of granulation fluid (0.3 moles of water per mole of theophylline anhydrate), water absorption first yielded NIR maxima (1475 and 1970 nm) that were characteristic of theophylline monohydrate. At higher quantities of granulation fluid (1.3–2.7 moles of water per mole of theophylline anhydrate), the absorption maxima (1410 and 1905 nm) of free water became evident. Owing to its greater ease of spectral acquisition, it was determined that NIR spectroscopy was the superior method for the detection of different states of water during the wet granulation process.

## SOLID-STATE NUCLEAR MAGNETIC RESONANCE SPECTROMETRY

### Principles

After X-ray crystallography, solid-state nuclear magnetic resonance (SS-NMR) spectroscopy can be considered as being the most powerful molecular level characterization technique for a pharmaceutical solid, since this spectroscopic method yields information regarding the individual chemical environments of each atom in the compound under study (53). Although effectively any nucleus that can be studied in the solution phase can also be studied in the solid state, most of the published work has involved on studies involving the $^{13}C$ nucleus. Although it is certainly possible to perform $^{1}H$-NMR work in the solid state, the main problem with such work is that $^{1}H$-NMR has one of the smallest isotropic chemical shift ranges (12 ppm), but is accompanied by peak broadening effects that can span several ppm in magnitude.

The local magnetic field ($B_{loc}$) at a $^{13}C$ nucleus in an organic solid is given by

$$B_{loc} = \pm \frac{h\gamma_H}{4\pi} \frac{3\cos^2\theta - 1}{r^3},$$

where $\gamma_H$ is the magnetogyric ratio of the proton, $r$ is the internuclear C–H distance to the bonded proton, and is the angle between the C–H bond and the external applied field ($B_o$). The $\pm$ sign results from the fact that the local field may add to or subtract from the applied field depending on whether the neighboring proton dipole is aligned with or against the direction of $B_o$. In a microcrystalline organic solid, there is a summation over many values of $\theta$ and $r$, resulting in a proton dipolar broadening of many kilohertz.

A rapid reorientation of the C–H internuclear vectors (such as those associated with the random molecular motions that take place in the liquid phase) would result in reduction of the dipolar broadening. In solids, such rapid isotropic tumbling is not possible, but if one spins the sample at the so-called "magic angle" of $54°44'$ with respect to direction of the applied magnetic field, the term $(3 \cos^2 \theta - 1)$ equals zero and one obtains an averaging of the chemical shift anisotropy. In a solid sample, the anisotropy reflects the chemical shift dependence of chemically identical nuclei on their spatial arrangement with respect to the applied field. Since it is this anisotropy that is primarily responsible for the spectral broadening associated with $^{13}C$ samples, spinning at the magic angle makes it possible to obtain high-resolution $^{13}C$-NMR spectra of solid materials.

An additional mechanism for the removal of $^{13}C-^1H$ dipolar broadening is to use a high-power proton-decoupling field, a process often referred to as dipolar decoupling. One irradiates the sample using high power at an appropriate frequency, which results in the complete collapse of all $^{13}C-^1H$ couplings. With proton dipolar coupling alone, the resonances in a typical solid-state $^{13}C$ spectrum will remain very broad (on the order of 10–200 ppm). This broadening arises from the fact that the chemical shift of a particular carbon is directional, depending on the orientation of the molecule with respect to the magnetic field.

Even though high-resolution spectra can be obtained on solids using the magic-angle spinning (MAS) technique, the data acquisition time is lengthy due to the low sensitivity of the nuclei and the long relaxation times exhibited by the nuclei. This problem is circumvented using cross-polarization (CP), where spin polarization is transferred from the high-abundance, high-frequency nucleus ($^1H$) to the rare, low-frequency nucleus ($^{13}C$). This process results in up to a fourfold enhancement of the normal $^{13}C$ magnetization and permits a shortening of the waiting periods between pulses. The CP experiment also allows the measurement of several relaxation parameters that can be used to study the dynamic properties of the solid under investigation.

When the crystallography of compounds related by polymorphism is such that nuclei in the two structures are magnetically nonequivalent, it will follow that the resonances of these nuclei will not be equivalent. Since it is normally not difficult to assign organic functional groups to observed resonances, SS-NMR spectra can be used to obtain information regarding the structural differences that become manifested in the existence of polymorphic or solvatomorphic variations. The technique is especially useful when the origin of the differing crystal structures arises from differences in molecular conformations in the different forms. Such information has proven to be extremely valuable during various stages in the development of numerous pharmaceutical substances (54,55).

## Representative Applications

During the development of fosinopril sodium, the single-crystal structure of the most stable polymorph was determined, but it was not possible to obtain crystallographic grade crystals of its metastable phase (56). As a result, it was necessary to employ solid-state spectroscopic methods to obtain a better understanding of the structural features that yielded the observed poly-morphism. As evident in Figure 7, the solid-state $^{13}$C-NMR spectra of many resonance bands of the two polymorphs were observed at the same chemical shifts, while others were substantially shifted (57). For example, two of the three carbonyl groups of fosinopril were effectively equivalent, while the third carbonyl (located on the acetal side chain) was found to resonate at different chemical shifts in the two crystal forms. This observation, combined with those derived from vibrational spectral studies, yielded the

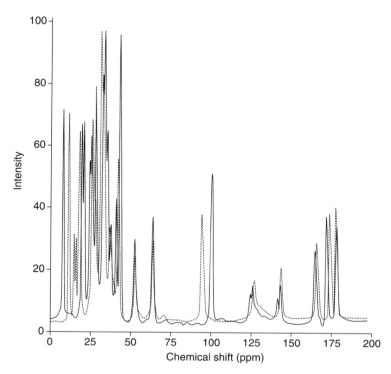

**Figure 7**   Solid-state $^{13}$C nuclear magnetic resonance spectra of fosinopril sodium form A (*solid trace*) and form B (*dashed trace*). *Source*: From Ref. 57.

deduction that the polymorphism of the compound was associated with different conformations of the acetal side chain. The NMR data also suggested that additional conformational differences between the two polymorphs were associated with *cis–trans* isomerization along the peptide bond, which in turn results in the presence of nonequivalent molecules existing in the unit cell.

The solid-state $^{13}$C-NMR spectra of the two polymorphs of furosemide revealed the existence of altered chemical shifts and peak splitting patterns indicative of differences in molecular conformations (58). Studies of $T_{1\rho}$ relaxation times were used to show the presence of more molecular mobility and disorder in form II, while the structure of form I was judged to be more rigid and uniformly ordered. During a solid-state spectroscopic study of the polymorphs of losartan, it was deduced that the spectral characteristics of form I implied the presence of multiple orientations for the *n*-butyl side chain and the imidazole ring (59). It was also concluded that losartan form II was characterized by the existence of a large molecular motion in the *n*-butyl side chain.

A significant number of polymorphic systems exist because different modes of molecular packing can result in the formation of differing solid-state structures, a situation very unlike that of conformational polymorphism. For example, the two polymorphs of enalapril maleate have been found to exhibit very similar molecular conformations (as evidenced by the similarity in spectral characteristics), and therefore the observed differences in crystal structure are attributed to different modes of crystal packing (60). Sufficient differences in the solid-state $^{13}$C-NMR spectra of the four polymorphs of sulfathiazole were observed that enabled the use of this technique as an analytical tool, but these differences could not be ascribed to differences in molecular conformations among the polymorphs (61).

Solid-state NMR spectroscopy can also be used to study the molecular environments of nuclei, as these vary in different solvatomorphic forms. Ampicillin is ordinarily obtained as its trihydrate solvatomorph, but is also capable of existing in an anhydrate form, and the physical properties of these have been exploited for studies of spectroscopy methods for characterization of water of hydration (62). Figure 8 shows the solid-state $^{13}$C-NMR spectra of the trihydrate and one of the anhydrate crystal forms, and the various resonance bands are seen to be grouped according to the functional groups of the differing carbons in the compounds (57). The effects of hydrogen bonding are seen most clearly in the bands associated with the three carbonyl groups, with these being fully resolved for the anhydrate and only partially resolved for the trihydrate. On the other hand, the trihydrate exhibits a well-resolved sequence of peaks for the carbons of the aromatic ring, while the degree of resolution is much worse for the aromatic carbons in the anhydrate structure.

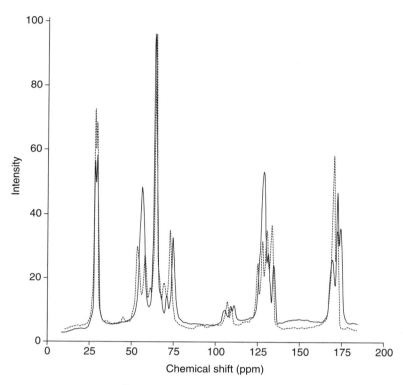

**Figure 8** Solid-state $^{13}$C nuclear magnetic resonance spectra of the anhydrate form of ampicillin (*solid trace*), and its trihydrate phase (*dashed trace*). *Source*: From Ref. 57.

One anhydrate and two polymorphic monohydrate phases of testosterone have been crystallographically characterized, and the solid-state $^{13}$C-NMR spectra obtained for each (63). The analysis of the spectra was complicated by the observation that many carbons of a given form were found to resonate as doublets, reflecting the situation of multiple occupancy within the unit cell. In another study, solid-state $^{13}$C-NMR spectra were obtained on the anhydrate and monohydrate phases of androstanolone, a known metabolite of testosterone (64). The spectrum obtained within the aliphatic carbon region for the anhydrate forms was found to consist of many doublets arising from incongruences in the unit cell. In the monohydrate phase, no such doubling was observed since the two molecules present in the unit cell were related by symmetry and consequently must be magnetically equivalent.

Owing to its ability to report on the chemical environment of nuclei within functional groups, solid-state NMR spectrometry can play an extremely useful role in the evaluation of interactions between drug substances and excipients in a formulation. For example, the interactions between ibuprofen free acid and its sodium salt with Eudragit RL-100 in solid dispersions have been evaluated using both $^1$H and $^{13}$C NMR spectrometries (65). After full assignment of the resonances for both forms of ibuprofen that permitted an understanding as to what was taking place in coevaporate formulations, it was determined that the degree of drug–polymer interaction was much strong for ibuprofen free acid as compared with that noted for its sodium salt. These results correlated with those obtained from in vitro dissolution testing, where the drug release of ibuprofen free acid was slowed and modulated by the Eudragit matrix.

Solid-state $^{13}$C-NMR spectrometry was used to investigate the effect of encapsulation on conformation of molecularly dispersed acylated esterified homologues of salicylic acid (i.e., acetylsalicylic acid, valerylsalicylic acid, or caprylsalicylic acid) (66). It was found that alteration of the microenvironment of the incorporated solutes had accompanied the formulation process. For example, increasing the aliphatic character of the acyl side chain resulted in an increase in the upfield shift of the acyl-bearing aromatic ring carbon of an incorporated substance relative to the resonance of the corresponding free compound. In addition, a downfield shift of the resonance of the free acid–bearing aromatic ring carbon was also observed. The electrostatic shielding within the microenvironment in the proximity of the ester carbonyl was attributed to an increase in the association of the probe molecule with the polymer subunits, suggesting that the incorporated compounds are essentially shielded from hydrolytic attack, being liberated into an aqueous environment.

Even though the mechanism of action of 2-*tert*-butyl-4-methoxyphenol (BHA) appears to proceed by a number of mechanisms, it is widely used as an antioxidant in numerous solid dosage forms. In order to evaluate the physical form of BHA subsequent to its wet granulation onto different excipients, solid-state $^{13}$C-NMR spectrometry was conducted on BHA for which a $^{13}$C label had been incorporated into the methoxy group (67). It was concluded that BHA could exist as either a crystalline or an amorphous component and that any amorphous material present was either bound to excipients or remained mobile during the lifetime of the NMR experiment. At a BHA loading level of 0.1% loading, BHA appeared to be amorphous and mobile in freshly prepared blends. At a loading of 0.5%, BHA was shown to be amorphous on microcrystalline cellulose and hydroxypropylmethyl cellulose, while remaining crystalline when deposited on lactose, mannitol, calcium phosphate dihydrate, or croscarmellose sodium.

## SUMMARY

There is little doubt that it is now abundantly clear that well-designed applications of spectroscopic techniques would be extraordinarily useful during the conduct of a preformulation program of investigation. Although the primary determinant of the existence of polymorphism or solvatomorphism must be crystallographic in nature, it is abundantly clear that the use of solid-state spectroscopy can yield information regarding the properties of individual functional groups. The same spectroscopic techniques can be equally useful during evaluations of the possible interactions between a drug substance and its excipients, especially since a large amount of information can usually be obtained in a nondestructive manner on small quantities of sample.

## REFERENCES

1.  Verma AR, Krishna P. Polymorphism and Polytypism in Crystals. New York: Wiley, 1966:1–7.
2.  Byrn S, Pfeiffer R, Ganey M, Hoiberg C, Poochikian G. Pharm Res 1995; 12: 945–54.
3.  Brittain HG. Pharm Tech 2000; 24(9):116–25.
4.  Byrn SR, Pfeiffer RR, Stowell JG. Solid State Chemistry of Drugs, 2nd ed. West Lafayette, IN: SSCI Inc., 1999.
5.  Brittain HG. Polymorphism in Pharmaceutical Solids. New York: Marcel Dekker, 1999.
6.  Bernstein J. Polymorphism in Molecular Crystals. London: Clarendon Press, 2002.
7.  Brittain HG. Physical Characterization of Pharmaceutical Solids. New York: Marcel Dekker, 1995.
8.  Threlfall TL. Analyst 1995; 120:2435–60.
9.  Brittain HG. "Methods for the characterization of polymorphs and solvates". In: Brittain HG, ed. Polymorphism in Pharmaceutical Solids. New York: Marcel Dekker, 1999:227–78.
10. Brittain HG. "Solid-state analysis". In: Ahuja S, Scypinski S, eds. Handbook of Pharmaceutical Analysis. New York: Marcel Dekker, 2001:57–84.
11. Markovich RJ, Pidgeon C. Pharm Res 1991; 8:663–75.
12. Bugay DE, Williams AC. "Vibrational spectroscopy". In: Brittain HG, ed. Physical Characterization of Pharmaceutical Solids. New York: Marcel Dekker, 1995:59–91.
13. Brittain HG. J Pharm Sci 1997; 86:405–12.
14. Findlay WP, Bugay DE. J Pharm Biomed Anal 1998; 16:921–30.
15. Coates J. "Instrumentation for infrared spectroscopy". In: Ewing GW, ed. Analytical Instrumentation Handbook. New York: Marcel Dekker, 1990: 233–79.
16. Bruno TJ. Appl Spect Rev 1999; 34:91–120.
17. Brimmer PJ, Griffiths PR. Anal Chem 1986; 58:2179–84.
18. Frei RW, MacNeil JD. Diffuse Reflectance Spectroscopy in Environmental Problem-Solving. Cleveland: CRC Press, 1973:3–19.
19. Urban MW. Attenuated Total Reflectance Spectroscopy of Polymers. Washington DC: American Chemical Society, 1996.

20. Brittain HG. Unpublished results for infrared spectra obtained at a resolution of 4 cm$^{-1}$, using a Shimadzu model 8400 Fourier-transform infrared spectrometer, and sampled against the ZnSe crystal of a Pike MIRacle™ single reflection horizontal ATR sampling accessory.

21. Brand HV, Rabie RL, Funk DJ, Diaz-Acousta I, Pulay P, Lippert TK. Phys Chem B 2002; 106:10594–604.

22. Takla PG, Dakas CJ. J Pharm Pharmacol 1989; 41:227–30.

23. Neville GA, Beckstead HD, Shurvell HF. J Pharm Sci 1992; 81:1141–6.

24. Hu T-C, Wang S-L, Chen T-F, Lin S-Y. J Pharm Sci 2002; 91:1351–7.

25. Alkhamis KA, Obaidat AA, Nuseirat AF. Pharm Dev Tech 2002; 7:491–503.

26. Caira MR, Alkhamis KA, Obaidat RM. J Pharm Sci 2004; 93:601–11.

27. Yamamura S, Gotoh H, Sakamoto Y, Momose Y. Int J Pharm 2002; 241: 213–21.

28. Yang R, Schulman SG, Zavala PJ. Anal Chim Acta 2003; 481:155–64.

29. Blaug SM, Huang W-T. Pharm Sci 1972; 61:1770–5.

30. Hartauer KJ, Guillory JK. Drug Dev Indust Pharm 1991; 17:617–30.

31. Grasselli JG, Snavely MK, Bulkin BJ. Chemical Applications of Raman Spectroscopy. New York: Wiley, 1981.

32. Lewis IR, Edwards HGM. Handbook of Raman Spectroscopy. New York: Marcel Dekker, 2001.

33. Huong PV. J Pharm Biomed Anal 1986; 4:811–23.

34. Frank CJ. "Review of pharmaceutical applications of Raman spectroscopy". In: Pelletier MJ, ed. Analytical Applications of Raman Spectroscopy. Oxford: Blackwell Science, 1999:224–75.

35. Brittain HG. Unpublished results for Raman spectra obtained at a resolution of 5 cm$^{-1}$, using an Ocean Optics model R-300–785 Raman spectrometer. Bulk powder samples were contained in aluminum sample cups, and then excited at 785 nm to obtain the spectrum.

36. Gu XJ, Jiang W. J Pharm Sci 1995; 84:1438–41.

37. Mehrens SM, Kale UJ, Qu X. J Pharm Sci 2005; 94:1354–67.

38. Kim T-S, Rousseau RW. Cryst Growth Des 2004; 4:1211–16.

39. Vogt FG, Cohen DE, Bowman JD, et al. J Pharm Sci 2005; 94:651–65.

40. Redman-Furey N, Dicks M, Bigalow-Kern A, et al. J Pharm Sci 2005; 94: 893–911.

41. Taylor LS, Zografi G. Pharm Res 1997; 14:1691–8.

42. Jones DS, Brown AF, Woolfson AD, Denis AC, Matchett LJ, Bell SEJ. J Pharm Sci 2000; 89:563–71.

43. Islam MT, Rodriguez-Hornedo N, Ciotti S, Ackermann C. Pharm Res 2004; 21:1844–51.

44. Davies MC, Binns JS, Melia CD, et al. Int J Pharm 1990; 66:223–32.

45. Stark E, Luchter K, Margoshes M. Appl Spect Rev 1986; 22:335–399.

46. Ciurczak EW. Appl Spect Rev 1987; 23:147–63.

47. Morisseau KM, Rhodes CT. Drug Dev Indust Pharm 1995; 21:1071–90.

48. Burns DA, Ciurczak EW. Handbook of Near-Infrared Analysis, 2nd ed. New York: Marcel Dekker, 2001.

49. MacDonald BF, Prebble KA. J Pharm Biomed Anal 1993; 11:1077–85.

50. Patel AD, Luner PE, Kemper MS. J Pharm Sci 2001; 90:360–70.

51. Norris T, Santafianos D. J Chem Soc Perkin Trans 2000; 2:2498–502.
52. Rasanen E, Rantanen J. Jorgensen A, Karjaalainen M, Paakkari T, Yliruusi J. J Pharm Sci 2001; 90:389–96.
53. Fyfe CA. Solid State NMR for Chemists. Guelph: CFC Press, 1983.
54. Bugay DE. Pharm Res 1993; 10:317–27.
55. Tichmack PA, Bugay DE, Byrn SR. J Pharm Sci 2003; 92:441–74.
56. Brittain HG, Morris KR, Bugay DE, Thakur AB, Serajuddin ATM. J Pharm Biomed Anal 1993; 11:1063–69.
57. Brittain HG. Unpublished results for solid-state $^{13}$C nuclear magnetic resonance spectra obtained at a frequency of 270 MHz, using a combination of magic-angle spinning and crosspolarization. The spectra were obtained using a contact time of one millisecond and a three-second recycle time.
58. Doherty C, York P. Int J Pharm 1988; 47:141–55.
59. Raghavan K, Dwivedi A, Campbell GC, et al. Pharm Res 1993; 10:900–12.
60. Ip DP, Brenner GS, Stevenson JM, et al. Int J Pharm 1989; 28:183–91.
61. Anwar J, Tarling SE, Barnes P. J Pharm Sci 1989; 78:337–42.
62. Brittain HG, Bugay DE, Bogdanowich SJ, DeVincentis J. Drug Dev Indust Pharm 1988; 14:2029–46.
63. Fletton RA, Harris RK, Kenwright AM, Lancaster RW, Packer KJ, Sheppard N. Spectrochim Acta 1987; 43A:1111–20.
64. Harris RK, Say BJ, Yeung RR, Fletton RA, Lancaster RW. Spectrochim Acta 1989; 45A:465–9.
65. Geppi M, Guccione S, Mollica G, Pignatello R, Veracini CA. Pharm Res 2005; 22:1544–55.
66. Vachon MG, Nairn JG. Eur J Pharm Biopharm 1998; 45:9–21.
67. Remenar JF, Wenslow R, Ostovic D, Peresypkin A. Pharm Res 2004; 21:185–8.

# 3.6

# Thermal Analysis and Calorimetric Methods for the Characterization of New Crystal Forms

**Denette K. Murphy**

*Bristol-Myers Squibb Company, New Brunswick, New Jersey, U.S.A.*

**Shelley Rabel**

*ALZA Corporation, Mountain View, California, U.S.A.*

## INTRODUCTION

Thermal analysis and calorimetric methods have demonstrated a wide array of applications in the pharmaceutical industry spanning drug discovery, preformulation, and formulation development (Table 1). One of the most critical tasks of the preformulation scientist in the evaluation of new crystal forms is to ensure that the most appropriate physical form is selected for development. A major facet of this task is to characterize the thermal properties of the solid form to determine if it demonstrates adequate physical and chemical stability to withstand the rigors of processing during drug substance manufacture, formulation development, and long-term storage. The compound should be characterized adequately so that there is a high degree of certainty that a physically and chemically stable, manufacturable, and registerable dosage form can be developed.

Thermal analysis and calorimetric techniques permit rapid characterization with small drug substance requirements. These techniques are critical in physical–chemical screening of early discovery leads, during salt form screening, and in the characterization of polymorphs to determine the

**Table 1** Thermal Applications in the Pharmaceutical Industry

| Thermal method | Measurement/mode of operation | Application/utility |
|---|---|---|
| Differential scanning calorimetry (DSC) | Heat flow/heat capacity, energy of transitions as a function of temperature | Crystallinity, polymorphism/ pseudopolymorphism, glass transitions, thermal decomposition/kinetics, melting point, purity, drug–excipient interactions |
| Thermogravimetric analysis | Weight change as function of temperature and/or time | Characterization of solvates/ hydrates, decomposition, loss on drying, sublimation, kinetics |
| Modulated DSC | Measurement of heat flow/ heat capacity as a function of a sinusoidal temperature fluctuation with underlying heat/cool ramp | Glass transitions, separation of reversible/nonreversible heat flows to deconvolute overlapping transitions, measurement of relaxation enthalpy stability |
| Thermomicroscopy (hot stage microscopy) | Photomicrography of a drug substance as a function of temperature | Melting point, decomposition, polymorphism, crystallization, desolvation |
| Isothermal microcalorimetry | Measurement of heat flows as a function of time/ temperature with a high degree of sensitivity | Stability, polymorphism, characterization of amorphous content |
| Solution calorimetry | Heat flow as a function of time and/or temperature | Polymorphism, amorphous content |
| Microthermal analysis | Surface topography, heat flow as a function of temperature | Melting, glass transition/ amorphous character in specific regions of the material surface |
| Thermomechanical analysis | Expansion coefficient (softening) | Glass transitions |
| Dynamic mechanical analysis | Mechanical strength/energy loss as a function of temperature | Glass transition, rheological properties |

thermodynamic relationships between the various crystal forms. Once the optimal form has been selected for development, the preformulation scientist continues to provide the interpretation of thermal behavior for the various lots of drug substance to ensure that the thermal properties are consistent from batch to batch. Careful monitoring of each lot is required given that the process for drug substance manufacture is continually scaled-up, with changes in equipment and process improvements to increase yield, purity, and ease of manufacture. These changes often result in lot-to-lot differences in physicochemical properties of drug substances and changes in product performance, which require research/interpretation by the preformulation scientist.

The objective of this chapter is not to focus on the theoretical considerations of each method, but rather to limit the discussion to those thermal analysis and calorimetric techniques that are most routinely used in preformulation and how they are applied in practice to address preformulation activities and issues that arise in the development of new crystalline forms.

## POLYMORPHS

There are many reviews on the principles of polymorphism and the impact of polymorphism in the pharmaceutical industry (1–6). Many molecular compounds can crystallize as two or more crystalline polymorphs that can differ in properties such as solubility, mechanical behavior, and chemical stability. The selection of a given polymorphic form for development will depend not only on its physical and chemical properties but also on whether the selected polymorph can be reproducibly crystallized and has adequate physical stability during formulation, processing, and storage. The latter two factors are largely governed by the relative thermodynamic stability relationship between the polymorphs and the kinetics and mechanism of interconversion. Thermal methods such as differential scanning calorimetry (DSC) and solution calorimetry can be invaluable in the characterization of polymorphic systems, and the application of these methods in determining the thermodynamic stability relationship between polymorphs is discussed below.

The thermodynamic stability relationship between polymorphs A and B is determined by the Gibbs free energy difference as a function of temperature, $\Delta G = G_B - G_A = \Delta H - T\Delta S$. The polymorph having the lowest free energy is the more stable form at a given temperature and pressure, and the two polymorphs are equally stable (i.e., in equilibrium) when the free energy difference is zero. As seen from the theoretical phase diagrams in Figure 1, the free energy versus temperature plots give rise to two thermodynamic relationships: enantiotropic and monotropic. If two polymorphs are monotropically related, one form is more stable at all temperatures below the melting point of either form, and the $\Delta G$ curves do not intersect below

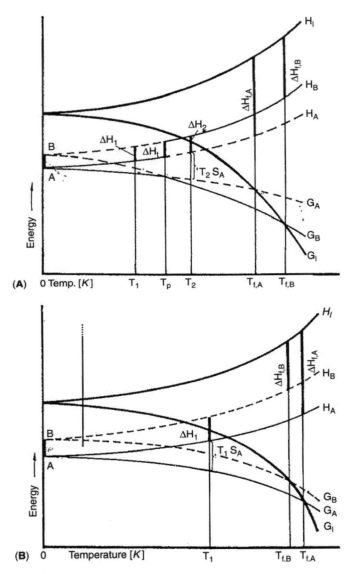

**Figure 1** Gibbs free energy $G$ and enthalpy $H$ versus absolute temperature $T$ at constant pressure for **(A)** enantiotropic and **(B)** monotropic polymorphs A and B and a liquid phase, l. For an enantiotropic system, the free energy curves cross at $T_p$ ($T_{eq}$ in text), the equilibrium temperature; while for a monotropic system, the free energy curves do not cross below the melting temperature $T_f$ of the lowest melting polymorph. The actual transition temperature ($T_1$ or $T_2$) that may be observed during a differential scanning calorimetry experiment usually does not coincide with $T_p$ ($T_{eq}$ in text). *Source:* From Ref. 7.

the melting point of the lowest melting polymorph. For enantiotropic systems, the $\Delta G$ curves intersect at the equilibrium temperature ($T_{eq}$). Below this temperature, one form is the more thermodynamically stable form, and above this temperature, the other form is more stable. In this chapter, the term "equilibrium temperature" instead of the more commonly used term "transition temperature" is used to describe the temperature at which the free energy difference between the two polymorphs is zero. For kinetic reasons, the temperature at which a polymorphic endothermic/exothermic transition is observed in DSC thermograms (denoted as $T_1$ and $T_2$ in Fig. 1) is often different from the equilibrium temperature $T_{eq}$.

The heat of transition rule (HTR) and heat of fusion rule (HFR) have been widely employed to establish the existence of monotropy or enantiotropy between polymorphs (7,8). Application of the HTR requires thermal measurements of the transition enthalpy between the two polymorphic forms. The transition enthalpy can be determined from DSC or solution calorimetry. The HTR states that if transition enthalpy is endothermic ($\Delta H > 0$), then the two polymorphs are enantiotropic, and if transition enthalpy is $\Delta H < 0$ (exothermic), then the two polymorphs are monotropic or the equilibrium temperature is higher than the exothermic transition temperature. The HFR has also been used to establish the stability relationship between two polymorphs and states that if the lower melting polymorph has the higher heat of fusion, then the two polymorphs are enantiotropic. Conversely, if the higher melting polymorph has the higher heat of fusion, the two polymorphs are monotropic. Application of the HFR requires thermal measurements of the heats of fusion and melting temperatures of each polymorph. Burger and Ramberger have applied the HTR and HFR to 228 transitions of 113 polymorphic systems of molecular crystals and found the HTR to give the right result in 99% of the cases, and the HFR was found to be invalid in only a few cases (8). Exceptions to these rules, particularly in cases of conformational polymorphism, have also been discussed (7–9).

Based on the HFR, the relative magnitude of the heat of fusion provides evidence for the relative stability of the polymorphs at absolute zero (10). However, for polymorphic systems that exhibit enantiotropy, the equilibrium temperature can only be determined from knowledge of the free energy differences as a function of temperature. The free energy difference between polymorphs can be determined directly from solubility measurements at different temperatures for each of the polymorphs using the following equation:

$$\Delta G = RT \ln \left( \frac{\gamma_B c_B}{\gamma_A c_A} \right) \cong RT \ln \left( \frac{c_B}{c_A} \right) \tag{1}$$

where $R$ is the gas constant, $T$ is temperature, $c_A$ and $c_B$ are the solubilities of polymorph A and B, respectively, and $\gamma_A$ and $\gamma_B$ are the activity coefficients at $c_A$ and $c_B$, respectively. For polymorphic systems that convert to another polymorphic/solvated form before equilibrium is achieved, and/or which form solvates in many different solvents, determination of the free energy difference from solubility measurements may not be possible.

Alternatively, thermal methods such as DSC (11–13) and adiabatic calorimetry (14) can be used to estimate the free energy differences between two polymorphic forms. Yu described a method for estimating the free energy difference between two polymorphs, A and B, from DSC measurements of the enthalpies of fusion ($H_{m,A}$ and $H_{m,B}$) and melting temperatures ($T_{m,A}$ and $T_{m,B}$) (12). The free energy difference between the polymorphs ($\Delta G_o$) at $T_{m,A}$, the melting temperature of the lowest melting polymorph, and the slope of the $\Delta G(T)$ curve is calculated from derived thermodynamic equations. These values are then used to estimate the free energy values at other temperatures through extrapolation. Extrapolating $\Delta G$ to zero gives an estimate of the equilibrium temperature (if it exists) from which the stability relationship (i.e., enantiotropy or monotropy) is inferred.

The entropy ($\Delta S_o$) and enthalpy ($\Delta H_o$) differences between polymorphs A and B (estimated over the temperature range $T_{m,A} - T_{m,B}$) and the free energy difference at $T_{m,A}$ ($\Delta G_o$) is calculated from Equations 2 to 4 (12):

$$\Delta G(T_{m,A}) = \Delta G_o = \Delta H_{m,B}\left(\frac{T_{m,A}}{T_{m,B}} - 1\right)$$
$$+ (C_{p,L} - C_{p,B})\left[T_{m,B} - T_{m,A} - T_{m,A}\ln\left(\frac{T_{m,B}}{T_{m,A}}\right)\right] \qquad (2)$$

$$\Delta S_o = \frac{\Delta H_{m,A}}{T_{m,A}} - \frac{\Delta H_{m,B}}{T_{m,B}} + (C_{p,L} - C_{p,B})\ln\left(\frac{T_{m,B}}{T_{m,A}}\right) \qquad (3)$$

$$\Delta H_o = \Delta H_{m,A} - \Delta H_{m,B} + (C_{p,L} - C_{p,B})(T_{m,B} - T_{m,A}) \qquad (4)$$

Equations 2 to 4 assume that the heat capacity difference between polymorph B and the supercooled liquid ($C_{p,L} - C_{p,B}$) is constant between $T_{m,A}$ and $T_{m,B}$. If $\Delta G$ is approximately linear with temperature (i.e., $\Delta H$ and $\Delta S$ are independent of temperature within the temperature range of extrapolation), then $\Delta G/dT = -\Delta S$, and the value of $\Delta G$ at other temperatures can be estimated from the following expression:

$$\Delta G(T) = \Delta G_o - \Delta S_o\left(T - T_{m,A}\right) \qquad (5)$$

Since $\Delta G = 0$ at $T_{eq}$, the equilibrium temperature, $T_{eq}$, can be calculated by setting Equations 5 to zero and by substituting $\Delta G_0 = \Delta H_0 - T_{m,A}\Delta S_0$:

$$T_{eq} = \frac{\Delta H_o}{\Delta S_o} \qquad (6)$$

Application of Equations 2 to 6 requires a value for $(C_{p,L} - C_{p,B})$. Yu has suggested that $(C_{p,L} - C_{p,B})$ at $T_{m,B} \approx k (\Delta H_{m,B})$ where $k = 0.003/K$ (12). The value of $(C_{p,L} - C_{p,B})$ can also be estimated if the heat of transition $(\Delta H_t)$ between polymorphs A and B is known either from solution calorimetry or from DSC measurements. In this case, $\Delta H_t$ can replace $\Delta H_o$ in Equation 4 and $(C_{p,L} - C_{p,B})$ can be estimated from the following (12):

$$(C_{p,L} - C_{P,B}) = \frac{(\Delta H_t - \Delta H_{m,A} + \Delta H_{m,B})}{T_{m,B} - T_{m,A}} \tag{7}$$

Alternatively, $(C_{p,L} - C_{p,B})$ can be determined by measuring the heat of crystallization, $\Delta H_{c,B}$ at $T_{c,B}$ (7,12).

$$(C_{p,L} - C_{p,B}) = \frac{(\Delta H_{m,B} - \Delta H_{c,B})}{T_{m,B} - T_{c,B}} \tag{8}$$

Equations 5 and 6 assume that $\Delta H_o$ and $\Delta S_o$ are independent of $T$ and therefore $\Delta G$ is linear with $T$ within the extrapolated temperature range [i.e., $T_{eq} - T_{m,A}$ for Equation 5]. If $\Delta G$ is nonlinear with $T$ within the extrapolated temperature range, then Equation 5 must be corrected for the heat capacity difference between the polymorphs, $C_{p,B} - C_{p,A}$ as described by Yu (12).

Based on the calculated equilibrium temperature from Equation 6, the thermodynamic relationship between polymorphs can be assigned as follows: (*i*) enantiotropic if $0 < T_{eq} < T_{m,A}$, (*ii*) monotropic if $T_{eq} > T_{m,A}$, and (*iii*) undecided if $T_{eq} < 0$. It is important to note that only in the first case does a true and definite equilibrium temperature exist. This treatment of the melting data has been applied to 96 pairs of polymorphs from the literature, and in most cases, it agreed well with previous determinations of the thermodynamic relationship and equilibrium temperature by other methods (12).

Yu et al. derived equations to determine the free energy differences between polymorphs based on eutectic melting data (11). This method may be useful for polymorphic systems that undergo chemical decomposition at temperatures close to the melting point. Collection of eutectic data involves measuring the eutectic temperatures and composition of each polymorph with several reference compounds that have melting points less than the polymorph evaluated. McCrone has described techniques to determine eutectic temperatures and compositions by hot stage microscopy (HSM) (15). In the selection of a reference compound, it must first be determined that the reference compound forms a eutectic with the polymorph, and the polymorph and reference compound do not form a solid solution or addition compound. Since the melting curve for each component can be estimated by the van't Hoff equation, intersection of the van't Hoff curves for the pure polymorph and reference compound can provide a reasonable estimate of the eutectic composition and temperature and serve as a good starting point for DSC measurements. Yu et al. used a combination of melting and eutectic data to determine the free energy differences between five polymorphs (R, Y, OP, ON, and YN) of 5-methyl-2-[(2-nitrophenyl) amino]-3-thiophenecarbonitirile (11). DSC was used to measure the temperature ($T_e$) and enthalpy of fusion ($\Delta H_{me}$) at the eutectic between each of the polymorphs and several reference compounds: acetanilide (mp 115°C), benzil (mp 95°C), azobenzene (mp 68°C), and thymol (mp 50°C). From these data, the differences in free energy were calculated using the following equation:

$$
\begin{aligned}
x_{e,B}(G_B - G_A)_{T_{eA}} \\
= \Delta H_{meB} \frac{(T_{eA} - T_{eB})}{T_{eB}} - \Delta C_{peB} \left[ T_{eA} - T_{eB} - T_{eA} \ln\left(\frac{T_{eA}}{T_{eB}}\right) \right] \\
+ RT_{eA} \left\{ x_{eB} \ln\left(\frac{x_{eB}}{x_{eA}}\right) + (1 - x_{eB}) \ln\left[\frac{(1 - x_{eB})}{(1 - x_{eA})}\right] \right\}
\end{aligned}
\tag{9}
$$

where $x_e$ is the eutectic composition of the specified polymorph and the reference compound and $\Delta C_{pe}$ is the heat capacity change upon melting at the eutectic. Equation 9 was derived by assuming ideal solution formation and by linking polymorphs A and B through intermediate steps involving eutectic melting, temperature change, and dissolution (11). Figure 2 shows the melting and eutectic data for polymorphs Y and ON. The DSC data in the lower half of Figure 2 show that $T_{e,ON} > T_{e,Y}$ for acetanilide, $T_{e,ON} \approx T_{e,Y}$ for benzil, and $T_{e,ON} < T_{e,Y}$ for azobenzene and thymol, suggesting that the stability order reverses and there is a equilibrium temperature close to ~70°C. The stability relationship between the polymorphs relative to Y as determined from the melting and eutectic data is shown in the top portion of Figure 2. The cluster of points near the melting temperature of the pure form was calculated using Equations 2 and 3 as described previously. The points < 90°C were calculated from the eutectic melting data. Since YN underwent a solid-state conversion prior to the eutectic temperature for the three highest melting reference compounds, only the data for the eutectic with thymol could be used in the relative stability estimations for YN. DSC traces of YN at 10°C/min showed an exothermic transition near 70°C, corresponding to the rapid solid-state conversion of YN to Y (and trace amounts of R). The enthalpy associated with the YN-to-Y conversion was determined from the DSC data and used to calculate the slope, $d(\Delta G_{YN} - \Delta G_Y)/dT = -(S_{YN} - S_Y) = -[(H_{YN} - H_Y) - (G_{YN} - G_Y)]/T$. This data combined with the thymol eutectic melting data was used to infer the stability relationship between YN and Y as shown in Figure 3. The monotropic relationship between YN and Y is consistent with the HTR and the observed exothermic transition.

The use of melting data from DSC measurements in determining the stability relationship between polymorphs and equilibrium temperatures

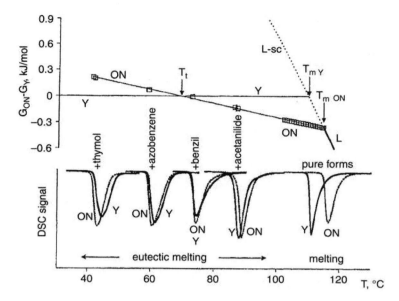

**Figure 2** Illustration of the use of melting and eutectic data for determining the stability relationship between polymorphs. (*Bottom*) Differential scanning calorimetry melting endotherms for polymorphs Y and ON as pure forms and in eutectics with four reference compounds. (*Top*) $\Delta G$ versus temperature curve for polymorphs ON and Y calculated using Equations 2, 3, and 9. *Abbreviations*: $T_{mY}$, $T_{mON}$, melting points of pure forms; $T_t$, equilibrium temperature; L, liquid phase; $L_{SC}$, supercooled liquid phase. *Source*: From Ref. 11.

assumes that there is no thermal decomposition and that the same conditions (i.e., heating rate, sample size, particle size, etc.) are used to obtain the melting data for all polymorphs. In cases in which thermal events overlap, sample conditions such as heating rate and sample size should be optimized to provide the most accurate melting data. Lower heating rates allow for the detection of solid–solid transformations as demonstrated for carbamazepine (CBZ) in which the enthalpy associated with the solid–solid transformation was used as an estimation of the heat of transition between the two enantiotropic polymorphs (16). Giron showed for temazepam that faster heating rates did not allow time for transformation to the higher melting polymorph, and only a single melting endotherm of the lower melting polymorph was observed at 10°C/min and 20°C/min (Fig. 4) (17). As shown in the lower half of Figure 4, small sample sizes provided better resolution and faster transitions (17).

Thermal methods have been used in combination with other techniques to determine the thermodynamic relationship and transition temperatures for polymorphic systems. For instance, Gu and Grant estimated the

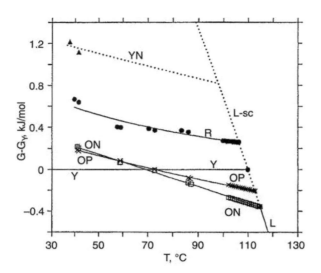

**Figure 3** Stability relationship between polymorphs of 5-methyl-2-[(2-nitrophenyl)amino]-3-thiophenecarbonitirile constructed from melting and eutectic data using Equations 2, 3, and 9. *Source*: From Ref. 11.

equilibrium temperatures of polymorphs from their heats of solution and solubility values (or intrinsic dissolution rates) at a given temperature (18). Behme and Brooke estimated the equilibrium temperature for enantiotropic polymorphs of CBZ from melting data and van't Hoff plots of the estimated solubilities of each of the polymorphs at various temperatures (16). In general, evaluating the free energy difference between polymorphic forms directly from both thermal and solubility measurements, as previously described, provides a much better understanding of the polymorphic system evaluated.

## SOLVATES

### Characterization and Identification

Solvated and hydrated crystal forms, commonly referred to as pseudopolymorphs and herein referred to as solvates, are crystals in which solvent molecules (i.e., water molecules in the case of hydrates) occupy regular positions in the crystal lattice (1). The solvent held within the crystal may be stoichiometric or nonstoichiometric. In some cases, the solvate is stoichiometric before isolation from the state in which it crystallized, and once placed in a nonequilibrium environment, it partially or completely desolvates, resulting in a nonstoichiometric solvate. Desolvation occurs as the solid attempts to reestablish equilibrium with the environment. The

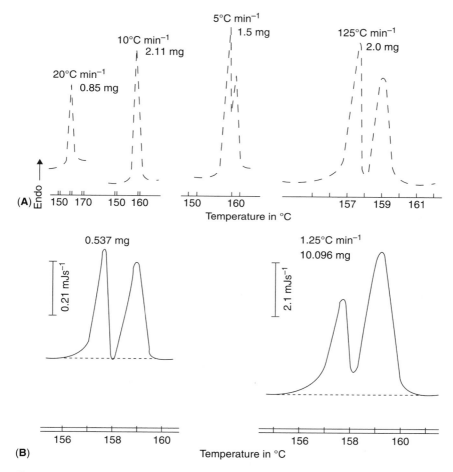

**Figure 4** Effect of (**A**) heating rate and (**B**) sample mass on the differential scanning calorimetry curve for a metastable polymorph of temazepam. *Source*: From Ref. 17.

tendency to desolvate is dependent on the environment (i.e., activity of the solvent in the vapor) and the activation energy for desolvation to occur. HSM, DSC, and thermogravimetric analysis (TGA) are used to detect transitions during the desolvation process and are therefore very useful thermal techniques for the characterization and identification of solvates. In the identification and characterization of solvates, thermal methods should be used with other techniques such as single crystal structure analysis, gas chromatography, solid-state/solution nuclear magnetic resonance (NMR), and Karl Fischer moisture determination to confirm the existence of solvent in the solid and to distinguish between desolvation events and other processes such as decomposition.

The use of HSM in the identification of hydrates and solvates has been extensively discussed by McCrone (15). A few crystals are immersed in mineral oil, placed on a hot stage, and observed during controlled heating. The dehydration can be directly observed as bubbles escaping from the crystalline solid. These bubbles may not be observed if the solid is a solvate comprised of a solvent that is miscible with mineral oil. In this case, the experiment can be repeated using a high-boiling liquid immiscible with the suspected solvent. In addition, HSM experiments conducted under cross-polarizers can be very useful in determining whether the solid remains crystalline or converts to an amorphous solid after desolvation. It is important to understand the desolvation behavior and the fate of a crystalline solvate after the desolvation process. These two factors are very helpful in evaluating the potential behavior of a solvate during processes such as drying and milling, which may result in desolvation.

HSM combined with knowledge of the crystal packing can provide very useful information on the desolvation mechanism. During HSM studies on several hydrates and solvates including caffeine (19,20) and theophylline (20), crystals became increasingly opaque from the outer ends to the center as the desolvation process progressed (1). Analyses of the single crystal structure revealed that these solvates are what are known as "channel solvates," in which the solvent interacts with other solvent molecules along an axis of the crystal, forming a channel or solvent tunnel within the crystalline lattice. For both caffeine and theophylline, desolvation occurs along a crystallographic direction that corresponds to the direction of the solvent channel, since this direction provides the path of least resistance for desolvation to occur (1). HSM of trehalose dihydrate particles $>425\,\mu m$ shows that dehydration occurs via a nucleation and growth mechanism in which needle-shaped crystals were observed to grow across the surface of the original crystals (21). X-ray diffraction and Fourier transformed (FT)–Raman spectroscopic studies confirmed that the phase transition corresponds to the conversion from the dihydrate to anhydrate. Smaller particles ($<45\,\mu m$) of trehalose dihydrate were shown to dehydrate by a different mechanism. HSM images show a change in birefringence as the crystals become increasingly opaque, presumably due to the formation of an amorphous solid. Further heating results in liquefaction of the solid followed by recrystallization and subsequent melting of the anhydrous form.

DSC and TGA are valuable techniques in the characterization of solvates by detecting the transition enthalpy and weight loss, respectively, that occur during desolvation. Desolvation in the solid state is an endothermic process since heat is absorbed to disrupt the interactions between the solvent–host and/or solvent–solvent molecules within the crystalline lattice. DSC can be used to measure the enthalpy and temperature range associated with the desolvation process, which can provide useful qualitative information on the state of association of the solvent molecules within the crystal lattice. For instance, more than one endotherm may be observed if the solvent molecules are in dissimilar crystal lattice sites with different solvent–host interactions. TGA measures the weight loss of a solvate as a function of temperature during the desolvation process and can be used to determine the stoichiometry of the crystalline solvate. TGA is typically coupled with DSC to confirm that the observed desolvation endothermic transitions are associated with a corresponding weight loss. Analysis of the TGA curve gives the sample weight loss as a percentage of the initial weight, which can be used to calculate the molar ratio, $n$, of solvent to drug using the following equation:

$$n = \frac{M_d m_d}{M_s(m_i - m_d)} \tag{10}$$

where $M_d$ and $M_s$ are the molecular weights of the desolvated material and solvent, respectively, and $m_i$ and $m_d$ are the initial sample mass and the mass of solvent lost (i.e., TGA weight loss). Coupled TGA instruments such as TGA/mass spectrometry (MS) and TGA/infrared (IR) are useful in the identification of the gaseous product evolved during a TGA weight loss event. These coupled instruments can be valuable in distinguishing desolvation events from other processes such as decomposition, as shown for aspartame in Figure 5 (22). Aspartame exhibits three endothermic transitions. The first endotherm is associated with a 3% weight loss and corresponds to the dehydration of the hemi-hydrate. The second endotherm is associated with a weight loss and results from the evolution of methanol due to the decomposition of aspartame to cyclic piperazine based on the IR spectra. The last DSC peak represents melting of the cyclic piperazine.

The rate and temperature of desolvation and the resulting shape of the DSC and TGA curves are greatly influenced by instrumental and sample variables (17,23). Depending on the type of information required, DSC samples can be run in crimped pans, hermetically sealed pans, or open pans without a lid. Compared to open pans, crimped pans and hermetically sealed pans provide better thermal contact between the sample and pan and a reduction in thermal gradients (24). Hermetically sealed sample pans have an airtight seal, which can result in high internal pressures during the release of solvent and therefore cause significant increases in the desolvation temperature. Crimped pans or hermetically sealed pans with a pinhole are the best choice for general purposes since they allow for pressure equilibration (23). The effect of pan type on the DSC and TGA curves for caffeine 4/5-hydrate is shown in Figure 6 (25). In a hermetically sealed pan with a pinhole, a sharp endotherm (*p*) at 80°C is observed; this can be attributed to the peritectic melting (26) of the hydrate. If a pan with a perforated cover is used, a sharp melting endotherm is observed corresponding to the peritectic

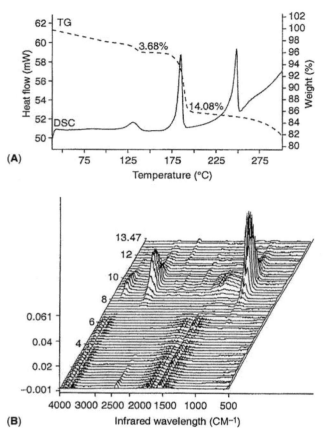

**Figure 5** (A) Differential scanning calorimetry (*solid line*) and thermogravimetric analysis (TGA) (*dashed line*) curves for aspartame and (B) the corresponding three-dimensional plot from TGA/infrared. *Source*: From Ref. 22.

melting (*p*) followed by a second endotherm (*e*), which can be attributed to the evaporation of water. The DSC and TGA curves C, for a sample run in an open pan, shows an endothermic dehydration transition at d1, which is associated with a 1% weight loss, and a second dehydration endotherm at 50°C (d2) coupled with the peritectic melting peak (p). In addition to pan type and atmospheric pressure, other factors such as heating rate can also influence the rate and temperature of desolvation. Faster heating rates generally give higher desolvation temperatures and reduce the resolution between adjacent peaks (23,27). DSC curves for caffeine hydrate run in an open pan show slow heating rates, resulting in a very broad dehydration endotherm due to the continuous loss of water over a broad temperature

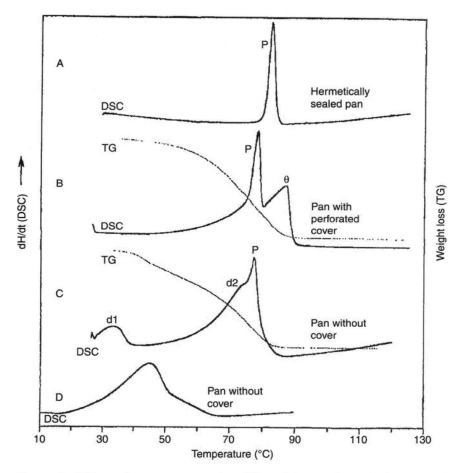

**Figure 6** Effect of pan type on the differential scanning calorimetry and thermogravimetric analysis curves of caffeine hydrate at a heating rate of 2.5 K/min. Curves A to C represent a batch having coarse crystals (at most 3 mm in length and an average of 50 μm in diameter), and curve D represents a batch having small crystals (< 100 μm in length and 5–10 μm in diameter). *Source*: From Ref. 25.

range (Fig. 7) (25). In some cases, if the heating rate is too slow, the DSC loses sensitivity to its detection of the desolvation event. Increasing the DSC heating rate for caffeine hydrate from 1.0 to 7.5 K/min both delayed dehydration and decreased the resolution between the dehydration and melting endotherms so that only a single endotherm is observed in the DSC curve at 7.5 K/min. Aside from instrumental variables, sample characteristics such as particle size (21), morphology (28), sample weight (29), and

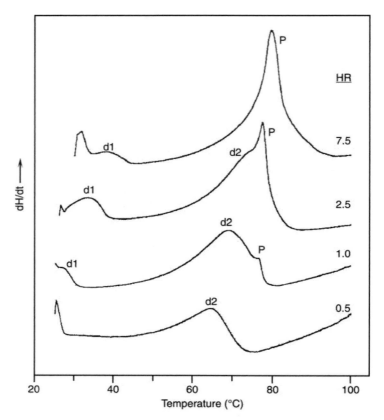

**Figure 7**  Effect of heating rate on the differential scanning calorimetry curves of caffeine hydrate under open conditions (sample pans without covers). The top three curves represent a batch having coarse crystals (at most 3 mm in length and an average of 50 μm in diameter), and the bottom curve represents a batch having small crystals (< 100 μm in length and 5–10 μm in diameter). *Source*: From Ref. 25.

crystal defects (1) can greatly influence the rate of desolvation and the resulting DSC and TGA curves.

## Kinetics and Mechanism of Desolvation

Extensive reviews have been written on the kinetic models and mechanisms of solid-state reactions (1,30,31). These models have been developed and applied to solid-state reactions involving desolvation, chemical decomposition, and polymorphic conversions. The application of these models involves monitoring the weight fraction of product phase with time. In the case of desolvation reactions, the formation of the product phase or the evolution of the solvent as a gas can be monitored isothermally by TGA from the weight loss versus time curves. The extent of conversion, $\alpha$, is then calculated using the following expression:

$$\alpha = \frac{m_i - m_t}{m_i - m_f} \tag{11}$$

where $m_i$ and $m_f$ are the initial and final sample masses and $m_t$ is the mass at time, $t$. The basic kinetic equation used in the treatment of isothermal kinetic data is

$$\frac{d\alpha}{dt} = k(T)f(\alpha) \tag{12}$$

where $k(T)$ is the temperature-dependent rate constant, and $f(\alpha)$ is the reaction model. Several examples of reaction models are shown in Table 2. In practice the integral form of Equation 12 is used:

$$g(\alpha) = \int_0^\alpha [f(\alpha)]^{-1} d\alpha = k(T)t \tag{13}$$

in which the slope of plots of the integral form of the reaction model $g(\alpha)$ versus time yields the reaction rate constant at the experimental temperature (Table 2). The kinetic model that best fits the data based on regression analysis is used to describe the mechanism of the reaction. However, while Equations 12 and 13 and the various kinetic models in Table 2 can be useful for gaining a mechanistic understanding of the reaction, a good fit to a kinetic model does not necessarily imply that the corresponding mechanism is correct. Other techniques such as HSM and powder X-ray diffraction should be used as further evidence of the mechanism of desolvation.

Han and Suryanarayanan studied the kinetics and mechanism of dehydration of CBZ dihydrate isothermally at controlled water vapor pressures (Fig. 8) (32). The dehydration of CBZ dihydrate at 44°C underwent a change in mechanism between 5.1 and 12 torr. At low water vapor pressures (≤5.1 torr), the dehydration kinetics was described by a two-dimensional phase boundary reaction, while at higher vapor pressures (≥12.0 torr), the dehydration kinetics was described by the Avrami-Erofeev model (also referred to as the three-dimensional nucleation and growth model). A single model could not explain the dehydration kinetics at an intermediate water vapor pressure of 7.6 torr. The dehydration process can be described by the following equation (32):

$$A(solid) \rightarrow B(solid) + H_2O(gas) \tag{14}$$

Consistent with Equation 14, low vapor pressures (≤5.1 torr) resulted in the fastest dehydration rate. The relationship between the dehydration kinetics

**Table 2**  Kinetic Equations in Differential Form and Corresponding Mechanism of Degradation in the Solid State

| Differential form, $f(\alpha)$ | Integral form, $g(\alpha)$ | Corresponding mechanisms |
|---|---|---|
| $2(1-\alpha)[-\ln(1-\alpha)]^{1/2}$ | $[-\ln(1-\alpha)]^{1/2}$ | Avrami-Erofeev, $n=2$ |
| $3(1-\alpha)[-\ln(1-\alpha)]^{2/3}$ | $[-\ln(1-\alpha)]^{1/3}$ | Avrami-Erofeev, $n=3$ |
| $4(1-\alpha)[-\ln(1-\alpha)]^{3/4}$ | $[-\ln(1-\alpha)]^{1/4}$ | Avrami-Erofeev, $n=3$ |
| $1/2\alpha$ | $\alpha^2$ | One-dimensional diffusion |
| $[-\ln(1-\alpha)]^{-1}$ | $(1-\alpha)\ln(1-\alpha)+\alpha$ | Two-dimensional diffusion |
| $1.5(1-\alpha)^{1/3}$ $\left[(1-\alpha)^{-1/3}-1\right]^{-1}$ | $\left[1-(1-\alpha)^{1/3}\right]^2$ | Three-dimensional diffusion (Jander) |
| $1.5\left[(1-\alpha)^{-1/3}-1\right]^{-1}$ | $1-2\alpha/3$ $-(1-\alpha)^{2/3}$ | Three-dimensional diffusion (Ginstlin-Brounshtein) |
| $1-\alpha$ | $-\ln(1-\alpha)$ | First-order reaction |
| $(1-\alpha)^2$ | $1/(1-\alpha)-1$ | Second-order reaction |
| $\alpha(1-\alpha)$ | $\ln[\alpha/(1-\alpha)]$ | Prout-Tompkins |
| $2\alpha^{1/2}$ | $\alpha^{1/2}$ | Power law ($n=1/2$) |
| $3\alpha^{2/3}$ | $\alpha^{1/3}$ | Power law ($n=1/3$) |
| $4\alpha^{3/4}$ | $\alpha^{1/4}$ | Power law ($n=1/4$) |
| $1$ | $\alpha$ | One-dimensional phase boundary |
| $2(1-\alpha)^{1/2}$ | $1(-1-\alpha)^{1/2}$ | Two-dimensional phase boundary |
| $3(1-\alpha)^{2/3}$ | $1-(1-\alpha)^{1/3}$ | Three-dimensional phase boundary |

and water vapor pressure is more complex at intermediate (7.6 torr) and higher water vapor pressures ($\geq$12.0 torr) when there is a change in the dehydration mechanism (Fig. 8). Variable-temperature X-ray diffraction (XRD) showed that at low water vapor pressures ($\leq$5.1 torr), the dehydrated phase was amorphous, while higher water vapor pressures ($\geq$12.0 torr) resulted in the formation of crystalline anhydrous γ-CBZ. Since water can act as a plasticizer, increasing the water vapor pressure resulted in an increase in the crystallization of γ-CBZ and a corresponding increase in the dehydration rate from 12 and 17 torr. Increasing the water vapor pressure further to 23 torr resulted in a decrease in the dehydration kinetics due to the

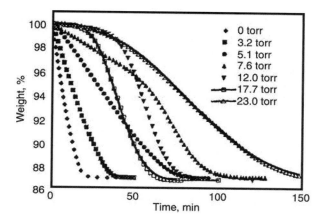

**Figure 8** Isothermal thermogravimetric analysis curves showing the dehydration of carbamazepine dihydrate at 44°C at controlled water vapor pressures. *Source*: From Ref. 32.

inhibitory effect of water vapor on the dehydration kinetics. The authors suggest that the direct crystallization of γ-CBZ is consistent with the Avrami-Erofeev model for nucleation and growth-controlled dehydration at higher vapor pressures. In this example, variable-temperature XRD nicely complemented the solid-state kinetic model in elucidating the dehydration reaction mechanism.

The temperature dependence of the reaction rate constant determined from Equation 13 is typically described by the Arrhenius equation:

$$\ln k = \ln A - \frac{E_a}{RT} \tag{15}$$

in which a plot of $\ln k$ versus $1/T$ yields the activation energy $E_a$ from the slope of the curve, and the frequency factor $A$ from the $y$-intercept. The Arrhenius plot may not be linear in cases in which the solvent is in different environments within the crystalline lattice or the mechanism of dehydration is temperature dependent. An example is Fenoprofen calcium dihydrate in which the activation energy was calculated to be 309 kJ/mol between 50°C and 60°C and 123 kJ/mol between 60°C and 80°C (33). The difference in activation energy was explained by differences in the location of the water molecules in the crystal lattice, the degree of hydrogen bonding between drug and water molecules, and the degree of crystallinity after loss of each mole of water. The dehydration of nedocromil magnesium pentahydrate also occurs in two steps associated with different activation energies (29). The first step corresponds to a loss of 4 mol of water and has an activation energy of 70 kJ/mol. The final mole of water is lost in the second step and has an activation energy of 121 kJ/mol.

Both dehydration steps were described by the Avrami-Erofeev equation, suggesting that the dehydration is nucleation controlled. Analysis of the single crystal structure showed that four of the water molecules were hydrogen bonded to each other, forming a tetrameric chain. The fifth water molecule was bonded to both a magnesium ion and a carboxylate oxygen atom and was thought to be more "tightly bound," thus requiring a higher activation barrier for dehydration. In addition, the activation energy for dehydration was found to decrease with decreasing particle size, presumably due to the greater surface area/volume ratio for smaller particles (29). Taylor and York reported a similar relationship between the activation energy and particle size fraction for the dehydration of trehalose dihydrate, which was thought to be attributed to the greater degree of disorder in the smaller particle size fraction since the material had been milled (34). Interestingly, for eprosartan mesylate dihydrate, the activation energy for dehydration was dependent not on particle size, but on the method of preparing the hydrated material (35).

As an alternative to the aforementioned kinetic analysis of isothermal data, additional methods based on nonisothermal DSC and TGA data have been developed, and there are several comprehensive reviews of these methods along with their shortcomings (27,30,31). Nonisothermal methods generally involve studying the desolvation reaction at various heating rates, $\phi$. The various methods used to calculate the Arrehenius parameters from nonisothermal data are an approximate form of the temperature integral that results from substituting

$$\frac{d\alpha}{dT} = \frac{1}{\phi}\frac{d\alpha}{dt}$$

and Equation 15 into Equation 13 (36,37):

$$g(\alpha) = \int_0^\alpha [f(\alpha)]^{-1}d\alpha = \frac{1}{\phi}\int_0^T k(T)dT = \frac{A}{\phi}\int_0^T \exp\left(-\frac{E}{RT}\right)dT \qquad (16)$$

Kinetic analyses from Equations 13 and 16 are called model-fitting approaches. Standard model-fitting approaches assume a constant mechanism throughout the reaction and therefore may not be applicable to solid-state reactions that can involve multiple reactions. As with many solid-state reactions, desolvation reactions can be complex, and in some cases, a single activation energy may not describe the process. Therefore, experimentally derived values for the Arrhenius parameters must be treated as empirical values unless there is auxiliary data to support the proposed mechanism (36). Model-free approaches to describing experimental kinetic data have also been developed. These model-free approaches have the advantage of being able to account for changes in the reaction mechanism during the course of the reaction (38) and have recently been applied to neotame monohydrate (39) and nedocromil sodium trihydrate (38).

## Characterization of the Amorphous (Glassy) State

Crystalline material consists of a highly structured lattice with a unit cell that repeats itself in three dimensions, whereas noncrystalline (amorphous) material is characterized by the absence of long-range order (40). Physical and chemical properties of amorphous material, such as solubility, vapor pressure, density, chemical stability, and hygroscopicity differ significantly from material in a crystalline state.

The characterization of a completely amorphous drug substance is important in those compounds for which the establishment of isolation conditions to give crystalline material is particularly difficult; therefore, the use of amorphous material in predevelopment or early development stages may be required. In some cases, development of the amorphous form of a compound may be of interest if the bioavailability of the crystalline form is unacceptably low due to solubility limitations. Compounds that are intended for development as a lyophilized or spray-dried product may also be totally amorphous. In these cases, characterization of the amorphous phase is critical to considerations of proper handling, storage, and processing conditions to ensure chemical and physical stabilization of the material.

One parameter used to characterize amorphous material is the glass transition ($T_g$), which represents the temperature below which the molecular mobility of a glassy amorphous solid is dramatically reduced and above which the amorphous material takes on a "rubbery" character with increases in the number and magnitude of molecular motions (41). Given that increased molecular mobility can lead to increased chemical reactivity and the propensity for a metastable amorphous material to crystallize over time, amorphous solids should be handled and stored well below the glass transition temperature, which makes accurate determinations of the $T_g$ imperative in preformulation and formulation development.

The glass transition can be determined using multiple thermal analysis techniques including DSC, modulated DSC (MDSC), thermal mechanical analysis, dynamic mechanical analysis, and dielectric analysis (40). However, DSC and MDSC are more commonly used in preformulation studies, and therefore their use will be the focus of this discussion.

The measurement of $T_g$ is based on changes in the material property that occur at the glass transition. DSC allows measurement of changes in the heat capacity of the amorphous material as it transitions from a glassy to a rubbery character. Often, the presence of extraneous thermal events such as enthalpic relaxation or moisture loss can confound the measurement of the $T_g$. Enthalpic relaxation originates from thermally induced atomic or molecular rearrangement at the glass transition, which results in structural relaxation toward equilibrium (42). Sample preparation for DSC requires a preconditioning step in which the material is heated to a temperature above its glass transition in order to remove any previous thermal history, followed by a cooling step to a temperature well below the $T_g$ and finally a subsequent heating step to measure the change in the heat capacity ($\Delta C_p$) and determine the $T_g$ (43). An example of this is shown in Figure 9, where the upper scan shows the change in heat capacity for a preconditioned sample. The lower scan represents an "aged" sample for which enthalpic relaxation that is obscuring the glass transition can be determined from the area under the endothermic transition.

Caution should be taken in the interpretation of DSC results in which a preconditioning step is used. Moisture in amorphous material can act as a plasticizer and profoundly reduce the apparent value for the $T_g$. Conventional DSC in which the sample is subjected to a heat/cool/reheat cycle can be used to determine the glass transition on material that has a significantly altered water content. Given the plasticizing effects of water and the fact that $T_g$ is lowered in the presence of water, determination of

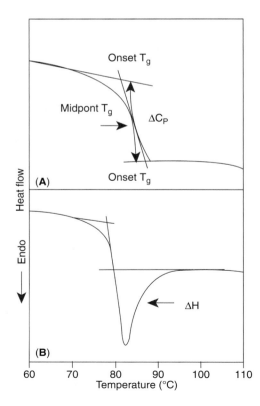

**Figure 9** The lower differential scanning calorimetry scan represents a sample that has not been preconditioned in which the $T_g$ is obscured by the enthalpic relaxation, while the upper scan shows the change in heat capacity at the $T_g$ for a preconditioned sample. *Source*: From Ref. 43.

$T_g$ in the absence of water may result in the actual values for $T_g$ being found. However, since amorphous materials are often hygroscopic and contain moisture, measurement of the $T_g$ without a preconditioning step may give a more relevant value.

MDSC offers a way of overcoming some of the limitations in the determination of $T_g$. Coleman and Craig have reviewed the use of MDSC in pharmaceutical thermal analysis (44). MDSC differs from conventional DSC wherein the sample is subjected to a more complex heating program incorporating a sinusoidal temperature modulation accompanied by an underlying linear heating ramp. Whereas DSC is only capable of measuring the total heat flow, MDSC provides the total heat flow, the nonreversible heat flow (kinetic component), and the reversible component (heat capacity component) heat flows. This results in improved resolution of overlapping transitions and increased sensitivity for the detection of weak transitions. Although MDSC is a powerful technique, it does come at the price of the number of experimental parameters (heating rate, oscillation amplitude, and period) that must be optimized to obtain accurate results. Underlying heating rates of 1°C/min to 5°C/min are typically used with the ideal heating rate, allowing at least four temperature oscillations to occur over the temperature range of the transition. The larger the magnitude of the oscillation temperature, the greater the sensitivity in detecting transitions; however, the oscillation amplitude must be small enough to allow adequate heat transfer within the sample. An oscillation period of 60 seconds is recommended, since longer periods require a lower heating rate to allow the minimum number of oscillations required for a transition and shorter periods often result in increased baseline noise.

Figures 10 and 11 illustrate the utility of MDSC in preformulation studies in which separation of thermal transitions into reversing and nonreversing signals allows the detection of overlapping thermal events. In Figure 10, the $T_g$, which is detected in the reversible signal, is separated from a broad dehydration endotherm, which is found in the nonreversing signal. The utility of MDSC in separating the $T_g$ from an overlapping enthalpic relaxation event can be seen in Figure 11, where the enthalpic relaxation transition occurs in the nonreversible signal and the glass transition is observed in the reversing signal. Above the glass transition, the increase in molecular mobility results in crystallization of the drug substance, as witnessed by the large nonreversible exotherm as confirmed by HSM.

Although characterization of partially amorphous materials is a considerable challenge, detection and quantification of amorphous content may be crucial to the understanding of drug product performance. Typical processing steps such as granulation, drying, milling, and compaction may give rise to partial or complete disruption of the crystal lattice. Additionally, the presence of impurities and the manner in which drug substance is recrystallized in the final step can also induce crystal defects, leading to

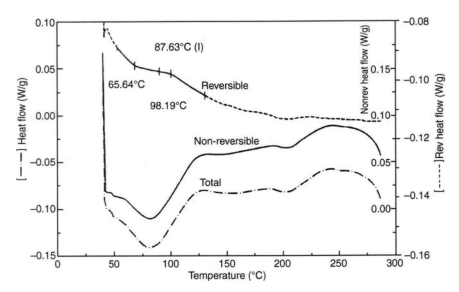

**Figure 10** The utility of modulated differential scanning calorimetry in separating out the glass transition from the dehydration thermal event in a single analysis is demonstrated. The glass transition is shown in the reversing heat signal and is clearly separated out from the dehydration endotherm seen in the total and nonreversing heat flows. *Source*: From Ref. 42.

amorphous regions. Lot-to-lot differences in amorphous content can lead to changes in processability and product performance, since the presence of amorphous material can potentially result in increased reactivity, increased dissolution rates, and the opportunity for solid-state transitions to occur. These physical changes in the drug product can lead to variability in bioavailability. Therefore the utility of thermal methods used to characterize the degree of crystallinity will be discussed along with some of the associated limitations.

DSC is a useful technique in which measurement of the heat of crystallization (45) or fusion (46) may be employed to quantitatively assess the amorphous content or the degree of crystal disruption. Several criteria need to be evaluated to determine whether DSC methods may be appropriate for a given compound. First, thermal events must be well resolved, and secondly, since heat flows in DSC are nonspecific and could be due, in part, to other processes such as decomposition or desolvation, a thorough understanding of the enthalpic events is essential for determining the source of the transition. If one is using the heat of crystallization in the calibration, one must also ensure that the compound undergoes 100% crystallization. In other words, for 100% amorphous material, the magnitude of the heat of crystallization should be equal but opposite in sign to the heat of fusion.

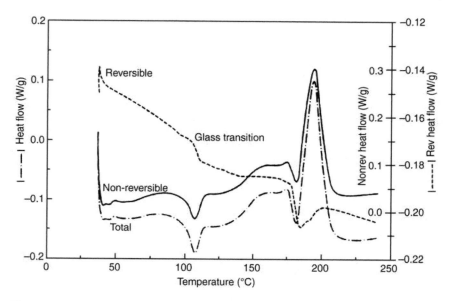

**Figure 11** Modulated differential scanning calorimetry is used to separate the $T_g$ from the enthalpic relaxation endotherm in a single analysis where the $T_g$ is shown in the reversing signal. The large exotherm shown in the nonreversing signal is attributed to crystallization of the amorphous material above its glass transition. *Source*: From Ref. 42.

Experimentally, one must establish DSC parameters such as sample weight, heating rate, and gas flow and consistently maintain these conditions for all analyses in order to obtain meaningful results. Using sucrose as a model compound, Saleki-Gerhardt et al. (45) were able to demonstrate a linear relationship between the percent disorder and the heat of crystallization (area under the exothermic recrystallization peak) for physical mixtures of amorphous and crystalline material. In applying the technique to quantitate the percentage of amorphous material in milled sucrose samples, there was a shift in the crystallization temperature, which required correction to allow a direct comparison between standards and sample. To make this correction, an equation describing free energy changes for crystallization processes that occur at temperatures other than at melting was modified to describe free energy changes for sucrose samples that recrystallized at a lower temperature than the standards. By making an assumption that entropy changes over the temperature range studied are negligible, the heat of crystallization could be corrected using the equation below:

$$\Delta H_{\mathrm{corr}} = (\Delta H_c \Delta T / T_c)(T / T_c) \tag{17}$$

where $\Delta H_{\mathrm{corr}}$ is the corrected heat of crystallization, $\Delta H_{\mathrm{c}}$ is the measured enthalpy of crystallization, $\Delta T$ is the temperature difference between the crystallization of standards and the milled samples, $T_{\mathrm{c}}$ is the crystallization temperature for standard mixtures, and $T$ is the crystallization temperature of milled samples. On utilizing this correction, the amorphous content determined from the DSC method was in good agreement with X-ray powder diffraction (XRPD).

In another application of DSC, Duddu and Grant (46) measured heats of fusion to establish a "disruption index" to quantitate the disorder introduced by the presence of an impurity as well as the "entropy of processing," which compared the amount of disorder of a processed sample to that of standard reference material (46).

Solution calorimetry represents another commonly used technique in the characterization of materials in which the heats of solution for amorphous and crystalline materials are used to quantitate the degree of crystallinity. This method takes advantage of the energy difference between crystalline and amorphous materials, with the sensitivity of the technique being dependent upon the magnitude of these energy differences. The percent crystallinity ($P_{\mathrm{c}}$) may be defined as

$$P_{\mathrm{c}} = 100 \left[ \frac{\Delta H_{\mathrm{S}}^{\mathrm{o}} - \Delta H_{\mathrm{a}}^{\mathrm{o}}}{\Delta H_{\mathrm{C}}^{\mathrm{o}} - \Delta H_{\mathrm{a}}^{\mathrm{o}}} \right] \tag{18}$$

where $\Delta H^{\circ}{}_{\mathrm{S}}$, $\Delta H^{\circ}{}_{\mathrm{C}}$, and $\Delta H^{\circ}{}_{\mathrm{a}}$ are the ideal heats of solution in a given solvent at infinite dilution for the sample, 100% crystalline standard and 100% amorphous standard, respectively. Several aspects must be considered when using heats of solution to characterize differences between amorphous and crystalline material. Heat of solution is a measure of total energy change, which may also include contributions from enthalpies associated with wetting or other physical processes that occur as a part of dissolution. One must assume that these contributions do not change as a function of crystal structure. In addition, one is faced with the challenge of obtaining 100% amorphous and crystalline materials where the heat of solution may vary from batch to batch depending on how the material was generated, the age of the material, and water content (47). One must identify an appropriate solvent in which solubility is not limiting and establish a linear relationship between the heat of solution and percent crystallinity. In situations where the relationship is nonlinear, getting a thorough understanding of the system one is characterizing cannot be overemphasized. For example, in solution calorimetry experiments of sodium warfarin, a nonlinear calibration curve relating the heat of solution to percent crystallinity for physical mixtures of crystalline and amorphous material was obtained (48). The nonlinearity was presumed to be due to the fact that the crystalline form of the compound exists as a clathrate containing isopropyl alcohol (IPA) and water, whereas these solvents are absent in amorphous form. It was suspected that there was a contribution to the heat of solution measurement from the interaction of IPA with water during the dissolution process. Indeed, corrections for the IPA content resulted in a linear relationship between the corrected heat of solution and percent crystallinity.

The limit of quantitation of amorphous material in predominantly crystalline solids is typically about 10% using methods such as DSC and XRPD. Since even minute quantities in amorphous content can influence the physical chemical properties of drug substance and hence product performance, analysis using these techniques does not always reveal lot-to-lot differences that may be due to small amounts of disorder. Several emerging thermal techniques are showing promising results with respect to sensitivity and may take on a greater role in the characterization of drug substances. Thermally stimulated current (TSC) has been used to characterize the amorphous phase by monitoring relaxations (molecular motions). Samples that have been compressed into a disk are subjected to an electric field at a fixed temperature, resulting in orientation of dipoles within the material. The dipoles are "trapped" in place by lowering the temperature, followed by a reheating step in which the thermal energy stimulates the relaxation of the trapped molecular segments, resulting in a depolarization current that can be measured as a function of temperature. Using TSC, the limit of detection for amorphous content in physical mixtures of amorphous and crystalline material has been demonstrated at approximately 1% (49).

Isothermal microcalorimetry is another highly sensitive technique that has demonstrated detection of amorphous material at or below 1% (50). Although microcalorimetry is $10^4$ times more sensitive than DSC and has the ability to detect temperature changes as small as $10^{-6}°C$, it does require that the material crystallize/recrystallize in the presence of elevated humidities or organic vapors and therefore may have limited applicability. From an experimental standpoint, the environment within the sample cell may be controlled by the use of ampoules containing saturated salt solutions or organic solvent, or alternatively the microcalorimeter may be fitted with a commercially available gas flow cell (51,52). The advantage of placing the vapor source within the sample cell is that the heat flow associated with the vaporization of solvent is approximately equal but opposite in sign to that of the heat of wetting of the sample. Therefore, these signals do not produce a large interference that otherwise might obscure the heat of crystallization response (53). The sample cell is first equilibrated to a constant temperature and then lowered into the measurement position within the microcalorimeter. The heat flow ($dQ/dt$) or power associated with the enthalpy of crystallization versus time is measured. Using standard mixtures of amorphous and crystalline material, the integrated area under the power versus time curve for the heat of crystallization may be used to determine the amorphous content in the sample. The sensitivity of isothermal microcalorimetry allows the detection of subtle energetic differences that may take place at the surface of particles due to processes such as milling. The rate and extent of recrystallization are dependent on the sample size (Fig. 12), temperature, and relative humidity. In the example of spray-dried lactose, a lag was observed during which time the powder in the cell is saturated, followed by a cooperative crystallization process. The delay in crystallization may be advantageous since the crystallization event is well resolved from any baseline perturbations due to the lowering of the sample cell into the measurement position and/or any signal due to wetting of the sample at the onset of the experiment.

Microthermal analysis presents another source to probe the nature of surface changes in drug substance. In this method, a combination of atomic force microscopy and thermal analysis allows the generation of the topological image and measurement of the thermal conductivity with thermal imaging at micron-to-submicron resolution. The technique was applied to a model compound, indometacin, in which amorphous regions could be differentiated from crystalline domains; however, there were some difficulties in the interpretation of data, partly due to the lack of experience with this emerging technique (54).

## CHARACTERIZATION OF THERMAL DECOMPOSITION

The combination of DSC, MDSC, TGA, and HSM is routinely used in preformulation studies in the characterization of thermally induced

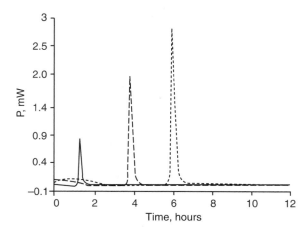

**Figure 12** Determination of amorphous content in spray-dried lactose by microcalorimetry shows that the rate and extent of recrystallization is dependent on sample size. With increasing sample size, the lag time for recrystallization to occur increases. *Source*: From Ref. 50.

decomposition/volatization processes. The ability to interface spectroscopic techniques such as FT-IR spectroscopy or MS to thermal instruments for structural confirmation adds a powerful element to these thermal analysis methods, allowing the generation of much information with very little expenditure of drug substance or time.

Generally, the first step is to obtain the DSC thermogram for a new chemical entity. The events observed in the DSC analysis were used to establish the temperature range for the TGA. The analyst looks for a temperature correlation between any weight loss events in the TGA scan versus the thermal transitions in the DSC thermogram. Often decomposition with volatization of the degradation products occurs in a step-wise fashion in the TGA analysis, and if the event occurs prior to compound melting, an exothermic transition is often observed in DSC. HSM may then be utilized to obtain a visual image of the events by placing a small amount of drug substance on a microscope slide, adding a drop of immersion oil, and placing a cover slip over the sample. The slide is positioned on a stage that is thermally controlled via a microprocessor and subjected to a heating program. The decomposition may be observed visually as discoloration of the material, or in the case of volatile decomposition byproducts, the evolution of gas from the crystals may be evident. A low heating rate such as 1°C/min to 5°C/min may be necessary to allow complete observation of the events. Technological advancements in HSM in the area of visual imaging have enhanced the capability to visualize rapid changes as a function of temperature and process, and store these images digitally (55). Given the different sample conditions in DSC, TGA, and HSM, such as pressure and atmosphere, there may be differences in the temperature at which decomposition occurs across methods. There are instruments that combine DSC and HSM, which will allow a single analysis and remove any differences due to experimental conditions.

As previously mentioned, the ability to interface thermal techniques with spectroscopic analysis has added significant value to these methods for the confirmation of structural changes. For example, DSC, TGA, and FT-IR microspectroscopy combined with a thermal analyzer was used to characterize the two-step dehydration process of lisinopril, which was followed by an intramolecular cyclization reaction, which was confirmed through structural information from FT-IR spectroscopy (56).

The use of MDSC provides insight into thermal events that are due solely to decomposition and also those transitions that may be a combination of decomposition and other processes. Figure 13 shows an MDSC thermogram of a compound that undergoes thermal decomposition with a large exothermic transition occurring at ca. 200°C in the total heat flow. Since the transition is due solely to decomposition, the transition occurs in the irreversible signal, with no significant events in the nonreversing signal. Alternatively, Figure 14 illustrates an example of a compound that

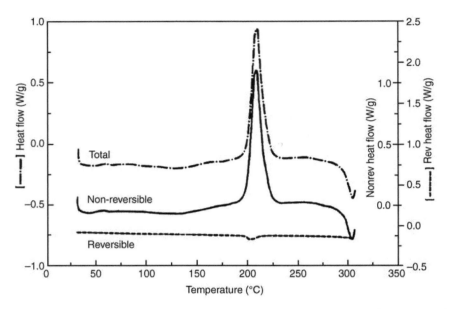

**Figure 13** Modulated differential scanning calorimetry thermogram of a compound that undergoes thermal decomposition at 200°C as demonstrated by the large exotherm in the nonreversing signal. *Source*: From Ref. 42.

undergoes simultaneous melting with decomposition where the endothermic melting event can be seen in the reversing signal and the exothermic decomposition is seen in the nonreversing heat flow. A combination of thermal techniques was used to characterize the compound shown in Figure 12. As shown in Figure 15, an overlay of the DSC analysis with the TGA thermogram shows a correlation between the exotherm at 216°C and a step-weight loss of 6.8% between 198°C and 240°C. HSM of the compound resulted in violent evolution of gas originating from the crystals also in the same temperature range. Analysis of the samples by TGA-FT-IR confirmed carbon dioxide and water as the evolved gases. Additional information on the heated samples obtained by NMR and liquid chromatography (LC)/MS indicated the formation of a dimeric species. This information coupled with the thermal data completed the picture and together helped confirm the mechanism of degradation. The proposed degradation route involves the loss of a water molecule followed by an intramolecular rearrangement and a series of reactions with loss of carbon dioxide prior to dimer formation. The TGA-FT-IR results were consistent with the loss of these gases, and in addition, the weight loss by TGA is consistent, since for every dimer formed, carbon dioxide and water totaling 62 mass units would be lost, which correlates with the 6.8% weight loss for that molecule. In this particular case,

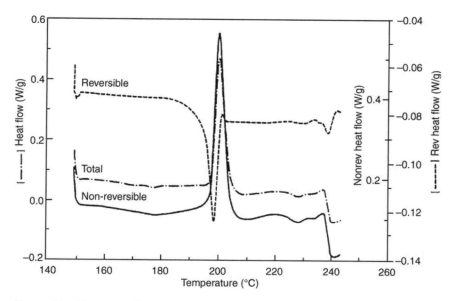

**Figure 14** Example of a compound that undergoes simultaneous melting with decomposition where the endothermic melting event can be seen in the reversing signal and the exothermic decomposition is seen in the nonreversing heat flow. *Source*: From Ref. 42.

useful information was gained in thermal analysis. However, these techniques alone did not solve the puzzle, but rather the use of thermal methods with complementary techniques was the key in the investigation.

## Chemical Stability Studies

Evaluation of chemical reactivity of new crystal forms in preformulation studies typically involves solution stability studies, and solid-state stability of drug substance alone and in the presence of excipients. Information gained from these studies, such as kinetic and thermodynamic parameters, is useful in the determination of reaction mechanisms and selection of formulation excipients and appropriate processing conditions to allow the manufacture of a stable product with an acceptable shelf life.

The traditional approach to stability studies involves preparation of numerous samples, which are stored at accelerated temperatures and/or humidity conditions. The stability of the samples may be monitored over a period of weeks to months, typically by using stability-indicating high performance liquid chromatography (HPLC) methods that allow the quantification of the loss of the parent compound and appearance of degradation products. In the case of excipient compatibility studies, there are often

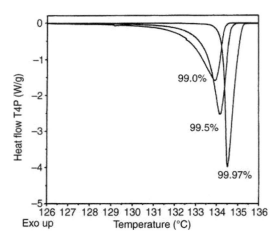

**Figure 15** DSC thermograms for phenacetin at three purity levels. *Source*: From Ref. 71, courtesy of TA Instruments.

difficulties in sample extraction, and in some cases, interferences of the excipient in the HPLC method may be problematic. In general, this approach to evaluating compound stability is very labor-and time-intensive and requires relatively large quantities of drug substance, which may not be readily available at an early stage of development. In addition, it is quite often the case that studies performed at accelerated conditions are not representative of processes at relevant temperatures. Changes in reaction mechanisms or competing reaction mechanisms often result in nonlinear Arrhenius relationships (log $k$ vs. $1/T$), making extrapolation across large temperature ranges invalid, leading to errors in predicting stability rate constants at ambient temperatures.

Furthermore, it is often impractical to store crystal forms that may be present as a hydrate or solvate at elevated temperatures due to the potential for loss of the solvent and thus physical instability. Thermal methods such as isothermal microcalorimetry and DSC can provide alternatives, or be used as complementary techniques, to traditional stability methods, with a much faster turnaround time and consumption of considerably less drug substance.

## Isothermal Microcalorimetry

Isothermal microcalorimetry, which can detect heat changes as small as 0.1 μW, has the sufficient sensitivity to allow slow reactions to be studied at ambient temperatures. The technique can be applied to both solution and solid-state stability studies and permits control of environmental conditions such as pH, oxygen, relative humidity, and light. Wilson et al. (57) presented general procedures to determine thermodynamic and kinetic parameters from power–time data from isothermal microcalorimetry experiments.

Transformation of kinetic equations as they may be used to fit microcalorimetric data is based on the premise that the total heat evolved ($Q$) during the reaction may be described by Equation 19:

$$Q = A_o \Delta H \tag{19}$$

where $A_o$ equals the total number of moles of material reacted and $\Delta H$ is equal to the molar change in enthalpy for the reaction. Therefore the heat evolved ($q$) at any time $t$ is determined by

$$q = x\Delta H \tag{20}$$

where $x$ equals the number of moles reacted at any time $t$. Equation 20 may be substituted into any general rate equation ($dx/dt$) to provide an expression in terms of the heat flow ($dq/dt$). Table 3 presents a summary of transformed equations that may typically apply to solid state and solution reactions

**Table 3**  Transformed Kinetic Expressions for Use in Microcalorimetry Stability Studies

| Reaction pathway | Kinetic rate equation | Transformed kinetic rate equation |
|---|---|---|
| $A - B$ | $\dfrac{dx}{dt} = k(A - x)^m$ | $\dfrac{dq}{dt} = \Delta Hk\left(A - \dfrac{q}{\Delta H}\right)^m$ |
| $A - B - C$ | $\dfrac{dx}{dt} = k(A - x)^m x$ $(B - x)^n$ | $\dfrac{dq}{dt} = \Delta Hk\left(A - \dfrac{q}{\Delta H}\right)^m$ $x\left(B - \dfrac{q}{\Delta H}\right)^n$ |
| $A \Longleftrightarrow B$ | $\dfrac{dx}{dt} = k\left(\dfrac{A}{x_e}\right)$ | $\dfrac{dq}{dt} = kA\left(\Delta H - \dfrac{q}{x_e}\right)$ |
| $A - B \Longleftrightarrow C$ | $\dfrac{dx}{dt} = k_1(A - x)^m$ $x(B - x)$ | $\dfrac{dq}{dt} = k_1(A\Delta H - q)$ $(B\Delta H - q)(k_{-1}q)$ |
| Ng equation | $\dfrac{dx}{dt} = Ak\left(\dfrac{x}{A}\right)^m$ $\left(1 - \dfrac{x}{A}\right)^n$ | $\dfrac{dq}{dt} = Ak\Delta H\left(\dfrac{q}{A\Delta H}\right)^m$ $\left(1 - \dfrac{q}{A\Delta H}\right)^n$ |
| Auto-catalytic | $\dfrac{dx}{dt} = k(A - x)$ $\times (x_c + x)$ | $\dfrac{dq}{dt} = k(A\Delta H - q)$ $\times (x_c\Delta H + q)$ |

studied using microcalorimetry. By using the integrated form of the transformed kinetic rate equation and an iterative process using mathematical worksheet software (e.g., Mathcad™ PTC, Needham, Massachusetts, U.S.A.), the reaction parameters may be obtained using the calorimetric data (57).

Solution reactions typically follow zero-, first-, or second-order kinetics. Therefore treatment and interpretation of solution kinetic data are typically more straightforward than solid-state kinetics, which are often described by fractional or autocatalytic rate constants (58). The Ng equation is used to describe solid–solid interactions in a two-phase system and is shown below:

$$\frac{d\alpha}{dt} = k\alpha^{1-x}(1 - \alpha_e)^{1-y} \tag{21}$$

where $\alpha$ is the fraction of the reaction that has occurred at time $t$, $k$ is the rate constant, and $x$ and $y$ are the constants that characterize the reaction mechanism. In the case where $x = 1$ and $y = 0$, the reaction is described by a first-order rate law; this and other reaction mechanisms are summarized in Table 2. The rate-determining step in solid-state reactions may be controlled by diffusion, chemical reaction, or nucleation. The Ng equation, once transformed into a calorimetric equation, was applied to study the solid-state degradation of L-ascorbic acid as a function of the quantity of water added (57). Results revealed useful mechanistic information from the microcalorimetry experiment. Additional work from the same group demonstrated the ability of microcalorimetry to study both chemical and physical transformations (e.g., complexation).

Isothermal calorimetry has clearly demonstrated its utility in the pharmaceutical industry, as in the early work of Pikal and Dellerman (59), who characterized the solution and solid-state reactions of cephalosporins with the ability to detect decomposition rates as low as 1%/yr over the course of a 24-hour experiment.

Microcalorimetry was successfully employed in excipient compatibility studies to characterize the solid-state browning reaction between lactose and the primary amine functionality of an HIV protease inhibitor (60). Results from the microcalorimetry experiment were obtained within a week and indicated an autocatalytic reaction mechanism. The photoreactivity of pharmaceutical solids and solutions of nifedipine and L-ascorbic acid was successfully studied using an isothermal microcalorimeter equipped with an irradiation cell (61).

While isothermal microcalorimetry has gained in popularity due to its high-sensitivity measurements and high throughput at relevant temperatures, it is more generally used as a complementary technique due to several limitations. The overall response (power output) from the instrument is a composite of the reaction concentration, the thermodynamic parameters, and kinetic rate constants. A reaction that may proceed very quickly from a kinetic perspective but having a low enthalpy of reaction may give a comparable response to a slow reaction with a large enthalpy value. Therefore caution must be exercised in not misinterpreting the information obtained and ensure that the results are relevant to the overall stability of the product/mixture.

## DSC and TGA

DSC, DTA, and TGA have also been used to monitor the kinetics and thermodynamics of decomposition processes for drug substance alone and in the presence of excipients. Various software packages are available to quantitatively evaluate kinetic studies performed using thermal analysis and to calculate the activation energy, preexponential factor, and rate constant from either dynamic or isothermal experiments (62). The Borchardt and Daniels (63,64) method is useful for simple first-order processes in which kinetic parameters may be obtained in a single run. Whereas the ASTM E698 kinetics approach based on the method of Ozawa (65) is more appropriate for complex reactions. Isothermal methods may be used in the case of *n*th order reactions and particularly autocatalytic exothermic reactions, and in general, data interpretation may be more straightforward since there are fewer experimental variables.

DSC, DTA, and TGA have been used to some extent in early screening studies to evaluate drug–excipient compatibility, with the goal of obtaining rapid results with minimal drug substance. Binary mixtures of drug–excipient are typically subjected to a programmed temperature ramp, and the resultant thermograms are compared to the thermograms of the individual components. If there are no interactions, one should observe a thermogram that is a combination of the contribution of the thermal transitions observed alone for each drug and excipient. However, if interactions do occur, new thermal events are observed that deviate from the original thermograms. While the lack of interactions is informative and would suggest that formulators may proceed with a particular excipient in formulation activities, the interpretation of data that suggest incompatibility is not nearly as straightforward. One assumes that the two components are not miscible with each other and other physical interactions are not present, which is rarely the case. Some degree of miscibility will typically result in melting point depression or the appearance of a new transition that may represent a eutectic mixture, solid solution, etc., making interpretation difficult. In these cases, supportive techniques such as XRPD, FT-IR, HSM, and HPLC may be required to aid in understanding the nature of the interactions and determine whether they are relevant in formulation development. Additionally, the sensitivity of

traditional DSC requires high temperatures in both scanning and isothermal modes in order to detect incompatibilities/decomposition, which is
neither realistic nor relevant to formulation processes and typical storage
conditions. Furthermore, environmental conditions such as humidity,
which may be important in the case of hydrolytic degradation processes,
cannot be controlled in a DSC experiment, and variables such as heating
rate, pan configuration, and particle size can also influence results
obtained by DSC. Given these limitations, DSC has not gained wide
acceptance as a stand-alone technique in early preformulation screening to
determine excipient incompatibilities.

More recently, high-sensitivity DSC has been used to evaluate drug
–excipient interactions using a step-wise temperature program to allow
evaluation under isothermal conditions for a period of time before ramping
up to the next temperature (66). Incompatibilities were detected as the heat
flow deviated from the baseline value. Results gave comparable results to
those obtained in long-term stability studies.

## Purity Determination

The use of DSC for purity determination has been reviewed extensively
(27,31,67–70). This method is based on the assumption that small amounts
of an impurity will depress the melting point of a material if the two components form a eutectic. Thus, with increasing amounts of impurity, the
melting range is broader and the liquidus temperature $(T_L)$ of an impure
solid decreases with respect to the melting temperature $(T_o)$ of a perfectly
pure material. The effect of increasing impurity concentration on the DSC
curves for phenacetin is shown in Figure 16. The "melting" point depression
that results from low impurity levels can be better understood by looking at
a theoretical phase diagram for a two-component system that forms a
eutectic (Fig. 17). Pure solid A and B melt at $T_{o,A}$ and $T_{o,B}$, respectively. At
$d$, the impure solid has composition $x_1$. As the solid is heated along isopleth
$abcd$ to $c$, the eutectic temperature, $T_e$, is reached. At this temperature, all of
component B "melts," leaving pure solid A in equilibrium with a liquid of
composition $x_e$. As the temperature increases toward $b$, the liquid in equilibrium with pure solid A becomes increasingly rich in A as more of solid A
"melts."

Above $b$, only liquid of composition $x_1$ exists. If it is assumed that $\Delta H_{o,A}$
is constant in the temperature range $T$ to $T_o$ (the melting temperature of the
pure component), then the equilibrium between pure solid and an ideal liquid
of mole fraction $X_A$ can be expressed by the following equation:

$$\ln(X_A) = -\frac{\Delta H_{o,A}}{R}\left(\frac{1}{T} - \frac{1}{T_o}\right) \tag{22}$$

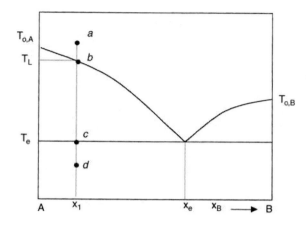

**Figure 16** Theoretical phase diagram showing a two-component system that forms a eutectic.

Equation 22 can be expressed as:

$$T = T_o - \frac{RT_o^2 X_B}{\Delta H_{o,A}} \tag{23}$$

if the following additional assumptions are made: (*i*) $X_A + X_B = 1$, therefore $\ln X_A = \ln (1 - X_B)$; (*ii*) the fraction of impurity is small, $X_B \ll 1$, therefore ln

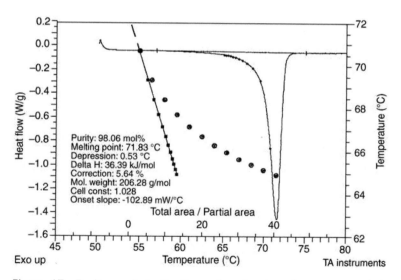

**Figure 17** Purity analysis for ibuprofen showing the uncorrected (*circles*) and corrected (*squares*) plots of temperature versus 1/F (total area/partial area) overlaid with the melting endotherm (head flow versus temperature). *Source*: From Ref. 71, courtesy of TA Instruments.

$(1 - X_B) \approx - X_B$; and (iii) $T$ approaches $T_o$ when $X_B \ll 1$, therefore

$$\frac{1}{T} - \frac{1}{T_o} = \frac{T_o - T}{T T_o} \approx \frac{T_o - T}{T_o^2}$$

In addition, it is assumed that the sample does not decompose during melting.

As shown for phenacetin, "melting" of an impure substance can occur over a broad temperature range and typically results in "tailing" in the DSC curve (Fig. 16). The conventional approach to purity determination by DSC requires an estimation of the molten liquid fraction, $F$, at various temperatures along the melting endotherm. The value of $F$ at a given $T$ is determined from the DSC trace as the partial area up to $T$ divided by the total area. In practice, only the first portion of the melting endotherm is used for analysis with $F$ values over a range of 0.1 to 0.5 (27,31). The impurity concentration, $X_B$, is determined from plots of $T$ versus $1/F$ according to the following relationship:

$$T = T_o - \frac{RT_o^2 X_B}{\Delta H_{o,A}} \frac{1}{F} \tag{24}$$

Eq. 24 is often referred to as the modified van't Hoff equation. A graphic plot of $T$ versus $1/F$ should in theory give a straight line with a slope of $(-RT_o^2 X_B/\Delta H_{o,A})$, from which $X_B$ can be determined if the values of $T_o$ and $\Delta H_{o,A}$ are known.

Despite the narrow range of temperature and $F$ values used in DSC purity analysis, plots of $T$ versus $1/F$ typically show an upward curvature, as shown for ibuprofen in Figure 17. The degree of departure from linearity increases with increasing levels of impurity (31). Factors such as errors in baseline estimation (or an underestimation of the amount of melting that has occurred), the formation of a solid solution, and nonequilibrium conditions have been given as reasons for the nonlinearity in $T$ versus $1/F$ plots. The latter two factors are a direct violation of the assumptions made in the derivation of Equations 23 and 24. Errors in baseline estimation can result from thermal lags or gradients between the sensor and sample (71).

Various methods have been developed to correct for the observed nonlinearity. These methods have been discussed in detail by others (31,67). One method applies a correction factor, $x$, to both the numerator and denominator in the calculation of $F$ as shown below:

$$\frac{1}{F_n} = \frac{A + x}{a_n + x} \tag{25}$$

where $A$ is the total area and $a$ and $F$ are the $n$th partial area and $F$ value, respectively. Various software programs frequently determine the value of $x$ that produces a linear profile. The correction is reported as $(100x/A)\%$. Figure 18 shows the correction for ibuprofen.

Joy et al. reviewed the accuracy of DSC purity measurements and found that there was $a \pm 20\%$ agreement in the impurity levels determined by DSC and impurity values determined by other methods or calculated from the composition of a known mixture (72). Samples suspected of solid solution formation or incomplete solubility in the melt were not included in the analysis.

Several experimental factors such as sample size and heating rate can be optimized to minimize the effects of nonequilibrium on the nonlinearity of the $T$ versus $1/F$ plots. In general, for best results, slow heating rates and small sample sizes should be used. Van Dooren found that the upper limit of heating rate is 3.0°C/min (68). TA Instruments suggests that for good purity measurements, optimal sample sizes of 1.7 mg ($\pm 0.3$ mg) and scan rates of 0.5°C/min should be used with even smaller sample sizes and slower heating rates if $\Delta H_{fus}$ is large and the purity levels are $> 99.5\%$, respectively (73). In addition, DSC purity determinations are limited to small amounts of impurity. The upper limit suggested by TA Instruments is $< 2$ mole% (73).

## ACKNOWLEDGMENTS

Denette K. Murphy would like to thank Drs. Raymond P. Scaringe, Rodrguez-Hornedo N, and Roxana Schlam for their many helpful comments and suggestions.

## REFERENCES

1. Byrn SR, Ralph PR, Joseph SG. Solid-state Chemistry of Drugs. 2nd ed. West Lafayette: SSCI Inc, 1999:574.
2. Brittain HG. Polymorphism in Pharmaceutical Solids. New York: Marcel Dekker, 1999.
3. Haleblian J, McCrone W. Pharmaceutical applications of polymorphism. J Pharm Sci 1969; 58(8):911–929.
4. Bernstein J. Polymorphism in Molecular Crystals. International Union of Crystallography Monographs on Crystallography 14. Oxford: Oxford University Press, 2002:410.
5. Yu L, Reutzel SM, Stephenson GA. Physical characterization of polymorphic drugs: an integrated characterization strategy. Pharm Sci Technol Today 1998; 1(3):118–27.
6. Rodríguez-Spong B, Price CP, Jayasankar A, Matzger AJ, Rodríguez-Hornedo N. General principles of pharmaceutical solid polymorphism: a supramolecular perspective. Adv Drug Delivery Rev 2004; 56(3):241–74.
7. Burger A, Ramberger R. On the polymorphism of pharmaceuticals and other molecular crystals. I. Theory of thermodynamic rules. Mikrochimica Acta 1979; 2(3–4):259–71.

8.  Burger A, Ramberger R. On the polymorphism of pharmaceuticals and other molecular crystals. II. Applicability of thermodynamic rules. Mikrochimica Acta 1979; 2(3–4):273–316.

9.  Burger A. Thermodynamic and other aspects of the polymorphism of drugs. Pharm Int 1982; 3(5):158–63.

10. Grunenberg A, Henck JO, Siesler HW. Theoretical derivation and practical application of energy/temperature diagrams as an instrument in preformulation studies of polymorphic drug substances. Int J Pharm 1996; 129 (147–58).

11. Yu L, Stephenson GA, Mitchell CA, et al. Thermochemistry and conformational polymorphism of a hexamorphic crystal system. J Am Chem Soc 2000; 122(4):585–91.

12. Yu L. Inferring thermodynamic stability relationship of polymorphs from melting data. J Pharm Sci 1995; 84(8):966–74.

13. Richardson MJ. The derivation of thermodynamic properties by DSC: free energy curves and phase stability. Thermochim Acta 1993; 229:1–14.

14. Van Hecke GR, Kaji K, Sorai M. Heat capacity of the discotic mesogen, 2,3,6,7,10,11–hexa-n-octanoyloxytriphenylene: a complex solid-state polymorphism. Mol Cryst Liq Cryst 1986; 136(2–4):197–220.

15. McCrone WC. Fusion Methods in Chemical Microscopy. New York: Interscience Publishers, Inc., 1957.

16. Behme RJ, Brooke D. Heat of fusion measurement of a low melting polymorph of carbamazepine that undergoes multiple-phase changes during differential scanning calorimetry analysis. J Pharm Sci 1991; 80(10):986–90.

17. Giron D. Thermal analysis and calorimetric methods in the characterisation of polymorphs and solvates. Thermochim Acta 1995; 248:1–59.

18. Gu CH, Grant DJW. Estimating the relative stability of polymorphs and hydrates from heats of solution and solubility data. J Pharm Sci 2001; 90(9): 1277–87.

19. Byrn SR, Lin CT. The effect of crystal packing and defects on desolvation of hydrate crystals of caffeine and L-(-)-1,4 cyclohexane-1–alanine. J Am Chem Soc 1976; 98:4004–5.

20. Lin CT, Byrn SR. Desolvation of solvated organic crystals. Mol Cryst Liq Cryst 1979; 50:99–104.

21. Taylor LS, York P. Characterization of the phase transitions of trehalose dihydrate on heating and subsequent dehydration. J Pharm Sci 1998; 87(3): 347–55.

22. Giron D. Contribution of thermal methods and related techniques to the rational development of pharmaceuticals part 1. Pharm Sci Technol Today 1998; 1(5):191–9.

23. Morris KR, Rodríguez-Hornedo N. Hydrates. In: Swarbrick J, ed. Encyclopedia of Pharmaceutical Technology. New York: Marcel Dekker, Inc., 1993.

24. TA Instruments. DSC 2920 Differential Scanning Calorimeter Operator's Manual. New Castle: TA Instruments, 1995.

25. Griesser UJ, Burger A. The effect of water vapor pressure on desolvation kinetics of caffeine 4/5-hydrate. Int J Pharm 1995; 120:83–93.

26. Suzuki E, Shirotani K, Tsuda Y, Sekiguchi K. Studies on methods of particle size reduction of medicinal compound: XXIII. Water content and dehydration behavior of crystalline caffeine hydrate. Chem Pharm Bull 1985; 33:5028–35.

27. Wendlandt WW. Thermal analysis. In: Winefordner IM, ed. Chemical Analysis: a Series on Monographs in Analytical Chemistry and Its Applications. 3rd ed. Vol. 19. New York: John Wiley & Sons, 1964:814.

28. Morris KR. Structural aspects of hydrates and solvates. In: Brittain HG, ed. Polymorphism in Pharmaceutical Solids. New York: Marcel Dekker, Inc., 1999.

29. Zhu H, Grant DJW. Dehydration behavior of nedocromil magnesium pentahydrate. Int J Pharm 2001; 215:251–62.

30. Monkhouse DC, Van Campen L. Solid-state reactions—theoretical and experimental aspects. Drug Dev Ind Pharm 1984; 10(8–9):1175–276.

31. Ford JL, Timmins P. Pharmaceutical thermal analysis techniques and applications. In: Rubinstein MH, ed. Ellis Horwood Series in Pharmaceutical Technology. Chichester: Ellis Horwood Limited, 1989:313.

32. Han J, Suryanarayanan R. Influence of environmental conditions on the kinetics and mechanism of dehydration of carbamazepine dihydrate. Pharm Dev Technol 1998; 3(4):587–96.

33. Zhu H, Xu J, Varlashkin P, Long S, Kidd C. Dehydration, hydration behavior, and structural analysis of fenoprofen calcium. J Pharm Sci 2001; 90(7):845–59.

34. Taylor LS, York P. Effect of particle size and temperature on the dehydration kinetics of trehalose dihydrate. Int J Pharm 1998; 167:215–21.

35. Sheng J, Venkatesh GM, Duddu SP, Grant DJW. Dehydration behavior of eprosartan dihydrate. J Pharm Sci 1999; 88(10):1021–29.

36. Vyazovkin S, Wight CA. Isothermal and noniosthermal reaction kinetics in solids: in search of ways toward consensus. J Phys Chem 1997; 101:8279–8284.

37. Vyazovkin S, Wight CA. Kinetics in solids. Annu Rev Phys Chem 1997; 48: 125–49.

38. Zhou D, Schmitt EA, Zhang GGZ, et al. Model-free treatment of the dehydration kinetics of nedocromil sodium trihydrate. J Pharm Sci 2003; 92(7): 1367–76.

39. Dong Z, Salsbury JS, Zhou D, et al. Dehydration kinetics of neotame monohydrate. J Pharm Sci 2002; 91(6):1423–31.

40. Foreman J, Sauerbrunn SR, Marcozzi CL. Exploring the sensitivity of thermal analysis techniques to the glass transition. TA Instruments, Application Note TA-082.

41. Hancock BC, Zografi G. Characterization and significance of the amorphous state in pharmaceutical systems. J Pharm Sci 1997; 86:1–11.

42. Rabel SR, JA Jona, Maurin MB. Applications of modulated differential scanning calorimetry in preformulation studies. J Pharm Biomed Anal 1999; 21: 339–45.

43. Shamblin SL, Zografi G. Enthalpy relaxation in binary amorphous mixtures containing sucrose. Pharm Res 1998; 15(12):1828–34.

44. Coleman NJ, Craig DQM. Modulated temperature differential scanning calorimetry: a novel approach to pharmaceutical thermal analysis. Int J Pharm 1996; 135:13–29.

45.  Saleki-Gerhardt A, Ahlneck C, Zografi G. Assessment of disorder in crystalline solids. Int J Pharm 1994; 101:237–47.

46.  Duddu SP, Grant DJW. The use of thermal analysis in the assessment of crystal disruption. Thermochim Acta 1995; 248:131–45.

47.  Pikal MJ, Lukes AL, Lang JE, Gaines K. Quantitative crystallinity determinations for β–lactam antibiotics by solution calorimetry: correlations with stability. J Pharm Sci 1978; 67(6):767–73.

48.  Gao D, Rytting JH. Use of solution calorimetry to determine the extent of crystallinity of drugs and excipients. Int J Pharm 1997; 151(2):183–92.

49.  Venkatesh GM, Barnett ME, Owusu-Fordjour C, Galop M. Detection of low levels of the amorphous phase in crystalline pharmaceutical materials by thermally stimulated current spectrometry. Pharm Res 2001; 18(1):98–103.

50.  Briggner LE, Buckton G, Bystrom K, Darcy P. The use of isothermal microcalorimetry in the study of changes in crystallinity induced during the processing of powders. Int J Pharm 1994; 105(2):125–35.

51.  Lehto VP, Laine E. Simultaneous determination of the heat and the quantity of vapor sorption using a novel microcalorimetric method. Pharm Res 2000; 17(6): 701–6.

52.  Buckton G, Dove JW, Davies P. Isothermal microcalorimetry and inverse phase gas chromatography to study small changes in powder surface properties. Int J Pharm 1999; 193(1):13–9.

53.  Ahmed H, Buckton G, Rawlins DA. The use of isothermal microcalorimetry in the study of small degrees of amorphous content of a hydrophobic powder. Int J Pharm 1996; 130(2):195–201.

54.  Royall PG, Kett VL, Andrews CS, Craig DQM. Identification of crystalline and amorphous regions in low molecular weight materials using microthermal analysis. J Phys Chem B 2001; 105(29):7021–6.

55.  Vitez IM, Newman AW, Davidovich M, Kiesnowski C. The evolution of hot-stage microscopy to aid solid-state characterizations of pharmaceutical solids. Thermochim Acta 1998; 324(1–2):187–96.

56.  Wang SL, Lin SY, Chen TF. Thermal-dependent dehydration process and intramolecular cyclization of lisinopril dihydrate in the solid state. Chem Pharm Bull 2000; 48(12):1890–3.

57.  Wilson RJ, Beezer AE, Mitchell JC, Loh W. Determination of thermodynamic and kinetic parameters from isothermal heat conduction microcalorimetry: application to long-term reaction studies. J Phys Chem 1995; 99:7108–13.

58.  Ng WL. Thermal decomposition in the solid state. Aust J Chem 1975; 281169–78.

59.  Pikal MJ, Dellerman KM. Stability testing of pharmaceuticals by high-sensitivity isothermal calorimetry at 25°C: cephalosporins in the solid and aqueous solution states. Int J Pharm 1989; 50(3):233–52.

60.  Vickery RD, Maurin MB. Utility of microcalorimetry in the characterization of the browning reaction. J Pharm Biomed Anal 1999; 20:385–8.

61.  Lehto VP, Salonen J, Laine E. Real time detection of photoreactivity in pharmaceutical solids and solutions with isothermal microcalorimetry. Pharm Res 1999; 16(3):368–73.

62. A review of DSC kinetics methods. New Castle: TA Instruments, Application Note TA-073.
63. Borchardt HJ, Daniels FJ. The application of differential thermal analysis to the study of reaction kinetics. J Am Chem Soc 1957; 79(1):41–6.
64. Swarin SJ, Wims AM. A method for determining reaction kinetics by differential scanning calorimetry. Anal Calorim 1977; 4:155–71.
65. Ozawa T. Kinetic analysis of derivative curves in thermal analysis. J Therm Anal 1970; 2(3):301–24.
66. McDaid FM, Barker SA, Fitzpatrick S, Petts CR, Craig DQM. Further investigations into the use of high sensitivity differential scanning calorimetry as a means of predicting drug–excipient interactions. Int J Pharm 2003; 252: 235–40.
67. Van Dooren AA, Mueller BW. Purity determinations of drugs with differential scanning calorimetry (DSC)—a critical review. Int J Pharm 1984; 20(3):217–33.
68. Van Dooren AA, Mueller BW. Effects of experimental variables on purity determinations with differential scanning calorimetry. Thermochim Acta 1983; 66(1–3):161–86.
69. Marti EE. Purity determination by differential scanning calorimetry. Thermochimica Acta 1972; 5:173–220.
70. Giron D. Thermal analysis of drugs and drug products. In: Swarbrick J, ed. Encyclopedia of Pharmaceutical Technology. New York: Marcel Dekker, 1996.
71. Cassel RB. Purity determination and DSC Tzero™ Technology. New Castle: TA Instruments:8.
72. Joy EF, Bonn JD, Bernard AJ Jr. Differential scanning calorimetric assessment of high purity. Thermochimica Acta 1971; 2(1):57–68.
73. Hints for good purity determination. New Castle: TA Instruments. Thermal Application Note.

# 3.7

# Solubility Methods for the Characterization of New Crystal Forms

### Harry G. Brittain

*Center for Pharmaceutical Physics, Milford, New Jersey, U.S.A.*

## CONCEPTS OF SOLUBILITY

The equilibrium solubility of a compound is defined as the maximum quantity of that substance which can be completely dissolved in a given amount of solvent. This quantity is of prime importance in many areas of pharmaceutical research, since the solubility of a potential drug substance can be the controlling factor in determining the bioavailability of that compound. As a result, studies of solubility phenomena assume a particularly important role in the preformulation aspect of drug development, and the degree of aqueous solubility, in particular, can be the defining quantity that kills a development program, alters its course, or provides a green light for continued development.

The solubility of a solid in a series of relevant solvent media is an intrinsic property of that substance and a defining characteristic of the solid. The solubility is defined as the concentration of the dissolved solid (i.e., the solute) in the solvent medium (i.e., the saturated solution), which is in equilibrium with the solid at a defined temperature and pressure. The solubility of a substance will depend on the physical form of the solid, the nature and composition of the solvent medium, the temperature, and the pressure (1). To the preformulation scientist, the most common encountered solvent media are liquids or liquid mixtures, which will therefore yield liquid solutions of the solute.

### Units of Solubility

The solubility of a substance may be defined in many different types of units, but each of these will represent an expression of the quantity of solute dissolved in a solution at a given temperature. Solutions are said to be "saturated" if the solvent has dissolved the maximal amount of solute permissible in a given solvent at a particular temperature, and clearly an "unsaturated" solution is one for which the concentration is less than the saturated concentration. Under special conditions, one can prepare meta-stable solutions that are "supersaturated," a situation existing when the actual solute concentration exceeds that of the saturated solution. In pre-formulation work, the most commonly encountered units are molarity, normality, mole fraction, and weight or volume percentages.

The "molarity" (abbreviated by the symbol "M") of a solution is defined as the number of moles of solute dissolved per liter of solution (often written as mol/L), where the number of moles equals the number of grams divided by the molecular weight. It follows that a given volume of different solutions that have the same molarity will necessarily contain the same number of moles of solute molecules. The use of molarity is especially important in equilibrium calculations, since substances react on a mole basis and not on a simple weight basis.

The "normality" (abbreviated by the symbol "N") of a solution is defined as the number of equivalents of solute dissolved per liter of solution (also written in units of eq/L), where the number of equivalents equals the number of grams divided by the equivalent weight. For nonelectrolytes such as organic compounds, the equivalent weight will equal the molecular weight, and therefore the normality of a given solution will equal its molarity. The use of normality as a concentration unit is particularly useful in describing the solubility of ionic compounds, as this unit takes into account the number of moles of each ion in the solution liberated upon dissolution of a given number of moles of solute.

The "mole fraction" of a given solute in a solution equals the number of moles of solute divided by the total number of moles of solute(s) and solvent in the solution. For a solution consisting of a single solute and a single solvent, the mole fraction of solvent ($X_A$) and solute ($X_B$) is expressed as

$$X_A = \frac{n_A}{n_A + n_B} \tag{1}$$

$$X_B = \frac{n_B}{n_A + n_B} \tag{2}$$

where $n_A$ and $n_B$ are the number of moles of solvent and solute, respectively. Obviously the sum of the mole fractions of the two components must equal unity. Since concentrations expressed in mole fractions provide quantitative information regarding a solution that can be readily translated down to the molecular level, this unit is most commonly used in thermodynamic studies of solubility behavior.

Owing to its ease in describing pharmaceutical processing steps, the use of "percentages" is widespread in pharmaceutical applications, being expressed as the quantity of solute dissolved in 100 equivalent units of solution. The "weight percentage" (expressed as % w/w) is defined as the number of grams of solute dissolved in 100 g of solution, while the "volume percentage" (expressed as % v/v) is defined as the number of milliliters of solute dissolved in 100 mL of solution. A frequently encountered unit, the "weight-volume percentage" (expressed as % w/v) is defined as the number of grams of solute dissolved in 100 mL of solution. For very dilute solutions, solubility is often expressed in units of "parts per million" (abbreviated as "ppm"), which is defined as the quantity of solute dissolved in 1,000,000 equivalent units of solution. As long as the same unit is used for both solute and solvent, the concentration in ppm is equivalent to the weight, volume, or weight-volume percentages multiplied by 10,000.

Each edition of the *United States Pharmacopeia* provides broad definitions of solubility. Compounds are said to be very soluble if less than 1 part of solvent is required to dissolve 1 part of solute, freely soluble if 1 part of solute dissolves in 1 to 10 parts of solvent, soluble if 1 part of solute dissolves in 10 to 30 parts of solvent, sparingly soluble if 1 part of solute dissolves in 30 to 100 parts of solvent, slightly soluble if 1 part of solute dissolves in 100 to 1000 parts of solvent, very slightly soluble if 1 part of solute dissolves in 1000 to 10,000 parts of solvent, and insoluble if more than 10,000 parts of solvent are required to dissolve 1 part of solute (2).

## Dissolution and Intrinsic Dissolution

Evaluation of the dissolution rates of solid drugs is extremely important in the development, formulation, and quality control of pharmaceutical solids (3,4). There are a multitude of methods available for determining the dissolution rates of solids, but the important ones among these may be categorized either as batch methods (Fig. 1) or as continuous-flow methods (Fig. 2). The common batch-type dissolution methods are derived from the beaker–stirrer method of Levy and Hayes (5) and include a number of thoroughly standardized procedures, especially those defined in the various editions of the *United States Pharmacopoeia*.

The dissolution rate of a solid may be defined as $dm/dt$, where $m$ is the mass of solid dissolved at time $t$. In a batch dissolution method, the analyzed concentration, $c_b$, in the solution (if well-stirred) is representative of the entire volume, $V$, of the dissolution medium, so that

$$m = V \cdot c_b \tag{3}$$

and

$$dm/dt = V(dc_b/dt) \tag{4}$$

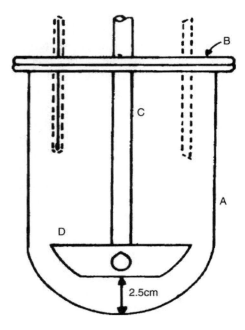

**Figure 1** Diagram of a batch-type dissolution apparatus, typified by the stirring paddle method.

If sufficient solvent is used to dissolve the solid solute, the dissolution profile will resemble the solid curve shown in Figure 3. However, if not all the added solute completely dissolves in the dissolution medium, the dissolution profile will instead resemble the dashed curve of Figure 3.

While batch dissolution methods are simple to set-up and operate, are widely used, and may be carefully and reproducibly standardized, they suffer from the following disadvantages: (*i*) the hydrodynamics are usually poorly characterized (with the notable exception of the rotating disc method); (*ii*) a small change in dissolution rate will often create an undetectable and hence immeasurable perturbation in the dissolution time curve; and (*iii*) the solute concentration may not be uniform throughout the solution volume.

By rotating sticks of benzoic acid or lead chloride (examples of sparingly soluble compounds) in water within a batch-type dissolution apparatus, Noyes and Whitney (6) found that the dissolved concentration of each solute increased with time according to first-order kinetics:

$$dm/dt = k_{NW} V(c_s - c_b) \tag{5}$$

where $k_{NW}$ is the first-order rate constant, and $c_s$ is the equilibrium solubility of the solute. From the onset of dissolution (i.e., $t = 0$) until the solute

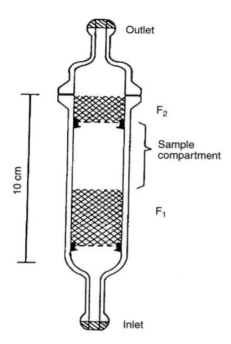

Outlet

F$_2$

Sample
compartment

F$_1$

10 cm

Inlet

**Figure 2** Diagram of a continuous-
flow dissolution apparatus.

concentration reaches a value of approximately 5% to 10% of the limiting concentration, one may make the assumption that $c_b \ll c_s$. This situation is typically referred to as the "sink condition." When the sink condition appropriately describes the dissolution condition, it follows that:

$$(dm/dt)_{t\to 0} = k_{NW}Vc_s \tag{6}$$

The dissolution rate of a given solid is usually strictly proportional to the wetted surface area ($A$) of the dissolving solid. The dissolution rate per unit surface area is the mass flux ($J$), which is usually termed the "intrinsic dissolution rate" in pharmaceutics. This quantity is given by

$$J = (dm/dt)(1/A) \tag{7}$$

It is not difficult to shown that under sink conditions,

$$J_{t\to 0} = (dm/dt)_{t\to 0}(1/A) \tag{8}$$

or that

$$J_{t\to 0} = = k'c_s \tag{9}$$

where $k'$ is the mass transfer coefficient, which has the units of length/time.

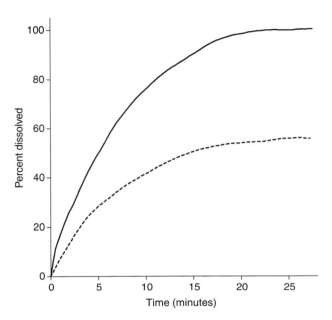

**Figure 3** Typical dissolution profiles for a substance achieving its anticipated complete solution (*solid trace*), and the profile of a substance for which incomplete solution was obtained (*dashed trace*).

## Effect of Particle Size on Dissolution Rate

Although it is effectively not possible for particle size to have an effect on the solubility of a substance, the effect of particle size on dissolution rate has been known since the pioneering work of Noyes and Whitney (6). Hixson and Crowell subsequently derived a highly useful equation that expresses the rate of dissolution based on the cube root of the weight of the particles (7). When the Hixson–Crowell model is applied to micronized particles, for which the thickness of the aqueous diffusion layer around the dissolving particles is comparable to or larger than the radius of the particle, the change in particle radius with time is given by

$$r^2 = r_0^2 - \frac{2Dc_s t}{\rho} \tag{10}$$

where $r_0$ is the initial radius of the particle, $r$ is the radius of the particle at time equal to $t$, $D$ is the diffusion coefficient of the molecules dissolving from the particle, $c_s$ is the equilibrium solubility of the substance, and $\rho$ is the density of the solution.

A very useful relation is obtained for the time, $T$, which would be required to achieve complete dissolution of the particle, or the condition, where $r^2 = 0$:

$$T = \frac{\rho r_0^2}{2 D c_s} \tag{11}$$

The value of $D$ in an aqueous solution is approximately equal to $5 \times 10^{-6}$ cm$^2$/sec, which was obtained for sucrose dissolved in water (8) and which is typically used for such computational purposes [see Ref. (9) for an example involving diazepam]. Since $\rho$ is approximately equal to 1.0 g/mL of aqueous solutions of low concentration, the calculation of Equation 11 can be performed if the equilibrium solubility of particles having a known initial particle size is known.

As an example, consider a substance whose equilibrium solubility is 1.0 mg/mL. For a particle whose initial diameter equals 10 μm, the time to achieve complete dissolution would be predicted to be 25 seconds (0.42 minutes). For the same substance, if the initial diameter instead equaled 50 μm, then the time to achieve complete dissolution would be predicted to be 625 seconds (10.4 minutes). For 100 μm particles of this substance, the time to achieve complete dissolution is calculated to be 2500 seconds (41.7 minutes). The relationship between particle size and the time required to completely dissolve particles of various sizes as defined in Equation 11 has been illustrated in Figure 4.

This effect of particle size on poorly soluble drug substances has been demonstrated in many instances by the superior dissolution rates observed after size reduction. Examples of compounds studied in such work include methylprednisolone (10), 1-isopropyl-7-methyl-4-phenylquinazolin-2(1H)-one (11), salicylic acid (12), griseofulvin (13), monophenylbutazone (14), nitrofurantoin (15), and piroxicam (16).

It has been mentioned that a deleterious effect on dissolution rate with decreasing particle size might be observed for systems where the finely divided drug substance particles clustered in agglomerates before dissolving (17), and this argument is often advanced to counter the more universally held view that decreasing particle size enhances dissolution rates. However, it has been known for a very long time that agglomeration effects can be easily overcome simply by adding surfactants to the dissolution medium to disrupt the agglomerates, and that under those conditions, one observes the correct correlation between particle size and dissolution rate (18).

## MEASUREMENT OF SOLUBILITY

Methods for the determination of solubility have been thoroughly reviewed (1,19,20), especially with respect to the characterization of pharmaceutical

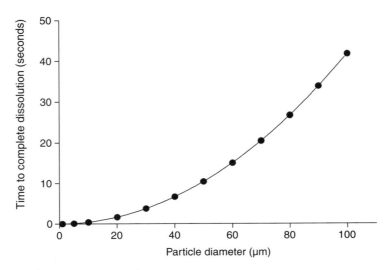

**Figure 4**   The relationship between particle size and the time required to completely dissolve particles of various sizes, as defined in Equation 11.

solids (21). Solubility is normally highly dependent on temperature, so the temperature must be recorded for each solubility measurement in addition to the precise nature of the solvent and the solid phase at equilibrium. Plots of solubility against temperature are commonly used for characterizing pharmaceutical solids, and have been extensively discussed (1,22). Frequently (especially over a relatively narrow temperature range), a linear relationship may be obtained using either the Van't Hoff equation

$$\ln X_2^{\text{sat}} = (-a/RT) + c' \tag{12}$$

or through the use of the Hildebrand equation:

$$\ln X_2^{\text{sat}} = (b/R)\ln T + c'' \tag{13}$$

In Equations 12 and 13, $X_2^{\text{sat}}$ is the mole fraction solubility of the solid solute at an absolute temperature $T$, $a$ is the apparent molar enthalpy of solution, $b$ is the apparent molar entropy of solution, and $c'$ and $c''$ are constants. The combined equation has been used by Grant et al. (22) in the form,

$$\ln X_2^{\text{sat}} = (-a/RT) + (b/R)\ln T + c''' \tag{14}$$

This three-parameter equation enables solubility to be simulated and correlated quite accurately over a wide temperature range. The relationship between a simple solubility plot and that generated through the use of the Van't Hoff equation is shown in Figure 5.

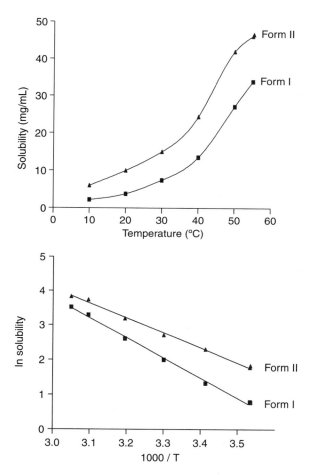

**Figure 5** Ordinary solubility plot for two crystal forms of a drug substance (*top*), and the same data plotted using the van't Hoff equation (*bottom*).

As implied in the previous paragraph, the validity of the afore-mentioned equations requires that each crystal phase be stable with respect to any phase conversion taking place during the determination of the equilibrium solubility.

Two general methods, the analytical method and the synthetic method (23,24), are available for determining solubility. In the analytical method, the temperature of equilibration is fixed, while the concentration of the solute in a saturated solution is determined at equilibrium by a suitable analytical procedure. The analytical method can be either the traditional "shake-flask" method, or the more recently developed flow column method. In the synthetic method, the composition of the solute–solvent system is fixed by appropriate addition and mixing of the solute and solvent, and then the temperature at which the solid solute just dissolves or just crystallizes is carefully determined.

## "Shake-Flask" or Batch Agitation Method

In what is probably the most commonly used method to determine solubility, the solvent is agitated or stirred in a suitable vessel with an excess of the solid solute. After sufficient time is allowed for the system to reach equilibrium, a solid-free aliquot of the saturated solution is removed from the system by an appropriate means, such as by centrifugation at the temperature of equilibration, filtration, straining through a plug of glass wool, or even decantation. The sample is usually diluted and analyzed by a method appropriate to the solute. As solubility is usually very temperature dependent, it is necessary to control the temperature of the system to the highest degree possible (typically $\pm 0.1°C$).

Equilibration is ordinarily asymptotically approached at a rate that depends on the volume of the solvent, the surface area of the solid solute, and on the nature and extent of the agitation. The method and time of equilibration can be established prior to the solubility determination by measuring the dissolved concentration of the solute as a function of time until no further change is noted. Analysis of the solution at times beyond the equilibration time is desirable so that one may verify that a state of true equilibrium has been achieved.

The equilibrium solubility value may be confirmed by creating a supersaturated solution by dissolving the solute at an elevated temperature, and then cooling with agitation until precipitation of the solute is observed. The temperature is decreased to the value of interest, whereupon the solution concentration will be constant. This solubility value should be the same as that obtained on approaching equilibrium from the usual unsaturated side. Supersaturation may be conveniently achieved by equilibrating the solid solute with the solvent at a higher temperature than required for solubility determination.

It is important to ascertain whether the solid phase of the solute changes during equilibration to produce a different polymorph or solvatomorph by analyzing the solid phase using X-ray powder diffraction. This procedure can be conveniently performed if one uses filtration to obtain a solid-free analyte solution, since the solute can be simply recovered off the filter. If a solid–solid phase transition occurs during equilibration, it follows that the measured equilibrium solubility would necessarily be that of the new solid phase of the solute. Methods of circumventing this problem have been proposed and evaluated (25).

It must be emphasized that genuine solubility values can only be obtained if one performs a rigorous phase separation of the saturated solution from the excess solid solute. Suspended solid particles surviving the phase separation can become solubilized during the dilution step of the analysis process, and would lead to the generation of excessively high solubility values. If a filter is employed, it must be inert to the solvent, it must not release plasticizers, and its pore size must be small enough to retain the smallest particles of the solid solute. Furthermore, steps must be taken to monitor, minimize, and preferably avoid losses of the dissolved solute by adsorption onto the filter material, and/or onto the vessels, pipettes, and syringes. Typically, the first small volume of filtrate is discarded until the surfaces of the filter and/or vessels are saturated with the adsorbed solute to ensure that the filtrate analyzed has not suffered significant adsorption losses. Adsorption can be a serious problem for hydrophobic solutes for which filtration would not be recommended. If decantation or centrifugation is employed for phase separation of the saturated solution, any disturbance and carry-over of the undissolved solid solute (whether precipitated or floating) must be monitored and avoided.

### Flow Column (Generator Column) Method

This more recent version of the analytical method has been developed by Wasik et al. (26,27). A suitable column, which may be made of glass or stainless steel, is packed with the solid solute, or with a suitable supporting material onto which the solute has previously been adsorbed by evaporation of a suitable solution. The solvent is pumped through the column or is forced through by applying gas pressure to the closed solvent vessel. The large area of contact between the solid solute and the solvent hastens the attainment of equilibrium so that the solution emerging from the column is saturated, which is analyzed in the typical manner.

The flow column method possesses useful advantages. Manipulation of the system prior to analysis is minimized, so that problems such as adsorption or evaporation that may arise from separation of the saturated solution and the undissolved solute are reduced. The method is rapid and precise (28,29), and is especially useful for solubility determinations of sparingly soluble solutes such as hydrophobic compounds in water.

If the solute is adsorbed onto a support material in the flow column method, certain problems may arise. The possibility that the polymorphic form, solvate form, or melting point may change on evaporating the solution for the coating process must be considered. Furthermore, a strong binding interaction between the adsorbed solute and the support material may reduce the thermodynamic activity of the adsorbed solute below that of the normal crystalline form, so that measured solubilities may be reduced below those determined by the common batch agitation method.

## Synthetic Method

In one embodiment of this method, an accurately weighed amount of the solute is placed in a suitable vessel. While agitating the system at a constant temperature, known amounts of the solvent are gradually added until the solid becomes completely dissolved. Knowledge of the initial mass of the solute and the added volume of solvent added permits one to calculate the solubility in that particular system. Appropriate checks must be carried out to ensure that the system is very close to equilibrium when the content of the system is recorded. In this method of measurement, attention is usually focused on the last small crystal. The equilibrium solubility is taken as the least amount of solvent necessary to completely dissolve the solute.

An alternative procedure is to place an accurately weighed amount of solute (anticipated to constitute a slight excess over the equilibrium solubility) and an accurately measured volume of solvent in a sealed container, and then to slowly raise the temperature. The temperature at which the solute becomes completely dissolved is recorded, and since one knew beforehand what the amounts of solid and solvent were, calculation of the solubility at that temperature is facile. If the experiment is performed at three different ratios of solute and solvent, then one may fit the data to the Van't Hoff equation to calculate the solubility at any intermediate value. This procedure may also be carried out at the microscale by examining a small volume of the system under a hot-stage microscope.

## IONIC EQUILIBRIA AND THE pH DEPENDENCE OF SOLUBILITY

As indicated above, the condition of dynamic equilibrium requires that excess solid phase be present in the solution in contact with the dissolved solute. The types of equilibria expected to exist for a weak acid can be separately considered by dividing a pH-solubility profile into the three zones shown in Figure 6. The processes taking place in zone-A are effectively those consisting of only the solid-free acid in equilibrium with its dissolved free acid, while the processes taking place in zone-C are effectively only those consisting of the solid salt of the acid in equilibrium with dissolved salt. zone-B is a buffer region, where the overall solubility would necessarily consist of the sum of dissolved free acid and salt. Continuing the example of the pH-solubility profile of a weak acid, the processes taking place in each zone will each be discussed in turn.

It is to be recognized, however, that the same general discussion would apply to the solubility processes associated with a weak base, except that the nature and definition of zone-A and zone-C would be reversed.

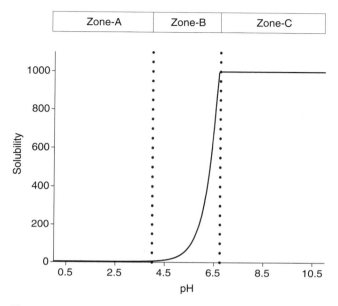

**Figure 6**  pH-solubility profile of a weak acid having a $pK_a$ value of 4.2, illustrating the three equilibrium zones of interest.

## Zone-A: Solubility of the Free Weak Acid

The equilibria existing in zone-A are very simple, consisting effectively of the equilibrium between solid free acid and the quantity dissolved in the aqueous phase:

$$HA_{(SOLID)} \longleftrightarrow HA_{(DISSOLVED)} \tag{15}$$

The concentration of dissolved HA is the intrinsic solubility of the free acid, which can be expressed as $S_{HA}$. The equilibrium constant expression for Equation 15 would be

$$K = \frac{A_{HA\text{-}DISS}}{A_{HA\text{-}SOL}} \tag{16}$$

where $A_{HA\text{-}DISS}$ is the activity of the dissolved free acid, and $A_{HA\text{-}SOL}$ is the activity of the solid salt. Recognizing that the activity of $MA_{(SOLID)}$ is a constant, expanding out the activities of Equation 16 in terms of concentrations and activity coefficients yields

$$K = [HA]\gamma_{HA} \tag{17}$$

As noted above, $S_{HA}$ values are typically fairly low in magnitude and would be independent of pH as long as no ionization of the acid takes place.

Consequently, the activity coefficient $\gamma_{HA}$ would be effectively equal to 1, making the value of the equilibrium constant approximately equal to the concentration of the dissolved free acid (i.e., $K = S_{HA}$). If more accuracy was required, however, the activity coefficient of the dissolved free acid could be approximated using any one of a number of theoretical approaches.

## Zone-C: Solubility of the Salt of the Weak Acid

In zone-C, the pH of the aqueous medium is such that all of the free acid, HA, has been converted into its salt form, MA, where $M^+$ will be a unipositive cation for the purposes of this discussion. The equilibria existing in this zone will therefore consist mainly of the equilibrium between the solid salt and its dissolved ions:

$$MA_{(SOLID)} \longleftrightarrow M^+ + A^- \tag{18}$$

In this zone, the concentration of dissolved MA is the intrinsic solubility of the salt of the free acid, which can be expressed as $S_{MA}$.

The equilibrium constant expression for Equation 18 would be

$$K = \frac{A_{M^+} A_{M^-}}{A_{MA-SOL}} \tag{19}$$

where $A_{M^+}$ is the activity of the cation, $A_{A^-}$ is the activity of the $A^-$ anion, and $A_{MA-SOL}$ is the activity of the solid salt. Recognizing that the activity of $MA_{(SOLID)}$ is a constant, expanding out the activities of Equation 19 in terms of concentrations and activity coefficients yields the solubility product constant:

$$K_{SP} = [M^+][A^-]\gamma_{M^+}\gamma_{A^-} \tag{20}$$

In the usual consideration for sparingly soluble salts, the activity coefficients $\gamma_{M^+}$ and $\gamma_{A^-}$ would each equal unity, and the solubility product constant can be derived using only the concentrations of the ions.

The condition of zone-C could be established in two different ways. The first is where a saturated solution of MA is established by equilibrating an excess amount of solid salt with water at a fixed temperature, and the second is where the weak acid has been exactly neutralized by the strong base MOH. In either case, it follows that $[M^+]$ must equal $[A^-]$, and therefore Equation 20 can be rearranged to yield an expression for the concentration of dissolved salt:

$$S_{MA} = \{K_{SP}/(\gamma_{M^+}\gamma_{A^-})\}^{1/2} \tag{21}$$

Since it is the usual situation that the solubility of the salt form is quite high, inclusion of the activity coefficient terms is necessary to obtain accurate results. These can be approximated as described above.

## Zone-B: Solubility of the Weak Acid and Its Salt Under Equilibrium Conditions

Inside the pH region enclosed by the limits of zone-B, one finds both the free acid and its salt form. The mass balance relationship in this zone defines the total solubility ($S_T$) at any particular pH value as the sum of the concentration of the free acid plus the concentration of its salt form:

$$S_T = [HA] + [A^-] \tag{22}$$

As long as the solubility of the generated salt is not exceeded, the concentration of $[A^-]$ generated by neutralization of HA by the strong base MA is calculated from knowledge of the acid ionization constant:

$$[A^-] = \frac{K_A[HA]}{[H_3O^+]} \tag{23}$$

or

$$[A^-] = \frac{K_A S_{HA}}{[H_3O^+]} \tag{24}$$

Therefore, as long as the formed salt is completely soluble, the total solubility in zone-B is given by

$$S_T = S_{HA}\{1 + (K_A/[H_3O^+])\} \tag{25}$$

In other words, Equation 25 is only valid for those pH conditions for which the solubility product constant of the salt is not exceeded.

A different set of equations holds when the solubility of the salt is exceeded, since the amount of solubilized $[A^-]$ will be limited by the solubility product constant. Recognizing that

$$[HA] = \frac{[H_3O^+][A^-]}{K_A} \tag{26}$$

Equation 22 becomes

$$S_T = \frac{[H_3O^+][A^-]}{K_A} + [A^-] \tag{27}$$

or

$$S_T = [A^-]\{1 + ([H_3O^+]/K_A)\} \tag{28}$$

However, since

$$[A^-] = \{K_{SP}/(\gamma_{M^+}\gamma_{A^-})\}^{1/2} \tag{29}$$

one obtains the equation that describes the solubility behavior for pH values where the solubility product constant of the salt is exceeded:

$$S_T = \{K_{SP}/(\gamma_{M^+}\gamma_{A^-})\}^{1/2}\{1 + ([H_3O^+]/K_A)\} \tag{30}$$

At the exact pH for which the solubility constant is exceeded, one may equate the $S_T$ relations of Equation 25 and 30, solve for the hydronium ion concentration and convert to the "p" scale. After solving the resulting quadratic equation, one obtains an expression for this critical pH value:

$$pH_{CRIT} = pK_A + \log\left\{S_{HA}/[K_{SP}/(\gamma_{M^+}\gamma_-)]^{1/2}\right\} \tag{31}$$

Several papers have been published that detail the equilibria associated with pH-dependent phenomena and solubility limitations (30–33).

## SOLUBILITY STUDIES OF POLYMORPHS AND SOLVATOMORPHS

One of the fundamental goals in a preformulation program is to discover the most crystal form of the drug substance in question, as this is almost always the form that should be developed. "Polymorphism" is defined as the ability of a substance to exist in two or more crystalline phases that differ in the arrangement and/or conformation of the molecules in the crystal structure, and it is understood that the empirical formulae of a polymorphic pair are identical. "Solvatomorphism" is defined as the ability of a substance to exist in two or more crystalline phases that differ in their empirical formulae, a property that arises from differences in their solvation states. Solvatomorphs are characterized by the presence of water molecules (i.e., hydrates) or other solvents (i.e., solvates) in the crystal structure, and it is entirely possible that solvatomorphs can also exhibit polymorphism if the arrangement and/or conformation of the molecules in the crystal structure can be achieved in different ways. How one goes about searching for such solid state forms is discussed elsewhere in this book, but in this chapter, the utility of solubility studies will be explored.

For any given system, it must be that one of the polymorphs or solvatomorphs will be more stable (i.e., be characterized by the lowest Gibbs free energy) than all of the others. As a result, the other crystal forms are metastable with respect to the stable form and over time will eventually convert to the more stable form. Pairs of polymorphic solids are classified as either being "enantiotropic" systems (where one polymorph is stable over one temperature and pressure range, and another polymorph is stable over a different temperature and pressure range) or monotropic systems (where only one polymorph is stable at all temperatures and pressures). Since the most stable polymorph under defined conditions of temperature and pressure has the lowest Gibbs free energy, it must also have the lowest thermodynamic activity, solubility in any given solvent, and intrinsic dissolution rate.

That the crystal structure of a solute can have a direct effect on its solubility can be understood using a simple model. For a solid to dissolve, the disruptive force of the solvent molecules must overcome the attractive forces holding the solid intact. In other words, the solvation free energy released upon dissolution must exceed the lattice free energy of the solid for the process to proceed spontaneously. The equilibrium solubility of the solid in question (which represents the free energy change of the system) will be determined by the relative balancing of the attractive and disruptive forces. The balance of these forces is determined by the enthalpy change and the increase in disorder of the system (i.e., the entropy change). Since different crystal structures are characterized by different lattice energies (and enthalpies), it follows that the solubility of different crystal polymorphs (or solvate species) must differ as well.

It should be emphasized that the solubility differences between polymorphs or solvates will be maintained only when a less stable form cannot convert to the most stable form. When such conversion takes place, the equilibrium solubility of all forms will approach a common value, namely that of the most stable form at room temperature.

The effect of polymorphism becomes especially critical on solubility since the rate of compound dissolution must also be dictated by the balance of attractive and disruptive forces existing at the crystal–solvent interface. A solid having a higher lattice free energy (i.e., a less-stable polymorph) will tend to dissolve faster, since the release of a higher amount of stored lattice free energy will increase the solubility and hence the driving force for dissolution. At the same time, each species would liberate (or consume) the same amount of solvation energy, since all dissolved species (of the same chemical identity) must be thermodynamically equivalent.

If the pressure of a system is fixed, then the Gibbs free energy difference between two polymorphic phases is determined by their relative fugacities:

$$\Delta G = RT \ln(f_2/f_1) \tag{32}$$

In a condensed phase, the fugacity is proportional to the activity, so the Gibbs free energy difference between the two phases is then determined by their relative activities:

$$\Delta G = RT \ln(A_2/A_1) \tag{33}$$

The most useful expression is obtained if one approximates the activity of each phase by its solubility:

$$\Delta G = \sim RT \ln(s_2/s_1) \tag{34}$$

The implication of Equation 34 is that in a noninteracting solvent system where phase conversion does not take place, the solubility ratio of a polymorphic pair is independent of temperature, and that one can calculate the free energy difference between the two phases from this ratio at a given temperature.

The use of solubility studies in the characterization of polymorphic systems can be illustrated using data published for the methylprednisolone system (34). This compound was found to crystallize in two polymorphic forms, each of which was characterized as having distinct X-ray powder diffraction patterns and infrared absorption spectra. The solubilities of each form were determined in water and in decyl alcohol, and the results are found in Table 1. The data indicate that form-I must be more stable than form-II over the range of temperatures studied, since its solubility in both solvent systems at a given temperature is always less. Over the temperature range of 30°C to 39°C, the solubility ratio for form-II/form-I is relatively constant and independent of the solvent, thus permitting the calculation that the free energy difference between the two forms at 30°C equals 1292 kJ/mol or 309 kcal/mol.

However, the solubility ratio is observed to decrease as the temperature is increased, and obviously will equal unity at some temperature. At that temperature, the two forms would be characterized by the same Gibbs free energy, making them of equal stability. Under those conditions, one form could convert into the other, making this temperature the transition point. Although the methylprednisolone data were not obtained over a sufficient temperature range to detect the transition point directly, one can plot the data using the Van't Hoff equation and extrapolate to the transition

**Table 1**   Solubility of Methylprednisolone in Various Solvents

| Temperature (°C) | Solubility (form-I) | Solubility (form-II) | Solubility ratio (form-II/ form-I) |
|---|---|---|---|
| *Solubility in water (mg/mL)* | | | |
| 30 | 0.09 | 0.15 | 1.67 |
| 39 | 0.12 | 0.20 | 1.67 |
| 49 | 0.16 | 0.26 | 1.63 |
| 60 | 0.21 | 0.33 | 1.57 |
| 72 | 0.30 | 0.43 | 1.43 |
| *Solubility in decyl alcohol (mg/mL)* | | | |
| 30 | 2.9 | 4.8 | 1.66 |
| 39 | 3.5 | 5.7 | 1.63 |
| 49 | 4.3 | 6.9 | 1.60 |
| 60 | 5.5 | 8.6 | 1.56 |
| 72 | 8.3 | 11.9 | 1.43 |

point. This is illustrated in Figure 7, where it can be seen that plots intersect at a reciprocal temperature of $1828 \, K^{-1}$, which is equivalent to a temperature of 274°C.

The Merck Index notes that methylprednisolone melts at 228°C to 237°C (35), a temperature that is less than the predicted transition point. Consequently, the transition point is virtual, and therefore the relationship between form-I and form-II would be classified as being monotropic.

Phenylbutazone has been found to be capable of existing in five different polymorphic structures, each of which exhibits a characteristic X-ray powder diffraction pattern and melting point (36). Form-I exhibits the highest melting point (implying the highest value for lattice energy at the elevated temperature), and its solubility is the lowest in each of the three solvent systems studied. This finding demonstrates that this particular crystal form is thermodynamically the most stable polymorph both at room

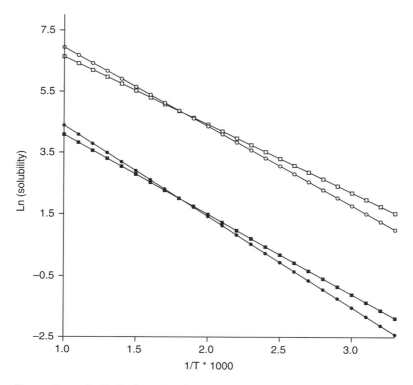

**Figure 7** van't Hoff plots describing the temperature dependence of the solubility of methylprednisolone in water (• = form-I and ■ = form-II) and in decyl alcohol (○ = form-I and □ = form-II). *Source*: From Ref. 34.

temperature and at the melting point. Identifying the sequence of stability for the other forms is not quite as simple. The polymorphs had been named in the order of decreasing melting points, but the solubility data do not follow this order, implying that the order of stability at room temperature is not equivalent to that which would exist at 100°C.

The effect of solvent composition on the solubility of polymorphs is illustrated by cimetidine (37). The onset of melting of the two forms is essentially indistinguishable, making it impossible to apply the conventional nomenclature to the labeling of the polymorphs. form-B was found to be less soluble than form-A, identifying it as the most stable polymorph at room temperature. The two forms were more soluble in mixed water–isopropanol solvents than in either of the pure solvents, reflecting the balance between solvation and lattice energies, and the entropy change in the various solvent systems.

Amiloride hydrochloride can be obtained in two polymorphic dihydrate forms (38). No distinction can be made between the two solvates, since each dehydrates around 115°C to 120°C, and the resulting anhydrous solids melt at the same temperature. However, form-B was found to be slightly less soluble than form-A between temperatures of 5°C and 45°C, suggesting it to be the thermodynamically stable form at room temperature. The temperature dependencies of the solubility data were processed by the van't Hoff equation to yield apparent enthalpies of solution for the two polymorphic dihydrates.

A very powerful method for the evaluation of solubility differences between polymorphs or solvates is that of intrinsic dissolution, which entails measurements of the initial rates of dissolution. One method for this work is to simply pour loose powder into a dissolution vessel, and to monitor the concentration of dissolved solute as a function of time. However, data obtained by this method are not readily interpretable unless they are corrected by factors relating to the surface area or particle size distribution of the powder. In the other approach, the material to be studied is filled into the cavity of a circular dissolution die, compressed until it exhibits the effective planar surface area of the circular disk, and then the dissolution rate is monitored off the surface of the rotating disk in the die (39).

The types of intrinsic dissolution profile obtainable through the loose powder and constant surface area methods are shown in Figure 8 for the crystalline anhydrate and monohydrate forms of oxyphenbutazone (the monohydrate is the less soluble) (40). The loose powder dissolution profiles consisted of sharp initial increases, which gradually leveled off as the equilibrium solubility was reached. In the absence of supporting information, the solubility difference between the two species cannot be adequately understood until equilibrium solubility conditions are reached. In addition, the shape of the data curves is not amenable to quantitative mathematical manipulation. The advantage of the constant surface area method is evident

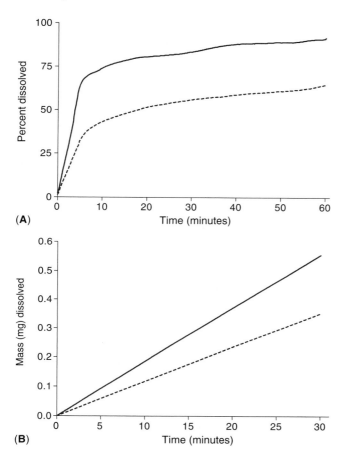

**Figure 8** (**A**) Loose powder dissolution profiles for the solubilization of oxyphenbutazone anhydrate (*solid trace*) and monohydrate (*dashed trace*). (**B**) Intrinsic dissolution profiles obtained using the constant surface area methods for oxyphenbutazone anhydrate (*solid trace*) and monohydrate (*dashed trace*). *Source*: From Ref. 40.

in that its dissolution profiles are linear with time and more easily compared. Additional information about the relative surface areas or particle size distributions of the two materials are not required since these differences were eliminated when the analyte disk was prepared.

Sulfathiazole has been found to crystallize in three distinct poly-morphic forms, all of which are kinetically stable in the solid state, but two of which are unstable in contact with water (41). The initial intrinsic dis-solution rates are different, but it was found that as form-I and form-II converted into form-III, the dissolved concentrations were seen to converge.

Only the dissolution rate of form-III was constant during the studies, which was taken to indicate it to be the thermodynamically stable form at room temperature. Aqueous suspensions of form-I and form-II were found to convert into form-III over time, supporting the finding of the dissolution studies. Interestingly, around the melting points of the three polymorphs, form-I exhibited the highest melting point and was thus assigned as being the most stable at the elevated temperature. This behavior would indicate an enantiotropic relationship between form-I and form-III.

When drug polymorphs cannot interconvert as a result of being suspended in aqueous solution, a different bioavailability of the two forms usually results (42). For instance, the peak concentration of chloramphenicol in blood serum was found to be roughly proportional to the percentage of the form-B polymorph present in a matrix of form-A (43). The same concept has been found to apply to hydrate species, where the higher solubility and dissolution rate of the anhydrous phase relative to the trihydrate phase resulted in measurably higher blood levels when using the anhydrate as the drug substance (44). However, when drug polymorphs can undergo phase transformations, no real difference in bioavailability parameters can be detected when administering the different polymorphic modifications. This situation has been realized with carbamazepine, where the rapid transformation of the anhydrate phase into the dihydrate ensures the bioequivalence of the two forms (45).

Auranofin (5-triethylphosphine gold-2,3,4,6-tetra-o-acetyl-1-thio-$\beta$-D-glyucopyranoside) has been found to crystallize in two anhydrate forms, with form-A melting at 112°C and form-B melting at 116°C (46). Using differential scanning calorimetry, the enthalpy of fusion for form-A was determined to be 9.04 kcal/mol, while the enthalpy of fusion for form-B was found to be 5.84 kcal/mol. Since the higher melting form exhibited the lower heat of fusion, one could use Burger's rule (47) to conclude that the two polymorphs were enantiotropically related. The equilibrium solubility of auranofin form-A in 25% aqueous polyethylene glycol 200 was found to be 0.65 mg/mL, and the solubility of form-B was 1.30 mg/mL. In addition, the intrinsic dissolution rate of form-B was significantly faster than that of form-A. While form-A is the most stable at room temperature (i.e., lowest solubility and dissolution rate), form-B is most stable at elevated temperature (i.e., highest melting point). This is classic enantiotropic behavior.

Pudipeddi and Serajuddin have examined a large number of literature reports on the solubility of polymorphic systems and have found that the ratio of polymorph solubility is typically less than 2 (48). A similar trend was noted for anhydrate/hydrate solubility ratios, although these appeared to be more spread out than the ratios for nonsolvated crystal forms. Morris et al. developed a quantitative model to evaluate the solubility relationships of polymorphs from their thermal properties and found that the free energy changes of the crystal forms permits one to predict the solubility ratio at any temperature (49). For monotropic systems, the solubility ratio estimate could be arrived at using the melting temperature and enthalpy of fusion of the two forms. For enantiotropic systems, only the temperature of the solid–solid transition and enthalpy of fusion were needed.

## REFERENCES

1. Grant DJW, Higuchi T. Solubility Behavior of Organic Compounds. New York: John Wiley and Sons, 1990.
2. United States Pharmacopeia, 30th ed. Vol. 1. Rockville, MD: United States Pharmacopeial Convention, 2007:9.
3. Abdou HM. Dissolution, Bioavailability and Bioequivalence. Easton PA: Mack, 1989.
4. Hanson R, Gray V. Handbook of Dissolution Testing. 3rd ed. Hockessin DE: Dissolution Technologies, Inc., 2004.
5. Levy G, Hayes BA. New Eng J Med 1960; 262:1053.
6. Noyes AA, Whitney WR. J Am Chem Soc 1897; 19:930–34.
7. Hixson AW, Crowell JH. Ind Eng Chem 1931; 23:923–31.
8. Adamson AW. A Textbook of Physical Chemistry. 2nd ed. New York: Academic Press, 1979:370.
9. Martin A. Physical Pharmacy. 4th ed. Philadelphia: Lippincott Williams & Wilkins, 1993:334.
10. Higuchi WI, Rowe EL, Hiestand EN. J Pharm Sci 1963; 52:162–4.
11. Kornblum SS, Hirschorn JO. J Pharm Sci 1970; 59:606–9.
12. Ullah I, Cadwallader DE. J Pharm Sci 1970; 59:979–84.
13. Ullah I, Cadwallader DE. J Pharm Sci 1971; 60:230–3.
14. Habib FS, Attia MA. Drug Dev Ind Pharm 1985; 11:2009–19.
15. Eyjolfsson R. Drug Dev Ind Pharm 1999; 25:105–6.
16. Swanepoel E, Liebenberg W, de Villiers MM, Dekker TG. Drug Dev Ind Pharm 2000; 26:1067–76.
17. Gibaldi M. Biopharmaceutics and Clinical Pharmacokinetics. 4th ed. Philadelphia: Lea & Febiger, 1991:52.
18. Wurster D, Seitz J. J Am Pharm Assoc Sci Edn 1960; 49:335–8.
19. Mader WJ, Vold RD, Vold MJ. Physical Methods of Organic Chemistry. 3rd ed. Vol. 1. Part I. Weissberger A, ed. New York, New York: Interscience Publishers, 1959:655–88.
20. Yalkowsky SH, Banerjee S. Aqueous Solubility Methods of Estimation for Organic Compounds. New York: Marcel Dekker, 1992:149–54.
21. Grant DJW, Brittain HG. Solubility of pharmaceutical solids. In: Brittain HG, ed. Physical Characterization of Pharmaceutical Solids. New York: Marcel Dekker, 1995:321–86.
22. Grant DJW, Mehdizadeh M, Chow AHL, Fairbrother JE. Int J Pharm 1984; 18:25.
23. Higuchi T, Shih FML, Kimura T, Rytting JH. J Pharm Sci 1979; 68:1267.
24. Bagley EB, Scigliano JM. Solutions and solubilities. Part II. In: Dack MRJ, ed. Techniques of Chemistry. Vol. VIII. New York: John Wiley, 1976:437–85.

25.  Ghosh S, Grant DJW. Int J Pharm 1995; 114, 185.
26.  De Voe H, Wasik SP. J Soln Chem 1984; 13:51.
27.  May WE, Wasik SP, Freeman DH. Anal Chem 1978; 50:175, 997.
28.  Friesen KJ, Sarna LP, Webster GRB. Chemosphere 1985; 14:1267.
29.  Dickhut RM, Andren AW, Armstrong DE. Environ Sci Technol 1986; 20: 807–10.
30.  Kramer SF, Flynn GL. J Pharm Sci 1972; 61:1896.
31.  Bogardus JB, Blackwood RK. J Pharm Sci 1979; 68:188.
32.  Streng WH, Hsi SK, Helms PE, Tan HGH. J Pharm Sci 1984; 73:1679.
33.  Pudipeddi M, Serajuddin ATM, Grant DJW, Stahl PH. Solubility and dissolution of weak acids, bases, and salts. In: Stahl PH, Wermuth CG, eds. Handbook of Pharmaceutical Salts. Weinheim, Germany: Wiley-VCH, 2002: 19–39.
34.  Higuchi WI, Lau PK, Higuchi T, Shell JW. J Pharm Sci 1963; 52:150.
35.  The Merck Index. 13th ed. O'Neil MJ, Smith A, Heckelman PE, eds. Whitehouse Station, NJ: Merck & Co., 2001:6137.
36.  Tuladhar MD, Carless JE, Summers MP. J Pharm Pharmacol 1983; 35:208.
37.  Sudo S, Sato K, Harano Y. J Chem Eng Japan 1991; 24:237.
38.  Jozwiakowski MJ, Williams SO, Hathaway RD. Int J Pharm 1993; 91:195.
39.  Jashnani RN, Byron PR, Dalby RN. J Pharm Sci 1993; 82:670.
40.  Stoltz M, Caira MR, Lotter AP, van der Watt JG. J Pharm Sci 1989; 78:758.
41.  Lagas M, Lerk CF. Int J Pharm 1981; 8:11.
42.  Habelian JK, McCrone W. J Pharm Sci 1969; 58:911.
43.  Aguiar AJ, Krc J Jr, Kinkel AW, Samyn JC. J Pharm Sci 1967; 56:847.
44.  Poole JW, Owen G, Silverio J, Freyhof JN, Rosenman SB. Current Therap Res 1968; 10:292.
45.  Kahela P, Aaltonen R, Lewing E, Anttila M, Kristoffersson E. Int J Pharm 1983; 14:103.
46.  Lindenbaum S, Rattie ES, Zuber GE, Miller ME, Ravin LJ. Int J Pharm 1985; 26:123.
47.  Burger A, Ramberger R, Mikrochimica Acta [Wien] 1979; 11:259, 273.
48.  Pudipeddi M, Serajuddin ATM. J Pharm Sci 2005; 94:929.
49.  Mao C, Pinal R, Morris KR. Pharm Res 2005; 22:1149.

# Part 4: Development of the Ideal Formulation

## 4.1

## Overview of the Solid Dosage Form Preformulation Program

**Harry G. Brittain**

*Center for Pharmaceutical Physics, Milford, New Jersey, U.S.A.*

### INTRODUCTION

Once a drug substance has been profiled, and a sufficient body of information acquired regarding its range of physical and chemical properties, the next stage in development is to acquire the scope of information necessary for the development of a stable and robust formulation. The nature of the formulation to be developed is obviously essential to the decision process, and in the present work the focus will be on solid dosage forms (i.e., tablets and capsules). Individual aspects of this work will be developed at greater length in succeeding chapters, but here the later stage of preformulation will be given an overview with the aim of setting up a rational design for the conduct of this work.

It is common to see works on preformulation encompass topics associated with the physical and chemical characterization of the active pharmaceutical ingredient (API), but which also end with that coverage. A more rational view is that the preformulation stage of drug development is really only half-complete at this stage, and that the program of drug development is not complete until it is fully understood how that API interacts with the excipients that will make up the remainder of its formulation.

According to Fiese and Hagen (1), API characterization can be divided into three main categories, beginning with bulk characterization. Here one is concerned with crystallinity and polymorphism, hygroscopicity, fine particle characterization, bulk density, and powder flow properties. The second category is solubility analysis, which covers ionization constants, the pH solubility profile, common ion effects, thermal effects, solubilization, partition coefficients, and dissolution. The final category is stability analysis, where one determines the stability of the API in solution as a function of pH, in the solid state when exposed to various stresses and in toxicology formulations. The subject of API characterization has been covered in depth in preceding chapters and in the literature (2–8).

In order to develop a pharmaceutical formulation, one has to identify the form of interest and all of the plausible components that might go into that formulation. The formulation will usually contain a number of additional ingredients that are not the API, but which carry out a variety of functions essential to the release of the API from the dosage form under the right conditions. These substances are, of course, excipients, and their role in a formulation precludes their being categorized as inactive ingredients, even though they have received that misnomer in the past. Excipients are formulated in a dosage form to achieve a certain result, and the functionality of these substances defines their physical and chemical characteristics of interest.

For a solid dosage form designed to rapidly release the API upon contact with a fluid, it is fairly likely that there would be no physical or chemical interaction between the API and the excipients. For such dosage forms, the existence of a physical or chemical interaction between the API and the excipients usually represents a bad situation, as the quality and stability of the dosage form will usually be adversely affected by the nature of those interactions. For solid dosage forms that are designed to release the API under controlled conditions, the excipients often exhibit a great deal of interaction with the API, which is usually of a benign and intended character. The mechanism of controlled release is often achieved by using the functional properties of the excipient to modify the delivery of the API into the environment of the dissolution fluid.

Finally, once the preformulation scientist has amassed the proper catalog of information regarding the API properties and its compatibility with intended excipients, then the design of prototype formulations becomes possible. Through acquisition of the appropriate range of knowledge, one should be able to propose several formulations that achieve the intended drug release profile, and which should exhibit the range of physical and chemical stability that would constitute pharmaceutical elegance. At that point, the project passes from the preformulation scientists to the formulation scientists, whose job is to evaluate the stability and utility of the formulation when it is produced at a much larger scale of manufacture.

## TYPES OF SOLID DOSAGE FORMS

Over the years, a substantial variety of solid dosage forms have been developed, each of which was chosen to optimally deliver an API so as to maximize its safety and efficacy. These dosage forms are typified by capsules and tablets, with tablets being subdivided into instant and controlled release types. Given the popularity of their use, tablet and capsule dosage forms have been the subject of many detailed reviews (10–14). It usually turns out that the actual identity of the dosage form eventually developed for a given API will represent a balance between what was desired and what actually worked. As will be discussed in a following section, the excipients that are used to produce each formulation type will depend critically on the identity and properties of the dosage form.

In the capsule dosage form, the API and excipients are enclosed in a gelatin shell, which may be either hard or soft in character. Capsule formulations are attractive in that their compositions are usually simpler than those of compressed tablets, and that the lack of compression can serve to minimize interaction between the formulation components. For low-potency drug substances, the API would represent practically the entire encapsulated formulation, with perhaps the addition of small amounts of an agent that would promote better powder flow. For high-potency drug substances, the API might be mixed with an inert diluent to fill the capsule contents, but relatively little else would be required.

The hard gelatin capsule consists of two sections, the longer of which is filled with the formulated API and the other is slipped over the first section to encapsulate the product. The two shells may be welded, or a locking mechanism may be used, to maintain the integrity of the finished dosage form. Soft gelatin capsules feature a globular shell that is generally thicker than a hard gelatin capsule shell, and the gelatin is usually plasticized to maintain its characteristics. Soft gelatin capsules represent the encapsulation method of choice when the API is formulated in the form of an oil. Once filled, the soft gelatin shells are heat sealed, the capsules usually open in the gastrointestinal tract along this seal.

Tablets are formed by the compaction of powdered solids and probably represent the most widely used method for the delivery of drug substances. The final dosage form may be obtained by simple compression and may or may not be coated. When more than one API is to be formulated, the dosage form may be obtained by the compression of multiple layers to form a layered product. If the API is supposed to be delivered via the buccal cavity, the tablet may be formulated so that it disintegrates completely in the mouth. Formulations designed to be tableted are necessarily more complex than those intended for encapsulation and will typically contain the API, a filler or a diluent, a binder or an adhesive, a disintegrant, and a lubricant.

Controlled or sustained release tablets are formulated so that the API is not instantly released, but instead is released over a prolonged period. Remington (9) categorizes these dosage forms into three groupings: (*i*) those responding to a physiological condition to release the API, (*ii*) those that release the API in a steady controlled manner, and (*iii*) those that combine release mechanisms to release repeated pulses of API. A controlled release of API can also be achieved by use of an enteric coating, where an instant release compressed tablet is coated with a polymer that resists dissolution in acidic gastric fluid but disintegrates in the higher pH environment of the intestine.

## EXCIPIENTS USED IN SOLID DOSAGE FORMS

As discussed above, the mode of drug delivery will determine the identity of the solid dosage form, and that choice of dosage form will in turn determine the types of excipient materials that are to be formulated. It is convenient to classify excipients by their intended functionality, as these materials are included in formulations primarily to execute a desirable physical effect. The excipient types of most interest to formulators of solid dosage forms can be classified as diluents, binders, disintegrants, lubricants, glidants, colors, and flavors, and a wealth of information is available in the continuing excipient handbook series (15).

A filler or a diluent is intended to make up the required bulk of capsule contents or a tablet when the physical magnitude of the bulk drug substance is not sufficient to achieve the desired volume. Examples of these substances include lactose, compressible starches, microcrystalline cellulose, calcium phosphates, and sugars. Full understanding of the compressibility of a filler requires knowledge of the bulk, tapped, and true densities of the substance. Since the function of a diluent is to provide bulk to a tablet, an important quantity to know is the volume that will be occupied by a given mass after compaction.

A binder is a material that is added during formulation to promote the formation of cohesive compacts during tableting. Examples of binders include cellulose derivatives, gelatin, processed starches, polyvinylpyrrolidone, and alginate derivatives. Binding agents play an important role during compaction, where they contribute to the overall plastic deformation during the consolidation process, generate or enhance interparticulate surface sites where bonding can take place, contribute to the plastic deformation during decompaction, and help to withstand the shear stress and strain during postcompaction (16).

A disintegrant is added to a formulation to facilitate breakup or disintegration of the tablet when it contacts water in the stomach. Some examples of disintegrants are starch and its derivatives, clays, cellulose and its derivatives, crosslinked polyvinylpyrrolidone, and alginates. These materials are used in formulations to overcome the cohesive forces introduced by the act of compression and by the presence of binders. The usual mechanism for disintegrant action entails a rapid water intake, followed by swelling of the particles that physically disrupts the tablet integrity.

Lubricants are materials intended to reduce friction between the powder compact and the walls or tooling during ejection of the tablet following compression. Examples of lubricants include stearic acid and its salts, talc, polyethylene glycols, and waxes. Since the function of lubricants is to reduce interfacial friction, it follows that an appropriate test for lubricity would entail a measurement of the mobility of a powder bed.

Glidants are excipients that are added to a formulation to improve the overall flowability of the bulk powder, and their use is very important when the powder properties of a formulation are insufficient for use in a high-speed tableting press. The most widely used glidant is colloidal silicon dioxide, but silica derivatives, talc, and cornstarch can be used for such purposes. Many pharmaceutical powders, especially those intended for use in direct compression formulations, do not exhibit adequate flowability properties; so a glidant is added to the formulation to enhance the bulk powder flow. It may be noted that lubricants can also exert a glidant effect, which is especially true in the case of magnesium stearate.

Colors and coloring agents are added to a formulation to achieve an intended color result, which may be derived from desirable product identification, manufacturing definition, or aesthetic value. Examples of coloring agents include FD&C and D&C dyes and lakes, iron oxides, titanium dioxide, and zinc oxide. The color of any solid material can be determined using reflectance spectroscopy and can be quantitatively specified using tristimulus colorimetry. Most often, one uses the CIE system for such determinations, derived from an $(x,y)$ chromaticity diagram set up to show the CIE coordinates (17).

For chewable solid dose formulations, user acceptance represents a key factor, since taste is a combination of perceptions that are usually subdivided between sweeteners and flavors. Sugars, saccharin, and aspartame represent common sweetening agents, and extracts of natural or synthetic sources are often used as flavoring agents. For obvious reasons, the choice of flavoring agents is usually correlated with the color of the formulation so as not to confuse the person taking the formulation. Quantitative definitions for flavors are difficult to obtain, since their response depends critically on the range of individual perceptions.

It should be noted that excipient monographs tend to be almost exclusively concerned with issues related to chemical purity, and that they generally have few requirements for the physical properties of the excipient. However, since excipients are included in solid dose formulations to achieve a desirable physical effect, it follows that formulators should devise appropriate types of physical testing that are related to the function of that excipient in a given formulation (18). Specifications for these functionality tests should be established on the basis of their ability to be correlated with batch production outcomes.

Of course, the situation is more complicated than this, since many excipients are able to act simultaneously in more than one capability in a formulation, and therefore the definition of an appropriate functionality test is often formulation dependent. Furthermore, a functionality test appropriate for one formulation may turn out to be entirely irrelevant when applied to another formulation. For these reasons, the choice of which functionality tests to apply to an excipient must be defined with respect to the action of that excipient in the formulation in question, and such issues can only be defined by the user of the excipient.

## COMPATIBILITY BETWEEN DRUG SUBSTANCES AND EXCIPIENTS

Once the dosage form for a given API has been identified, and the formulator believes that he or she has identified the possible excipient categories that need to be included in the formulation of that API, the next step in the process is to determine whether deleterious interactions can take place between the API and the proposed excipients. Elucidation of possible chemical and/or physical reactions in a formulation is an absolute requirement to establish the stability of a given dosage form (19,20). An understanding as to the plausible range of solid–solid reactions available to a drug substance should be established once a full preformulation study is completed.

In a solid dosage form under suitable conditions, a drug substance may undergo a variety of interactions or transformations through either one or more solid–solid chemical or physical reactions. It is important to understand the full range of solid–solid interactions that can take place in a proposed formulation, as these can lead to the formation of new impurities, an incomplete mass balance, destruction of the dosage form, changes in physicochemical properties (such as stability, solubility, dissolution profile, degree of crystallinity, and hygroscopicity). All of these problems can ultimately result in the inability to obtain a successful registration and approval of the API for clinical purposes.

Once the characteristics of the bulk drug substance have been evaluated, its compatibility with the excipients that would potentially be used in its dosage form must be studied. In this work, the substance is blended with excipients at levels that are realistic with respect to the proposed formulation. For example, if a lubricant is to be used at a level of 0.5% in a formulation, then the evaluation of a 50% substance:excipient mixture is not appropriate. Each blend is stored at accelerated stress conditions (elevated temperature and humidity) and is tested for drug substance stability and release after an appropriate equilibration period.

The purity and impurity profiling of the API in the blend mixtures is ordinarily conducted using a chromatographic procedure, such as high-performance liquid chromatography, capillary electrophoresis, or gas chromatography, or through the coupling of a separation method with mass spectrometric detection. The physical characteristics associated with the API and its formulation blends are followed by means of appropriate physical analysis methodology, such as microscopy (optical or electron), X-ray powder diffraction, thermal methods of analysis (differential scanning calorimetry or thermogravimetry), ultraviolet, visible, or near-infrared diffuse reflectance spectroscopy, solid-state nuclear magnetic resonance, and solid-state vibrational spectroscopy (Raman or infrared absorption spectroscopies).

It is important to note that a wide variety of reactions can take place in the solid state, and that these all need to be recognized and investigated when they occur. The scope of solid–solid reactivity spans chemical and physical interactions that can be broadly identified as association [e.g., the interaction between indomethacin and polyvinylpyrrolidone (21)], adsorption [e.g., the interaction between ketotifen and Acdisol (22)], solubilization [e.g., the interaction between quinine and phenobarbital (23)], addition [e.g., the interaction between fluoxetine hydrochloride and various forms of lactose (24)], desolvation [e.g., the evolution of isopropanol from its loracarbef solvatomorph (25)], decomposition [e.g., reactions taking place in a suboptimal formulation of flucloxin (26)], and phase transformation [e.g., the effect of microcrystalline cellulose on the form-II to form-I conversion of fostedil (27)] reactions. A wide variety of methodologies that exist make it possible for the preformulation scientist to effectively study whatever needs to be studied.

It is essential to establish a catalog of the plausible solid-state reactions accessible to a drug substance. This information should be obtained as early in the development process as possible, preferably during the preformulation stage of drug development. The degree of concern associated with each possibility should be roughly proportional to its likelihood of actually being encountered, so studies need to be performed at appropriate concentration levels. It is worth noting that although regulatory agencies want to review real-time data, the discovery of drug–excipient interactions is greatly aided through the use of accelerated studies.

## CONCLUSION

The final stage of the preformulation program is the proposal of two or three trial formulations for the API. These should be formulations suitable for conduct of the phase I or II clinical studies and ideally would represent the formulation upon which phase III studies could be based. If the work is performed properly, then the proposed formulations would be free from all undesirable physical and chemical interactions. Then, with any luck, the formulation would prove to be able to be scaled up to the desired manufacturing level. However, all of this requires a broad basis of understanding regarding the API and its possible interactions with excipient materials and a thorough understanding of the range of excipients required to achieve the pharmacological profile that is sought for the API. These areas will be developed at greater length in the following chapters.

## REFERENCES

1. Fiese EF, Hagen TA. Preformulation. In: Lachman L, Lieberman HA, Kanig JL, eds. The Theory and Practice of Industrial Pharmacy, 3rd ed. Philadelphia: Lea and Febiger, 1986:171–96.
2. Sinko PJ, ed. Martin's Physical Pharmacy and Pharmaceutical Sciences, 5th ed. Philadelphia: Lippincott Williams and Wilkins, 2006.
3. Florence AT, Attwood D. Physicochemical Principles of Pharmacy, 4th ed. London: Pharmaceutical Press, 2006.
4. Aulton ME. Pharmaceutics: The Science of Dosage Form Design. Edinburgh: Churchill Livingstone, 1988.
5. Byrn SR, Pfeiffer RR, Stowell JG. Solid State Chemistry of Drugs, 2nd ed. West Lafayette, IN: SSCI Inc., 1999.
6. Carstensen JT, Rhodes CT. Drug Stability: Principles and Practices, 3rd ed. New York: Marcel Dekker, 2000.
7. Wells JT. Pharmaceutical Preformulation: The Physicochemical Properties of Drug Substances. New York: Halsted Press, 1988.
8. Carstensen JT. Pharmaceutical Preformulation. Boca Raton: CRC Press, 1998.
9. Rudnic EM, Schwartz JB. Oral solid dosage forms. In: Troy DB, ed. Remington: The Science and Practice of Pharmacy, 21st ed., Philadelphia: Lippincott Williams and Wilkins, 2006:889–928.
10. Lieberman HA, Lachman L, Schwartz JB, eds. Pharmaceutical Dosage Forms: Tablets, 2nd ed. New York: Marcel Dekker, 1989 (Vol. 1), 1990 (Vol. 2), 1990 (Vol. 3).
11. Ansel HC, Popovich NG, Allen LV. Pharmaceutical Dosage Forms and Drug Delivery Systems, 6th ed. Baltimore: Williams and Wilkins, 1995.
12. Podczeck F, Jones BE. Pharmaceutical Capsules, 2nd ed. London: Pharmaceutical Press, 2004.
13. Banker GS, Rhodes CT. Modern Pharmaceutics, 4th ed. New York: Marcel Dekker, 2002.
14. Gibson M. Pharmaceutical Preformulation and Formulation. Boca Raton: CRC Press, 2001.
15. Rowe RC, Sheskey PJ, Owen SC. Handbook of Pharmaceutical Excipients, 5th ed. London: Pharmaceutical Press, 2006.
16. Symecko CW, Rhodes CT. Drug Dev Indust Pharm 1995; 21:1091–114.
17. Bogdansky FM. J Pharm Sci 1975; 64:323–8.
18. Brittain HG. Physical Characterization of Pharmaceutical Solids. New York: Marcel Dekker, 1994.
19. Ahuja S, Scypinski S. Handbook of Modern Pharmaceutical Analysis. San Diego: Academic Press, 2001.
20. Ohannesian L, Streeter AJ. Handbook of Pharmaceutical Analysis. New York: Marcel Dekker, 2002.
21. Taylor LS, Zografi G. Pharm Res 1997; 12:1691–8.
22. Al-Nimry SS, Assaf SM, Jalal IM, Najib NM. Int J Pharm 1997; 149:115–21.

23. Guillory JK, Hwang SC, Lach JL. J Pharm Sci 1969; 58:301–8.
24. Wirth DD, Baertschi SW, Johnson RA, et al. J Pharm Sci 1998; 87:31–9.
25. Forbes RA, McGarvey BM, Smith DR. Anal Chem 1999; 71:1232–9.
26. Stark G, Fawcett JP, Tucker IG, Weatherall IL. Int J Pharm 1996; 143:93–100.
27. Takahashi Y, Nakashima K, Ishihara T, Nakagawa H, Sugimoto I. Drug Dev Indust Pharm 1985; 11:1543–63.

# 4.2

# Drug–Excipient Interaction Occurrences During Solid Dosage Form Development

Moji Christianah Adeyeye

*School of Pharmacy, Duquesne University, Pittsburgh, Pennsylvania, U.S.A.*

## INTRODUCTION

Preformulation is a critical phase in drug development where the physico-chemical profiling of the active pharmaceutical ingredients (APIs) and excipients are determined and prototype formulations are made. The performance of a solid dosage form is dependent on the physicochemical properties of the active ingredient and the excipients. It is at this crucial stage, usually preceding the phase I clinical formulation, that suitable excipients are identified. Concomitant with the choice of excipients is an exhaustive evaluation of drug–excipient interaction and compatibility. The goal is to eventually prevent unnecessary and very costly changes involving time and overall development cost in subsequent steps. The process is part of what the Food and Drug Administration (FDA) refers to as quality by design, in which quality is built into the product and not added. The ultimate goal is to identify the critical properties that are considered important in the formulation of a stable, effective, and safe drug delivery system or dosage form.

Drug–excipient interaction is one of the most important considerations in solid dosage form development and in drug discovery programs. It is a derived preformulation parameter that encapsulates the application of fundamental characteristics such as the spectral nature of the components, solubility, particle size distribution (size and shape), partition coefficient, melting point, and stability. At the point when the scientist embarks on drug–excipient interaction testing, all these fundamental data should have been gathered, ready to be used as a template for the interaction evaluation.

357

The importance of a robust drug–excipient interaction study at the preformulation stage is underscored when the consequences of inadequacy of the study are viewed critically. Such consequences include formation of new impurities, incomplete mass balance, destruction of the dosage form, unnecessary multiplicity of prototype formulations, changes in physicochemical properties (stability, solubility, dissolution profile, degree of crystallinity, hygroscopicity) and inability to obtain successful drug registration (1).

*General considerations*: The evaluation of drug–excipient compatibility is based on the inherent properties of the excipients and their importance in the delivery of the active ingredients to the target site. Excipients or "inert ingredients" are substances added to pharmacologically active compounds to facilitate dosage form production, enhance drug stability and absorption, and improve palatability for the patient (2). The definition appears to be contradictory based on the functionalities stated; therefore, excipients are not truly inert and can be defined as "enabling."

Physical/chemical interaction studies must be approached rationally to avoid unnecessary setting-up of experiments (stability studies) that either are not practical or may not yield the necessary information that could reveal interaction or incompatibility. At the point of studying these interactions (which is early in the development phase), there may not be enough bulk drug for such studies and time may not also be available to the extent which the investigations may require. The overall focus of interaction studies should be on the parameters stated below and the impact of these on the integrity of the dosage form:

- Nature of the drug and excipients
- Excipient–drug ratio necessary for meaningful evaluation
- Role of moisture
- Influence of heat
- Effect of pH of the microenvironment
- Processing effect on formulation
- Role of light

## THE ACTIVE PHARMACEUTICAL INGREDIENT

The intrinsic or inherent reactivity of the APIs in the solid state is very important, because it can be accentuated by the presence of excipients or water. The basic solid-state reactions include polymorphic transformations and loss or gain of solvent of crystallization. The reactivity of the drug is made possible through a four-step process: (*i*) molecular loosening or mobility that allows for the next step; (*ii*) molecular change: this involves breaking of chemical bonds of the reactant (drugs and/or excipients) and formation of the new one in the product; (*iii*) solid solution formation; and (*iv*) separation of product (3). These reactions start at the crystal defects or nucleation sites and spread through the crystal. According to some reports (4), it can be assumed that the reactions are solid state instead of solution state if some of the following observations are made: the liquid reaction does not occur or is very slow, the degradative products are significantly different in the liquid state, and the solid-state reaction occurs below the eutectic point of a mixture of the starting materials and products.

The mobility of groups in a solid state is enhanced by water absorption, and this underscores the role of water in the reactivity of solid APIs. For example, water has been reported to enhance the mobility of an amorphous solid or a crystalline solid with small amounts of amorphous entities as a result of plasticization. The onset of this mobility in the amorphous regions progresses to degradation via the formation of eutectic melts of the degradative product and starting material (5).

Knowledge of the nature of the drug's susceptibility to mobility and means of prediction could become valuable in the choice of the most stable crystal form prior to further development and stability evaluation. The consequence of some of the reactions highlighted may be oxidation, cyclization, hydrolysis, and deamidation of the drug substance. Anticipation of such reactions early in the development phase will reduce unwanted trials and expedite the process. Some examples are discussed below.

## Oxidation

### Vitamin A

Esters of vitamin A degrade via oxidation and polymerization (6,7). Generally, vitamin A breakdown is influenced by free radical reaction, oxygen, pressure, and temperature. It is known that vitamin A is also light sensitive. Diluents or excipients such as aluminium salts of fatty acids such as stearic acid, gelatin, and dextrin can stabilize vitamin A.

### Peptides

Due to the reactive side chains or amino acid groups on some peptides and proteins, oxidation can occur in the solid state. This reaction is complicated by the different degradative products that usually result. An example is methionine, which degrades to methionine sulfoxide and methionine sulfone. Xu (8) investigated this using three model peptides—DL-Ala-DL-Met (a zwitterionic peptide), *N*-formyl-Met-Leu-Phe methyl ester (a neutral peptide), and Met-enkephalin acetate salt (a weakly acidic pentapeptide). The structures are shown in Figures 1 and 2.

The peptides were chosen because they exist in both amorphous and crystalline states. Oxidation was induced using ultraviolet (UV) radiation (254 nm). The authors observed that the amorphous forms of DL-Ala-DL-Met and *N*-formyl-Met-Leu-Phe methyl ester degraded faster than the

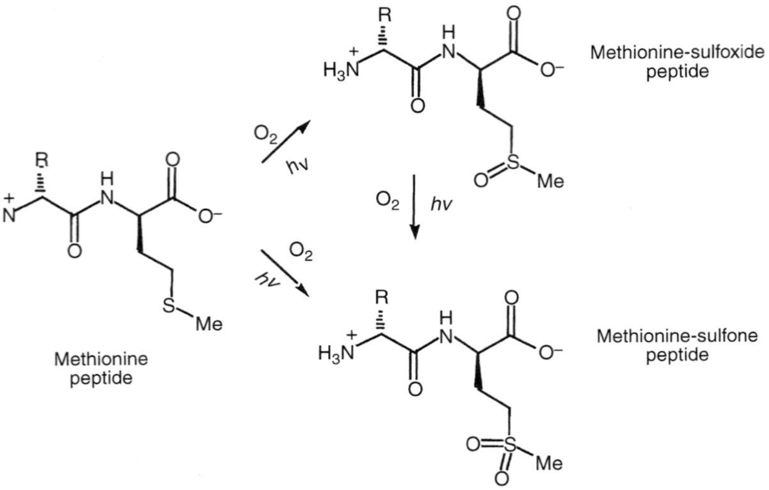

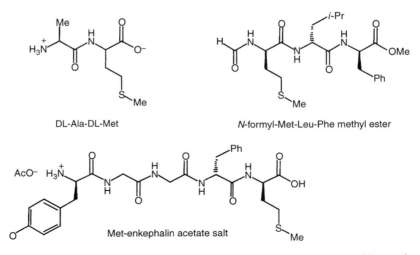

**Figure 1**   Methionine oxidation reactions. *Source*: From Ref. 8.

crystalline materials (Fig. 3). The effect of particle size was ruled out by studying the degradation of different size fractions. They concluded that the particle size was not a factor in the reactivity of the crystalline forms of the peptides (Fig. 4).

DL-Ala-DL-Met

N-formyl-Met-Leu-Phe methyl ester

Met-enkephalin acetate salt

**Figure 2**   Model peptides DL-Ala-DL-Met (a zwitterionic dipeptide), *N*-formyl-Met-Leu-Phe methyl ester (a neutral tripeptide), and Met-enkephalin acetate salt (a weakly acidic pentapeptide). *Source*: From Ref. 8.

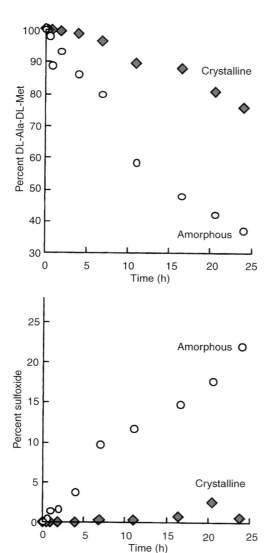

**Figure 3** Ultraviolet-induced degradation (*top*) and oxidation (*bottom*) of crystalline and amorphous DL-Ala-DL-Met at ambient conditions. *Source*: From Ref. 8.

## Steroids

A significant number of steroids are known to exist as polymorphs, and these different crystalline forms could potentially display different reactivities. Hydrocortisone 21-*tert*-butylacetate was investigated by Lin et al. (9) and found to exist as five polymorphs (forms I, II, III, IV, and V) depending on the solvents used to crystallize the drug. Using UV irradiation in air, form I was oxidized to cortisone 21-*tert*-butylacetate (Fig. 5). The

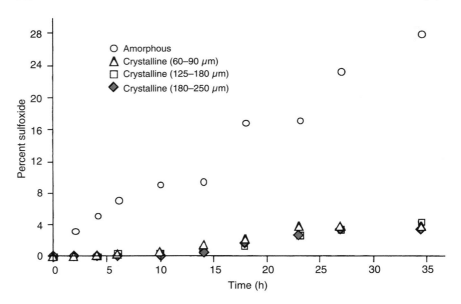

**Figure 4** The effect of particle size on the ultraviolet-induced Met oxidation of DL-Ala-DL-Met at ambient conditions. *Source*: From Ref. 8.

extent of degradation was monitored using nuclear magnetic resonance (NMR) while the desolvation of ethanol was measured using gas chromatography.

Another steroid, prednisolone (Fig. 6), was reported to exist in five crystalline polymorphic forms (10), and form V was found to be reactive. Form V had a hexagonal crystal form in which the steroid molecules form tunnels running down the sixfold axis. The nonstoichiometric solvent of crystallization is located in the center of the tunnels, and the authors

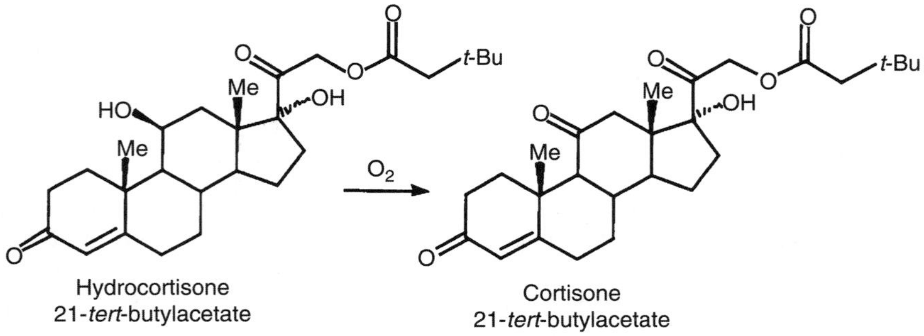

**Figure 5** Oxidation of hydrocortisone 21-*tert*-butylacetate. *Source*: From Ref. 9

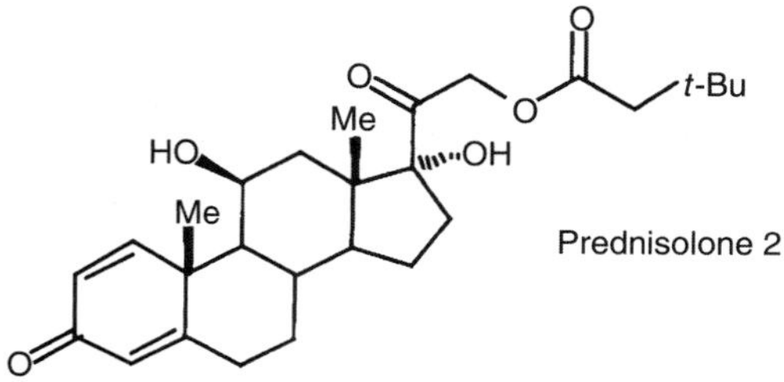

**Figure 6** Structure of prednisolone 21-*tert*-butylacetate. *Source*: From Ref. 10.

postulated that the reactivity or susceptibility to degradation was due to the location of the solvent and consequent vulnerability to penetration of oxygen down the axis.

## Cyclization

These reactions were reported by Xu (8) in his study of some angiotensin-converting enzyme (ACE) inhibitors—spirapril HCL and quinapril HCL (Fig. 7). Both drugs cyclize to form diketopiperazines as water is lost by the intermediate product. The cyclization mechanism is shown in Figure 7. From the study of Xu (8) and Hausin and Codding (11), it was found that the reacting nitrogen atoms (nitrogen of the alanine residue and the carbonyl of the adjacent carboxylic acid) in spirapril HCL and quinapril HCL (Fig. 8) are $> 5$ Å apart and the conformation must be disturbed in a

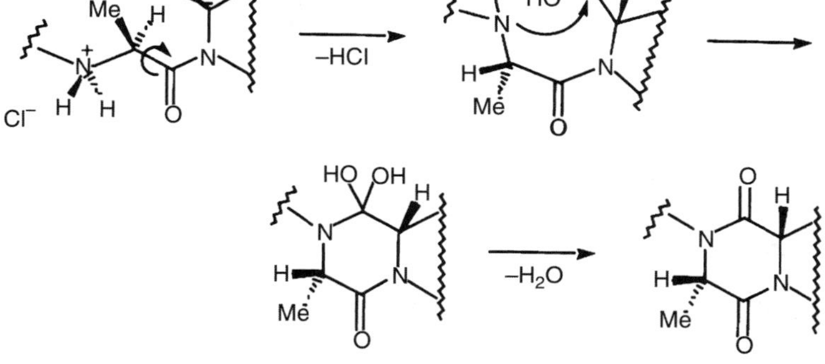

A diketopiperazine

**Figure 7** Mechanism scheme for the cyclization of an angiotensin-converting enzyme inhibitor to the corresponding diketopiperazine product. *Source*: From Ref. 8.

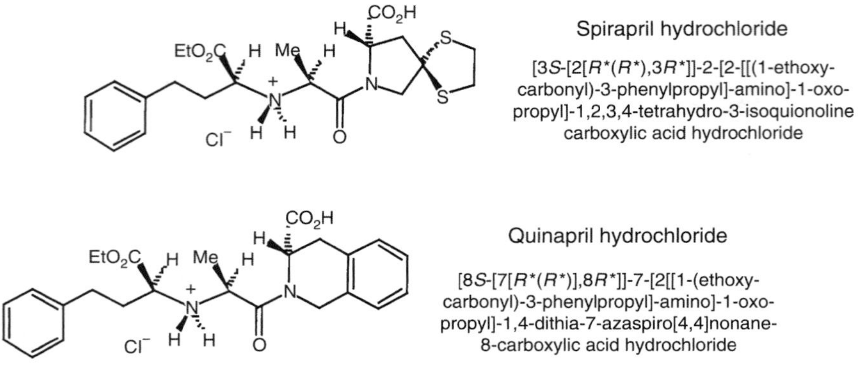

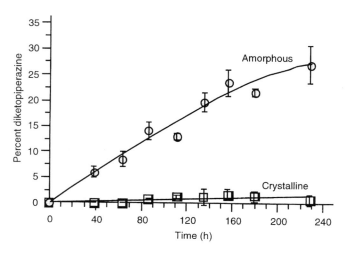

Spirapril hydrochloride
[3S-[2[R*(R*),3R*]]-2-[2-[[(1-ethoxy-carbonyl)-3-phenylpropyl]-amino]-1-oxo-propyl]-1,2,3,4-tetrahydro-3-isoquionoline carboxylic acid hydrochloride
Quinapril hydrochloride
[8S-[7[R*(R*)],8R*]]-7-[2[[1-(ethoxy-carbonyl)-3-phenylpropyl]-amino]-1-oxo-propyl]-1,4-dithia-7-azaspiro[4,4]nonane-8-carboxylic acid hydrochloride

**Figure 8** Structures of spirapril hydrochloride and quinapril hydrochloride. *Source*: From Ref. 8.

solid-state reaction. Therefore, Xu studied the crystalline and amorphous spirapril at different relative humidity (RH) conditions (1, 75, 80, 90, 95, and 100% RH). As shown in Figure 9, the author observed that the amorphous drug was more susceptible to degradation into the diketopiperazine than the crystalline. This was confirmed using interrupted-decoupled solid-state NMR, which indicated that the amorphous drug had more mobility than the crystalline. The presence of water on the two amorphous drugs was studied, and it was reported that water (with a lower glass transition temperature $T_g$) lowers the $T_g$ of the drugs. The decrease in $T_g$ correlated with the increase in reactivity due to a corresponding increase in mobility (Fig. 10).

Percent diketopiperazine
35
30
25
20
15
10
5
0
Amorphous
Crystalline
0
40
80
120
160
200
240
Time (h)

**Figure 9** Rates of degradation of crystalline and amorphous spirapril hydrochloride at 75°C. *Source*: From Ref. 8.

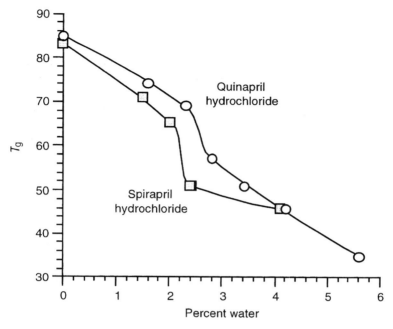

**Figure 10** The effect of water content on the $T_g$ of quinapril hydrochloride and spirapril hydrochloride. *Source*: From Ref. 8.

The author concluded that mobility is related to reactivity and that amorphous materials must be kept at temperatures below their $T_g$ values in order to maintain the stability of the drugs.

## Deamidation/Hydrolysis

These are chemical degradation pathways that are often observed in the solid state in proteins and peptides. Unfolding of proteins could also occur in the solid state due to factors such as processing (e.g., shear and lyophilization) and storage conditions. In order to mitigate the instability, excipients such as sucrose, trehalose, glucose, polyvinyl alcohol (PVA), and polyvinylpyrrolidone (PVP) are added. The presence of water is very critical in protein formulation because both the drug and the excipients are amorphous, and the potential for mobility increases in the presence of water. Water can affect the stability of a protein or peptide either by increasing its mobility, acting as a direct reactant or indirectly as a solvent. Therefore, it is important at the preformulation stage to identify other critical parameters that could affect the stability of these biomolecules. For example, the temperature of storage should be lower than the $T_g$ because molecular mobility increases with increased $T_g$. An example is the deamidation of a model hexapeptide (Val-Tyr-Pro-Asn-Gly-Ala) in the presence of water. Lai et al. (12,13) studied the role of water in the stability of the peptide using lyophilized formulations made with PVA, PVP, and glycerol. The author observed degradation with cyclic imide-hexapeptide, iso-Asp hexapeptide, and the Asp-hexapeptide as the degradative products. The mechanism of degradation involves intramolecular cyclization to form the cyclic imide, which is then hydrolyzed to form the iso-Asp and Asp-hexapeptide. Water was found to enhance the mobility, acting as both a reactant and a solvent. All these observations underscore the critical role water plays in the reactivity of the active ingredient and the stability and performance of the drugs.

## SOLID DOSAGE FORM EXCIPIENTS

Excipients are usually present in levels ranging between 10% and 99% of the formulation. Despite this, the components are not usually adequately characterized compared to the API. Although over 1000 excipients are currently being used in various solid dosage forms, only about 200 are commonly used in dosage form development. The majority of excipients are classified as follows, based on their functionality:

1. Diluents
2. Binders
3. Disintegrants
4. Lubricants
5. Glidant/adherents
6. Others:
    a. Film-coating agents
    b. Colors
    c. Flavors
    d. Sweeteners
    e. Surfactants and wetting agents

Examples of such excipients plus others in minor categories referenced in this chapter are shown in Table 1. Some of these materials have a dual role, depending on the level in a formulation.

The functionality of an excipient is often modified unintentionally due to drug–excipient or excipient–excipient interactions. Sometimes, these interactions are exploited to achieve a predetermined formulation objective, the usual being bioavailability. A few examples of some interactions that were not anticipated will be mentioned briefly in this section and discussed in detail later in the chapter.

Diluents are traditionally used to bulk the formulation and make the dosage form size practical, e.g., tablet. However, the physical form of the excipient could significantly affect the dissolution and bioavailability

**Table 1**   Examples of Commonly Used Excipients

Binders/adhesives
  Pregelatinize starch
  Starch
  Polyvinylpyrrolidone (povidone)—different grades
Coatings/polishing agents
  Shellac
Colors/flavors/sweeteners
  Titanium dioxide
Cryoprotectants
  Trehalose
  Cellobiose
  Lactose
  Sorbitol
  Mannitol
Cyclodextrins
  β-cyclodextrin
  α-cyclodextrin
  γ-cyclodextrin
  Hydroxypropyl-β-cyclodextrin
  Sulfobutylether-β-cyclodextrin
Diluents/fillers/bulking agents
  Lactose (hydrated, anhydrous, spray-dried)
  Calcium stearate
  Microcrystalline cellulose (various grades)
  Hydroxypropyl methylcellulose
  Calcium phosphate
  Sucrose
  Glucose
  Trehalose
  Mannitol
  Sodium chloride
  Sorbitol
  Sodium carboxymethylcellulose
  Hydroxypropyl methylcellulose
  Croscarmellose sodium
  Maltose
Disintegrants
  Croscarmellose sodium
  Sodium starch glycolate
  Starch
  Acacia
  Cross-linked polyvinylpyrrolidone
Lubricants/glidants
  Magnesium stearate
  Talc

*(Continued)*

**Table 1** Examples of Commonly Used Excipients
(*Continued*)

Stearic acid
Colloidal silicon dioxide
Magnesium oxide
Colloidal magnesium aluminum silicate
Polymers/waxes
  Microcrystalline wax
  Beeswax
  Cellulose acetate
  Ethyl cellulose
  Polycaprolactone
  Poly(*d,l*-lactide-PLA)
  Poly(glycolide)
  Eudragit® (different grades)
Solubilizers
  Tris buffer
  Meglumine
Surfactants
  Sodium lauryl sulfate
  Lauryl sacrospinale
  Sodium stearate

outcomes. For example, microcrystalline cellulose, a diluent, was reported to interact with and degrade a calcium channel blocker formulation (14). Although a lubricant-like magnesium stearate is included to prevent adhesion of the granules or powder blend during tableting and improve flow, it was reported in the same study to degrade the drug. Therefore, the choice of the excipients from a category becomes critical due to the propensity for interaction.

The choice of excipients in a formulation development program is determined by many factors, e.g., origin and source, functionality, quality and purity, extent of characterization, batch-to-batch consistency of basic properties, compatibility with actives and packaging materials, toxicity, and regulatory status. These factors add up to safety of the excipient or the status generally regarded as safe (GRAS).

If rational excipient selection is made earlier in the preclinical phase, the drug development program can be accelerated. Serajuddin et al. (14) expressed this in their investigation on the selection of solid dose formulation components. The authors reported that rational drug–excipient compatibility testing of dosage form composition at the outset of a developmental program (design of phase I clinical formulations) would help accelerate the development program in phases II and III and reduce time and cost significantly.

## SCREENING METHODS USED FOR DRUG–EXCIPIENT INTERACTION STUDIES

There is no universally accepted protocol in literature or by regulatory agencies for evaluating drug–excipient interactions or compatibility. Methods for robust characterization of drug–excipient interactions are limited, very time consuming, and labor intensive due to the number of variables that will need to be incorporated into the study. There have been suggestions in the literature on how to improve on this apparent limitation. Monkhouse and Maderich (15) suggested that excipients should be selected based on the physical and chemical characteristics of the actives and literature data on the excipients. They recommended that the final composition should be selected based on accelerated stability testing of one or several target formulations at high temperature and humidity conditions.

### Differential Scanning Calorimetry

A rapid method for selection of excipients should be included in the interaction study program because meaningful differences in the stability of the sample or formulations being tested may not be observed even at the International Conference on Harmonization (ICH) recommended conditions such as 40°C/75% RH. Differential scanning calorimetry (DSC) has been suggested by many authors (16–23) for evaluating drug–excipient interactions. Despite the apparent advantages of DSC, such as the use of small samples and rapid evaluation, the higher temperatures (up to 300°C) used in the analysis could introduce an added variable into the techniques that is not usually encountered in real-life situations. This is because the increased temperature increases the kinetics of reaction, which may consequently change the physicochemical properties of the components or reaction product. Therefore, the data must be interpreted carefully.

### Isothermal Stress Testing

Aging of drug–excipient blends in the presence of moisture under a constant temperature for a specific period or isothermal stress testing (IST) has been used by many authors (24–26). IST could reveal both drug–excipient interaction and compatibility. IST involves storage of drug–excipient blends with or without moisture at high temperature for a specified time to accelerate the aging and interaction with excipients. The samples are observed visually and the potency of the active ingredient determined using high-performance liquid chromatography (HPLC).

Serajuddin et al. (14) used a drug–excipient interaction study model that consisted of multicomponent blends of drug substances with excipients that were mixed with 20% added water and stored in closed vials at 50°C/75% RH. Examples of drugs used included fosinopril, pravastatin, and sorivudine (Fig. 11). The samples were analyzed for chemical and physical (appearance, color) stability. Drug–excipient blends without water and stored in a refrigerator or at room temperature served as controls. For photodegradable drugs, clear glass vials were used and the samples were exposed to room or high-intensity fluorescent light. For comparison, similar vials were wrapped in aluminum foil and stored under the same light

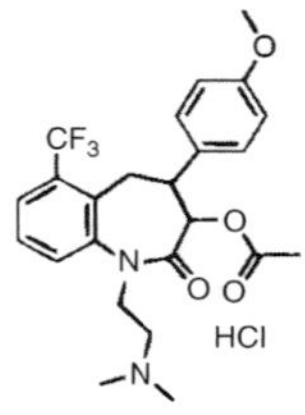

I

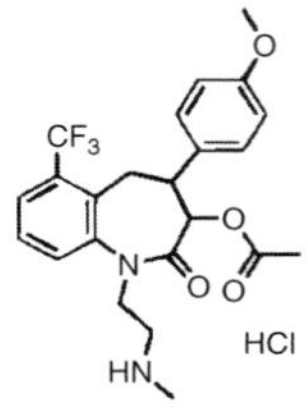

II

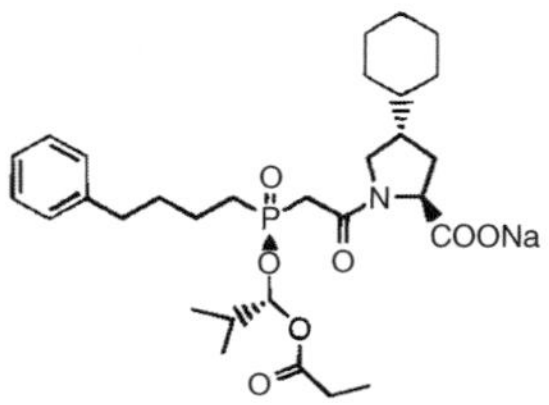

Fosinopril sodium (III)

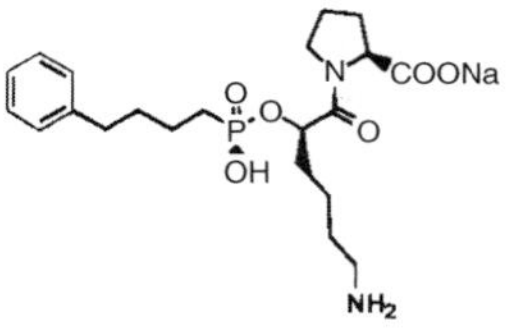

Ceronapril (IV)

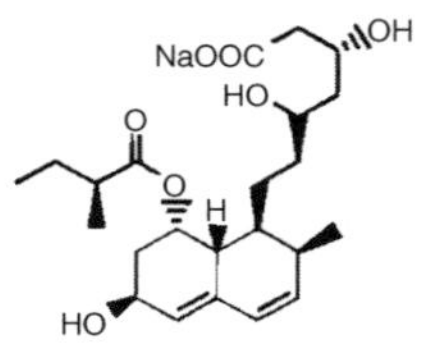

Pravastatin sodium (V)

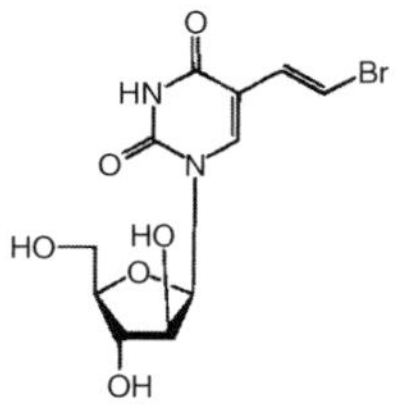

Sorivudine (VI)

Ifetroban sodium (VII)

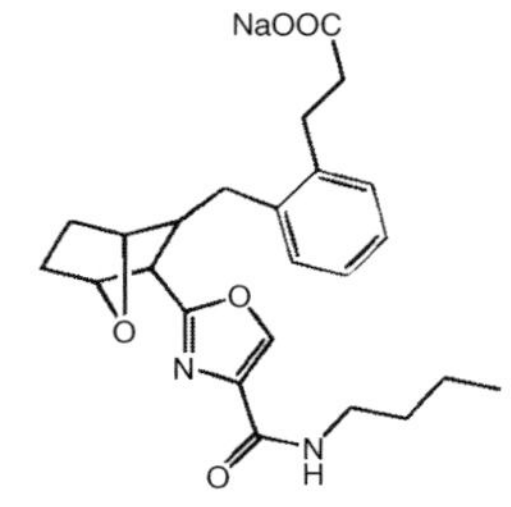

**Figure 11** Names and chemical names of drugs used. *Source*: From Ref. 14.

conditions. The number of blends could be determined using a statistical design. However, in a multicomponent solid dosage formulation, where excipients such as diluents, lubricants, disintegrants, and binders are usually screened for a particular formulation, the number of blends that would be needed for an interaction study may be high. The authors suggested that the drug–excipient interaction study could be performed in two stages:

1. Stage I: Compatibility testing of drug with diluents and lubricants. The goal is to identify one primary diluent and one primary lubricant.
2. Stage II: Compatibility testing of the drug–diluent–lubricant mixture with other excipients, such as binders and disintegrants.

The mixtures could be placed in gelatin capsules, since capsules are used for initial clinical studies. The total weight of the drug–excipient blend (200 mg) was based on the expected drug-to-excipient ratio in the final formulation. The lowest and the highest expected ratios were used to bracket drug concentrations in a formulation. The design used by the authors is shown in Table 2. Although this screening method is more practical, it can be time consuming and usually involves a lot of HPLC studies.

## Combination of DSC and IST

In general, a lot of drug–excipient studies involve the combination of DSC and IST plus other relevant analytical techniques. Verma and Garg (27) used the combination in their investigation of interaction between isosorbide mononitrate (IMN) and selected excipients such as cellulose acetate, colloidal silicon dioxide, ethyl cellulose, and magnesium stearate. The investigators vortexed drug–excipient blends with 10% w/w water in vials followed by additional mixing with a glass capillary (with sealed ends), which was broken and left inside the vial to prevent loss of material. The drug–excipient ratio was 1:1 ratio for all excipients except for drug–silicon dioxide blend, which was 4:1. The vials sealed with Teflon®-lined caps were stored at 50°C. Blends without water were stored similarly and used as controls. The blends were examined periodically for color change and analyzed for potency by HPLC after three weeks of storage.

Their results, as observed in the HPLC analysis, showed that there was interaction and incompatibility between IMN and cellulose acetate (Fig. 12). For some excipients, interaction was observed but not incompatibility. For example, drug–microcrystalline cellulose (MCC) blend, analyzed with DSC, showed a shift of the endothermic peak to lower temperature (80.9°C) from the characteristic IMN peak at 91.08°C (Fig. 13). There was also a significant decrease in the enthalpy value (Table 3). However, the incompatibility was not characterized. Drug–excipient interaction should be distinguished from drug–excipient incompatibility. The latter is a consequence of interaction and can be rapidly determined using DSC, whereas

**Table 2** Composition of Drug–Excipient Blends Used for Compound I after Three Weeks of Storage at 50°C in Closed Vials with 20% Added Water[a]

| | | | | | | | | | Experiments | | | | | | | | |
|---|---|---|---|---|---|---|---|---|---|---|---|---|---|---|---|---|---|
| | 1 | 2 | 3 | 4 | 5 | 6 | 7 | 8 | 9 | 10 | 11 | 12 | 13 | 14 | 15 | 16 | 17 |
| Drug substance (I) | 200 | 25 | 25 | 25 | 25 | 25 | 25 | 25 | 25 | 25 | 25 | 25 | 25 | 25 | 25 | 25 | 25 |
| Lactose | | 175 | | | | 170 | | | | 170 | | | | 170 | | | |
| Mannitol | | | 175 | | | | 170 | | | | 170 | | | | 170 | | |
| Microcrystalline cellulose | | | | 175 | | | | 170 | | | | 170 | | | | 170 | |
| Dibasic calcium phosphate dehydrate | | | | | 175 | | | | 170 | | | | 170 | | | | 170 |
| Magnesium stearate | | | | | | 5 | 5 | 5 | 5 | | | | | | | | |
| Sodium stearyl fumarate | | | | | | | | | | 5 | 5 | 5 | 5 | | | | |
| Stearic acid | | | | | | | | | | | | | | 5 | 5 | 5 | 5 |
| Potency remaining | 96.4 | 95.7 | 95.8 | 93.9 | 85.0 | 64.3 | 65.4 | 65.3 | 68.1 | 77.9 | 81.9 | 77.6 | 81.8 | 90.0 | 92.9 | 88.1 | 78.3 |
| Hydrolysis product formed | 3.3 | 4.1 | 4.0 | 5.8 | 16.7 | 37.0 | 36.7 | 36.3 | 33.7 | 21.8 | 15.4 | 20.1 | 15.3 | 9.7 | 6.9 | 11.7 | 21.6 |

[a]Weights of all ingredients are in milligrams.
*Source:* From Ref. 14.

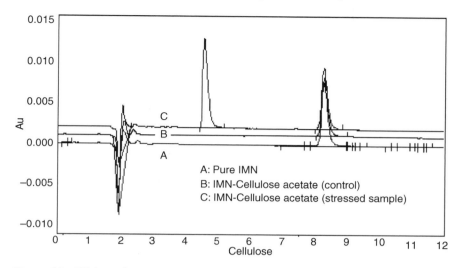

**Figure 12**  High performance liquid chromatography chromatogram of IMN with cellulose acetate. *Abbreviation*: IMN, isosorbide mononitrate. *Source*: From Ref. 28.

the incompatibility is better studied using IST. Interaction between drugs and excipients could be tolerated within reasonable limits if there are no possible alternative excipients. In contrast, if solid-state evaluation reveals incompatibility, the excipients should be eliminated in the development process. On the basis of the incompatibility of the drug with IMN, the excipient was not included in further formulation development.

In another study, Verma and Garg (28) examined compatibility between glipizide and many excipients such as microcrystalline cellulose acetate, magnesium stearate, sodium chloride, lactose, mannitol, meglumine, and Tris buffer. DSC, infrared (IR), and IST were used to evaluate the interaction. They reported that there was no incompatibility between the drug and some excipients such as MCC, sodium chloride, and magnesium stearate. Incompatibility (yellow discoloration of blend) was observed with meglumine/Tris buffer (used as solubilizer in the formulation) in the presence of lactose. This was reported to be due to reaction of the amine group of meglumine and lactose.

In a diclofenac–excipient interaction study, Adeyeye et al. (29) also used an IST technique in which a slurry of drug–excipient liquid binary and ternary mixtures and ratios expected in the formulation were used (Table 4). The mixtures were dried overnight and then analyzed using X-ray diffraction (XRD) and DSC. A comparison was made with individual components. This will be discussed further in the section titled *Charge Interaction*).

Brittain (1) emphasized the IST or combination with other screening techniques in his overview of drug–excipient interactions. He remarked that

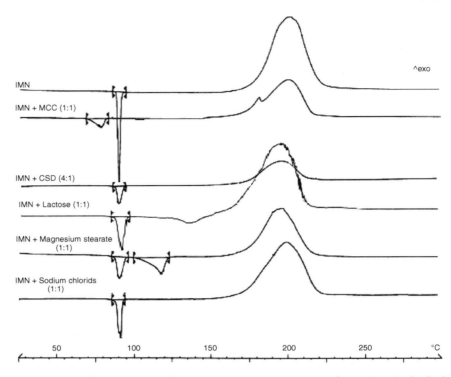

**Figure 13**  Differential scanning calorimetry thermogram of IMN and physical mixtures of IMN with different excipients. *Abbreviations*: IMN, isosorbide mononitrate; CSD, colloidal silicon dioxide; MCC, microcrystalline cellulose. *Source*: From Ref. 28.

the drug should be blended with excipients at levels that are realistic with respect to the proposed formulation (1). For example, if a lubricant is to be used at the 0.5% level in a formulation, the evaluation of a 50% substance: excipient (or binary) mixture is not appropriate or practical. Instead, each blend should be stored at accelerated stress conditions (elevated temperature and humidity), and tested for drug substance stability after an appropriate equilibration period. The purity and impurity profiling is then performed using a chromatographic procedure, while the physical characteristics are studied using appropriate physical analysis methodology. Some of these will be discussed later in the chapter.

## Solubility Parameter

This method can be used to study polymer–drug miscibility and evaluate incompatibility and/or predict polymer–drug, polymer–polymer interactions. The author addressed incompatibility as miscibility and/or interaction

**Table 3** Peak Temperature and Enthalpy Values of IMN in Various Drug–Excipient Mixtures

| Sample | Ratio (drug–excipient) | $T_{onset}$ (°C) | $T_{peak}$ (°C) | $\Delta H_{fcorr}$ (J/g)[a] |
|---|---|---|---|---|
| IMN | – | 90.42 | 91.08 | 125.32 |
| IMN + cellulose acetate | 1:1 | 68.01 | 74.82 | 34.10 |
| IMN + colloidal silicon dioxide | 4:1 | 89.10 | 91.09 | 69.22 |
| IMN + ethyl cellulose | 1:1 | 89.24 | 93.35 | 131.48 |
| IMN + hydroxypropylmethyl cellulose | 1:1 | 87.55 | 89.88 | 71.51 |
| IMN + lactose | 1:1 | 89.10 | 92.39 | 123.48 |
| IMN + MCC | 1:1 | 73.40 | 80.91 | 73.03 |
| IMN + magnesium stearate | 1:1 | 88.98 | 91.50 | 89.65 |
| IMN + polyvinylpyrrolidone | 1:1 | 53.17 | 71.41 | 140.53[b] |
| IMN + sodium chloride | 1:1 | 89.45 | 92.00 | 128.24 |
| IMN + sorbitol | 1:1 | 87.25 | 92.89 | 253.67[c] |

[a] $\Delta H_f = \Delta H_{fobs}/\%\text{drug in sample} \times 100$ (2).
[b] Total value (IMN melting + polymer dehydration).
[c] Total value (IMN melting + excipient melting).
*Abbreviations*: IMN, isosorbide mononitrate; MCC, microcrystalline cellulose.
*Source*: From Ref. 27.

with no alteration in the chemical nature of the polymer or drug (30). There is generally no template or set parameters used in the study of drug–polymer interactions because of the uniqueness of the physical and chemical properties of the drug. The use of the traditional methods stated above can sometimes be costly and prolonged. Therefore, the use of a solubility parameter accompanied by thermal and spectroscopic analysis has been considered. Hildebrand solubility parameter (δ) is defined as the square root of a molecule's cohesive energy (CED).

$$\delta = (\text{CED})^{0.5} = (\Delta E_v/V_m)^{0.5}$$

$\Delta E_v$ is the energy of vaporization and $V_m$ is the molar volume of the compound. CED is the minimum energy required to physically separate the constituent atoms of a molecule. The total solubility parameter is a sum of different components that account for different interatomic and intermolecular forces:

$$\delta = \left(\delta_d^2 + \delta_p^2 + \delta_h^2\right)^{1/2}$$

$\delta_d$, $\delta_p$, and $\delta_h$ are the partial solubility parameters indicating contributions from Van der Waal's dispersion forces, dipole–dipole interactions, and hydrogen bonding, respectively.

**Table 4** Mixtures of Diclofenac and Respective Components

| System | Composition |
|---|---|
| Single | Diclofenac |
| | Eudragit L100 |
| | Eudragit RS PO |
| | Calcium carbonate |
| | Avicel Cl-611 |
| Binary mixture (dry powder) | Eudragit L100 + drug |
| | Eudragit RS PO + drug |
| | Avicel CL-611 + drug |
| | Calcium carbonate + drug |
| Binary mixture (liquid, codried) | Eudragit RS30D + drug |
| | Eudragit L30D-55 + drug |
| | Avicel Cl-611 + drug |
| | Calcium carbonate + drug |
| | Suspending medium + drug |
| Ternary (liquid, codried) | L30D + RS30D + drug |
| Ternary (dry powder) | RS PO + L100D + drug |
| Multicomponent | Formulation comp. + Avicel |
| | Suspending medium + physical admix of components |
| | Suspending medium + drug microcapsules |

*Source*: From Ref. 29.

The solubility parameter is usually measured using the functional group contribution method. This is based on the assumption that the total CED of a molecule is a sum of the contributions from the individual functional groups:

$$\delta = \left(\sum F\right)/V = \left(\sum F\right)\rho/M_o$$

$F$ is the molar attraction constant for individual functional groups, $V$ is the molar volume of the repeat unit, $M_o$ is the molar mass, and $\rho$ is the polymer density. The energy of mixing ($\Delta G_M$) between two molecules is determined by the enthalpy ($\Delta H_M$) and entropy of mixing ($\Delta S_M$) at a particular temperature of mixing as shown below:

$$\Delta G_M = \Delta H_M - T\Delta S_M$$

$$\Delta H_M = \phi_1\phi_2(\delta_1 - \delta_2)^2$$

$\phi_1$ and $\phi_2$ are the volume fractions of drug and polymer. From the equation, it is seen that as the solubility parameters of the drug and polymer approach each other, or as $\Delta H_M$ approaches zero, miscibility or interaction is promoted.

The use of the solubility parameter to predict drug–polymer interaction may not always be accurate because of the fact that sometimes, differences in total solubility are considered whereas differences in partial solubility could have been more predictive. However, a logical approach is to first consider the physical and chemical properties of the drug and match these with a suitable polymer.

Liu et al. (30) considered the properties of ellipticine and then calculated the total and partial solubility parameters for various polymer–ellipticine pairs. The polymers used included poly-β-benzyl-L-aspartate (PBLA), polycaprolactone (PCL), poly(D,L-lactide-PLA-), and poly(glycolide). Fourier transform IR (FTIR) and X-ray analyses of the pairs were performed, and compatible polymers were consequently identified. Based on the solubility parameter and enthalpy of mixing ($\Delta H_M$) studies, it was demonstrated that the suitability of the polymers decreased in this order: PBLA > PCL > PLA > Poly (glycolide) (PGA). The total solubility parameters for ellipticine and various polymers are shown in Table 5. The authors used the polymers to formulate the drug using a solvent casting method, and their studies showed a good correlation between drug formulation characteristics and the drug–polymer compatibility studies.

The solubility parameter approach was also used by Greenhalgh et al. (31) to study compatibility between solid dispersions of ibuprofen and

**Table 5** Difference Between Total and Partial Solubility Parameters and Enthalpy of Mixing for Ellipticine and Various Polymers (Mpa ½)

| Polymer | $\Delta\delta_d{}^a$ | $\Delta\delta_p{}^a$ | $\Delta\delta_h{}^a$ | $\Delta\delta_t{}^a$ | $\Delta H_m$ |
|---|---|---|---|---|---|
| Poly (β-benzyl-L-aspartate) | 2.0 | −1.2 | −2.0 | 0.8 | 2.2 |
| Poly (β-benzyl-L-glutamate) | 2.6 | −0.4 | −1.4 | 1.8 | 2.2 |
| Poly (5-benzyloxy-trimethylene carbonate) | 4.0 | −0.4 | −1.8 | 2.9 | 4.9 |
| Poly [(3S)-sec-butylmorpholine-2,5-dione] | 5.0 | −1.4 | −2.2 | 3.3 | 8.0 |
| Poly (δ-valerolactone) | 6.3 | 0.1 | −1.5 | 5.2 | 10.0 |
| Poly (ε-caprolactone) | 6.5 | 1.1 | −0.7 | 5.9 | 10.8 |
| Poly (β-butyrolactone) | 6.8 | −1.3 | −2.6 | 4.6 | 11.9 |
| Poly (propylene oxide) | 7.6 | −1.5 | 0.1 | 6.3 | 12.0 |
| Poly (β-propiolactone) | 5.7 | −3.7 | −4.1 | 2.1 | 12.2 |
| Poly (β-methyl-δ-valerolactone) | 7.0 | 1.1 | −0.7 | 6.3 | 12.3 |
| Poly (α-allyl-valerolactone) | 6.8 | 2.1 | 0.2 | 6.7 | 12.5 |
| Poly (trimethylene carbonate) | 5.7 | −2.9 | −4.2 | 2.3 | 13.2 |
| Poly (ethylene oxide) | 6.4 | −5.0 | −1.4 | 3.2 | 13.7 |
| Poly (d,l-lactide) | 6.6 | −3.6 | −4.1 | 2.8 | 14.3 |
| Poly (glycolide) | 4.8 | −8.3 | −6.6 | −1.9 | 21.7 |

$^a \Delta\delta$ ¼, δEllipticine- δPolymer

hydrophilic carriers such as xylitol, lutrol F68, sugars (sucrose, maltose sorbitol), and sugar–polymer (dextran). The authors used analytical techniques such as DSC, powder XRD, and UV analyses. They observed that there was incompatibility between the drug and some sugar carriers and there was a trend between large differences in drug/carrier solubility parameters and increasing degree of immiscibility or incompatibilities between ibuprofen and carrier. There was miscibility or compatibility between the drug and carriers such as PVP and lutrol F68, where the $\Delta\delta$ were 1.6 and 1.9, respectively. In contrast, there was immiscibility between the drug and maltose, sorbitol, and xylitol. The $\Delta\delta$ were 18.0, 17.3, and 16.2, respectively. They remarked that Hildebrand parameters gave an indication of incompatibilities and concluded that partial solubility parameters may provide more accurate predictions of interactions. Despite the limitations, solubility parameters may provide a simple and generic means for rational selection of carriers in the preparation of solid dispersions.

Susuki and Sunada (32) also used the Hildebrand solubility parameters to select suitable polymers for nifedipine solid dispersions.

## Microcalorimetry

### Isothermal Titration Microcalorimetry

The technique can be used to study drug–excipient interactions (complexation) in solution at a controlled temperature. At the same time, the thermodynamic parameters such as the binding constant ($K$) and enthalpy ($\Delta H$) can be measured. The values can then be used to calculate the free energy of binding ($\Delta G$) and the change in entropy ($\Delta S$). It has an advantage over phase solubility techniques, where the equilibration of the sample takes longer time and the subsequent handling cannot be easily performed at constant temperature. The latter technique often results in inaccurate binding constants at temperatures other than those around the room temperature. Katpally et al. (33) used the method to study interaction between sulfobutyl ether cyclodextrin (SBE-7$\beta$-CD) and four bile salts to establish the differences in the binding thermodynamics of the dihydroxy bile salts (e.g., ursodeoxycholic acid and chenodeoxycholic acid) versus trihydroxy bile salts (e.g., cholic acid and glycocholic acid). They concluded that the bile salt complexation or interaction with SBE-7$\beta$-CD was greatly influenced by the degree of hydroxylation, functional groups, and stereochemistry of the bile salts. The thermodynamic data revealed that several forces such as Van der Waal's forces, hydrogen bonds, hydrophobic interactions, and changes in the environment of water molecules in the SBE-7$\beta$-CD cavity contributed to the inclusion complexation. One of the bile salts, ursodeoxycholate, had a strong tendency to form complexes with SBE-7$\beta$-CD.

High-Sensitivity DSC

The method's high sensitivity (± 0.5 μW), due to its capacity for larger sample and slower scan rates, made it suitable for studies such as drug–excipient compatibility where small changes in reaction enthalpy often take place. The instrument was operated at the isothermal mode, and temperature scanning was used to raise the temperature in 5°C steps between the isothermal phases. The thermal behavior of the individual drug and excipient components were compared with that of the drug–excipient mixture. The difference in heat flow is used as the index of possible interaction. Investigators who have used the method to study drug–excipient interactions include Wissing et al. (34) and Beezer et al. (35). Wissing et al. (34) used the method to study the interaction between aspirin and magnesium stearate. They observed a shift in the baseline (endothermic signals) during isothermal stages above 55°C, indicative of interaction between aspirin and magnesium stearate (Fig. 14).

## Use of Experimental Design

A statistical experimental design is sometimes used to develop a more robust model during the evaluation of interactions or incompatibilities in different

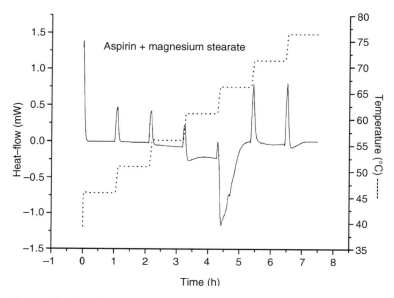

**Figure 14**  HSDC trace for a binary mixture of aspirin and magnesium stearate in 5°C steps. *Abbreviation*: HSDC, high sensitivity scanning calorimetry. *Source*: From Ref. 34.

drug–excipient mixtures. This should be preceded by a rapid excipient–drug screening on binary mixtures using DSC techniques. The use of experimental design will ensure that only necessary experiments are run and the results are as precise as possible for optimization of the formulation. An experimental mixture design that is predicated on the assumption that the measured response depends only on the proportions of the ingredients present can be used.

Mura et al. (36) used a 20-run D-optimal design (Table 6) to evaluate the compatibility of glibenclamide (a model drug) in a tablet formulation. A preliminary experiment using a binary mixture was set followed by the use of a statistical matrix. The designed relative amounts of excipients such as natrosol (a binding agent), stearic acid (lubricant), sorbitol as diluent, and cross-linked PVP as disintegrant. The goal was to identify the proportions of the mixture components that would give the optimal formulation parameter—maximum stability. The authors kept the total amount of the mixture or weight of tablet constant. The tablet was prepared using a hydraulic

**Table 6**   20-Run D-Optimal Experimental Plan

| Experiment number | Mixture component proportions (% w/w) | | | |
|---|---|---|---|---|
| | Binder | Diluent | Lubricant | Disintegrant |
| 1 | 42.19 | 46.87 | 0.94 | 3.75 |
| 2 | 42.19 | 45.00 | 2.81 | 3.75 |
| 3 | 42.19 | 43.12 | 0.94 | 7.50 |
| 4 | 42.19 | 41.25 | 2.81 | 7.50 |
| 5 | 46.87 | 42.19 | 0.94 | 3.75 |
| 6 | 46.87 | 40.32 | 2.81 | 3.75 |
| 7 | 46.87 | 38.44 | 0.94 | 7.50 |
| 8 | 46.87 | 36.57 | 2.81 | 7.50 |
| 9 | 42.19 | 45.94 | 1.88 | 3.75 |
| 10 | 42.19 | 44.99 | 0.94 | 5.62 |
| 11 | 44.53 | 44.53 | 0.94 | 3.75 |
| 12 | 42.19 | 43.13 | 2.81 | 5.62 |
| 13 | 44.53 | 42.66 | 2.81 | 3.75 |
| 14 | 42.19 | 42.19 | 1.88 | 7.50 |
| 15 | 44.53 | 40.78 | 0.94 | 7.50 |
| 16 | 44.53 | 38.91 | 2.81 | 7.50 |
| 18 | 46.87 | 40.31 | 0.94 | 5.62 |
| 19 | 46.87 | 38.45 | 2.81 | 5.62 |
| 20 | 46.87 | 37.51 | 1.88 | 7.50 |
| 27 | 44.53 | 41.72 | 1.88 | 5.62 |

The number of experiments is a subset of the original mixture design.
*Source*: From Ref. 36.

press at a fixed pressure. The compacts were then broken and sieved and a size faction was collected for DSC analysis. The DSC responses (which represent drug stability and compatibility of the drug–excipients mixture), i.e., difference between the melting point of pure drug and that of each analyzed mixture ($\Delta T_{fusion}$) and the enthalpy ($\Delta H$) were used. The authors concluded there was no incompatibility, as shown in Table 7.

## NATURE OF DRUG–EXCIPIENT INTERACTIONS

Understanding of drug–excipient interactions is based on the knowledge of the reactivity of the excipient (physically or chemically) in the presence of drug, other components, or environmental factors. The reactivity could be positive or negative in terms of the effect on the performance of the dosage form. For example, grinding can cause polymorphic changes or a change in the crystalline

**Table 7** Comparison Between the Observed and Predicted Responses by the Calculated Model

| Experiment number | $Y_{observed}$ | $Y_{calculated}$ |
|---|---|---|
| 1 | 39.980 | 38.264 |
| 2 | 75.200 | 77.243 |
| 3 | 56.490 | 59.011 |
| 4 | 69.480 | 71.050 |
| 5 | 66.150 | 65.490 |
| 6 | 61.690 | 61.921 |
| 7 | 85.000 | 86.932 |
| 8 | 54.540 | 52.634 |
| 9 | 63.150 | 63.421 |
| 10 | 51.890 | 52.008 |
| 11 | 39.210 | 41.754 |
| 12 | 90.150 | 88.013 |
| 13 | 60.500 | 57.770 |
| 14 | 78.630 | 75.962 |
| 15 | 63.510 | 60.507 |
| 16 | 46.500 | 47.662 |
| 18 | 79.420 | 77.685 |
| 19 | 67.480 | 69.247 |
| 20 | 79.630 | 80.003 |
| 27 | 65.510 | 67.534 |
| — | — | — |
| 17[a] | 57.455 | 56.532 |
| 21[a] | 60.447 | 64.596 |
| 22[a] | 63.328 | 63.862 |

[a] Test point.
*Source*: From Ref. 36.

state that could improve solubility but negatively affect flowability, stability, packing or, consolidation during compression. Since often times, the API cannot be easily modified, formulators have to identify an excipient or group of excipients that will be compatible with the drug or best suit. Sometimes, it is the processing technique that will need modification to accommodate the peculiarities of the drug and/or excipients. Therefore, the reactivity of the active ingredient becomes the basis for the choice. Whatever the case, it is early in the development phase or at the preformulation phase that the scientist must confront these issues and rationally determine components that will eventually lead to a robust and stable formulation. Some of the different types of interactions—physical and chemical—will now be considered.

## Physical Interaction

The reactivity between drug and excipient could be initiated via milling, phase transformation, addition, or adsorption. Phase transformation or polymorphic transformation of fostedil (in the presence of microcrystalline cellulose) was reported by Takahashi et al. in which form I polymorph of the drug converted to form II as a result of the interaction with the excipient (37).

### Milling

The effects of milling and compression on the physical stability of metoclopramide hydrochloride and various crystal forms of lactose blends were investigated by Qiu et al. (38). Spray-dried lactose monohydrate (LMH), lactose anhydrate, and LMH were used. The milling was expected to increase the surface area, produce more amorphous entities in the solid, and create defects in the solid. Milling was done using an electric motor grinder and a methacrylate ball. The impact of milling was tested by checking the propensity of the milled product (with increased surface area) toward a Maillard reaction. Unmilled samples were used as control. Annealing of milled samples was done (by exposure to the vapor of 25% ethanol and dimethyl formamide solution) to recover the crystallinity of the drug lost by milling. The study revealed that the increase in surface area produced by milling as well as the presence of amorphous content in the mixture makes the system more sensitive to pressure and promotes chemical degradation via Maillard reaction. Figure 15 shows the effect of milling time on the reactivity of metoclopramide and amorphous lactose at a specified temperature and humidity. The annealed product showed less degradation (Fig. 16).

### Compression

Similarly, unmilled and milled samples were compressed and studied for relative reactivity toward the Maillard reaction. There was no reactivity with the lactose forms except for amorphous lactose, in which the reaction rate increased with increase in compression pressure (Fig. 17—open triangle symbol).

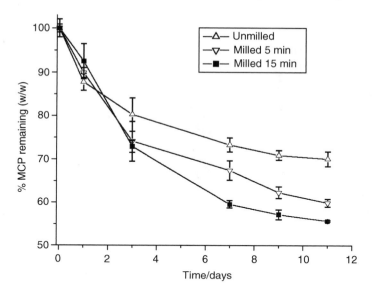

**Figure 15** Effect of milling time on the reactivity of metoclopramide and amorphous lactose stored at 105°C and 0% relative humidity. *Abbreviation*: MCP, metoclopramide hydrochloride. *Source*: From Ref. 38.

Effect of compression pressure on the polymorphs of sulfamerazine (SMZ I and SMZ II) was investigated by Roy et al. (39). In an earlier report, SMZ I was reported by Sun and Grant (40) to have slip planes, which imparts plasticity to the polymorph, thus rendering it more compressible and with better tablettability. Excipients such as microcrystalline cellulose (Avicel 101) and magnesium stearate were each used in a 1:1 ratio with the drug. DSC curves of the binary mixture of SMZ I and SMZ I + MCC did not reveal any interaction (Fig. 18).

However, at increased elevated humidity conditions (e.g., 100% RH), there was a peak that appeared at 145°C that was not observed in freshly prepared samples and room temperature (Fig. 19). The authors reported that the observation could be due to the effect of both humidity and temperature. This could not be confirmed by powder XRD. The authors suggested that variable temperature XRD, IR, and proton NMR techniques could confirm the drug–excipient interaction.

### Solid-on-Solid Adsorption

Interaction between magnesium stearate and a surfactant, sodium lauryl sulfate, was reported by Wang and Chowhan (41). The results suggested a strong interaction between magnesium stearate and the surfactant during solid-state powder mixing process. The interaction allowed adsorbed magnesium stearate to be freed from surfaces of the drug particles. This

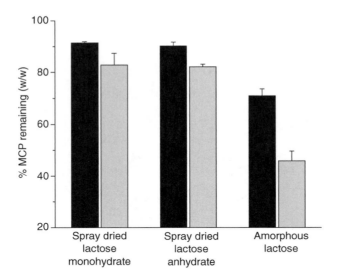

**Figure 16** Effect of compression on the reaction rate of Maillard reaction between metoclopramide hydrochloride and lactose compressed at 350 MPa for five seconds and incubated at 105°C at 0% for nine days. Annealed product represented as dark bar graph. *Abbreviation*: MCP, metoclopramide hydrochloride. *Source*: From Ref. 38.

resulted in the prevention of the deleterious effect of magnesium stearate (retarding effect on dissolution and unmixing) on the dissolution rate of the drug. In another study, Ong et al. (42) reported a similar interaction between magnesium stearate and various hydrophilic surfactants such as sodium-*N*-lauryl sacrospinale, sodium stearoyl-2-lactylate, and sodium stearate.

Solid phase interaction was reported by Mura et al. (20) in their study of ibuproxam and various excipients. The excipients included PVP K-30, polyvinylpolypyrolidone (PVPP), polyethyleneglycol (PEG) 4000, sodium carboxymethylcellulose (NaCMC), microcrystalline cellulose (Avicel PH 101), palmitic acid, and magnesium stearate. The apparent drug–excipient interaction was observed for some of the excipients using DSC analysis. For example, there was an interaction between the drug and PVP K30 and PVPP (Fig. 20). However, further elucidation using hot stage microscopy and scanning electron microscopy (SEM) excluded incompatibility. This underscores the importance of using more than one analytical method to establish compatibility.

### Liquid-on-Solid Adsorption (Role of Moisture)

Interaction between moisture and solid materials in a formulation could involve adsorption of the moisture as monolayers or multilayers or may be

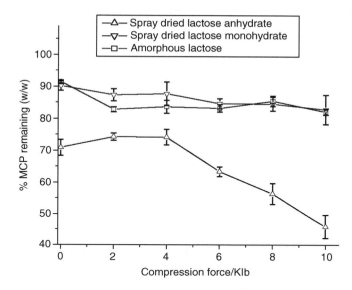

**Figure 17** Effect of compression pressure on the reaction rate of tablets made from metoclopramide hydrochloride and various forms of lactose. Tablets were incubated at 105°C at 0% for nine days. *Abbreviation*: MCP, metoclopramide hydrochloride. *Source*: From Ref. 38.

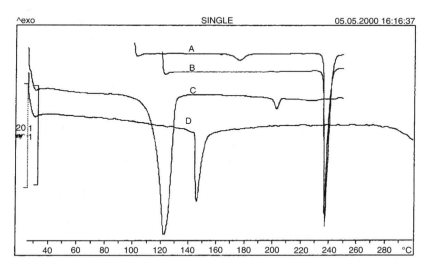

**Figure 18** Overlaid differential scanning calorimetry profiles of the freshly prepared binary mixtures: (**A**) SMZ I + MCC; (**B**) SMZ I + MgSt; (**C**) SMZ II + MgSt; (**D**) SMZ II + MCC. *Abbreviations*: MCC, microcrystalline cellulose; MgSt, magnesium stearate; SMZ, sulfamerazine. *Source*: From Ref. 39.

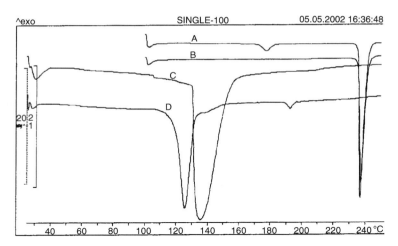

^exo                        SINGLE-100              05.05.2002 16:36:48

**Figure 19** Overlaid differential scanning calorimetry profiles of the binary mixtures stored at 100% relative humidity for a period of 10 days: (**A**) SMZ I + MCC; (**B**) SMZ I + MgSt; (**C**) SMZ II + MgSt; (**D**) SMZ II + MCC. *Abbreviations*: MCC, microcrystalline cellulose; MgSt, magnesium stearate; SMZ, sulfamerazine. *Source*: From Ref. 39.

present as condensed water at the surface (43). Adsorption of moisture on crystalline solids could result in crystal hydrate formation, deliquescence, and capillary condensation. On the other hand, amorphous materials have a high capacity for water vapor sorption that far exceeds what can be accounted for by adsorption. Instead of adsorption, water can be absorbed through incorporation into the crystal lattice of a hydrate former via hydrogen bonding or coordinate covalent bonds with other water molecules and/or drug molecules. This is possible due to the small size of water and its ability to act as hydrogen bond donor and acceptor, thereby stabilizing hydrate structures.

The water interacts with the bulk solid and this could lead to significant changes in the bulk properties of the solid. The amount of moisture sorbed depends on particle size distribution of the solid, specific surface area, nature of the adsorbent, porosity of the solid, and deliquescence. The moisture sorption mechanism will need to be established using the vapor sorption isotherm.

The Brunauer-Emmett-Teller's multilayer adsorption theory was developed to depict the different mechanisms. There are six different models (I–VI) for different mechanisms of water adsorption. Types I, III, V, and VI are not commonly observed. Type II isotherms (sigmoid or S-shaped) are the normal forms of isotherms that are observed with nonporous and macroporous adsorbents, classes of adsorbents under which many pharmaceutical drugs and excipients fall (44,45). It also represents unrestricted

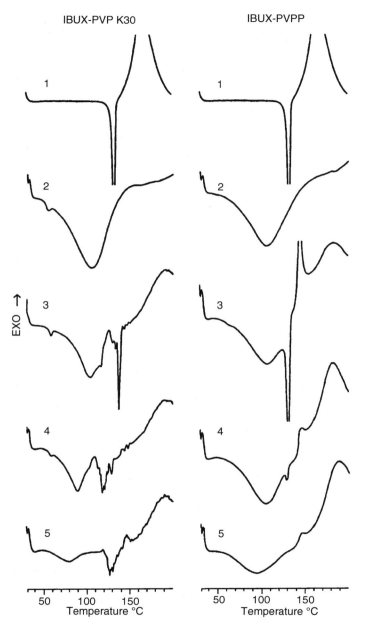

**Figure 20** Differential scanning calorimetry curves of ibuproxam (IBUX) and its 1:1 w/w mixed systems with PVP K30 and PVPP: (*1*) Ibuproxam; (*2*) excipient; (*3*) physical mixture; (*4*) coground mixture; (*5*) kneaded mixture. *Abbreviation*: PVP, polyvinylpyrrolidone. *Source*: From Ref. 20.

monolayer–multilayer sorption. Monolayer adsorption occurs at lower pressures compared to multilayer adsorption. Moisture sorption on drug in the presence of excipients could result in phase transformation of the active ingredient that could change the solid-state properties and consequently properties such as physical or chemical stability, manufacturability, and bioavailability. Crystalline excipients could accelerate and the amorphous excipients could delay the phase transformation.

Phase Transformation

The transformation resulting from adsorbed or absorbed water usually leads to hydrate formation via hydrogen bonding or coordinate covalent bonds as stated earlier. The pharmaceutical hydrates thus formed can be classified into three categories. These are (*i*) isolated lattice sites, (*ii*) lattice channels that could be either nonstoichiometric expanded channels lattice planes or dehydrated hydrates, and (*iii*) metal ion coordinated water hydrates (46).

Phase transformation was reported by Otsuka and Matsuda (47) for nitrofurantoin anhydrate in the presence of α-LMH or MCC under high humidity conditions. They observed that the hydrate formation of nitrofurantoin was accelerated by LMH in the formulation but not by MCC. Salameh and Taylor (46) also reported moisture-induced hydrate–anhydrate transformation of theophylline monohydrate (MT) and carbamazepine dihydrate (DC) by some excipients such as mannitol, MCC, and PVP (PVP K12 and PVP K90). Mannitol and PVP K90 enhanced the dehydration of MT (Fig. 21) but had a retarding effect on transformation of the anhydrous (AT) to the hydrate (Fig. 22). The phase transformation was monitored using AT-Raman spectroscopy and bivariate analysis.

The effect of various excipients on carbamazepine was also studied. The authors concluded that PVP K12 and PVP K90 enhanced dehydration; mannitol showed some increase in dehydration, while MCC had a stabilizing effect (Fig. 23). These excipients functioned as molecular dessicants where the uptake of moisture by the more hygroscopic component (excipient) and shielding of hydrate former (drug) from moisture took place. Including such excipients as dessicants can delay hydration kinetics or the transformation tendency of the drug. The effect of the PVP K90 on DC is in contrast to the little or no dehydrating effect it had on MT.

This phase transformation was due to a complex process that involves partial dissolution of the drug (under high RH condition), thus changing the hydration process form a solid state to a solution-mediated transformation. The effect of compaction on phase transformation was also reported for theophylline. This will be further discussed under the section titled Chemical Changes. Other analytical methods used to evaluate such physical interactions include XRD, near-IR spectroscopy, specific surface area, SEM, and particle size distribution. The preformulation implications highlighted by the authors (46) are summarized below:

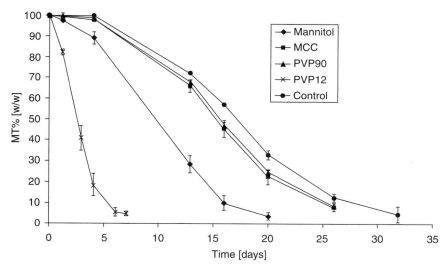

**Figure 21** Effect of excipients on the dehydration of MT at 33% relative humidity. *Abbreviations*: MCC, microcrystalline cellulose; MT, theophylline monohydrate; PVP, polyvinylpyrrolidone. *Source*: From Ref. 47.

- Drying of multicomponent formulations, following or during wet granulation, may make formulations susceptible to dehydration/hydration at different rates.

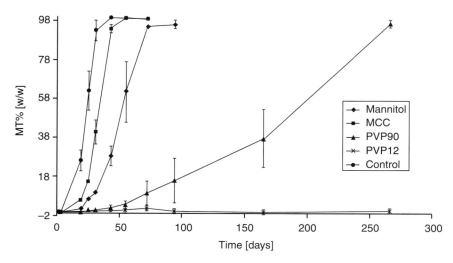

**Figure 22** Effect of excipients on the hydration of MT at 75% relative humidity. *Abbreviations*: MCC, microcrystalline cellulose; MT, theophylline monohydrate; PVP, polyvinylpyrrolidone. *Source*: From Ref. 47.

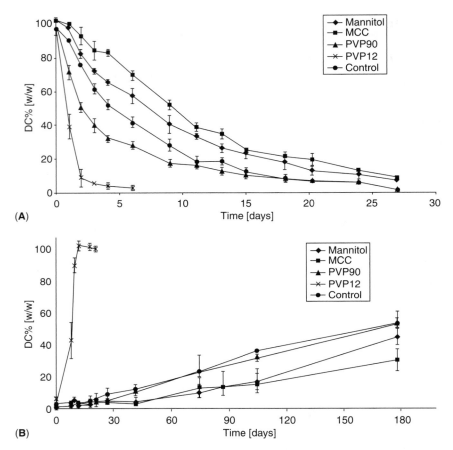

**Figure 23** Effect of excipients on the (**A**) dehydration of DC at 33% relative humidity; (**B**) hydration of DC at 94% relative humidity. *Abbreviations*: DC, carbamazepine dihydrate; MCC, microcrystalline cellulose; PVP, polyvinylpyrrolidone. *Source*: From Ref. 47.

- Some excipients can interact with the surface of the API particles, increase the number of defects, facilitate dehydration, or act as molecular dessicants.
- Phase transformation could take place during direct compression of formulation blends containing susceptible hydrates.

Adeyeye et al. also investigated the role of moisture in the phase transformation of theophylline anhydrate in the presence of hydroxypropylmethylcellulose, an excipient that is hygroscopic (48). The relative water sorption of the tablets compressed at different pressures are shown in Figure 24. Transformation of the anhydrate to the hydrated form was

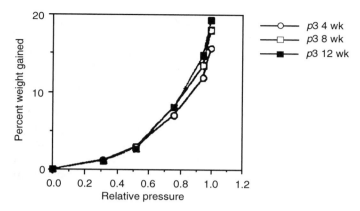

**Figure 24**  Moisture sorption isotherms of directly compressed anhydrous theophylline tablets during storage. Compression pressure $p3 = 274.4$ MPa. *Source*: From Ref. 48.

observed as indicated by XRD and dissolution studies. More crystalline peaks for the formed hydrated theophylline were observed (Fig. 25). DSC study revealed an additional endothermic peak resulting from either the conversion of magnesium stearate to it pseudopolymorph. It could also be

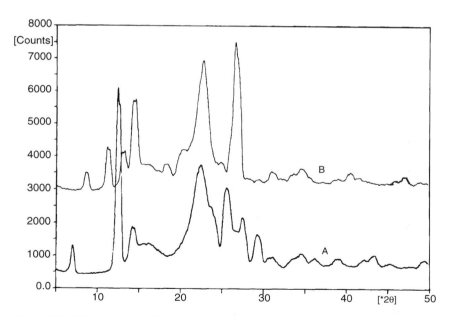

**Figure 25**  X-ray powder diffraction pattern of directly compressed theophylline tablets stored at $\leq 52\%$ relative humidity (*A*) and at $> 52\%$ relative humidity (*B*) for three months. *Source*: From Ref. 48.

an interaction between the hydrated microcrystalline cellulose (another excipient) and the magnesium stearate (Fig. 26). The drug dissolution rate decreased significantly consequent to the formation of the hydrated theophylline (Figs. 27 and Fig. 28). The methods used in the evaluation were also used by Airaksinen et al. in their investigation of the water sorption properties of the different excipients (43).

In crystalline materials such as theophylline in which hydrogen bonding is relatively weak, water molecules can produce hydrate stabilization primarily due to their space-filling roles. Nonhydrating amorphous excipients such as hydroxypropylmethylcellulose (HPMC) can sorb enough moisture to cause phase transformations that can affect physicochemical properties and bioavailability.

## Chemical Interaction

Chemical interactions occur in potential drug–excipient mixtures or formulations. As stated earlier, the nature of the chemical interaction depends on factors such as the nature of the drug and excipient, relative ratio of the drug–excipient, which could cause instability, role of moisture, influence of heat, effect of pH of the microenvironment, processing effect on formulation, and the role of light. The awareness or knowledge of the

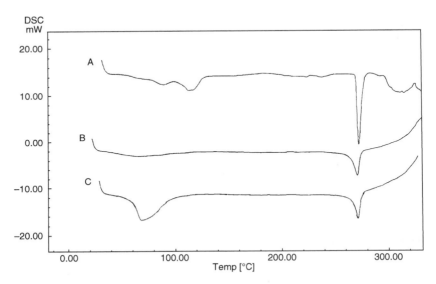

**Figure 26** Differential scanning thermograms of the physical mixture of the tablet components (*A*), tablet stored at relative humidity < 52% (*B*), and tablets stored at relative humidity > 52% (*C*). *Abbreviation*: DSC, differential scanning calorimetry. *Source*: From Ref. 48.

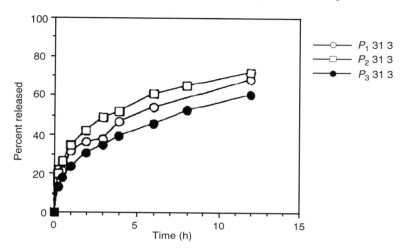

**Figure 27** Drug-release profiles of tablets compressed at different pressures after three months of storage at 31% relative humidity: $P_1 = 137.2$ MPa; $P_2 = 194.8$ MPa; $P_3 = 274.4$ MPa. *Source*: From Ref. 48.

chemical nature of the drug and possible consequent reactivity and that of the excipients is very critical in establishing drug–excipient interaction or incompatibility. If an API is inherently unstable (e.g., sensitive to moisture, heat, or light), its presence in a formulation induces interaction. Solid-state chemical interactions that cause degradation are often related to molecular

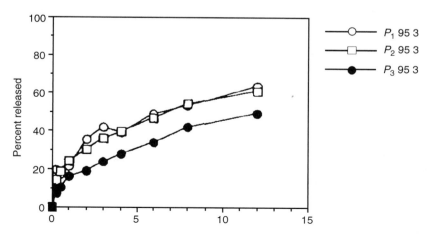

**Figure 28** Drug-release profiles of tablets compressed at different pressures and stored at 95% relative humidity for three months: $P_1 = 137.2$ MPa; $P_2 = 194.8$ MPa; $P_3 = 274.4$ MPa. *Source*: From Ref. 48.

mobility and water (10,49); the presence of moisture has also been reported to enhance this mobility (5). Examples of common chemical interactions that have been reported are discussed here.

Acid–Base Reactions

Many pharmaceutical drugs are weak acids and bases; 75% of APIs are weak bases while 20% are weak acids (50). About 45% to 50% of the marketed drugs are salts, and the majority of these are either weakly acidic or basic. Acid–base reactions are a common type of drug–excipient inter-action, and many such reactions occur in the solid state. Screening for these is very critical order to avoid unexpected consequences resulting from incompatibility. The screening of acid–base reactions requires analytical techniques that do not involve solvent extraction. This is because the free form and salt form of the analyte may have different solubilities in a given solvent, especially an organic solvent. Therefore, it will be impractical and impossible to avoid proton transfer from the acidic or basic excipient during sample preparation. Residual moisture in the solvent may also cause proton transfer. In addition, solvent extraction can disrupt the physical interaction involved when such a reaction takes place in the solid state, thus con-founding the results. Moreover, the ionized and free forms will be difficult to analyze using HPLC.

Consequently, analytical techniques such as powder XRD, IR spec-troscopy, and solid-state $^{13}C$ NMR have been used as alternatives.

Chen et al. (51) used the techniques to study acid–base reactions between a model drug, α-indomethacin, 1-(-4-chlorobenzoyl)-5-methoxy-2-methyl-1H-indole-3-acetic acid, and sodium bicarbonate in the solid state. The samples were prepared by grinding a 1:1 ratio of the drug and excipient in an agate mortar and stored at 40°C over 80%, 66%, and 11% RH conditions created using saturated solutions of potassium bromide, potas-sium iodide, and lithium chloride, respectively.

XRD, IR spectroscopy, and solid-state $^{13}C$ NMR all revealed that sodium indomethacin trihydrate was formed for the mixture kept at 40°C. The reaction reached completion at 300 hours. At 66% RH, the reaction was 86% complete at 500 hours, whereas no interaction was observed at 11% RH. IR spectra of the reference samples (prepared using potassium bromide pellet), α-indomethacin, γ-indomethacin, sodium indomethacin trihydrate, and sodium bicarbonate are shown in Figure 29A. IR spectra of samples placed at 80% RH are shown in Figure 29B.

The characteristic absorption band at $1717 \, cm^{-1}$ in γ-indomethacin corresponds to the carbonyl stretch of the carboxylic acid dimer. The $1692 \, cm^{-1}$ is assumed to be the carbonyl stretch of the nonprotonated amide. The absorption bands at 1735, 1692, and $1680 \, cm^{-1}$ in α-indomethacin are related to its crystal structure. It contains three molecules with three dif-ferent conformations. Two of the molecules form the carboxylic acid dimer,

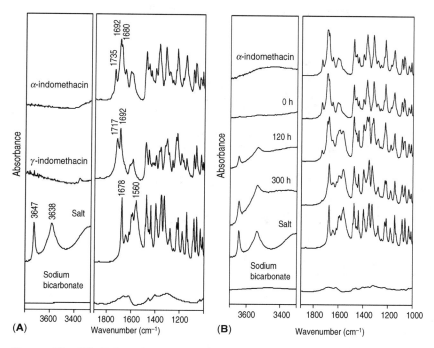

**Figure 29** (**A**) Infrared spectra of α-indomethacin, γ-indomethacin, sodium indomethacin trihydrate, and sodium bicarbonate. (**B**) The spectra of indomethacin, sodium bicarbonate, and physical mixture stored at 40°C and 80% relative humidity for 0, 120, and 300 hours. *Source*: From Ref. 51.

while the carboxylic acid of the third molecule forms a hydrogen bond with the amide carbonyl of the dimer. The $1735 \text{ cm}^{-1}$ band and the $1692 \text{ cm}^{-1}$ band were assigned to the nondimer-involved carboxylic acid and the carbonyl stretch of the nonprotonated amide, respectively. The $1680 \text{ cm}^{-1}$ is assigned to the protonated amide of the third molecule.

The spectra for the samples stored at 40°C at 80% RH showed a decrease in intensities at 1725 and $1692 \text{ cm}^{-1}$ and new bands at 1678 and $1560 \text{ cm}^{-1}$. The new peaks are for sodium indomethacin while the α-indomethacin peak completely disappeared. Two hydroxyl peaks of water at 3647 and $3438 \text{ cm}^{-1}$, typical of a hydrate, were also observed in the stored samples. This is indicative of the formation of sodium indomethacin trihydrate at 40°C and 80% RH.

XRD patterns of the drug, excipient, and the physical mixtures before and after storage gave further indications of the reaction's progress and the formation of sodium indomethacin trihydrate as observed in the IR spectra. The diffraction pattern is shown below (Fig. 30).

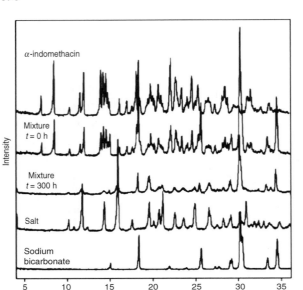

**Figure 30** Powder X-ray diffraction patterns of pure indomethacin and a physical mixture of indomethacin and sodium bicarbonate before and after storage at 40°C and 80% relative humidity. *Source*: From Ref. 51.

Solid-state NMR further confirms the identity of the reaction product (Fig. 31). The crystal structure of α-indomethacin contains molecules in three conformations. Hence, the solid-state NMR consists of multiple resonances for some carbon atoms, such as the carboxylic acid carbon and methyl carbon attached to $C_2$ of the indole ring (Figs. 31 and 32). Solid-state acid–base reactions have also been reported for effervescent tablets, which contain edible acids such as citric and tartaric acids and a bicarbonate (52,53).

Charge Interaction

This is a common drug–excipient interaction that occurs in excipients and drugs with ionizable groups such as carboxylic acid and amino acids that can generate corresponding anions and cations. The interaction is dependent on the pH of the environment. If a charged excipient is formulated with an ionizable oppositely charged drug, an ionic interaction can occur, forming an insoluble complex. This may cause the drug to be retained with the excipient, leading to problems with solubility, disintegration, dissolution, and bioavailability. The extent of interaction is dependent on the inherent properties of the drug and excipient, the ratio of the components in the formulation, and strength of interaction.

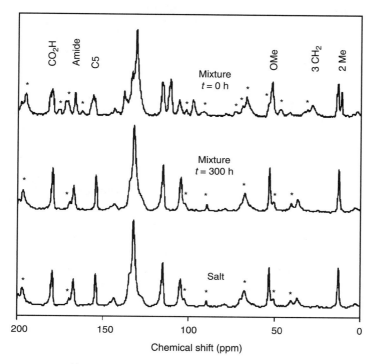

**Figure 31** $^{13}$CCP/MAS spectra of indomethacin and sodium bicarbonate physical mixtures before and after storing at 40°C and 80% relative humidity for 300 hours as well as sodium indomethacin trihydrate. *Source*: From Ref. 51.

Charge interaction was observed and reported by Haung et al. (54), who studied the interaction between metformin and croscarmellose sodium. Metformin is a strong base with a p$K$a of 12.4 that easily protonates and

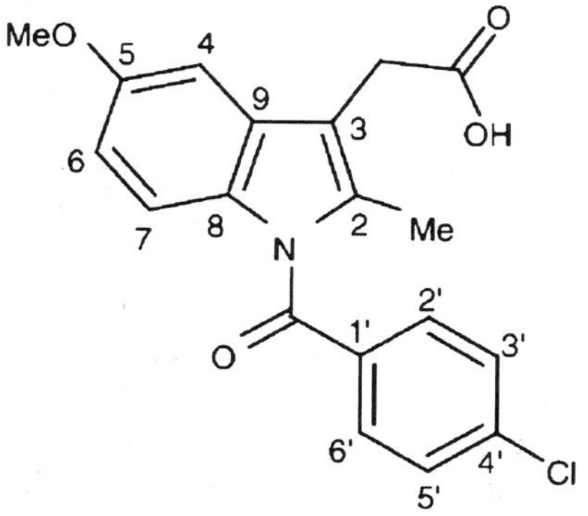

**Figure 32** Chemical structure of indomethacin and the numbering scheme. *Source*: From Ref. 51.

carries a positively charged amino ($=NH_2^+$). Croscarmellose sodium, a cross-linked polymer of NaCMC, can be ionized in water due to the carboxylic acid groups, thus carrying a negative charge ($COO^-$). Charge interaction was also observed in earlier reports of Hollenbeck (1983) (55) and Crowley and Martini (2001) (56). The study was performed based on the low percent recovery during analytical method development and validation of the combination bilayer product, Metformin/Starlix®, which is intended for treating type II diabetes. The bilayer is meant to separate the metformin from the croscarmellose sodium, and in the solid-state, charge interaction is not expected due to the low moisture content (<2%) in the tablet. However, in solution, the positively charged metformin and the negatively charged croscarmellose sodium occurred, and this led to a 4% to 8% loss in metformin recovery from the tablets. In solution, the recovery was very low (55.6–73%), indicative of interaction.

The authors studied this interaction by using a competition method involving the use of four basic amino acids (arginine, lysine, glutamic acid, and histidine) chosen to compete with metformin for the $COO^-$ of the croscarmellose sodium. The drug–excipient interactions and equilibrium constants for metformin and arginine are shown below.

$$[C^-] + [M^+] \Leftrightarrow [CM] \qquad\qquad [C^-] + [A^+] \Leftrightarrow [CA]$$

$$K_{CM} = \frac{[CM]}{[C^-][M^+]} \qquad\qquad K_{CA} = \frac{[CA]}{[C^-][A^+]}$$

$$\text{Metformin-croscarmellose} \qquad \text{Arginine-croscarmellose}$$

$[C^-]$ and $[M^+]$ represent the molar concentrations of the negatively charged croscarmellose sodium and positively charged metformin in the solution at equilibrium, respectively. $[CM]$ is the molar concentration of the metformin–croscarmellose complex at equilibrium. Similarly, for arginine–croscarmellose interaction, the molar concentration of negatively charged croscarmellose is $[C^-]$ while the positively charged arginine is represented with $[A^+]$. The scheme for interactions between metformin or arginine and croscarmellose sodium competition and their respective equilibrium constants $K_{CM}$ and $K_{CA}$ are shown in Figure 33.

The scheme for interaction between metformin or arginine and croscarmellose sodium is shown in Figure 33.

Arginine, being an ideal competitor for metformin, would be expected to interact with croscarmellose sodium with a greater affinity compared to the interaction between metformin and croscarmellose sodium. The authors reported that a strong charged interaction between metformin and croscarmellose sodium was successfully eliminated by arginine competition.

Drug–excipient interactions or excipient–excipient charge interactions have been reported in some formulations containing Eudragit®. Electrostatic ionic interaction via adsorption of drug (salicylic acid) onto the

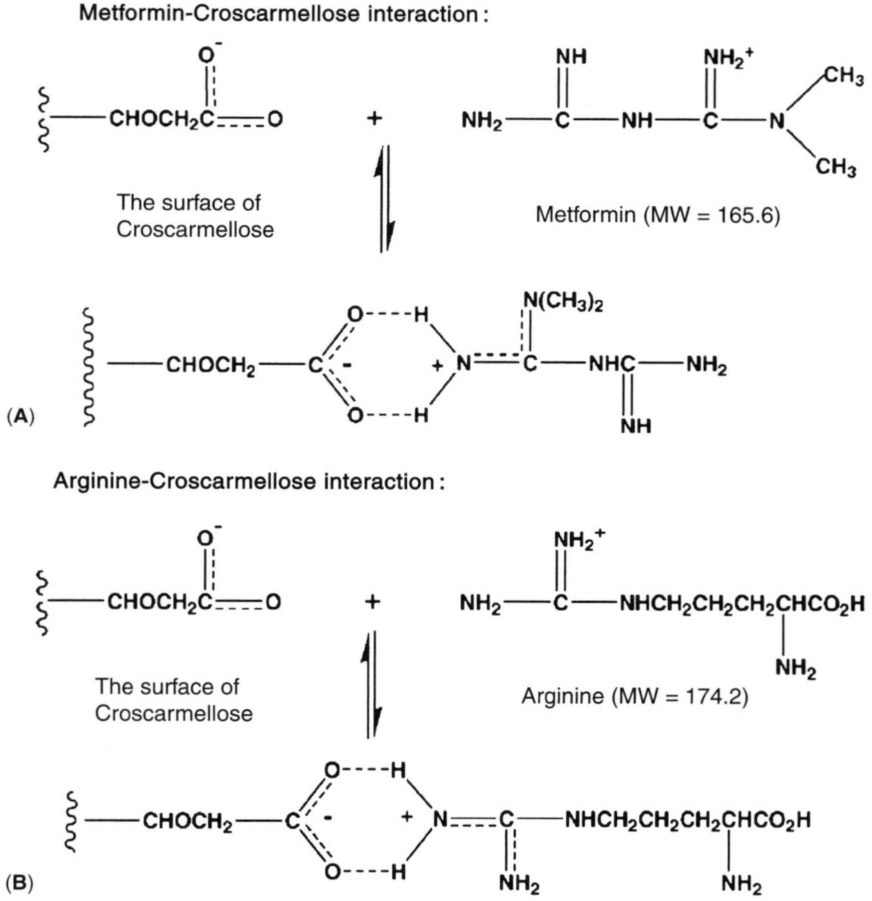

**Metformin-Croscarmellose interaction:**

(A)

**Arginine-Croscarmellose interaction:**

(B)

**Figure 33** Scheme for possible charge interactions: (**A**) metformin–croscarmellose interaction; (**B**) arginine–croscarmellose. *Abbreviation*: MW, molecular weight. *Source*: From Ref. 54.

polymer and ionic strength were reported to be causes of some interactions (57). Khalil and Sallam (58) also reported that negatively charged diclofenac molecules in a dissolution medium interacted with the positively charged quaternary ammonium groups of the polymer. Increasing the pH of the dissolution medium (buffer solution) decreased the drug release, a result of decrease in dissociation of the quaternary ammonium groups.

As reported earlier, under IST, Adeyeye et al. (29) reported an inter-action between diclofenac–excipient and polymers such as Eudragit L30D and RS30D in a microcapsule dosage form (29). The authors used a slurry of drug–excipient liquid binary and ternary mixtures in ratios expected in the formulation (Table 4). As mentioned, the mixtures were dried for 48 hours at 60°C and then analyzed using XRD and DSC. A comparison was made with individual dry components.

The thermal event parameters such as enthalpy values were used to conclude that there was an interaction between diclofenac and the Eudragit RS30D and L30D-55 used as suspending agents (Table 8). As shown in Table 9, the DSC curves of the binary mixture of diclofenac codried with liquid forms of Eudragit (i.e., RS30D or L30D-55) revealed a greater interaction compared to the curves of drug and powdered forms of Eudragit (L100-55 or RS PO). This was depicted by a greater shift in the fusion points of the mixtures relative to the drug. When the RS and L-type Eudragit were compared, the latter generally showed a greater interaction with the drug.

Powder XRD of the binary or ternary mixtures of diclofenac and the Eudragit polymers indicated reduction, shift, or modification of the crystalline peaks of the drug or excipients at $2\theta$ of 12° and 18°, suggesting more interaction between diclofenac and L30D-55 Eudragit (Figs. 34 and 35). Some changes, though not significant, in drug peak characteristics at 18° and 23° were observed for Avicel/drug mixture (figure not shown).

The presence of ammonium groups on the RS polymers (Fig. 36) could also have caused interaction between the carboxyl groups of the drug and the positively charged ions of the ammonium groups (58). The microcapsule formulation contained PEG, which might have also caused interaction in an acidic medium (the suitable pH medium used for suspending the particles). This was probably due to hydrogen bonding between the ether oxygen of the oxyethylene groups of PEG 4000 (7), causing faster dissolution of the suspended microcapsules. PEG usually strongly interacts with molecules that

**Table 8**  Thermal (Differential Scanning Calorimetry) Characteristics of Diclofenac and Respective Powder Components

| Material | Fusion point (°C) | $\Delta$°C | $\Delta H$ (J/g) |
|---|---|---|---|
| Diclofenac sodium | 287.4 | – | 130.4 |
| Eudragit® L100-55 | 247.4 | – | 43.1 |
| Eudragit RS PO | – | – | – |
| Calcium carbonate | – | – | – |
| Avicel® CL-611 | 202.7 | – | 100.2 |
| Drug + Eudragit L100-55 | 257.9 | 29.5 | 12.4 |
| Drug + Eudragit RS PO | 263.7 | 23.7 | 15.5 |
| Drug + Avicel CL-611 | 284.6 | 2.8 | 23.7 |
| Drug + calcium carbonate | 286.8 | 0.6 | 55.4 |
| Components (formulation ratio) | – | – | – |
| Microcapsules | – | – | – |

*Source*: From Ref. 29.

**Table 9** Thermal (Differential Scanning Calorimetry) Characteristics of Diclofenac and Respective Codried Component Mixtures

| Material | Fusion point (°C) | Δ°C | ΔH (J/g) |
|---|---|---|---|
| Diclofenac sodium | 287.4 | – | 130.4 |
| Drug + Eudragit L30D-55 | 244.6 | 42.8 | 23.5 |
| Drug + Eudragit RS30D | 266.9 | 20.5 | 15.5 |
| Drug + Avicel CL-611 | 282.8 | 4.6 | 93.2 |
| Drug + suspending medium | 268.1, 282.3 | 21.3, 5.1 | 1.2, 22.0 |
| Components + suspending medium | – | – | |
| Microcapsules + suspending medium | – | – | |

*Source*: From Ref. 29.

have hydrogen bonding donor or acceptor functions such as the poly-methacrylic acid polymers (59).

### Hydrolysis Reaction (Interactions Involving Magnesium Stearate with Some Amines)

A model of testing drug–diluent–lubricant as a first-phase study in a drug interaction was used by Serajuddin et al. (14). The authors argued that this

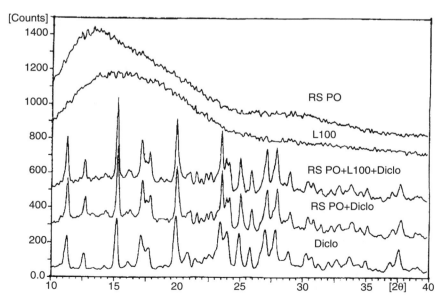

**Figure 34** Powder X-ray diffraction profiles of binary mixture of diclofenac and Eudragit L100-55 or RS PO and a ternary mixture (Eudragit L100-55 + RS PO). *Source*: From Ref. 29.

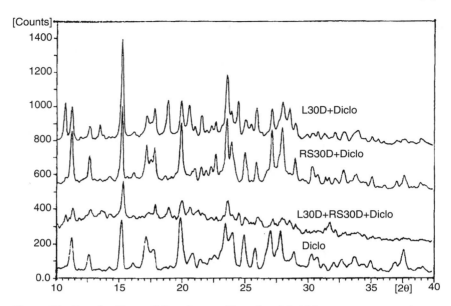

**Figure 35** Powder X-ray diffraction profiles of codried binary or ternary mixtures of diclofenac and Eudragit L30D or RS30D. *Source*: From Ref. 29.

simple three-component model can be used followed by examination of incompatibility of other excipients such as binders and disintegrants in a second phase. The method used for screening was discussed in the section titled "Screening Methods." Briefly, various blends were made with and without water (20% w/w) and samples were stored at 50°C at 75% RH. Moisture was added to facilitate drug–excipient interaction since it has been established that presence of moisture facilitates formation of disorderliness or amorphousness.

The study was based on an earlier interaction study in aqueous medium that revealed hydrolysis of the *O*-acetyl group of two calcium channel blockers, tertiary (compound I) and secondary amine (compound II), that belong to the benzazepine series (Fig. 37).

The drug–microcrystalline cellulose–magnesium stearate or drug–dicalcium phosphate–magnesium stearate mixture showed degradation of the ester bond in compound I to compound VIII. In contrast, mixtures containing either lactose or mannitol as diluent did not show the interaction. Formation of the degradation product was confirmed by an HPLC analysis. Other lubricants, stearic acid and sodium stearyl fumarate, had less effect on degradation, with the former being the most stable.

The reactivity of the mixture containing magnesium stearate could be attributed to the pH of the microenvironment, which was about 5.5,

Diclofenac sodium

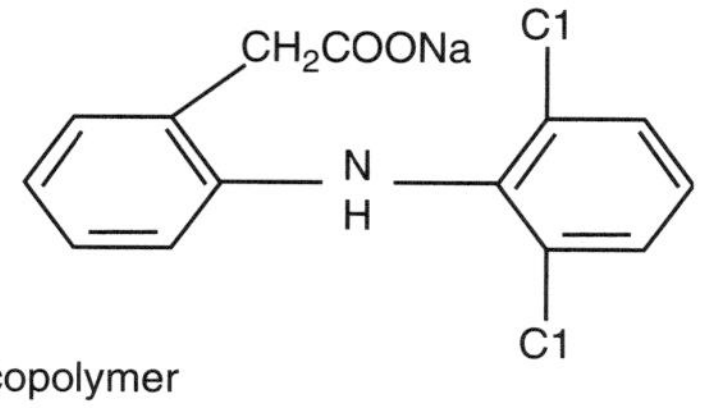

Ammoniomethacrylate copolymer

**A**

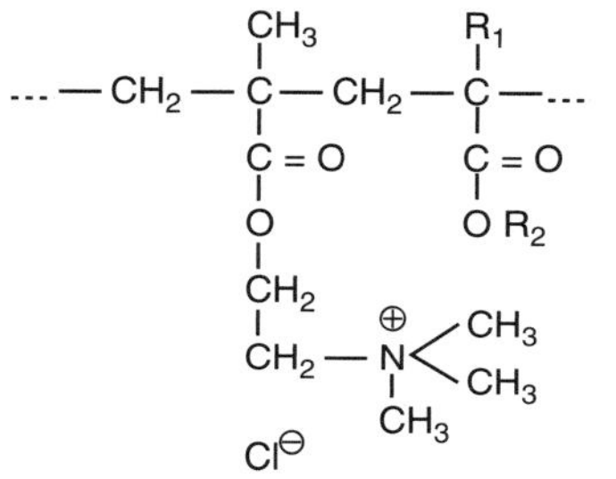

Methacrylic acid copolymer

**B**

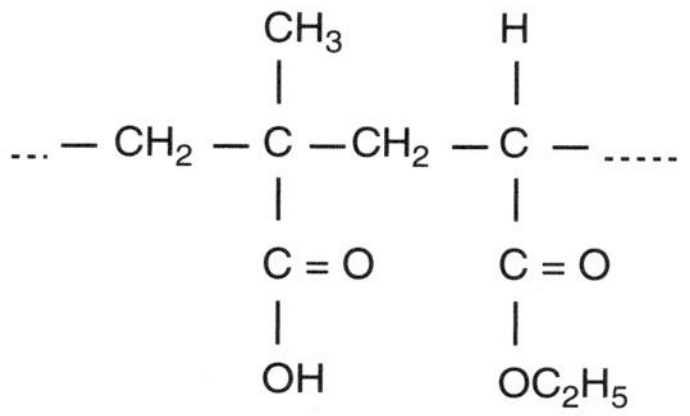

$R_1 = H_1, CH_3 ; R_2 = CH_3, C_2H_5$

**Figure 36**  Eudragit RS30D or RS PO (*A*) and Eudragit L30D-55 or L100 55 (*B*). *Source*: From Ref. 29.

compared to the microenvironment of the mixtures containing stearic acid, which was 3.8. The surface acidity of the dicalcium phosphate and formation of phosphoric acid upon hydrolysis also contributed to the degradation. Compound II, the secondary amine, also showed similar hydrolytic degradation, with the resultant formation of compound IX (Fig. 37). Stearic acid did not have a significant effect on degradation while magnesium stearate had the most significant effect.

Another drug that showed reactivity with magnesium stearate is fosinopril sodium (compound III), a prodrug of an ACE inhibitor that coverts in vivo to fosinoprilat (compound X) by hydrolysis of the phosphonic acid ester side chain. Compound X was observed as a degradative product in a drug–excipient interaction study of fosinopril sodium with excipients (Fig. 38). HPLC was used in the identification of the degradants, which were further elucidated by the NMR technique. The latter method

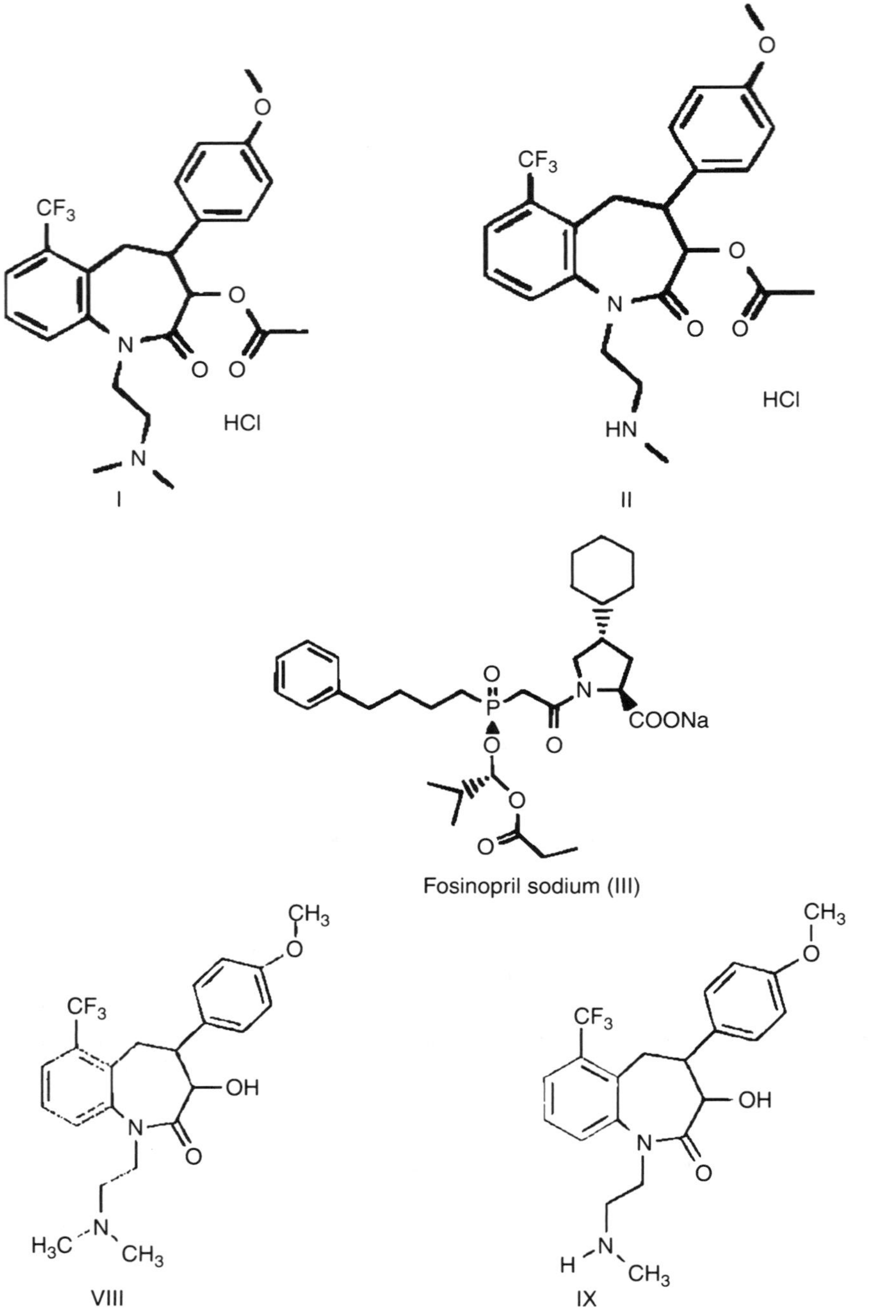

**Figure 37**  Structures of compounds I, II, III, VIII, and IX. *Source*: From Ref. 14.

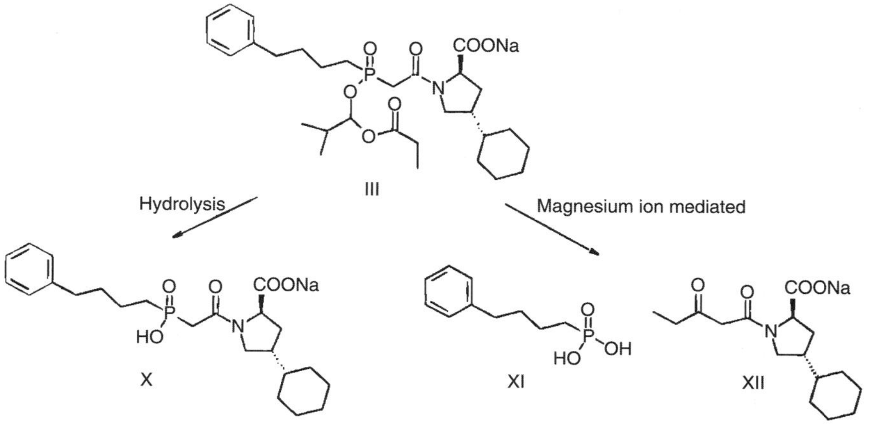

**Figure 38** Magnesium stearate–induced degradative products of compound III. *Source*: From Ref. 14.

indicated that ~90% of the drug degraded within a week (Fig. 39A). In contrast, degradation of a 1:1 mixture of compound III and magnesium stearate was less than 1% after three weeks (Fig. 39B). This is because the two compounds were nonhygroscopic.

The interaction was earlier reported by Thakur et al. (60) to be due to metal ion (magnesium stearate) mediated rearrangement in addition to the hydrolysis of the side chain. The authors concluded that the prodrug would require protection from moisture in order to prevent its conversion into the active drug during processing. Magnesium stearate accelerated the formation of compound X and two other major degradation products, compound XI and compound XII.

Although the model used included water, the drastic condition revealed what could happen in a real situation (tablets and capsules) where the presence of excipients such as lactose, starch, and gelatin shell could result in moisture absorption. From the drug–excipient interaction, the investigators made a decision to exclude magnesium stearate from the formulations and recommended that the dosage forms must be protected from moisture.

## Maillard Reaction

Maillard reaction, reported over 80 years ago by Louis Maillard, involves the reaction of reducing carbohydrates and some amines to produce brown pigments. Reducing sugars such as glucose, maltose, and lactose are subject to Maillard reaction because their cyclic tautomers are in equilibrium with their more reactive aldehyde forms. On the other hand, nonreducing sugars such as mannitol, sucrose, and trehalose are not substrates for the Maillard

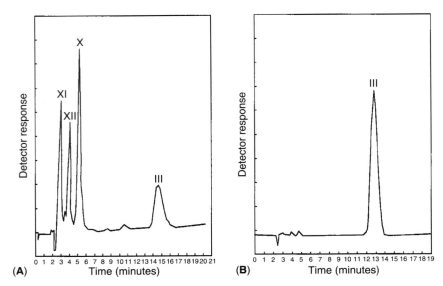

**Figure 39** (**A**) High performance liquid chromatography chromatogram of a fosinopril sodium (III)–lactose–magnesium stearate mixture (40:150:10) containing 20% added water stored at 50°C for one week. (**B**) Chromatogram of fosinopril sodium (III)–magnesium stearate (1:1) mixture stored at 50°C under 75% relative humidity for three weeks. Compounds X, XI, and XII were the major degradation products. *Source*: From Ref. 14.

reaction. In pharmaceutical development, these reactions could become critical in the functionality of excipients, the stability of the products, and in vivo performance. Indeed, many reports have been made in the pharmaceutical literature of these reactions from intended and unintended outcomes.

Prozac®, fluoxetine hydrochloride (I), a secondary amine, is an antidepressant innovator product that had starch as the diluent. However, as the patent expired, many generics of the drug were developed. However, some of these were found to contain lactose as the primary diluent and to be less stable than the branded product. Lactose is one of the most widely used excipients in the pharmaceutical industry because of its excellent compressibility, stability, low price, and high purity. However, it has also been known to undergo nonenzymatic browning or Maillard reaction in the presence of primary amines. But it has been accepted that secondary amines such as fluoxetine are also subject to the browning effect in the presence of lactose. The first product of this reaction is glycosylation followed by the Amadori rearrangement (ARP) as shown in Figure 40.

The dissimilarity in stability between the innovator and generic products was then investigated by Wirth et al. (61) using a solid-state screening

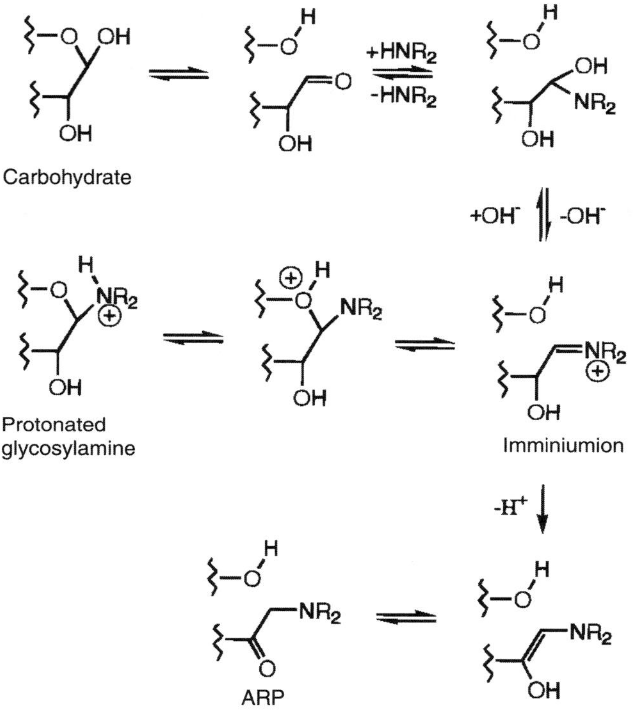

**Figure 40** Mechanism of glycosylation and Amadori rearrangement with secondary amines. *Source*: From Ref. 61.

method. Various blends of lactose and fluoxetine HCL were made by either the tumbling, grinding, or wet grinding method as shown in Table 10. These blends were repeated with the addition of magnesium stearate but before the blending and mixing operation. Four grades of lactose were used: crystalline monohydrate, two particle-size grades of anhydrous lactose (granular and finely milled), and a mixture of crystalline and spray-dried lactose. The blends were then subjected to heating at 98°C in an oven for 24 hours. Analysis of the drug and suspected degradation products 2 and 3 shown in Figures 41A and B was done using HPLC (Fig. 42). The relatively high temperature was chosen for its expediency and not for prediction of decomposition reaction rates of drug mixtures stored at normal storage conditions.

Maillard reaction (accelerated by water) was observed in all experiments, and the rate was slightly faster with spray-dried lactose than the LMH (Fig. 43A and B). The rate of formation of ARP was similar with the anhydrous and monohydrate lactose. The anhydrous was less sensitive to water, possibly due to conversion to the monohydrate, while there was no

**Table 10** Solid Phase Screening Experiments for Mixtures Heated at 98°C for 24 Hrs

| | | | Impurities (%) | | |
|---|---|---|---|---|---|
| Lactose type | Mixing mode | Mg stearate | Total | Amadori rearrangement, 2 | N-formyl fluoxetine, 3 |
| Monohydrate | Tumble | N | 0.48 | 0.073 | |
| | | Y | 0.46 | 0.16 | 0.023 |
| | Grind | N | 0.48 | 0.089 | |
| | | Y | 0.6 | 0.21 | 0.039 |
| | Wet grind | N | 6.13 | 3.23 | 0.02 |
| | | Y | 17.3 | 8.56 | 0.4 |
| Spray-dried | Tumble | N | 1.2 | 0.26 | |
| | | Y | 0.92 | 0.4 | 0.036 |
| | Grind | N | 1.48 | 0.45 | 0.02 |
| | | Y | 1.44 | 0.41 | 0.12 |
| | Wet grind | N | 22.8 | 5.1 | 0.078 |
| | | Y | 24.2 | 13 | 0.48 |
| Anhydrous granular | Tumble | N | 0.46 | 0.072 | |
| | Grind | N | 0.5 | 0.079 | |
| | Wet grind | N | 3.11 | 1.51 | 0.014 |
| Anhydrous milled | Tumble | N | 0.44 | 0.079 | |
| | Grind | N | 0.53 | 0.107 | |
| | Wet grind | N | 2.06 | 0.86 | 0.011 |

*Source*: From Ref. 61.

remarkable difference between the blended and grounded mixtures. Magnesium stearate catalyzed the reaction. These observations were earlier made in the same study using a solution state study. The relative amounts of the impurities as detected by HPLC were shown in Figures 38A and B. The levels of impurities in the generic and innovator fluoxetine (Prozac) differed accordingly, as shown in Table 11.

Transacylation

Tablet formulations containing aspirin (acetylsalicyclic acid) or drugs with easily acylated functionalities react to give acyl compounds and salicylic acid (3). Troup and Mitchner (62) reported the reaction between acetylsalicyclic acid and phenylephrine as shown in Figure 44. An acetyl group is transferred from the acetylsalicyclic acid to the phenylephrine. Storing the formulation at 70°C showed that the mixture contained 80% acylated phenylephrine after 34 days. Addition of starch and magnesium stearate slowed the acylation to about 1% after 34 days, whereas addition of magnesium stearate alone resulted in complete degradation in 16 days.

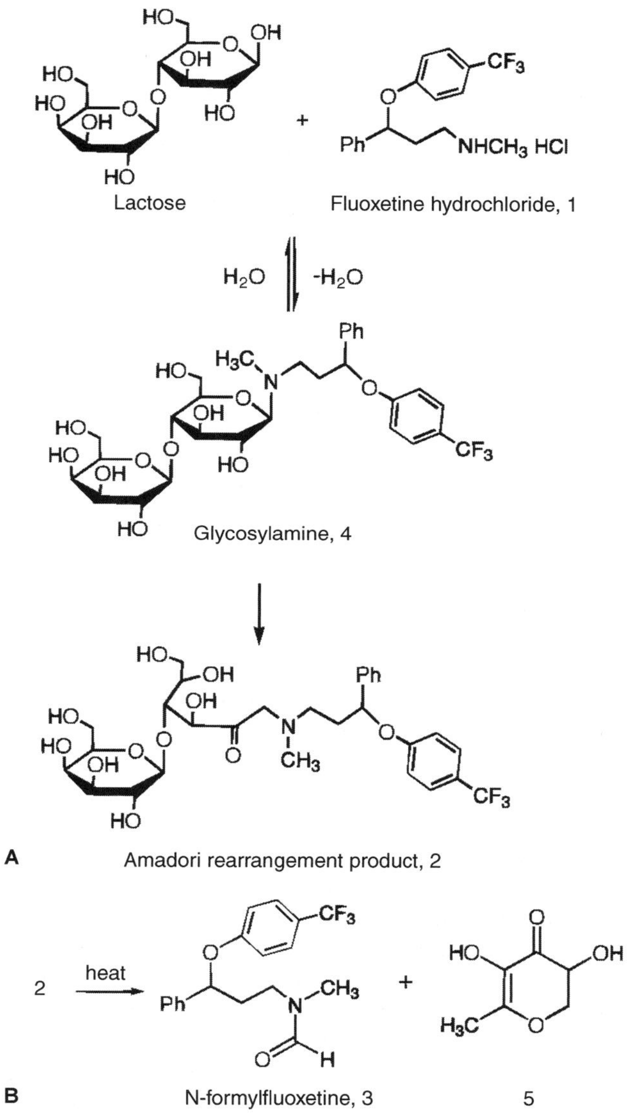

**Figure 41** (*A*) Maillard reaction of lactose and fluoxetine HCL; (*B*) decomposition of Amadori rearrangement, 2. *Source*: From Ref. 61.

Jacobs et al. (63) and Koshy et al. (64) also reported acylation reaction in aspirin tablets containing codeine or acetaminophen upon heating, as shown in Figure 45.

*410*    *Adeyeye*

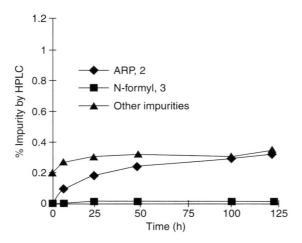

**Figure 42**  Lactose monohydrate and fluoxetine HCL at 85°C. *Abbreviation*: HPLC, high performance liquid chromatography. *Source*: From Ref. 61.

## PEPTIDE/PROTEIN–EXCIPIENT INTERACTION

### Sugar–Peptide/Protein Interactions

Peptide and protein drugs are highly susceptible to degradation during processing or preparation; however, the presence of excipients and the interaction have been exploited in the stabilization of such drugs. Aside from the interaction with excipients, the presence of moisture is very critical in maintaining the stability of the protein or drug. Processes such as spray drying (65,66), spray freeze-drying (67), ball or jet milling, and precipitation in supercritical fluids (68) could change the conformational arrangements, causing irreversible aggregation of the protein drug.

Tzannis and Prestrelski (69) studied the effects of sucrose on the stability of a model protein, trypsinogen prepared using the spray drying technique. They reported that in the absence of sucrose, spray drying destabilizes the protein, as indicated by the decrease in the denaturation temperature to 143.5°C. Addition of sucrose to the trypsinogen solution (optimized 1:1 ratio) before processing resulted in induced structural stabilization, shown by the increase in the denaturation temperature to 190.6°C. Examination by size exclusion chromatography revealed that the extent of aggregation decreased via reduction in dimerization (Fig. 46). The ratio of sucrose to protein was found to be critical because high concentrations of sucrose (>2:1 ratio) caused destabilization or decreased activity. This was reported to be possible deviation from the native state conformation.

In order to examine the secondary structure integrity of the protein, FTIR study was performed, and it revealed that in the absence of sucrose,

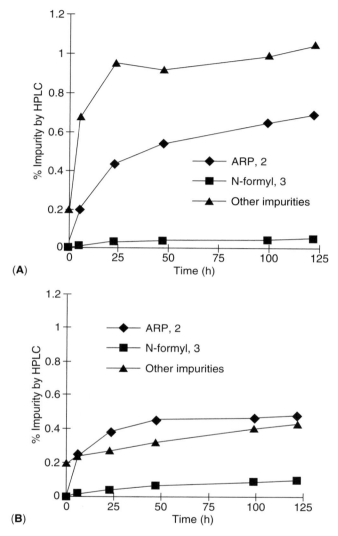

**Figure 43** (**A**) Spray-dried lactose and fluoxetine HCL 85° C. (**B**) Lactose monohydrate, fluoxetine HCL, and magnesium stearate 85° C. *Abbreviation*: HPLC, high performance liquid chromatography. *Source*: From Ref. 61.

spray drying resulted in the departure from the native structure of the protein. As shown in Figure 47, the second derivative of the amide I band (denoting the presence of a major β-sheet), seen in the native structure around 1636 cm$^{-1}$, has lost its sharp features in the sample without sucrose.

The major bands such as the characteristic β-sheet band shifted from 1636 to 1642 cm$^{-1}$, indicating rearrangement of the β-sheet of the native

**Table 11** Stability of Fluoxetine HCL Products at 40°C, 75% Relative Humidity

| Product | Impurity | Impurity by high performance liquid chromatography (%) | | | | |
|---|---|---|---|---|---|---|
| | | Initial | 1 mo | 3 mo | 6 mo | 9 mo |
| Prozac (starch) | Total | 0.17 | 0.19 | 0.21 | 0.23 | 0.23 |
| | 2 | | | | | |
| | 3 | | 0.01 | 0.01 | 0.01 | 0.02 |
| Generic A (lactose) | Total | 0.43 | 0.47 | 0.60 | 0.90 | 1.10 |
| | 2 | 0.03 | 0.01 | 0.01 | 0.05 | 0.05 |
| | 3 | | 0.02 | 0.03 | 0.13 | 0.22 |
| Generic Z (lactose) | Total | 0.30 | 0.35 | 0.45 | 0.63 | 0.74 |
| | 2 | | 0.01 | 0.02 | 0.03 | 0.02 |
| | 3 | | 0.01 | 0.04 | 0.08 | 0.13 |

*Source*: From Ref. 61.

protein. The overall conformational change relative to the native protein is shown in the low value of the correlation coefficient of $0.54 \pm 0.05$ (Table 12).

In another study conducted by Costantino et al. (70), the influence of different sugars and the derivatives such as mannitol, sorbitol, lactose, trehalose, and cellobiose on the stability of lyophilized recombinant human growth hormone (rhGH) was investigated. The rhGH, somatropin, is susceptible to aggregation in the solid state. The authors prepared lyophilized rhGH without and with various excipients in molar ratios of 31:1, 131:1, 300:1, and 1000:1. The formation of soluble and insoluble aggregates was monitored with size-exclusion HPLC following incubation at the accelerated storage condition of 50°C.

In the absence of excipients, soluble aggregate formation was very small, but after a four-week storage, the formation of insoluble aggregates was significant (Fig. 48A and B). Formation of aggregates in a protein such as human growth hormone can be detrimental due to bioactivity and immunogenic reactions. Soluble and insoluble aggregates were formed with

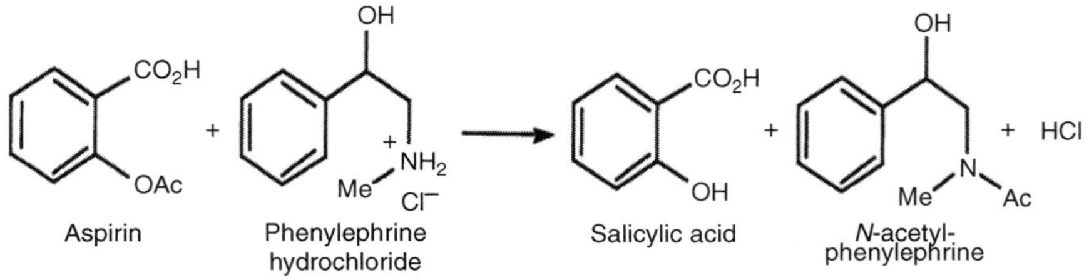

**Figure 44** Reaction of aspirin with phenylephrine hydrochloride. *Source*: From Ref. 62.

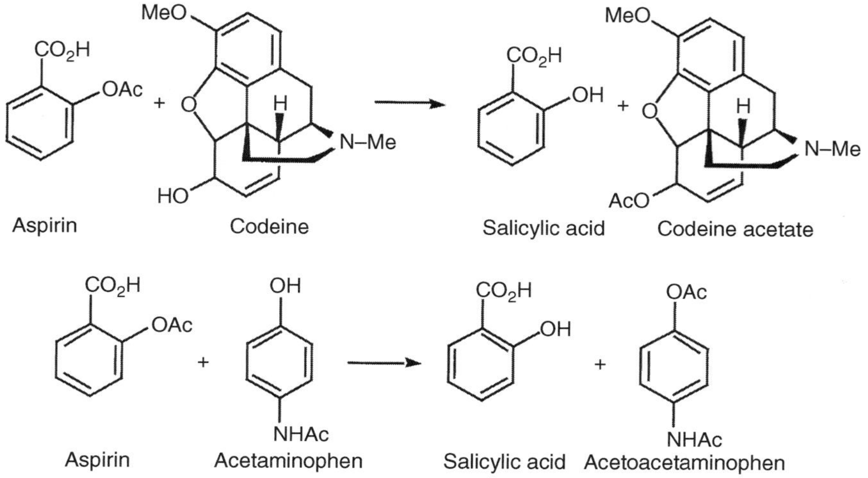

**Figure 45** Reactions of aspirin with codeine and acetaminophen. *Source*: From Ref. 64.

the lyophilized products made with mannitol, sorbitol, and methyl α D-mannopyranoside. A 131:1 excipient to rhGH ratio was found to be most stabilizing against solid-state insoluble aggregate formation (Fig. 49). Lyophilized products made with lactose, trehalose, and cellobiose were also found to be protected against insoluble aggregates at a ratio of 131:1. Cellobiose–rhGH lyophilized products were well stabilized with little or no insoluble aggregates.

The use of XRD to characterize the products revealed that all the lyophilized excipient–protein samples were amorphous except for the 300:1 and 1000:1 mannitol:rhGH ratios. The influence of moderately high temperature (50°C) and storage effect on the product (especially with low protein content) was investigated. The authors reported that all except sorbitol:rhGH (1000:1) and 300:1 methyl α D-mannopyranoside:rhGH (Fig. 50D– F) remained amorphous at the conditions studied. The other three products had undergone crystallization (Fig. 50A–C).

FTIR spectroscopy was also used, and the authors reported that there was lyophilization-induced denaturation. The resolution was enhanced by Fourier self-deconvolution. On comparing the spectra of the lyophilized powder to the protein-rich rhGH aqueous solution, the characteristic sharp α-helix band (the predominant element of native structure) with a peak at $1655 \, \text{cm}^{-1}$ of the protein in solution was found to be very broad (Fig. 51). The spectra for the colyophilizates showed that rhGH had a more native secondary structure than lyophilized proteins without excipients. The α-helix band for the excipients was prominent at $1655 \, \text{cm}^{-1}$, indicating that the

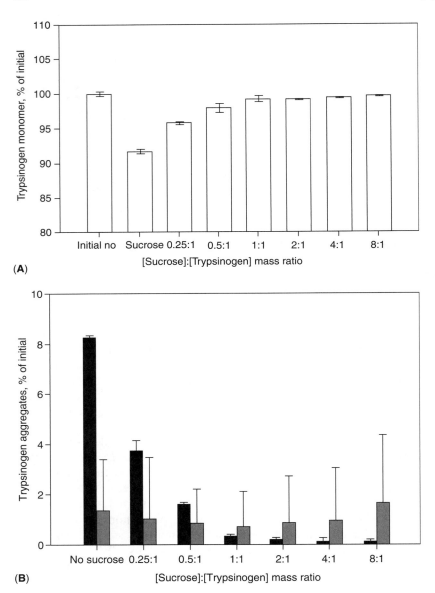

**(A)**

**(B)**

**Figure 46**  Aggregation status of trypsinogen following spray drying at different sucrose mass ratios and subsequent reconstitution at 5 mg/mL in 1 mM HCl: (**A**) relative amount of monomer; (**B**) relative amounts of dimer (*black bars*) and insoluble aggregates (*grey bars*). Error bars represent (±) one standard deviation based on triplicate determinations. *Source*: From Ref. 69.

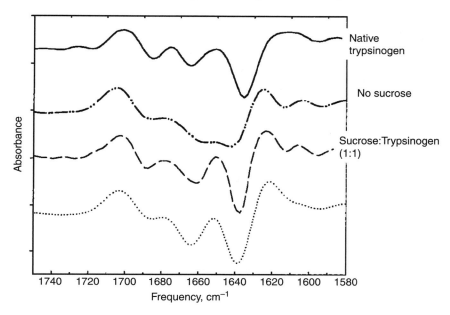

**Figure 47** Amide I second derivatives of native trypsinogen in solution (*solid line*) and in the solid state after spray drying: in the absence of sucrose (-·····-), and with sucrose at 1:1 (- -) and 8:1 (... ....) mass ratios. *Source*: From Ref. 69.

excipients were lyoprotectants. Mannitol:rhGH (31:1) gave the least α-helix content of 35% (Fig. 52). Lactose and trehalose produced an α-helix content of 48% and 46% in the lyophilized powder, respectively (Fig. 53).

The β-sheet content of the colyophilizates was significantly higher than in the aqueous solution. This is due to the formation of both inter- and

**Table 12** Correlation Coefficient Analysis of the Second Derivative Spectra of Spray-Dried Trypsinogen–Sucrose Powders

| Sucrose:trypsinogen mass ratio | Correlation coefficient[a] |
|---|---|
| No sucrose | $0.54 \pm 0.05$ |
| 0.25:1 | $0.74 \pm 0.04$ |
| 0.5:1 | $0.88 \pm 0.01$ |
| 1:1 | $0.93 \pm 0.01$ |
| 2:1 | $0.87 \pm 0.06$ |
| 4:1 | $0.78 \pm 0.06$ |

[a] Values represent averages and standard deviation of triplicate measurements.
*Source*: From Ref. 69.

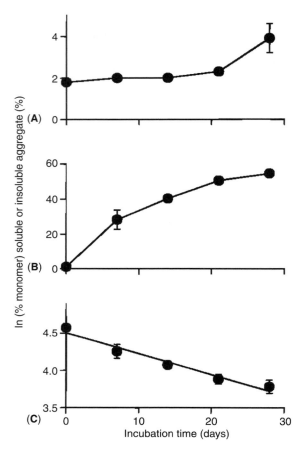

**Figure 48** Solid-state stability of excipient-free recombinant human growth hormone (rhGH). (**A**) Formation of soluble aggregates. (**B**) Formation of insoluble aggregates. (**C**) Loss of monomeric rhGH modeled as a pseudo first-order deterioration (calculated rate constant of $4.5 \pm 0.1$ day-1). *Source*: From Ref. 70.

intramolecular β-sheets as a result of the loss of water and consequent close molecular proximity of the individual protein molecules (70). The increase in β-sheet content may not be an indication of structural alterations or loss of α-helix. In the report, there was no correlation between the β-sheet and α-helix content.

The authors concluded that lyophilization subjects rhGH to a loss in α-helix and an increase in a β-sheet content. Their studies also revealed that samples with the greatest structural preservation (retention of α-helix) and least degree of protein–protein contacts (lowest β-sheet formation) tended to have superior stability.

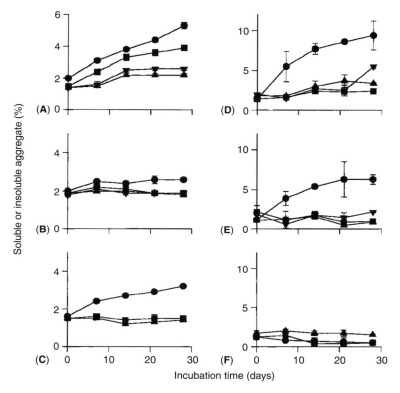

**Figure 49** Soluble aggregate formation of recombinant human growth hormone (rhGH) colyophilized with (**A**) lactose, (**B**) trehalose, and (**C**) cellobiose. Insoluble aggregate formation of rhGH colyophilized with (**D**) lactose, (**E**) trehalose, and (**F**) cellobiose. Ratios of excipient-to-protein (mol:mol) were 31:1 (•), 131:1 (■), 300:1 (2), and 1000:1 (▼). *Source*: From Ref. 70.

## Amide Bond Formation (Peptide and PVP)

Covalent interaction between primary amines in peptides/protein and carbonyl functional groups could occur during product development. An example is the reported interaction between the electrophilic carbonyl group of PVP and the reactive peptide amino group, forming an amide bond (71). A reaction scheme is depicted in Figure 54. This solid-state reaction is similar to Maillard reaction, in which the carbonyl functional group of a reducing sugar reacts with the free amine of a peptide or protein. It is important that this type of reaction be identified early in the development phase or in preformulation. Excipients containing carbonyl functional groups should be eliminated as early as possible or not considered at all in the solid-state formulation of peptides and proteins. The authors also

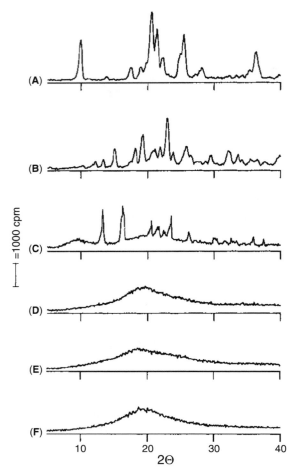

**Figure 50** X-ray powder diffraction patterns for various lyophilizates following a four-week incubation at 50°C: (**A**) 1000:1 mannitol:rhGH; (**B**) 1000:1 sorbitol:rhGH; (**C**) 300:1 methyl R-D-mannopyranoside:rhGH; (**D**) 1000:1 lactose:rhGH; (**E**) 1000:1 trehalose:rhGH; and (**F**) 1000:1 cellobiose:rhGH. *Abbreviation*: rhGH, recombinant human growth hormone. *Source*: From Ref. 70.

remarked that hydrogen bonding may facilitate the reaction via increased proximity and susceptibility of the terminal amino group to become nucleophilic enough to react (Fig. 55). To prove this, lyophilized PVP-Asn-hexapeptide was prepared using a constant peptide concentration, but it decreased the peptide-to-PVP ratio. The extent of reaction increased accordingly. The authors also used solid-state NMR spectroscopy to elucidate the peptide–polymer interaction in the solid matrix. The spectra of

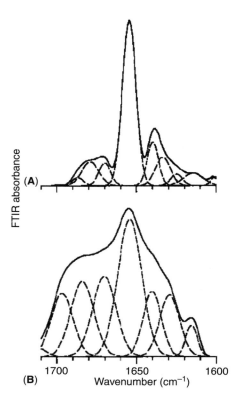

FTIR absorbance

(A)

(B) 1700    1650    1600
Wavenumber (cm⁻¹)

**Figure 51** FTIR spectra of recombinant human growth hormone (**A**) in aqueous solution at pH 7.8 and (**B**) the lyophilized powder. The solid lines represent the superimposed Fourier self-deconvolution and the curve-fit, and the dashed curves represent the individual Gaussian bands. *Abbreviation*: FTIR, Fourier transform infrared. *Source*: From Ref. 70.

the lyophilized product (containing $^{15}$N-labeled valine as a model of the peptide N-terminus), stored for varying periods, indicated the formation of a peptide–PVP complex.

## DELIBERATELY DESIGNED INTERACTIONS (POSITIVE DRUG–EXCIPIENT INTERACTIONS)

### Dicoumarol-Magnesium Oxide Interaction

Dicoumarol–excipient interactions could be used intentionally to an advantage; i.e., positive changes such as faster solubility and bioavailability could result. Akers et al. (72) observed increased plasma levels of dicoumarol with magnesium oxide as an excipient in the physical mixture with the drug. On the other hand, talc, colloidal magnesium aluminum silicate, aluminum or magnesium hydroxide, or starch caused a reduction in plasma levels (Figs. 56–58). The mechanism of the interaction was reported to be magnesium chelation with dicoumarol, causing an increase in the pH of the microenvironment of the drug. Another mechanism reported by the

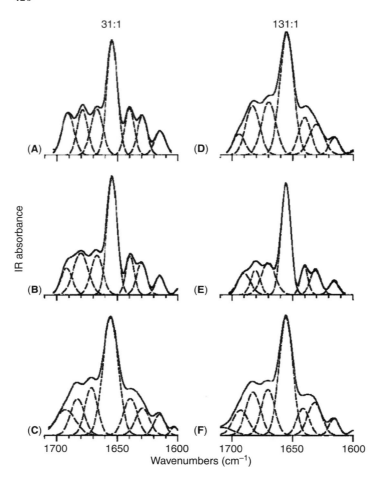

**Figure 52** Fourier transform infrared spectra of recombinant human growth hormone colyophilized at a excipient-to-protein mole ratio of 31:1 with (**A**) mannitol, (**B**) sorbitol, and (**C**) methyl R-D-mannopyranoside, and at 131:1 with (**D**) mannitol, (**E**) sorbitol, and (**F**) methyl R-D-mannopyranoside. The solid lines represent the superimposed Fourier self-deconvolution and the curve-fit, and the dashed curves represent the individual Gaussian bands. *Abbreviation*: IR, infrared. *Source*: From Ref. 70.

authors was an acid base reaction that resulted in the complex and the increase in solubility and dissolution.

## Danazol–Cyclodextrin Interaction

Another good example is the interaction between different drugs and cyclodextrins (CDs). CDs are hydrophilic, cyclic, nonreducing oligosaccharides,

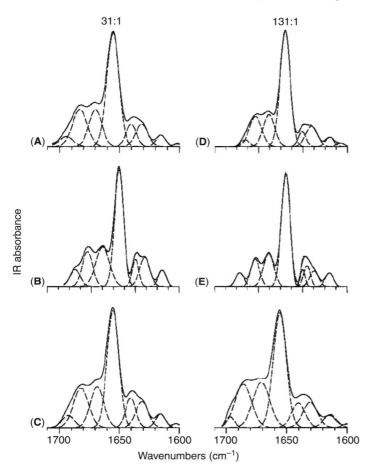

**Figure 53** Fourier transform infrared spectra of recombinant human growth hormone colyophilized at an excipient-to-protein mole ratio of 31:1 with (**A**) lactose, (**B**) trehalose, and (**C**) cellobiose, and at 131:1 with (**D**) lactose, (**E**) trehalose, and (**F**) cellobiose. The solid lines represent the superimposed Fourier self-deconvolution and the curve-fit, and the dashed curves represent the individual Gaussian bands. *Abbreviation*: IR, infrared. *Source*: From Ref. 70.

composed of six to eight glucopyranose units (73) and have been extensively used to increase the solubility of many poorly water-soluble drugs (74). CDs have the ability to form inclusion complexes with many organic molecules, in which the guest molecule is entrapped within its hydrophobic cavity, as seen in Figure 59, thus resulting in an enhancement of solubility of the guest molecule.

Badawy et al. (75) reported a great improvement in the solubility and bioavailability of an otherwise poorly soluble drug, danazol. The solubility

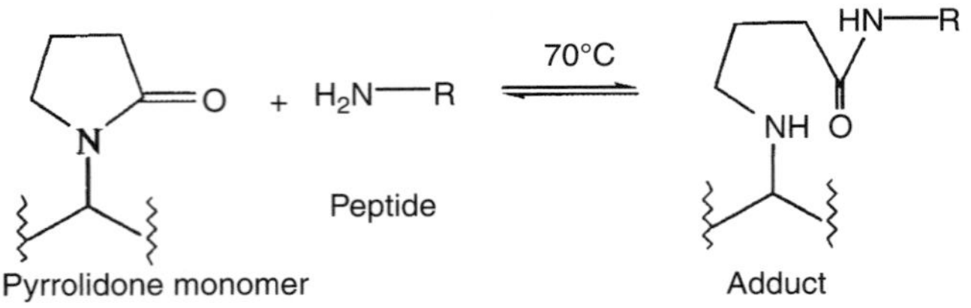

**Figure 54** Proposed mechanism of reaction. *Source*: From Ref. 71.

of danazol is 0.61 or 0.32 mg/L at 37°C and 22°C, respectively. It is also a drug that undergoes first-pass metabolism. Improved solubility, dissolution, and bioavailability were observed using hydroxypropyl β-cyclodextrin (HPCD).

The authors interacted HPCD with danazol via a solvent evaporation method in w/w drug–excipient ratios ranging between 1:1 and 1:10. Coprecipitates formed were characterized using various techniques such as XRD, proton NMR, IR, solubility, and dissolution analysis. The solubility of the coprecipitate or complex increased significantly especially at higher drug:excipient ratios (Fig. 60). The bioavailability in rats also improved significantly ($p < 0.05$) when compared with the commercial formulation (Danocrine®) as shown by the higher area under the curve (AUC) depicted in Figure 61. Another study of danazol by Jain et al. (76), in which a buccal controlled-release danazol-SBE-CD tablet was used, yielded plasma concentration 20 times higher than the commercial formulation of the drug and SBE-CD.

### Ibuprofen–CD In Situ Interaction

In another investigation, Ghorab and Adeyeye (77) exploited the in situ interaction between β-CD and ibuprofen to enhance the dissolution and bioavailability of the drug. β-CD is a high-molecular-weight (MW) hydrophilic compound (MW = 1135) that does not cross the gastrointestinal (GI) membrane to any significant extent (78). In another study, it was reported that after oral administration of high dose (313.5 mg/kg) to rats, there was

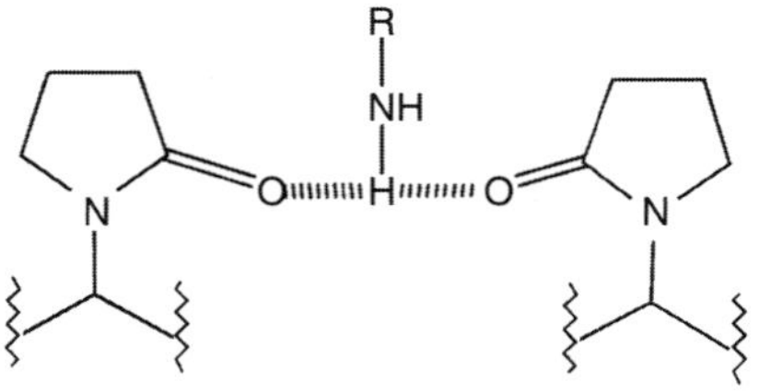

**Figure 55** Proposed hydrogen bonding of the terminal amino group. *Source*: From Ref. 71.

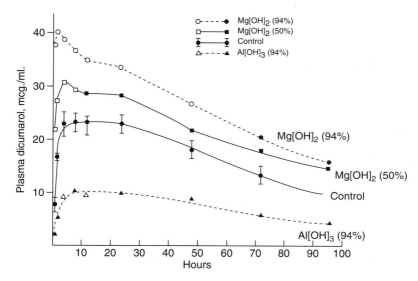

**Figure 56** Plasma–concentration time profiles of dicoumarol and its physical mixtures with some excipients. *Source*: From Ref. 72.

no more than 3 to 50 ppm of β-CD detected in the blood (79). Therefore, in the GI tract (GIT), the release of any drug from its complex with β-CD has to occur for the drug to reach the systemic circulation. Thus, the equilibrium

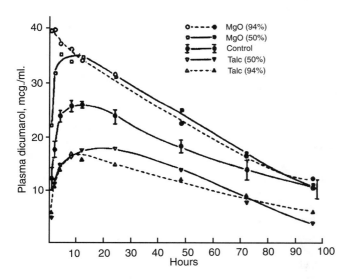

**Figure 57** Plasma–concentration time profiles of dicoumarol and physical mixtures with some excipients. *Source*: From Ref. 72.

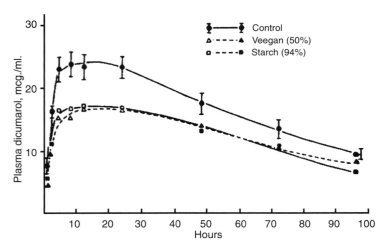

**Figure 58** Plasma–concentration time profiles of dicoumarol and physical mixtures with some excipients. *Source*: From Ref. 72.

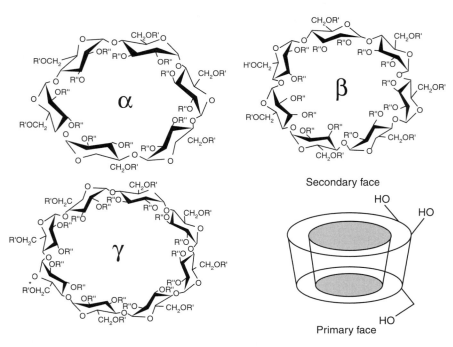

**Figure 59** Structures of different cyclodextrins. *Source*: From Ref. 73.

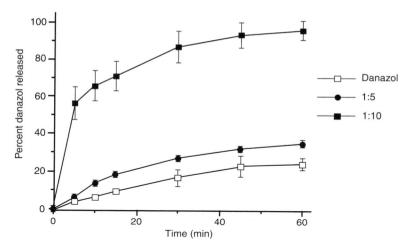

**Figure 60** Dissolution profiles of crystalline danazol and its coprecipitates. Error bars represent 1 S.D. *Source*: From Ref. 75.

constant of the complex becomes a very important parameter in determining the rate of drug absorption, especially for poorly water-soluble drugs. For drugs that possess low stability constants or that dissociate easily high

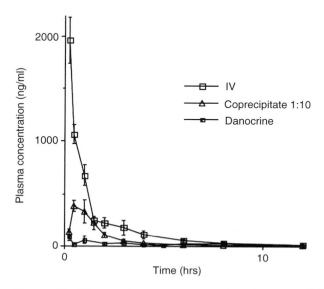

**Figure 61** Plasma danazol concentration (mean + S.E.M., $n = 5$) following intravenous administration, oral administration of coprecipitate and Danocrine (mean + S.E.M., $n = 6$). *Source*: From Ref. 75.

free drug concentration (greater than the saturation concentration) could result and ultimately cause drug precipitation. In contrast, a very high stability constant could result in low concentration of free drug available for absorption. The concentration of drug could further decrease as the relative amount of the free CD increases, due to its insignificant absorption from the GIT. Therefore, a moderate dissociation of the complex is important for drug absorption. According to Stella and Rajewski, release of drug from the complex could be facilitated by dilution and presence of competing agents especially for complexes with high stability constants (80).

Ghorab and Adeyeye (77) made a wet granulation of ibuprofen–β-CD blend (in 2:1 molar ratio) using different solvents such as water and isopropanol. The granules were dried for two hours in a convection oven followed by characterization using various solid-state techniques such as XRD, DSC, FTIR, and proton NMR spectroscopy. This is an interaction that had planned positive outcomes. The authors used a nontraditional method, cogranulation, to interact the drug with the excipients instead of the traditional solvent evaporation technique. They observed improved dissolution and bioavailability from the co-granulated product compared with the physical mixture of the excipient and drug (Figs. 62 and 63). Usual processing conditions (water as binder, drying at 60°C for two hours) were used; therefore, the interaction was the driving factor in the observations made.

In some cases, enhancement in solubility and bioavailability might not have been planned, in which case, unexpected higher levels of the drug in the blood would be observed. This is underscored if a high-potency drug was used in the formulation, such high blood levels could lead to toxicity or unwanted side effects.

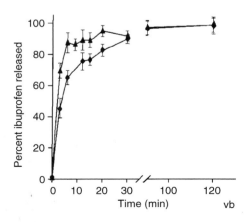

**Figure 62** Dissolution profiles of ibuprofen from oven-dried physical mixture (♦) and oven-dried granules prepared using water (▲). *Source:* From Ref. 77.

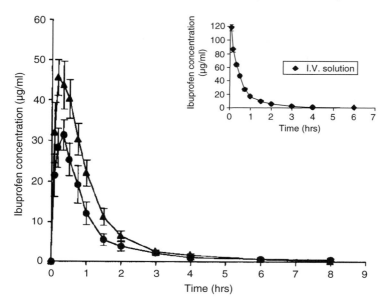

**Figure 63** Mean plasma concentration–time profiles of intravenous solution and orally administered ibuprofen from oven-dried physical mixtures (•) and oven-dried granules (▲) in bile duct–nonligated rats ($n = 5$). *Source*: From Ref. 77.

## DRUG–EXCIPIENT INTERACTION AND ABSORPTION

Excipients can interact with drugs to influence the absorption and bioavailability. The reports in the literature of drug–excipient interactions resulting in the modification of absorption or bioavailability may be a small segment of the actual occurrence, since other interactions may be classified as confidential by the pharmaceutical industry. In the previous section, emphasis was placed on formulations that were deliberately designed to interact with excipients such as CDs with the goal of positively influencing the in vivo disposition. Sometimes, the interaction may result in reduced bioavailability as reported by Jackson et al. (81). For example, interaction of tetracycline with calcium carbonate resulted in an insoluble complex with consequent reduction in bioavailability (82). Similarly, a complex that led to reduced dissolution and bioavailability was reported for the interaction of phenobarbital with PEG 4000 (83).

The functionalities of different classes of excipients on physical characteristics may become modified due to interaction with unexpected consequences on absorption. Diluents in solid dosage forms are usually used as bulking agents to make the size practical, and the tablet compressible and compactable as referred to earlier. However, the outcome may be far outreaching than the basic function of the excipient. For example, the drug triamterene was shown to dissolve faster when formulated with hydrophilic fillers such as lactose and starch compared to water-insoluble diluents such as terra alba (84).

Disintegrants and superdisintegrants are present in formulations to facilitate the break-up and rapid deaggregation of the solid dosage form, respectively. However, the superdisintegrant croscarmellose sodium was reported to extensively bind to oxymorphone, resulting in slower drug release (85). Lubricants and/or glidants in tablet formulations improve flow of the powder blends by preventing interparticulate friction or adhesion to tablet dies and punches via coating of the particle or metal surfaces, respectively. These excipients are usually hydrophobic and present in very low concentrations (0.5–1% w/w), and excessive amounts can lead to a decrease in dissolution. However, increased bioavailability was observed in the amoxycillin-synthetic fat derivative of glycerin formulation as a result of interaction of the drug with colloidal silica present as the lubricant (86–88).

Many drug–excipient interactions have also been found to occur during processing affecting disintegration and dissolution, with the outcome being a positive effect on bioavailability. A cogrounded mixture of nifedipine, a calcium-channel blocker, PEG 6000, and HPMC was reported to increase the bioavailability of the product (89). This was concluded to be due to hydrophobic interactions between the drug and the polymer during the grinding process. The $C_{max}$ of the product increased 10-fold while the AUC increased threefold when compared to the physical mixture (Fig. 64).

The bioavailability can also be influenced by physiological processes and factors such as pH of the microenvironment, protein binding, GI transit time, stability in the GIT, effects on the flora, and so on. Chlorpromazine, an antipsychotic that usually undergoes presystemic transformation or degradation, was reported to have improved stability after complex formation with β-CD, leading to improved bioavailability.

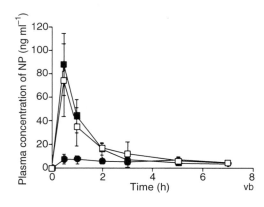

**Figure 64** Mean plasma–concentration–time profiles of nifedipine (NP) after the oral administration of various preparations equivalent to 10 mg of NP to beagle dogs. Physical mixture (●); coground mixture prepared in the presence of water (■); NP solution of PEG 400 (□). *Source*: From Ref. 82.

Solid dispersions formed as a result of drug–excipient reaction have been extensively reported by many authors to increase the bioavailability (90–92). Other investigations involving several drugs and excipients such as PEG 4000 or 6000 revealed no change in bioavailability (93–96).

An acid–base reaction can lead to a change in the microenvironment in a biological medium, thus favoring absorption. The antibiotic erythromycin acistrate is a derivative of erythromycin that converts to anhydroery-thromycin in an acidic pH medium. In the presence of sodium bicarbonate (an excipient), an acid–base reaction takes place, resulting in an increase in the pH of the stomach. The product, which otherwise would not absorb in the stomach, had a better absorption due to the increase in the pH of the stomach. Another example was given in the section titled Positive Drug–Excipient Interactions, where dicoumarol was reported to absorb better in the presence of an excipient, magnesium oxide (72).

## REGULATORY OUTCOMES OF DRUG–EXCIPIENT INTERACTIONS

Biowaiver of in vivo bioequivalence testing of a new or reformulated immediate-release solid oral dosage form by the FDA is usually based on the Biopharmaceutical Classification System (BCS) (97). According to the FDA, the solubility class should be determined by calculating the volume of an aqueous medium sufficient to dissolve the highest dose strength in the pH range of 1 to 7.5. A drug substance should be classified as highly soluble when the highest dose strength is soluble in $\leq 250$ mL of aqueous media over the pH range of 1 to 7.5 at $37°C$. However, to assess if the definition of high solubility as proposed in the FDA guidance on BCS is too strict for "highly permeable acidic drugs," or in case of drug–excipient interactions, many researchers have argued in support of the strictness or the inappropriateness of the FDA biowaiver. There are reports that have focused on these aspects and relevance in early preformulation studies. The solubility of ranitidine hydrochloride, a histamine $H_2$-antagonist (used for the treatment of gastric and duodenal ulcer), in pH range of 1–7.4 was experimentally found to be over 550 mg/ml. It is classified as a Class III drug, i.e., a highly soluble, low-permeability drug. However, the solubility ratio at the highest dose, 300 mg, is less than 0.55 mL at room temperature, which is far below the critical value of 250 mL. It is expected to meet the highly soluble drug definition at $37°C$.

However, depending on the excipients used and the product that was developed and registered from such formulation, the Caco-2 permeability may be significantly different. For example, excipients such as lactose, HPMC, docusate sodium EDTA, PEG 400, and propyleneglycol did not affect the Caco-2 permeability of ranitidine. In contrast, other excipients such as sodium lauryl sulfate, sodium caprate, deoxycholate, glycocholate, and taurodyhydrofusidate increased the Caco-2 permeability. This is because some excipients may open the tight junctions and affect absorption via the paracellular route (98,99). Earlier, a Caco-2 permeability study had concluded that the presence of calcium ions can aid permeability. Therefore, this implies that ranitidine is absorbed by diffusion via the paracellular route. Considering the positive influence of some excipients on the Caco-2 permeability of ranitidine and what the corresponding increase in absorption could be, the drug product can qualify for a biowaiver as a Class I drug, i.e., highly soluble and highly permeable. In general, the authors agreed with the other group of investigators [Yu et al. (100)] that there may be very little or no clinical risks if excipients are present only in the expected amounts in respective formulations.

## CONCLUSIONS

Incidences of drug–excipient interactions or incompatibilities in solid dosage form development could be more than reported. Consideration should always be given to the reactivity of the API in the presence of excipients. Moisture, pH of the microenvironment, processing, and heat are some of the factors that could trigger drug–excipient interactions and incompatibilities. The criteria for evaluation must be rational and meaningful. These include the use of a drug:excipient ratio similar to that present in the formulation, appropriate screening methods such as IST (accompanied by use of statistical design), and combination analytical techniques. Recognition of the consequences of drug–excipient interactions early in the development or preformulation phase will lead to the avoidance of unnecessary impurities or degradants, needless multiplicity of prototype formulations, and unwanted changes in the physicochemical properties of the formulation. The outcomes of the awareness are robust formulation, overall achievement of quality by design, successful drug product registration, and faster time to get the product to the market.

## ACKNOWLEDGMENTS

I am grateful to my graduate students—Vishal Bijlani, Fred Esseku, Uday Kotreka, and Anjali Joshi—for their assistance in various capacities during the preparation of the manuscript.

## REFERENCES

1. Brittain HG. Overview of drug-excipient interactions in pharmaceutical solid dosage forms. Presentation at AAPS Meeting.
2. Committee on Drugs; American Academy of Pediatrics. "Inactive" ingredients in pharmaceutical products. Pediatrics 1997; 99(2):268–7.
3. Byrn SR, Xu W, Eewman AW. Chemical reactivity in solid state pharmaceuticals: formulation implications. Adv Drug Deliv Rev 2001; 48:115–36.

4.  Paul IC, Curtin DY. Thermally induced organic reactions in the solid-state. Acc Chem Res 1973; 6:217–25.
5.  Ahlneck C, Zografi G. The molecular basis of moisture effects on the physical and chemical stability of drugs in the solid-state. Int J Pharm 1990; 62:87–95.
6.  Baxter JG, Robeson CE. Crystalline aliphatic esters of vitamin A. J Am Chem Soc 1942; 64:2407–10.
7.  Guillory JK, Higuchi T. Solid-state stability of some crystalline vitamin A compounds. J Pharm Sci 1962; 5:100–5.
8.  Xu W. Investigation of Solid-State Stability of Selected Bioactive Compounds. Ph.D. thesis, Purdue University, West Lafayette, IN, 1997:47 907–1333.
9.  Lin CT, Perrier P, Clay GG, Sutton PA, Byrn SR. Solid-state photooxidation of 21-cortisol *tert*-butylacetate to 21-cortisone *tert*-butylacetate. J Org Chem 1982; 47:2978–81.
10. Byrn SR, Sutton PA, Tobias B, Frye J, Main P. Crystal structure, solid-state NMR spectra, and oxygen reactivity of five crystal forms of prednisolone tertbutylacetate. J Am Chem Soc 1988; 110:1609–14.
11. Hausin RJ, Codding PW. Molecular and crystal structures of MDL27,467A hydrochloride and quinapril hydrochloride, two ester derivatives of potent angiotensin converting enzyme inhibitors. J Med Chem 1991; 34:511–7.
12. Lai MC, Hageman MJ, Schowen RL, Borchardt RL, Topp EM. Chemical stability of peptides in polymers. 1. Effect of water on peptide deamidation in poly(vinyl alcohol) and poly(vinyl pyrrolidone) matrixes. J Pharm Sci 2000; 88:1073–80.
13. Lai MC, Hageman MJ, Schowen RL, Borchardt RL, Laird BB, Topp EM. Chemical stability of peptides in polymers. 2. Discriminating between solvent and plasticizing effects of water on peptide deamination in poly(vinylpyrrolidone). J Pharm Sci 2000; 88:1081–9.
14. Serajuddin ATM, Thakur AB, Ghoshal RN, et al. Selection of solid dosage form composition through drug-excipient compatibility testing. J Pharm Sci 1999; 88:696–704.
15. Monkhouse DC, Maderich A. Whither compatibility testing? Drug Dev Ind Pharm 1989; 15:2115–30.
16. Botha SA, Lotter AP. Compatibility study between atenolol and tablet excipients using differential scanning calorimetry. Drug Dev Ind Pharm 1990; 16(12):1945.
17. Venkataram S, Khohlokwane M, Wallis SH. Evaluation of the compatibility of ketorolac tromethamine with selected polymers and common tablet excipients by thermal and isothermal stress testing. Drug Dev Ind Pharm 1995; 21:847–55.
18. Kandarapu R, Grover V, Chawla HPS, Garg S. Evaluation of the compatibility of ketorolac tromethamine with selected polymers and common tablet excipients by thermal and isothermal stress testing. STP Pharm Sci 2001; 11:449–57.
19. Mura P, Manderioli A, Bramanti G, Furlanetto S, Pinzauti S. Utilization of differential scanning calorimetry as a screening technique to determine the compatibility of ketoprofen with excipients. Int J Pharm 1995; 119:71–9.
20. Mura P, Faucci MT, Manderioli A, Bramanti G, Ceccarelli L. Compatibility study between ibuproxam and pharmaceutical excipients using differential

scanning calorimetry, hot-stage microscopy and scanning electron microscopy. J Pharm Biom Anal 1998; 18:151–63.

21. Botha SA, Lotter AP. Compatibility study between naproxen and tablet excipients using differential scanning calorimetry. Drug Dev Ind Pharm 1990; 16(4):673.

22. McDaid FM, Barker SA, Fitzpatrick S, Petts CR, Craig DQM. Further investigations into the use of high sensitivity differential scanning calorimetry as a means of predicting drug–excipient interactions. Int J Pharm 2003; 252: 235–40.

23. Balestrieri F, Magri AD, Magri AL, Marini D, Sacchini A. Application of differential scanning calorimetry to the study of drug-excipient compatibility, Thermochimica Acta 1996; 285:337.

24. Morris KR, Newman AW, Bugay DE, et al. Characterization of humidity-dependent changes in crystal properties of a new HMG-CoA reductase inhibitor in support of its dosage form development. Int J Pharm 1994; 108: 195–206.

25. Carstensen JT, Johnson JB, Valentine W, Vance JJ. Extrapolation of appearance of tablets and powders from accelerated storage tests. J Pharm Sci 1964; 53:1050–4.

26. Gu L, Strickley RG, Chi L, Chowhan ZT. Drug-excipient incompatibility studies of the dipeptide angiotensin-converting enzyme inhibitor, moexipril hydrochloride: dry powder vs wet granulation. Pharm Res 1990; 7:379–83.

27. Verma RK, Garg S. Compatibility studies between isosorbide mononitrate and selected excipients used in the development of extended release formulations. J Pharm Biomed Anal 2004; 35:449–58.

28. Verma RK, Garg S. Selection of excipients for extended release formulations of glipizide through drug–excipient compatibility testing. J Pharma Biomed Anal 2005; 38:633–44.

29. Adeyeye MC, Mwangi E, Katondo B, Jain A, Ichikawa H, Fukumori Y. Dissolution stability studies of suspensions of prolonged-release diclofenac microcapsules prepared by the Wurster process: I. Eudragit-based formulation and possible drug-excipient interaction. J Microencapsul 2005; 22(4): 333–42.

30. Liu J, Xiao Y, Allen C. Polymer–drug compatibility: a guide to the development of delivery systems for the anticancer agent, ellipticine. J Pharm Sci 2004; 93(1):132–43.

31. Greenhalgh D, Williams A, York TP. Solubility parameters as predictors of miscibility in solid disperisons. J Pharm Sci 1999; 88:1182–90.

32. Suzuki H, Sunada H. Influence of water-soluble polymers on the dissolution of nifedipine solid dispersions with combined carriers. Chem Pharm Bull 1998; 46:6(3):482–7.

33. Katpally S, Ghorab S, Madura MK, Mosher JD, Thompson JD, Adeyeye MC. Characterization of Bile Salt/SBE-7 β-Cyclodextrin Interactions Using Isothermal Microcalorimetry. MS thesis, Duquesne University.

34. Wissing S, Craig DQM, Barker SA, Moore WD. An investigation into the use of stepwise isothermal high sensitivity DSC as a means of detecting drug-excipient incompatibility. Int J Pharm 2000; 199:141–50.

35. Beezer AE, Loch W, Mitchell JC, et al. An investigation of dilute aqueous solution behavior of poly(oxyethylene) + poly(oxypropylene) + poly (oxyethylene) block copolymers. Langmuir 1994; 10:4001–5.
36. Mura P, Furlanetto S, Cirri M, Maestrelli F, Marras AM, Pinzauti S. Optimization of glibenclamide tablet composition through the combined use of differential scanning calorimetry and d-optimal mixture experimental design. J Pharm Biomed Anal 2005; 37:65–71.
37. Takahashi Y, Nakashima K, Ishihara T, Nakagawa H. Polymorphism of fostedil: characterization and polymorphic change by mechanical treatments. Drug Dev Indust Pharm 1985; 11:1543–63.
38. Qiu Z, Stowell JG, Cao W, Morris KR, Byrn SR, Carvajal MT. Effect of milling and compression on the solid-state Maillard reaction. J Pharm Sci 2005; 94(11):2568–80.
39. Roy S, Alexander KS, Riga AT, Chatterjee K. Characterization of physical mixtures and directly compressed tablets of sulfamerazine polymorphs: implications on in vitro release characteristics. J Pharm Sci 2003; 92(4):747–59.
40. Sun C, Grant DJ. Influences of crystal structure on the tableting properties of sulfamerazine polymorphs. Pharm Res 2001; 18:274–80.
41. Wang LH, Chowhan ZT. Drug-excipient interactions resulting from powder mixing. Part 5. Role of sodium lauryl sulfate. Int J Pharm 1990; 60: 61–78.
42. Ong JT, Chowhan ZT, Samuels GJ. Drug-excipient interactions resulting from powder mixing. Part 6. Role of various surfactants. Int J Pharm 1993; 96: 231–42.
43. Airaksinen S, Karjalainen M, Shevchenko A, et al. Role of water in the physical stability of solid dosage formulations. J Pharm Sci 2005; 94(10): 2147–65.
44. Sing KSW, Everett DH, Haul RAW, et al. Reporting physisorption data for gas/solid systems with special reference to the determination of surface area and porosity (recommendations). Pure Appl Chem 1985; 57:603–19.
45. Rouquerol F, Rouquerol J, Sing K. Introduction, assessment of mesoporosity and general conclusions and recommendations. In: Rouquerol F, Rouquerol J, Sing K, eds. Adsorption by Powders and Porous Solids. London, Great Britain: Academic Press, 1999:1–26, 191–218, 439–47.
46. Salameh AK, Taylor LS. Physical stability of crystal hydrates and their anhydrates in the presence of excipients. J Pharm Sci 2006; 95(2):446–61.
47. Otsuka M, Matsuda Y. The effect of humidity on hydration kinetics of mixtures of nitrofurantoin anhydride and diluents. Chem Pharm Bull 1994; 42: 156–9.
48. Adeyeye, et al. Evaluation of crystallinity and drug release stability of directly compressed theophylline hydrophilic matrix tablets stored under varied moisture conditions. Int J Pharm 1995; 116:65–75.
49. Byrn SR, Lin CT. The effect of crystal packing and defects on desolvation of hydrate crystals of caffeine and L-(2)-1,4-cyclohexadiene-1-alanine. J Am Chem Soc 1976; 98:4004–5.
50. Wells JI. Pharmaceutical Preformulation: the Physical and Chemical Properties of Drug Substances. Chichester: Ellis Horwood, 1988.

51. Chen X, Ulrich J, Griesser J, et al. Analysis of the acid–base reaction between solid indomethacin and sodium bicarbonate using infrared spectroscopy, X-ray powder diffraction, and solid state nuclear magnetic resonance spectroscopy. J Pharm Biomed Anal 2005; 38:670–7.

52. Usui F, Carstensen JT. Interactions in the solid-state. I. Interactions of sodium bicarbonate and tartaric acid under compressed conditions. J Pharm Sci 1985; 74:1293–7.

53. Wright L, Carstensen JT. Interactions in the solid-state. II. Interaction of sodium bicarbonate with substituted benzoic acids in the presence of moisture. J Pharm Sci 1986; 75:546–51.

54. Huang WX, Desai M, Tang Q, Yang R, Vivilecchia RV, Joshi Y. Elimination of metformin–croscarmellose sodium interaction by competition. Int J Pharm 2006; 27:311(1–2):33–9.

55. Hollenbeck RG, Mitrevej KT, Fan AC. Estimation of the extent of drug–excipient interactions involving croscarmellose sodium. J Pharm Sci 1983; 72:325–7.

56. Crowley P, Martini L. Drug–excipient interactions. Pharm Tech Eur 2001; 26–34.

57. Jenquin MR, Liebowitz SM, Sarabia RE, McGinity JW. Physical and chemical factors influencing the release of drugs from acrylic resin films, J Pharm Sci 1990; 79(9):811–6.

58. Khalil E, Sallam A. Interaction of two diclofenac acid salts with copolymers of ammoniomethacrylate: effect of additives and release profiles. Drug Dev Ind Pharm 1999; 25(4):419–27.

59. Breitkreutz J. Leakage of enteric (Eudragit® L)-coated dosage forms in simulated gastric juice in the presence of poly(ethylene glycol). J Control Rel 2000; 67:79–88.

60. Thakur AB, Morris K, Grosso JA, et al. Mechanism and kinetics of metal ion-mediated degradation of fosinopril sodium. Pharm Res 1993; 10(6): 800–9.

61. Wirth DD, Baertschi SW, Johnson RA, et al. Maillard reaction of lactose and fluoxetine hydrochloride, a secondary amine. J Pharm Sci 1998; 87: 31–9.

62. Troup AE, Mitchner H. Degradation of phenylephrine hydrochloride in tablet formulations containing aspirin. J Pharm Sci 1964; 53:375–9.

63. Jacobs AL, Dilatush AE, Weinstein S, Windheuser JJ. Formation of acetylcodeine from aspirin and codeine. J Pharm Sci 1966; 55:893–5.

64. Koshy KT, Troup AE, Duvall RN, Conwell RN, Shankle LL. Acetylation of acetaminophen in tablet formulations containing aspirin. J Pharm Sci 1967; 56:1117–21.

65. Broadhead J, Edmond-Rouan SK, Rhodes CT. The spray drying of pharmaceuticals. Drug Dev Ind Pharm 1996; 22:813–22.

66. Mumenthaler M, Hsu CC, Pearlman R. Feasibility study on spray-drying protein pharmaceuticals: recombinant human growth hormone and tissue plasminogen activator. Pharm Res 1994; 11:12–20.

67. Mumenthaler M, Leuenberger H. Atmospheric spray-freeze-drying: a suitable alternative in freeze-drying technology. Int J Pharm 1991; 72:97–110.

68. Winters MA, Knutson BL, Debenedetti PG, et al. Precipitation of proteins in supercritical carbon dioxide. J Pharm Sci 1996; 85:586–94.
69. Tzannis ST, Prestrelski SJ. Activity-stability considerations of trypsinogen during spray drying: effects of sucrose. J Pharm Sci 1999; 88(3):351–9.
70. Costantino HR, Carrasquillo KG, Cordero RA, Mumenthaler M, Hsu C, Griebenow K. Effect of excipients on the stability and structure of lyophilized recombinant human growth hormone. J Pharm Sci 1998; 87(11): 1412–20.
71. D'Souza AJM, Schowen RL, Borchardt RT, Salisbury JS, Munson EJ, Topp EM. Reaction of a peptide with polyvinylpyrrolidone in the solid state. J Pharm Sci 2003; 92(3):585–93.
72. Akers MJ, Lach JL, Fischer LJ. Alterations in the absorption of dicoumarol by various excipient materials. J Pharm Sci 1973; 62:391–5.
73. Ghorab MK. A Dissertation Presented to Graduate School of Pharmaceutical Sciences. Duquesne University, Sept 2001:7.
74. Krenn M, Gamcsik MP, Vogelsang GB, Colvin OM, Leong KW. Improvements in solubility and stability of thalidomide upon complexation with hydroxypropyl-β-cyclodextrin. J Pharm Sci 1992; 81:685–9.
75. Badawy SIF, Ghorab MM, Adeyeye CM. Characterization and biovailability of danazol-hydroxypropyl-β-cyclodextrin. Int J Pharm 1996; 128:45–54.
76. Jain AC, Aungst BJ, Adeyeye CM. Development and in vivo evaluation of buccal tablets prepared using danazol-sulfobutylether-cyclodextrin (SBE 7 cyclodextrin) complexes. J Pharm Sci 2002; 91(7):1659–68.
77. Ghorab MK, Adeyeye MC. Enhanced bioavailability of process-induced fast-dissolving ibuprofen cogranulated with β-cyclodextrin. J Pharm Sci 2003; 92(8):1691–7.
78. Irie T, Uekama K. Pharmaceutical applications of cyclodextrins. III. Toxicological issues and safety evaluation. J Pharm Sci 1997; 86(2):147–62.
79. Gerloczy A, Fonagy A, Keresztes P, Perlaky L, Szejtli J. Absorption, distribution, excretion and metabolism of orally administered [14]C-betacyclo-dextrin in rat. Arzneim-Forsch 1985; 35(7):1042–47.
80. Stella VJ, Rajewski RA. Cyclodextrins: their future in drug formulation and delivery. Pharm Res 1997; 14:556–67.
81. Jackson K, Young D, Pant S. Drug–excipient interactions and their effect on absorption. Research focus: reviews. PSTT 2000; 3(10):336–45.
82. Shargel L, Yu ABC, eds. Applied Biopharmaceutics and Pharmacokinetics. 2nd ed. Norwalk, CT: Appleton–Century–Crofts, 1985.
83. Singh P, et al. Effect of inert tablet ingredients on drug absorption, I. Effect of polyethylene glycol 4000 on the intestinal absorption of four barbiturates. J Pharm Sci 1966; 55:63–8.
84. Yen JKC. The dissolution rate principle in practical tablet formulation. Can Pharm J 1964; 26:493–9.
85. Asakawa Y, et al. Drug–disintegrant interactions: binding of oxymorphone derivatives. J Pharm Sci 1981; 70:709–11.
86. Llabres M, et al. Quantification of the effect of excipients on bioavailability by means of response surfaces, I: amoxicillin in fat matrix. J Pharm Sci 1982; 71:924–7.

87.  Llabres M, et al. Quantification of the effect of excipients on bioavailability by means of response surfaces, II: amoxicillin in fat–silica matrix. J Pharm Sci 1982; 71:927–30.

88.  Llabres M, et al. Quantification of the effect of excipients on bioavailability by means of response surfaces, III: in vivo–in vitro correlations. J Pharm Sci 1982; 71:930–2.

89.  Sugimoto M, et al. Improvement of dissolution characteristics and bioavailability of poorly water-soluble drugs by novel cogrinding method using water-soluble polymer. Int J Pharm 1998; 160:11–9.

90.  Bhattacharyya M, et al. Formulation and in vitro–in vivo characterization of solid dispersions of piroxicam. Drug Dev Ind Pharm 1993; 19:739–47.

91.  Fawaz F, et al. Bioavailability of norfloxacin from PEG 6000 solid dispersion and cyclodextrin inclusion complexes in rabbits. Int J Pharm 1996; 132:271–5.

92.  Guyot M, et al. Physicochemical characterization and dissolution of norfloxacin/cyclodextrin inclusion compounds and PEG solid dispersions. Int J Pharm 1995; 123:53–63.

93.  Veiga MD, et al. Dissolution behaviour of drugs from binary and ternary systems. Int J Pharm 1993; 93:215–20.

94.  Ghosh LK, et al. Product development studies on the tablet formulation of ibuprofen to improve bioavailability. Drug Dev Ind Pharm 1998; 24:473–7.

95.  Owusu-Ababio G, et al. Comparative dissolution studies for mefenamic acid–polyethylene glycol solid dispersion systems and tablets. Pharm Dev Technol 1998; 3:405–12.

96.  Chowdary KPR, Suresh Babu KVV. Dissolution, bioavailability and ulcerogenic studies on solid dispersions of indomethacin in water soluble cellulose polymers. Drug Dev Ind Pharm 1994; 20:799–813.

97.  Kortejarvi H, Yliperttula M, Dressman JB, et al. Biowaiver monographs for immediate release solid oral dosage forms: ranitidine hydrochloride. J Pharm Sci 2005; 94(8):1617–35.

98.  Aungst BJ. Intestinal permeation enhancers. J Pharm Sci 2000; 89:429–42.

99.  Rege BD, Yu LX, Hussain AS, Polli JE. Effect of common excipients on Caco-2 transport of lowpermeability drugs. J Pharm Sci 2001; 90:1776–86.

100. Yu LX, Wang JT, Hussain AS. Evaluation of USP apparatus 3 for dissolution testing of immediate-release products. AAPS PharmSci 2002; 4:E1.

# 4.3

# Methodology for the Evaluation of Chemical and Physical Interactions Between Drug Substances and Excipients

Harry G. Brittain

*Center for Pharmaceutical Physics, Milford, New Jersey, U.S.A.*

## INTRODUCTION

As discussed in previous chapters, preformulation scientists must determine whether the bulk drug substance will be developed as a salt form or not, they must decide which of the known polymorphs or solvatomorphs is the most desirable physical form, and then catalog all of the physical and chemical characteristics of this form. Once the profiling of the drug substance is complete, one can begin to design appropriate prototype formulations that will meet the needs set down by the pharmacologists regarding the particulars of drug availability. After considering the range of possible solid–solid reactions, the preformulation scientist is able to propose several trial formulations that hopefully will achieve the desired drug release profile.

Of course, before congratulations on the development of the new formulation are in order, one must first prove that the new formulations actually exhibit the range of physical and chemical stabilities that constitute a pharmaceutically acceptable product. This requires that drug–excipient mixtures be prepared, and then stressed to allow whatever physical or chemical reactions that might take place to actually take place. Finally, the formulations must be tested by some type of analytical methodology in order to determine whether a reaction has taken place or not.

Given the vast array of techniques available for the evaluation of the chemical and physical properties of materials, several questions become immediately obvious. One of these can be phrased as: "What analytical methodology is most suitable for the study of chemical reactions among the ingredients in a prototype formulation?"; and the second question parallels the first except that it pertains to physical reactions. The third essential question to be answered is: "How do I know that the analytical methods I use are reliable and will provide information that can be trusted?" Topics related to these three questions constitute the focus of the present chapter.

Another question that is often raised concerns sources of information that workers in the field would find to be most useful. As will be seen from the magnitude of the reference list, the number of works pertaining to analytical methodology is simply overwhelming. However, anyone needing knowledge in a hurry would be well advised to consult the latest edition of the *Analytical Instrumentation Handbook* (1) as a starting position. A second valuable and indispensable reference source is the *Handbook of Modern Pharmaceutical Analysis* by Ahuja and Scypinski (2).

## TECHNIQUES FOR THE STUDY OF CHEMICAL COMPATIBILITY

In any study of formulation stability, the most important information to be developed concerns the chemical compatibility of the drug substance and the excipients in the formulation. Although the safety profile of the active pharmaceutical ingredient (API) will be established long before the preformulation work begins, and knowledge will even be available regarding the safety profiles of known process impurities and degradants, one must be prepared for the possibility that a drug–excipient reaction might produce a new impurity or degradant of unknown character. Clearly, the best formulation will be one where such reactions do not occur, but one must still develop appropriate methodologies to prove that undesirable reactions do not take place. Equally clear is the need for analytical methodology that is oriented toward the detection and quantification of impurity species (3,4).

The range of analytical methodology suitable for the evaluation of chemical compatibility between a drug substance and proposed excipients is extremely large, and methods can range from the relatively simple to the extremely complex. The most frequently used methods for obtaining chemical composition information in the preformulation stage of development are based on various types of separation science, such as thin-layer chromatography (TLC) or high-pressure liquid chromatography (LC), with the occasional use of gas chromatography. The latter two methods are often coupled with mass spectrometry (MS) when the identity of degradant species is required.

Although chromatographic methods usually dominate investigations of chemical compatibility, applications for ultraviolet (UV)/visible (VIS) or near-infrared (IR) diffuse reflectance spectroscopy, vibrational spectroscopy (either Raman or IR absorption), or nuclear magnetic resonance can be valuable under appropriate circumstances. Since most preformulation scientists will exclusively use chromatographic methods in their work, only such methodologies will be discussed in this section.

## Fundamentals of Separation Science

While detailed expositions of the science underlying chromatographic separations are available (5), a brief outline of the fundamentals is appropriate here. The equilibration of substance-A between phases 1 and 2 is defined by its "partition coefficient," $P_A$:

$$P_A = C_{1A}/C_{2A} \tag{1}$$

where $C_{1A}$ and $C_{2A}$ are the respective concentrations of substance-A in the two phases. To separate substance-A from substance-B, the partition coefficients of the two solutes should be as different as possible.

The "separation factor," $\alpha$, is defined as the ratio of the partition coefficients:

$$\alpha = P_A/P_B \tag{2}$$

Eq. 2 may also be defined in concentration units:

$$\alpha = \frac{C_{1A} \cdot C_{2B}}{C_{2A} \cdot C_{1B}} \tag{3}$$

An efficient separation can be obtained when $\alpha$ is either much larger or much smaller than unity, and is most effective when $P_A$ is approximately equal to $1/P_B$. The practice of chromatography may be viewed as a continuous sequence of an equilibrium of solutes between phases, although theoretical treatments of the phenomena make use of the theoretical plate concept that originates in fractional distillation theory.

Chromatography is often considered as being a "countercurrent extraction" method, where the phases involved are continuously replenished with fresh solvent. This can be visualized as a situation where the sample is stationary while both phases move by it in opposite directions. This is obviously not convenient, so in practice, one phase is fixed in place (the "stationary phase") while the other phase (the "mobile phase") moves over the first phase. In this arrangement, the sample will move as well, but it will travel at a much slower rate than does the mobile phase, since the affinity of the solutes for the stationary phase will retard their motion.

Chromatographic systems therefore consist of a mobile phase passing over a stationary phase, and the sample is injected in a as small and compact a form as possible at or near the point where contact is first made between the two phases. As the experiment proceeds, the sample will move with reference to the stationary phase, and its zone will broaden over time.

If substance-A travels a distance of $X_A$, and if substance-B travels a distance of $X_B$, then it can be shown that

$$W_A / W_B = \{X_A / X_B\}^{1/2} \tag{4}$$

where $W_A$ and $W_B$ are the respective peak widths for substance-A and substance-B when measured at the base of the peaks. The consequences of Eq. 4 are that the separation between the peaks corresponding to two substances increases in proportion to the distance traveled, while the width of the peak increases only as the square root of the distance. In principle, one could therefore achieve any desired degree of separation simply by increasing the length of the stationary phase, but practical considerations would necessarily limit this approach.

Chromatographic separation is based on the repeated transfer of solute molecules between the mobile and stationary phases. Any given solute molecule will spend part of its time attached to the stationary phase, and the other part of its time moving along with the mobile phase, so that the relative magnitudes of these time events determine how quickly the solute moves through the system.

The various factors that contribute to the efficiency of a separation are frequently treated through the use of a "theoretical plate" concept. This quantity is defined as the length of stationary phase that will yield an effluent that is in a condition of equilibrium with the solute over that length of stationary phase. To achieve a high degree of separation, a large number of theoretical plates is desirable, and for a stationary phase of practical length, this means that the height equivalent to a theoretical plate must be as short as possible. If $H$ is the height equivalent to a theoretical plate over the distance $X$, then the number of theoretical plates ($N_X$) existing within the distance $X$ along the stationary phase equals

$$N_X = X/H \tag{5}$$

or:

$$N_X = 16\{X/H\}^2 \tag{6}$$

where $W$ is the width of the peak. For a chromatographic column having a length equal to $L$, the height equivalent to a theoretical plate is given by

$$H = L/N_X \tag{7}$$

or:

$$H = LW^2/16X^2 \tag{8}$$

In actual practice, one does not actually measure the distances for which solutes travel, but instead one measures the time elapsed between the injection of a sample onto the column and the time at which the peak corresponding to that sample is observed. This quantity is known as the "retention time" of the solute. A typical practice is to divide the retention times of analytes by the retention time of a suitable reference, quantities that are known as "relative retention times." The degree of separation between adjacent peaks is known as "resolution," and is defined by

$$R = \frac{X_A - X_B}{(0.5)(W_A + W_B)} \tag{9}$$

The resolution between two peaks has been shown to be proportional to the square root of the number of theoretical plates. A good chromatographic separation is one for which the resolution, as calculated by Eq. 9, exceeds unity.

Additional references that expound on the fundamentals of separation science are available in Refs. (6–12).

## Thin-Layer Chromatography

TLC was once one of the most important and valuable techniques available to the analytical scientist (13), but its use has gone somewhat out of vogue owing to the development of newer instrumental methods. Nevertheless, TLC still can play an important role in preformulation characterization studies and has undergone a steady evolution in technology and capability over the years (14–19). Although other separation methods are more widely used, TLC still possesses the powerful advantage that whatever is introduced into the system is ultimately detected, and hence its use permits visualization and quantitation of all separated species in an analyzed mixture.

Performance of a TLC analysis can be broken down into five main steps, which can be identified as preparation of the stationary phase, preparation of the mobile phase, application of the sample, development of the plate through elution with the solvent system, and visualization of the final chromatogram.

The stationary phase is typically a rigid plate, onto which is coated a material capable of interaction with the analyte through adsorption. At one time, practitioners of the art prepared their own TLC plates by spreading a slurry of the adsorbent onto rectangular glass plates, but now one typically obtains commercially prepared plates that have already been coated with the stationary phase. The most common stationary phase is silica gel ($SiO_2 \cdot xH_2O$), where the pore size, surface area, and surface pH will be determined by details of the substance preparation. Silica gel is weakly acidic, and therefore interacts most strongly with basic solutes. Alumina ($Al_2O_3 \cdot xH_2O$) is the other most commonly used adsorbent, and is slightly basic. Strongly acidic analytes will interact strongly with alumina, but the stationary phase appears to contain other additional sites of different chemical character, which provide an ability to interact with unsaturated compounds as well. Plates are often activated through heating, which modifies the water content and the adsorption capability.

In TLC, the solvent system will compete with the analytes for active adsorption onto the stationary phase, and hence the ability of a solvent to interact with a given stationary phase is independent of the presence of analytes. The consequence of this is that the elution of analytes during a TLC analysis is a displacement of the analytes from the adsorbent rather than a partitioning of the analytes between the mobile phase and the stationary phase. Elutropic series have been developed for various stationary phases, where solvents are listed by the relative abilities to displace solutes from the adsorbent. An example of an elutropic series is shown in Table 1, where data for alumina were derived from the literature [Ref. (5), p. 385].

In general, the greater the strength of the solvent, the more rapidly will analytes be eluted. To develop a TLC method of analysis, the analyst will typically attempt separations with a variety of pure or mixed solvents in an effort to determine the proper composition that completely separates all of the analytes of interest in an appropriate amount of time.

The application of a dissolved sample onto the plate is performed simply by placing an aliquot using a capillary tube or micropipette. The use

**Table 1**  Elutropic Series for Alumina

| Solvent | Eluent strength |
|---|---|
| n-Pentane | 0.00 |
| Cyclohexane | 0.04 |
| Carbon disulfide | 0.15 |
| Diisopropyl ether | 0.28 |
| Toluene | 0.29 |
| Diethyl ether | 0.38 |
| Methylene chloride | 0.42 |
| Acetone | 0.56 |
| Dioxane | 0.56 |
| Tetrahydrofuran | 0.57 |
| Ethyl acetate | 0.58 |
| Acetonitrile | 0.65 |
| Pyridine | 0.71 |
| Dimethyl sulfoxide | 0.75 |
| Isopropanol | 0.82 |
| Ethanol | 0.88 |
| Methanol | 0.95 |

Source: From Ref. 12.

of a micropipette to spot the sample is superior, as its use facilitates semi-quantitative control of the sample size. Typically, one places a spot of sample solution near the bottom of the place, and then the plate is placed in a pool of solvent in a closed chamber. The elution and separation process is facilitated when the liquid of the solvent system slowly creeps up the plate due to capillary action, thus performing an ascending chromatographic separation. When the solvent front nears the top of the plate, the plate is removed from the solvent and dried.

Visualization of the separated spots can be effected by placing the plate in a warm chamber containing molecular iodine crystals. The $I_2$ vapor is reversibly adsorbed on most substances, and its adsorption will create a dark spot wherever an analyte appears on the plate. An alternative viewing method is to use commercially available TLC plates that contain a fluorescent material whose emission is quenched by adsorbed solutes. After the plate is developed and the solvent evaporates, the plate is viewed under a UV (irradiation wavelength of either 254 or 365 nm) source. When viewed under these conditions, analyte spots will appear dark while the rest of the plate exhibits bright fluorescence.

The practice of TLC analysis can be demonstrated through the use of a practical example. A TLC method for the analysis of process impurities and degradants in nalmefene hydrochloride has been described, where the solvent system is 10:75:15 v/v/v cyclohexane:chloroform:diethylamine, and the separation is effected on silica gel $GC_{254}$ (20). The analyte solution was prepared by dissolving 10 mg of drug substance in 10 mL of methanol, and then 10 μL of this solution was spotted on the plate. The plate was allowed to develop to a height of approximately 12 cm and then dried. As illustrated in Figure 1, the relative retention time (Rf) for nalmefene was 0.41, the Rf for naltrexone (a process impurity) was 0.28, and the Rf for *bis*-nalmefene (a degradant) was 0.07.

The amount of material in each spot was visualized using short-wave UV (254 nm) irradiation, and quantitated by densitometry.

The possible acetylation of acetaminophen by acetylsalicylic acid in solid dosage forms was studied by using TLC to monitor any formation of the *O, N*-diacetyl-*p*-aminophenol degradant (21). Using silica gel $GC_{254}$ as the stationary phase, plates were developed using either 80:18:2 v/v/v chloroform:acetone:acetic acid or 88:10:2 chloroform:ethanol:acetic acid as the solvent systems, with the products being visualized by irradiation of the plate at 254 nm. While the postulated acetylation product was not detected in the formulations, it was determined that the stability of preparations containing acetaminophen decreased rapidly with increasing moisture content and temperature.

The impurity profiles of meperidine in various formulations has been studied using TLC analysis, where the separations were conducted using filter paper as the stationary phase and a rather complicated solvent system

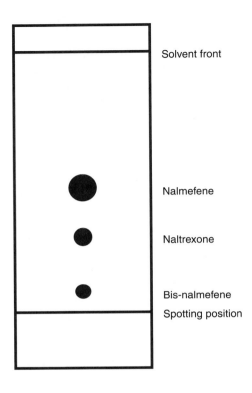

Solvent front

Nalmefene

Naltrexone

Bis-nalmefene

Spotting position

**Figure 1** Thin-layer chromatogram of nalmefene hydrochloride, illustrating the position where the sample was spotted, the spot corresponding to *bis*-nalmefene (Rf = 0.07), naltrexone (Rf = 0.28), nalmefene (Rf = 0.41), and the solvent front. *Source*: From Ref. 20.

consisting of 50:50:20:10:1:1 v/v/v/v/v/v ethyl acetate:cyclohexane:methanol:dioxane water:concentrated ammonium hydroxide (22). An extraction procedure was developed to dissolve the drug substance from powdered tablets so that the solubilized components could be spotted on the stationary phase. The developed sheets were sprayed with a dilute potassium iodobismuthate solution, which enabled visualization of the analytes upon irradiation with UV light having a wavelength of 254 nm.

TLC can be used as a separation method to obtain impurities from dosage forms in a state suitable for further analysis. For example, impurity species developed in solid dosage forms of fusidic acid were first separated on silica gel plates using 160:20:20:5 v/v/v/v chloroform:acetic acid:cyclohexane:methanol, and then the spots were scraped off (23). The analytes contained in the scrapings were eluted off the silica gel with ethanol and subsequently quantitated using a spectrophotometric method. The method proved to be sufficiently rugged that it could be used in a routine control of sodium fusidate in dosage forms.

A vast improvement in planar chromatography came about with the introduction of commercially available plates that were layered with fine and uniform stationary phase particles, coupled with the increased use of instrumental densitometry methods for the quantitation of analyte spots. The modern practice of TLC is now distinguished as high-performance TLC (HPTLC), and one can use the methodology to achieve accuracy and precision performance parameters that rival those achievable with other chromatographic methods.

Nifedipine has been determined in its tablet and capsule dosage forms using an HPTLC method based on the use of silica gel $60_{F254}$ as the stationary phase and 19:2:2 v/v/v chloroform:ethyl acetate:cyclohexane as the mobile phase (24). Tablets were crushed, the contents extracted with methanol, and then streaked onto the plate. Quantitation of the bands on the developed plate was effected using densitometric analysis, and precision values exceeding 99% were obtained. In a similar study, HPTLC was used to determine trimetazidine in formulations after being spotted on a silica gel plate and eluted with 70:1:1:10 v/v/v/v *n*-butanol:water:methanol:20% aqueous ammonium hydroxide (25). In this latter study, the limit of detection was found to be 50 ng on the plate.

HPTLC analysis has been shown to be capable of separating the components of multicomponent tablets. For example, using a mobile phase consisting of 88:13:1 v/v/v methylene chloride:methanol:25% aqueous ammonium hydroxide and silica gel $60_{F254}$ plates, the composition of atenolol–amlodipine combination tablets was established (26).

Gorman and Jiang have summarized the advantages of TLC analysis, and why one would want to make use of the methodology (27). The reasons can be summarized as open format of stationary phase and evaluation of the whole sample, simple sample preparation, high sample throughput, flexible and versatile dissolving solvent and mobile phase, general and specific detection methods, and one-dimensional multiple development and two-dimensional development.

## High-Performance Liquid Chromatography

As discussed above, the theoretical place height of a chromatography column decreases as the size of the particles making up the stationary phase decreases, and hence one can achieve high-resolution conditions by using particles whose size is less than 10 μm. However, such columns offer a considerable degree of resistance to the mobile phase, and consequently one must use high pressures in the range of 7 to 35 MPa (or 70–350 atm) to achieve reasonable flow rates in the range of 0.5 to 5.0 mL/min. However, these instrumental problems have been entirely overcome, and as a result, most studies of chemical composition in preformulation studies make use of high-performance LC (HPLC).

HPLC methodology is unique in that the analytical separation step is coupled with on-line analysis instrumentation that senses all analytes as they elute out of the chromatographic system (28). The science underlying HPLC separation methods and associated methods of detection is highly developed, and the literature published on the subject is exceedingly large. A number of books on the general methodology of HPLC analysis are available (29–35), as are books devoted to the development of HPLC analysis methods (36,37). More specialized monographs have been published that cover stationary phases (38–40), mobile phases (41,42), and detection technology (43,44). In addition to these sources, compilations of stability-indicating methods for drug substances are even available (45,46).

Figure 2 shows a block diagram for a typical HPLC system.

The bulk mobile phase is contained in a reservoir, and is pulled at a steady rate through a prefilter or precolumn by the solvent pump. The sample is injected into the flowing mobile phase stream, immediately passed through a column containing the stationary phase, and finally passed through a flow cell whose design facilitates detection of the analytes. The flow cell is an integral part of the detector, where most often, a spectroscopic technique is used to detect analytes in the mobile phase stream. The effluent from the detector is passed into a waste container, while the output from the

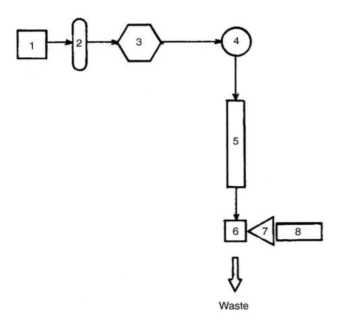

Waste

**Figure 2**  Block diagram of a typical high-performance liquid chromatography system, illustrating the relative placement of the (*1*) mobile phase reservoir, (*2*) prefilter or precolumn, (*3*) solvent pump, (*4*) sample injector, (*5*) column containing stationary phase, (*6*) flow cell, (*7*) detection system, and (*8*) electronic entry into the data acquisition system.

detection system is usually digitized to facilitate electronic entry into a data acquisition system.

The most commonly encountered form of HPLC uses microporous silica particles that have been overcoated with a covalently bonded stationary phase (47). The particles are typically $5\,\mu m$ in diameter, and contain an extensive pore system that provides a large degree of surface area to the mobile phase. Since the surface of silica particles is composed of acidic silanols and siloxane bridges, one may prepare the bonded phase by covalently reacting the surface of the particles with an alkoxysilane:

$$(\text{particle}) - \text{Si} - \text{OH} + (CH_3CH_2O)_3\text{Si} - \mathbf{R} \rightarrow (\text{particle}) - \text{Si} - \text{O}$$
$$- \text{Si}(\mathbf{R})(CH_3CH_2O) + CH_3CH_2OH \tag{10}$$

The surfaces of the particles making up the resulting stationary phase can be polar in nature if the $\mathbf{R}$ group is $-CH_2-CH_2-CH_2-NH_2$ (typically known as an amino phase) or $-CH_2-CH_2-CH_2-CN$ (typically known as a cyano phase). Alternatively, the particles can be nonpolar if the $\mathbf{R}$ group is $-(-CH_2-)_7-CH_3$ (typically known as a $C_8$ phase), $-(-CH_2-)_{17}-CH_3$ (typically known as a $C_{18}$ phase), or $-CH_2-CH_2-C_6H_5$ (typically known as a phenyl phase). The latter hydrocarbon bonded phases are used in "reversed-phase" chromatography, which is probably the most widespread type of HPLC analysis.

While the majority of HPLC methods will make use of silica-based packings, the use of polymer particles represents a viable alternative. Examples of such stationary phases include those made by the polymerization of divinylbenzene or styrene-divinylbenzene, or the polymers prepared from a methacrylate and an appropriate cross-linking agent. The advantage of polymeric stationary phases is that they tend not to be affected by mobile phases having extreme pH values, whereas such mobile phases can degrade silica-based stationary phases.

Most compounds of pharmaceutical interest are relatively nonpolar in character, and as such are eminently suited for separation using reversed-phase HPLC analysis. The mobile phases typically used in this mode are relatively polar, but the solubility of analytes does not generally present an issue, as the concentrations used in the analysis are quite low. As discussed above, HPLC is effectively a continuous partitioning of the analytes between the polar mobile phase and the nonpolar stationary phase, so that the retention time of the analytes is critically dependent on the nature of their interaction with the column packing. In general, the order of elution of analytes in a reversed-phase HPLC analysis is from the most hydrophilic down to the most hydrophobic.

Mobile phases will typically be a mixture of organic solvents and water, with the latter often containing a buffering agent. Scales of mobile phase strength have been proposed that enable investigators to provide rough guides to the separation efficiency of different systems (48). For example, the mobile phase strength of a 50% acetonitrile–water mobile phase is predicted to be approximately equal to that of a 60% methanol–water mobile phase. Owing to its low absorptivity in the 185 to 220 nm region, which permits ready measurement of the absorbance of analytes, sacetonitrile is probably the solvent of choice for reversed-phase HPLC work. For systems where acetonitrile-based mobile phases fail to provide adequate performance, methanol-based solvent systems would constitute the next choice.

When the degree of hydrophobicity of all of the analytes is roughly similar, the species may be separated using a mobile phase having a constant composition to effect the separation. Such procedures are known as "isocratic" HPLC methods and represent the simplest type of analysis method. However, when the analytes differ significantly in their degree of hydrophobicity, the strength of the mobile phase might have to be continually increased during the analysis to ensure that all species eventually elute off the column. These latter methods are known as gradient methods, and their use requires a more sophisticated type of solvent pump capable of real-time mixing of multiple types of solvents.

Once the separation of analytes has been accomplished, detection and quantitation of the various species as they pass through the flow cell is required. The most common method of detection is based on the inherent UV absorption of the analytes, but detectors based on measurement of refractive index, fluorescence, electrical conductivity, or light scattering have also been used. UV detection can be used for any analyte possessing a chromophore, but for molecules that lack this functionality, one might have to derivatize the analytes prior to their injection onto the column (49).

An isocratic, stability-indicating HPLC method has been used to determine the impurity profile of nalmefene hydrochloride bulk drug substance, as well as the impurity profiles in drug products (20). The separation was effected using a $C_{18}$ column, and a mobile phase consisting of 20:80 v/v acetonitrile:0.05 M phosphate buffer (pH = 4.2). Using a mobile phase flow rate of 1.0 mL/min, analytes were detected on the basis of their UV absorption at 210 nm. As depicted in Figure 3, excellent separation of nalmefene was obtained from its process impurities (naltrexone and $\Delta^7$-nalmefene) and the sole degradant (*bis*-nalmefene).

The well-known Maillard reaction between amines and lactose has been studied using fluoxetine hydrochloride as the drug substance, with the compatibility between the drug substance and a variety of lactose materials being evaluated using HPLC analysis (50). The method was based on the use of a $C_8$ column, and gradient elution using solvent-A as 0.07% v/v trifluoroacetic acid in water and solvent-B as 0.07% v/v trifluoroacetic acid in acetonitrile. The elution program began with a mobile phase consisting of

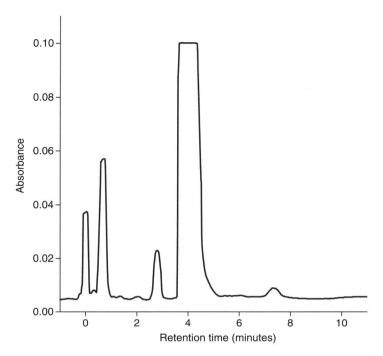

**Figure 3**  High-performance liquid chromatogram of nalmefene hydrochloride, illustrating the peak due to the solvent front (time = 0.0 minutes), and the peaks corresponding to naltrexone (time = 0.7 minutes), $\Delta^7$-nalmefene (time = 2.8 minutes), nalmefene (time = 4.0 minutes), and *bis*-nalmefene (time = 7.0 minutes). *Source*: From Ref. 20.

80:20 solvent-A:solvent-B that was eluted for five minutes, followed by a linear ramping to 15:85 solvent-A:solvent-B over a 30-minute period, isocratically held at 15:85 solvent-A:solvent-B for five minutes, and then returned to the initial 80:20 solvent-A:solvent-B mobile phase after another five minutes. It was reported that this method enabled the detection and quantitation of impurities that were not eluted using the isocratic method described in the *United States Pharmacopoeia* (USP).

It has been found that the potency of hydralazine hydrochloride that has been formulated in tablets containing starch decreases over time (51). An isocratic method was developed to study the degree of degradation and to identify the degradants resulting from the reaction between the drug substance and starch excipients. Tablet contents were extracted from the ground powder using 150:850 v/v acetonitrile:5 mM $C_8H_{17}SO_3Na$, and separated on a $C_{18}$ column using a mobile phase consisting of 150:850:0.45 v/v/v acetonitrile:5 mM $C_8H_{17}SO_3Na$:phosphoric acid. All eluted compounds were detected on the basis of their UV absorbance at 220 nm.

The utility of HPLC analysis in a program of preformulation testing was demonstrated for a number of compounds, including fosinopril sodium, ceronapril, pravastatin sodium, sorivudine, and ifetroban sodium (52). In this work, a general program for drug–excipient testing was outlined, where multicomponent blends were prepared with 20% added water, and then isothermally stressed at 50°C for various periods of time prior to analysis. To cut down on the number of prepared samples, a statistical design was developed where the studies were conducted in two phases. In the first phase, the compatibility of the drug substance with various diluents and lubricants was determined, with the results being used to select one primary diluent and one primary lubricant. The second phase of the program consisted of testing one drug–diluent–lubricant mixture with other excipients, such as binders and disintegrants, to complete the scope of materials that could be used in formulations.

A reversed-phase method for the determination of nicotine in immediate- and extended-release formulations has been reported that also was used in the analysis of drug–excipient compatibility samples (53). Elution of the analytes on a $C_{18}$ column was effected using a mobile phase consisting of 65:35 v/v methanol:phosphate buffer (5 mM, pH 6.8), and detection was made on the basis of the UV absorbance at 259 nm. The compatibility samples were prepared by mixing 1:1 w/w ratios of nicotine and various excipients in glass vials, adding sufficient water to achieve a 5% w/w level, and then storing at 40°C and 75% relative humidity for three weeks. Control samples were prepared to have identical compositions, but were stored at 4°C in a refrigerator. At the end of the storage period, the samples were dissolved in methanol, diluted with phosphate buffer, filtered, and analyzed by the HPLC method.

A relatively simple HPLC method consisting of separation on $C_{18}$ column, a mobile phase consisting of 80:20 v/v water:methanol and at 220 nm was used to study the compatibility between isosorbide mononitrate and extended-release excipients (54). In this work, samples were mixed in glass vials at ratios comparable to those anticipated in the actual formulations, water equivalent to 10% w/w was added, and then the samples were isothermally stressed at 50°C. At the end of the storage period, the samples were dissolved in the mobile phase prior to analysis by the HPLC method, and their composition was compared to analogous reference samples stored in a refrigerator to which no water had been added.

The compatibility between glucosamine, chondroitin sulfate, and formulation excipients was demonstrated using an HPLC system based on an amino column and elution with 75:25 v/v acetonitrile:phosphate buffer (20 mM, pH 7.5) (55). The glucosamine analyte presented analytical difficulties as it did not possess any chromophores, and it could only be detected on the basis of its UV end-absorption around 200 nm. This limited the mobile phase composition to aqueous phosphate buffer and acetonitrile combinations, as other solvents possessed too much inherent absorption at the analysis wavelength. Glucosamine was only weakly retained on $C_{18}$, $C_8$, or phenyl columns in the absence of ion-pairing reagents, and while cyano, diol, strong cation exchange, and porous graphitic carbon columns showed potential, only use of the amino stationary phase proved to be acceptable.

As will be discussed in a subsequent section, many drug–excipient compatibility studies use differential scanning calorimetry (DSC) to evaluate possible interactions between drug substances and excipients, and a number of studies have used DSC in conjunction with HPLC to acquire a more complete picture of the compatibility landscape. Drug–excipient compatibility investigations along these lines have been reported for niclosamide (56), albendazole and closantel (57), acetylsalicylic acid (58), and glipizide (59). In many instances, the suggestion of a particular drug–excipient interaction deduced from DSC studies could not be confirmed using the HPLC method.

It is to be recognized that the conduct of a drug–excipient compatibility study will generate large numbers of samples and a considerable degree of analytical testing. One of the ways to deal with the workload is to automate the process as much as possible, and a system for automated chemical analysis has been integrated into the automated determinations of drug substance solubilities, ionization constants, and partition coefficients (60). The HPLC system was built around a liquid-handling robot equipped with a dilution system, and multiple solvent pumps and injector valves. A $C_{18}$ column was used to effect the analytical separations, where the mobile phase was a linear gradient beginning with 20:80:0.05 v/v/v acetonitrile: water:trifluoroacetic acid and ending with 90:10:0.05 v/v/v acetonitrile: water:trifluoroacetic acid. Chemical stability was evaluated at pH values of 2, 7, and 12, and in 3% hydrogen peroxide, and the system was described as being able to screen approximately 100 compounds/wk.

## MS (Coupled with HPLC)

In the majority of preformulation studies, one merely seeks to establish the existence or absence of drug–excipient interactions. Typically, when an interaction is observed between a drug substance and an excipient of interest, the formulation scientist will simply eliminate that excipient from further consideration as a formulation ingredient.

However, instances can arise when one needs to learn the identity of a particular drug–excipient interaction product, which requires that one combine the separation step with an identification step rather than a quantitation step (61). Since the first HPLC methods are usually developed during the preformulation stage of development, the combination of this technology with MS probably represents the ideal combination of technologies for the detection and identification of drug–excipient interaction products (62).

In usual practice, one must vaporize the analytes, convert these into charged species, allow the ions to undergo fragmentation, and finally separate and detect the ion fragments on the basis of their mass-to-charge ($m/e$) ratio. Instrumentation that enables these steps to be performed will typically consist of an inlet system that facilitates the transfer of analytes into the vapor phase, a source that serves to ionize the analytes and retain the ions so that they may undergo fragmentation, a system that separates the ions according to the $m/e$ ratio, and a detection method. One of the more valuable sources of information regarding the technology associated with MS analysis is available in the four volumes of the *Encyclopedia of Mass Spectrometry* (63–66).

The coupling of HPLC technology to that of MS is accompanied by a number of requirements (67). The key element in developing an HPLC-MS method is that all components must be volatile and capable of carrying the analytes into the vapor phase. This limits the composition of mobile phases to include volatile solvents and buffering agents that can be vaporized (such as ammonium acetate). As would be imagined, it is vitally important to eliminate the solvent from a nebulized spray in order to achieve the high-vacuum conditions necessary for MS analysis, and this has been achieved using electrospray, thermospray, ion spray, or laser desorption interfaces. When the analytes have been appropriately processed, they are eventually detected and quantitated using conventional instrumentation (68). More information on the instrumentation and conduct of LC/MS analysis is available in specialized reference texts (69–72).

As an example of the structure elucidation power of MS, the $m/e$ values for the six most intense peaks observed in the electron-impact mass spectrum of nalmefene hydrochloride are shown in Figure 4 along with the proposed structures of the molecular fragments (20).

The $m/e$ value of the molecular ion confirms the formula weight of the compound, while the structures of the various fragments are consistent with the structure of the compound.

The oxidative degradants formed by the tromethamine salt of a 5,6,7,8-tetrahydro-1,8-naphthyridine derivative and mannitol were identified by HPLC and MS analysis (73). For on-line LC/MS and LC/MS/MS analyses of stressed formulations, samples were eluted on a $C_{18}$ column using a gradient profile where the initial mobile phase consisted of 10% v/v 0.1% aqueous trifluoroacetic acid, and which was ramped up to 90% v/v aqueous acetonitrile. It was found that the thermal stressing of the trial formulations led to the formation of two isomeric condensation products between the drug substance and mannitol, although the degree of degradant formation was not extensive at lower temperatures.

Seven degradation products arising from the reaction of pregabalin with lactose via the Maillard reaction and Amadori rearrangement in formulated products have been isolated using LC, and the structures of the

m/e Ratio          Structure of Ion

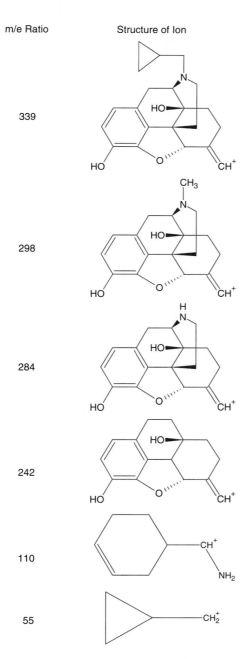

339

298

284

242

110

55

**Figure 4** Structures of the molecular fragments observed in the electron-impact mass spectrum of nalmefene hydrochloride. *Source*: From Ref. 20.

degradants determined using MS (74). Samples were introduced in the system and ionized using the electrospray mode, and it was found that the conjugates contained pregabalin in its lactam form. The identity of the structures was confirmed using nuclear magnetic resonance, demonstrating the strong appeal of multidisciplinary studies.

## TECHNIQUES FOR THE STUDY OF PHYSICAL COMPATIBILITY

Although it is always possible to detect a new chemical reaction of the drug substance under study with one or more excipients in a proposed formulation, more often than not, drug–excipient interactions are manifested in a change of one of the physical properties. When the study of physical interactions between drug substances and excipients is neglected, one often detects the first signs of incompatibility when the dissolution profile of the API in the formulation begins to change. However, one should be able to determine the existence of possible interactions that would affect formulation performance through the conduct of appropriately designed studies.

As might be anticipated, the range of physical characterization methodology is large, and appropriate technology can be differentiated on the basis of the desired scale of scrutiny (75,76). Physical properties can be classified as being associated with the molecular level (those associated with individual molecules), the particulate level (those pertaining to individual solid particles), or the bulk level (those associated with an assembly of particulate species). The properties of most interest to the preformulation scientist will generally be crystallography (studied by X-ray diffraction methods), thermally induced phase transitions [studied by DSC and thermogravimetry (TG)], color (studied by UV/VIS diffuse reflectance), and molecular motion of functional groups (studied by vibrational spectroscopy).

### X-Ray Powder Diffraction

The technique of X-ray powder diffraction (XRPD) is of the highest importance to the preformulation scientist since it represents the method that enables one to determine whether changes in the crystalline form of a drug substance have taken place as a result of excipient interactions. The technique is based on the diffraction of X-rays by crystals, where the atoms in a solid act as scattering centers arranged in a plane so that constructive interference occurs for the direction of specular reflection (77–83). Within a given family of planes, defined by a Miller index of $(h\ k\ l)$ and each plane being separated by the distance $d$, each plane produces a specular reflectance of the incident beam. If the incident X-rays are monochromatic (having wavelength equal to $\lambda$), then for an arbitrary glancing angle of $\theta$, the reflections from successive planes are out of phase with one another. This yields destructive interference in the scattered beams. However, by varying $\theta$, a set of values for $\theta$ can be found so that the path difference between X-rays reflected by successive planes will be an integral number ($n$) of wavelengths, and then constructive interference will occurs. These relationships are summarized in the expression known as Bragg's law:

$$2d \, \sin\theta = n\lambda \tag{11}$$

Unlike the case of diffraction of light by a ruled grating, the diffraction of X-rays by a crystalline solid leads to observation of constructive interference (i.e., reflection) occurs only the critical Bragg angles. When reflection does occur, it is stated that the plane in question is reflecting in the $n$th order, or that one observes $n$th order diffraction for that particular crystal plane. Therefore one will observe an X-ray scattering response for every plane defined by a unique Miller index of ($h \, k \, l$).

While single crystal X-ray diffraction is the most powerful technique available for the study of crystalline solids, this methodology is suitable for the routine evaluation of the crystalline state of powdered solids. Such work falls exactly within the scope of preformulation studies, and hence XRPD becomes the most useful crystallographic technique (84,85). Since a powdered sample will present all possible crystal faces at a given interface, and the diffraction off this powdered surface will therefore provide information on all possible atomic spacings (i.e., defined by the crystal lattice). The powder pattern will therefore consist of a series of peaks having varying intensities that are detected at various scattering angles. These angles, and their relative intensities, are correlated with computed $d$-spacings to provide a full crystallographic characterization of the powdered sample (86,87).

To measure a powder pattern, a randomly oriented powdered sample is prepared so as to expose all the planes of a sample. The scattering angle is determined by slowly rotating the sample and measuring the angle of diffracted X-rays (typically using a scintillation detector) with respect to the angle of the incident beam. Alternatively, the angle between sample and source can be kept fixed, while moving the detector to determine the angles of the scattered radiation. Knowing the wavelength of the incident beam, the spacing between the planes (identified as the $d$-spacings) is calculated using Bragg's Law.

The main drawbacks associated with the use of XRPD as a routine method of analysis are that the accuracy of the results depends critically on the quality of the sample preparation procedure, and that the measurement simply takes time to run. As a result, many screenings of drug–excipient interactions are made using other methods, and then XRPD is brought in to confirm or disprove the findings. For example, thermal analysis studies indicated a number of possible interactions between sulfamerazine polymorphs and various excipients in stressed samples, while XRPD analysis demonstrated that the crystal structures of the drug substance and the excipients remained unchanged in either physical mixtures or in compressed tablets (88).

To illustrate the utility of XRPD analysis in drug–excipient studies, famotidine Form-A and Form-B were blended with microcrystalline cellulose in a 28:72 w/w ratio. The two samples were then spiked with 5% water, isothermally heated in sealed vials at 50°C for 12 hours, and then allowed to air-dry. It had been previously established that for pure bulk drug substance subjected to this procedure, no change in the polymorphic composition took place for either form. As seen in the XRPD patterns of Figure 5 [Brittain HG. Unpublished results obtained using a Rigaku MiniFlex powder diffraction system, equipped with a horizontal goniometer in the $\theta/2\theta$ mode. The X-ray source was nickel-filtered $K\alpha$ emission of copper (1.54184 Å).

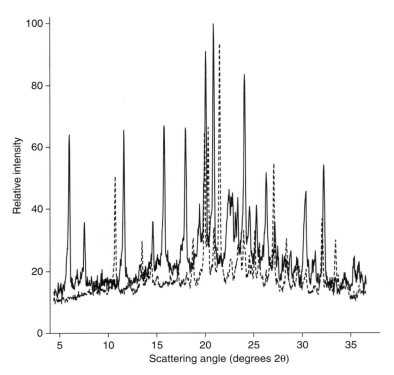

**Figure 5**  X-ray powder diffraction pattern of a 28:72 w/w mixture of famotidine form-B and microcrystalline cellulose, after isothermal stressing of a sample spiked with 5% water (*solid trace*), and the X-ray powder diffraction pattern of a similarly stressed 28:72 w/w mixture of famotidine form-A and microcrystalline cellulose (*dashed trace*).

Samples were packed into a zero-background sample holder using a back-fill procedure, and were scanned over the range of 4° to 50° $2\theta$, at a scan rate of 0.5° $2\theta$/min, and a step size of 0.0084° $2\theta$], while no polymorphic change was observed in the form-A sample, a significant amount of the famotidine form-B in its sample had converted to form-A.

This finding indicates that microcrystalline cellulose can facilitate the phase transformation of form-B to form-A. Were one seeking to develop a formulation with famotidine form-B, one would necessarily avoid the use of microcrystalline cellulose in the formulation.

During the course of a formulation optimization project, the crystalline state of the drug substance 3,9-*bis*(*N*, *N*-dimethylcarbamoy-loxy)-5*H*-benzo-fural[3,2-*c*]quinoline-6-one was determined by XRPD after it had been dispersed in hydroxypropylcellulose or poly(vinylpyrrolidone) (PVP) (89). In the formulations, the polymers appeared to inhibit the crystallization of the drug substance in a new polymorph described in the work, and instead appeared to convert the drug substance into an amorphous form that was formed during preparation of the solid dispersions. This stabilization of the amorphous form yielded a dissolution enhancement that was more pronounced for hydro-xypropylcellulose than for PVP.

A study was undertaken to determine if excipients could be used to retard the formation of the monohydrate phase of theophylline during the wet granulation of the anhydrate (90). Since the XRPD of both solvatomorphs of the drug substance were substantially different from each other and from the excipients, XRPD analysis was used to deduce the phase composition after the secondary processing had been completed. Granulations containing lactose monohydrate (which had minimal water sorption capability) not only prevented transformation to the hydrate, but instead promoted its formation. Even though silicified microcrystalline cellulose has appreciable water sorption properties, it was only able to prevent the phase transformation at water levels that would be insufficient to form granules.

The compatibility between diflunisal and polyethylene glycol 4000 was studied by using XRPD to examine the solid dispersions prepared by melting, solvent, and melting–solvent methods (91). It was found that polymorphic form-I of the drug substance was obtained at high concentrations of the drug substance in the polymer matrix, while at lower ratios, form-III was formed. Variable-temperature XRPD was found to be an extremely useful tool for the characterization of solid dispersions formed with erythromycin and poly-ethylene glycol 6000, where the API was observed to undergo multiple phase transformations during hot-melt processing (92).

## Thermal Methods of Analysis

Historically, the techniques of differential thermal analysis (DTA), DSC, and TG have played important roles in the study of drug–excipient interactions (93–96). Thermal methods of analysis are defined as those techniques in which a property of the analyte is determined as a function of an externally applied temperature (97). The sample temperature is increased in a linear fashion, while the property in question is evaluated on a continuous basis. Thermal analysis methods are normally used to monitor endothermic processes (melting, boiling, sublimation, vaporization, desolvation, solid–solid phase transitions, and chemical degradation) as well as exothermic processes (crystallization and oxidative decomposition). Access to this methodology is extremely useful during the conduct of preformulation studies, since carefully planned studies can be used to indicate the existence of possible drug–excipient interactions in a prototype formulation (98).

DTA was developed to provide an instrumental improvement over the performance of simple melting point determinations, where one monitored the difference in temperature between the sample and a reference as a function of applied temperature (99). As long as no thermally induced transitions were to take place, the temperature of the sample and reference would necessarily be the same since the two heat capacities would be effectively equivalent. When a transition takes place that requires a finite heat of reaction, a measurable difference in temperature between the sample and reference will develop. If the enthalpy change for the transition is positive (an endothermic reaction), the temperature of the sample will lag behind that of the reference since more heat will be absorbed by the sample than by the reference. If the enthalpy change is negative (an exothermic reaction), the temperature of the sample will exceed that of the reference (since the sample itself will be a source of additional heat). DTA analysis proved to be an excellent qualitative technique for the deduction of temperature ranges associated with thermally induced transitions, and it could also be used to assign the endothermic or exothermic nature of these reactions.

Once introduced, the technique of DSC completely replaced DTA analysis, and it has become the thermoanalytical method of choice. In the DSC method, the sample and reference are kept at the same temperature, and the heat flow necessary to maintain the equality in temperature between the two is measured. In power-compensation DSC, one places separate heating elements in the sample and reference cells, and then controls and measures the rate of heating by these elements. In heat-flux DSC, the sample and reference cells are heated by the same element, and one then monitors the direction and magnitude of the heat being transferred between the two. DSC thermograms are typically plotted as the differential rate of heating (in units of watts/sec, cal/sec, or J/sec) against temperature, and thus represent direct measures of the heat capacity of the sample. The area contained within a DSC peak is directly proportional to the heat absorbed or evolved by the thermal event, and integration of these peak areas yields the enthalpy of reaction (in units of cal/sec g or J/sec g). Additional information regarding DSC instrumentation is available in Refs. (93–101).

TG is another important method of thermal analysis, where one continually measures the thermally induced weight loss of a material as a function of the applied temperature (102). TG analysis is typically restricted to studies that involve the loss in mass during the process, and is therefore commonly used to study desolvation processes and compound decomposition. In preformulation work, the major use of TG analysis will be in the quantitative determination of the total volatile content of a solid. When a solid can decompose by means of several discrete, sequential reactions, the magnitude of each step can often be separately evaluated, and in suitable systems, one can deduce the existence of multiple solvatomorphs on the basis of patterns in the thermally induced weight loss.

To illustrate the utility of DSC analysis in drug–excipient studies, the samples of famotidine form-A and form-B that were used in the XRPD illustration of the preceding section were also analyzed by DSC. Pure form-B exhibits a lower endotherm maximum (166.2°C) and enthalpy of fusion (144.3 J/g) than does form-A (174.5°C and 149.3 J/g, respectively), and thus form-B is a metastable crystal form that bears a monotropic relationship to form-A. In addition, form-B does not undergo phase transformation to form-A during the conduct of a DSC scan, and therefore DSC analysis can be used as a reliable measure of phase composition. The partial conversion of form-B to form-A in the stressed binary mixture is evident in the DSC thermograms of Figure 6 (Brittain HG. Unpublished results obtained using a TA Instruments 2910 thermal analysis system. Samples of approximately 1–2 mg were accurately weighed into an aluminum DSC pan, and crimped with an aluminum lid. The samples were then heated at a rate of 10°C/min), and integration of the endothermic transitions indicated that only 21% of the initial form-B remained in the stressed sample.

The results of the DSC study provide additional evidence that microcrystalline cellulose facilitates the phase transformation of form-B to form-A in isothermally stressed samples.

During the course of a DSC study of the compatibility of sulfamethoxazole with carbohydrates, it was found that the drug substance could form a eutectic mixture with mannitol that contained 90.3% of the API (103). The establishment of the full phase diagram proved difficult, owing to the similarities in the melting points of the two components, but the system could be mapped since straight-line relationships were found to exist between the composition in the mixtures and the enthalpies so fusion for both the eutectic component and the excess mannitol.

The compatibility between pryidoxal hydrochloride and various excipients has been studied by the isothermal stressing of multicomponent mixtures and by DSC analysis of binary drug–excipient mixtures (104). Incompatibilities were noted between the drug substance and mannitol,

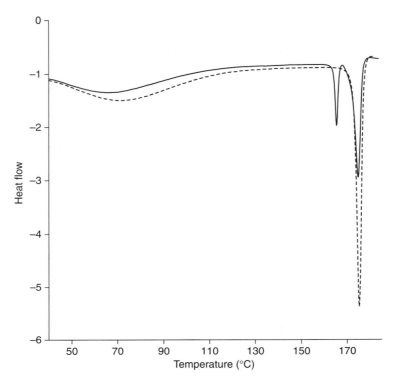

**Figure 6** Differential scanning calorimetry (DSC) thermogram of a 28:72 w/w mixture of famotidine form-B and microcrystalline cellulose, after isothermal stressing of a sample spiked with 5% water (*solid trace*), and the DSC thermogram of a similarly stressed 28:72 w/w mixture of famotidine form-A and microcrystalline cellulose (*dashed trace*).

lactose, and cornstarch, while microcrystalline cellulose, cellulose derivatives, and silicon dioxide were wont to induce a stabilizing effect. Of course, DSC analyses alone could not be used to deduce whether the incompatibilities originated from physical or chemical reactions, but DSC was deduced to be a useful adjunct method to the standard method of isothermal stress testing.

A combined DSC and TG approach was used to study the possible interactions between acetaminophen and various excipients in binary mixtures and in solid dosage forms, where thermodynamic data on drug substance melting and vaporization were determined for the pure API and in its mixtures (105). Compatibility between components was reported as long as a high ratio of drug substance to excipient was used, as evidenced by the additivity in the features attributed to various thermal events in the mixtures. However, interaction between acetaminophen and mannitol was noted for samples containing appreciable quantities of excipient.

Mura et al. have published the results of a number of investigations where DSC analysis was used as the primary tool for establishing the compatibility of various excipients with ketoprofen (106) and with picotamide (107,108). In another study (109), DSC investigations were combined with scanning electron and hot-stage microscopies to obtain data required to interpret some of the DSC thermograms. It was noted that misinterpretation of DSC results could lead to conclusions regarding incompatibilities that might in fact actually exist, and that the supporting microscopic methods could present one such means to deduce only the genuine incompatibilities.

The question of false-positive drug–excipient interactions is always a possibility when DSC analysis is used as the sole method of analysis, and the problem is exacerbated when investigators use 1:1 w/w binary mixtures. In drug–excipient interaction studies conducted on mixtures containing niclosamide (56), albendazole, and closantel (57), HPLC analysis of samples that had exhibited incompatibility via DSC could not confirm the existence of an incompatibility. It was concluded that DSC screening of mixtures and formulations remains a viable method of detecting reactions between drug substances and excipients, but that any conclusion reached upon completion of that work should be tested using a referee method. This will be addressed in more detail in a subsequent section.

## Vibrational Spectroscopy

Owing to the sensitivity of molecular vibrations to changes in their chemical or physical environments, and the ease with which such properties can be studied, techniques of vibrational spectroscopy can be extremely important in the study of drug–excipient interactions. The energies characterizing the fundamental vibrational modes of drug substances lie within the range of 400 to $4000\,cm^{-1}$, and this spectral region corresponds to what is referred to as mid-IR electromagnetic radiation (110). Transitions among vibrational energy levels can therefore be observed directly through their absorbance in the IR region of the spectrum, or indirectly through an inelastic scattering of incident energy via the Raman effect. Although not as useful to the preformulation scientist, overtones and combination bands of vibrational modes are observed in the near-IR region of the spectrum ($4,000–13,350\,cm^{-1}$).

IR absorption spectroscopy, especially when measured by means of the Fourier-transform IR method (FTIR), has been shown to be a powerful technique for the physical characterization of pharmaceutical solids. Once a molecule is placed within the confines of a crystalline material, the structural characteristics of the solid sufficiently perturb the pattern of vibrational motion so that one can use these alterations as a means to study the solid-state chemistry of the system. FTIR spectra are often used to evaluate the type of polymorphism existing in a drug substance, and can be very useful in obtaining information regarding the physical or chemical reactions associated with drug–excipient interactions.

The vibrational energy levels of a molecule in its solid form can also be studied using Raman spectroscopy. Since most compounds of pharmaceutical interest are characterized by low molecular symmetry, the same bands observed in the IR absorption spectrum would necessarily be observed in the Raman spectrum. However, the fundamentally different nature of the selection rules associated with the Raman effect leads to the observation of significant differences in peak intensity between the two methods. In general, symmetric vibrations and nonpolar groups will yield the most intense Raman scattering bands, while antisymmetric vibrations and polar groups yield the most intense IR absorption bands.

As would be expected, a considerably higher degree of complexity in theoretical interpretation is available in the literature, with the two books by Herzberg forming the best references (111,112). Discussions of the quantum mechanical foundation of vibrational spectroscopy are available in Refs. 113–118, and more specific details of molecular spectroscopy can be found in Refs. 119–123. A listing of significant books covering vibrational spectroscopy is located in Refs. 124–134, and a detailed exposition of the instrumentation suitable for measurement of IR absorption and Raman spectra can be found in the Ewing's *Analytical Instrumentation Handbook* (135).

The utility of vibrational spectroscopy for obtaining information on systems of pharmaceutical interest is well documented (136–141), and an excellent compilation of spectra of excipient materials is available (142). To illustrate the point, the samples of famotidine form-A and form-B that were used in the XRPD and DSC illustrations of preceding sections were also analyzed by FTIR, using the attenuated total reflectance sampling mode [Brittain HG. Unpublished results obtained at a resolution of $4\,cm^{-1}$ using a Shimadzu model 8400S FTIR spectrometer, with each spectrum being acquired by the averaging of 50 individual spectra. The data were acquired using the attenuated total reflectance sampling mode, where the samples were clamped against the ZnSe crystal of a Pike MIRacle™ single reflection horizontal attenuated total reflectance (ATR) sampling accessory]. The spectra shown in Figure 7 are dominated by the absorption spectrum of the microcrystalline cellulose excipient, but they do demonstrate the appearance of absorption bands attributable to famotidine form-A in the form-B sample.

Digital subtraction of the microcrystalline cellulose absorption from the FTIR spectrum of the stressed form-A sample yielded a spectrum that contained all of the anticipated peaks. Digital subtraction of the microcrystalline cellulose absorption from the FTIR spectrum of the stressed form-B sample yielded a spectrum that contained peaks associated with form-B as well as peaks due to the form-A that resulted from the partial

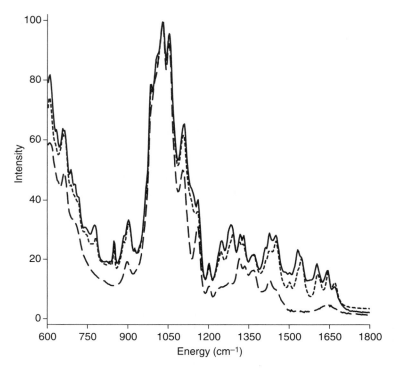

**Figure 7** Infrared absorption spectrum of a 28:72 w/w mixture of famotidine form-B and microcrystalline cellulose, after isothermal stressing of a sample spiked with 5% water (*solid trace*), and the Fourier-transform IR (FTIR) spectrum of a similarly stressed 28:72 w/w mixture of famotidine form-A and microcrystalline cellulose (*short dashed trace*). Also shown is the FTIR spectrum of similarly treated microcrystalline cellulose (*long dashed trace*).

conversion. The results of the FTIR-ATR study confirm that microcrystalline cellulose can facilitate the phase transformation of famotidine form-B to form-A in isothermally stressed samples.

The use of Raman spectroscopy for the characterization of solid-state characteristics of drug substances in dosage forms has been explored, where spectra were obtained from tablets and capsules containing enalapril maleate, prednisolone, ranitidine, theophylline, and warfarin sodium (143). In this work, it was shown that information on the properties of the API could be detected even when the levels of the drug substance were quite low, demonstrating that the technique would be well suited for the evaluation of the physical or chemical reactions that might be encountered during the performance of a drug–excipient screening study. Of particular importance was the observation that nonaromatic, noncrystalline, hydrophilic excipients tend to exhibit low degrees of Raman scattering in comparison with drug substances, making the API peaks particularly easy to observe in formulation mixtures.

The Raman spectra shown in Figure 8 demonstrate the preceding point.

Unlike the FTIR spectra of Figure 7, which consisted largely of the absorption spectrum of the microcrystalline cellulose excipient, the Raman spectra of the same samples are instead dominated by the spectra of the famotidine form-A and form-B peaks (Brittain HG. Unpublished results) obtained using a Raman systems model R-3000HR spectrometer, operated at a resolution of $5\,cm^{-1}$ and using a laser wavelength of 785 nm. The data were acquired using front-face scattering from a thick powder bed contained

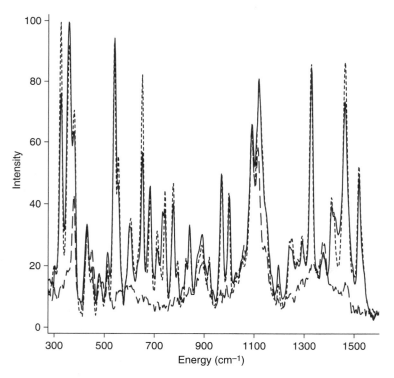

**Figure 8**  Raman spectrum of a 28:72 w/w mixture of famotidine form-B and microcrystalline cellulose, after isothermal stressing of a sample spiked with 5% water (*solid trace*), and the Raman spectrum of a similarly stressed 28:72 w/w mixture of famotidine form-A and microcrystalline cellulose (*short dashed trace*). Also shown is the Raman spectrum of similarly treated microcrystalline cellulose (*long dashed trace*).

in an aluminum sample holder). In fact, the effect of the excipient is so minor that digital subtraction of the microcrystalline cellulose contribution from the spectra was not necessary to conclude that the Raman spectrum of the stressed form-B sample contained peaks associated with form-B as well as peaks due to the form-A resulting from the partial phase conversion.

The interactions between erythromycin and film-forming polymers were studied using a number of techniques, including vibrational spectroscopy (144). The drug substance was dispersed in Eudragit® L100, shellac, polyvinyl acetate phthalate, cellulose acetate phthalate, hydroxypropylmethyl cellulose, and hydroxypropylmethyl cellulose acetate phthalate, and the results of the spectroscopic studies indicated that the amino group of erythromycin could be protonated by the carboxylic acid groups of the polymers. This finding was not viewed unfavorably, as there was no evidence of drug decomposition in the mixtures and the interaction probably aided in the dispersion of the drug substance in the polymer film.

A critical analysis of the relative merits of DSC and FTIR analysis in the evaluation of drug–excipient interactions has been conducted, where the two techniques were used to study the reaction of aminophylline and lactose (145). DSC analysis indicated that the two components would interact, and this observation was corroborated by the brown discoloration observed after samples formulated at a 1:5 w/w aminophylline:lactose ratio were stored for three weeks of storage at 60°C. While the DSC work correctly predicted the incompatibility, only the spectroscopic analysis could provide information regarding the nature of the interaction. It was deduced that ethylenediamine was liberated from the aminophylline drug substance, which then reacted with the lactose through a Schiff base intermediate.

Vibrational spectroscopy has played an important role in several studies where the interaction between PVP and drug substances was studied. Ibuprofen was found to become amorphous when being blended with PVP, and it was deduced that proton transfer from the drug to the excipient took place at the ketone group rather than at the nitrogen atom of the heterocycle (146). A combination of IR absorption and Raman spectroscopy was used to study the interaction between PVP and indomethacin in amorphous dispersions, with the association taking place between the hydroxyl group of the API and the carbonyl group of the polymer (147). Coprecipitates of diflunisal and PVP were studied by a number of techniques, and the FTIR spectra of 70:30 w/w drug–polymer blends suggested the existence of hydrogen bonding between the two components (148). In the latter study, the API could be obtained in either a crystalline or amorphous state, depending on the magnitude of the drug–excipient ratio.

A cautionary tale regarding overdependence on the use of DSC in compatibility testing has been published for carbamazepine and various tablet excipients (149). DSC analysis indicated that mannitol, microcrystalline cellulose, starch, and stearic acid were incompatible with the drug substance, but these findings could not be confirmed by either X-ray diffraction or IR absorption spectroscopy. The FTIR spectra of most stressed samples (storage at 55°C for three weeks) did not contain any new absorption bands, and no shifting in characteristic peaks was observed. Some shifting in the carbonyl band of carbamazepine was noted in its mixtures with stearic acid, but XRPD studies showed that this interaction was due to the formation of a solid solution between the two and not a chemical incompatibility.

## VALIDATION OF ANALYTICAL METHODOLOGY IN THE PREFORMULATION PROGRAM

The validation of any type of analytical methodology is extremely important during all stages of drug development, and it becomes critical as drug substances progress closer and closer toward registration with regulatory authorities. The topic is so important that entire books have been devoted to the validation of analytical methods (150–154), and the *Journal of Validation Technology* covers developments in the field. The current practice is that analytical methods are to be validated according to the current pharmacopoeial standard, and USP general test < 1225 > contains the overall guidelines for the validation of compendial methods together with a summary of the particular performance parameters required for various types of assay methods (155).

Validation can be defined as the process by which laboratory studies are used to establish that the method in question can meet the requirements for its intended use. The need for validation of analytical methodology is not as great during preformulation work as it would be later on in development, but it is always essential for an analyst to prove that the method being used actually is capable of producing information that can be relied upon. The need to appropriately validate methods is obvious since one will base the development of a particular drug substance on results obtained from preformulation studies.

The characteristics associated with an analytical method are expressed in terms of analytical performance parameters, and the validation procedure is designed to yield information, which enables one to judge the reliability of the analytical method in question. According to the USP general test, the full set of analytical performance parameters to be evaluated are precision, accuracy, specificity, limits of detection and quantitation, linearity and range, ruggedness, and robustness. For the preformulation stage of work, one can suffice by conducting a minimal validation that entails measurement of precision, accuracy, and linearity. For those instances where impurity species are to be measured, determination of the limits of detection and quantitation become important.

The "precision" of an analytical procedure expresses the closeness of agreement between a series of results obtained from the multiple sampling of the same homogeneous sample under the exact conditions required for performance of the method. This quantity is normally expressed in terms of the relative standard deviation measured during the multiple series of measurements. To evaluate the precision of an analytical method, one conducts assays of a sufficient number of independently prepared samples so as to be able to calculate a statistically valid estimate of the relative standard deviation. An example of typical precision data, and a suggestion as to the format for its presentation, is given in Table 2.

The "accuracy" of an analytical procedure expresses the closeness of agreement between the value found using the assay and the value, which is accepted either as a conventional true value or as an accepted reference value. As such, it is a measure of the exactness of the analytical method. Accuracy is typically expressed as the percent recovery by the assay of a known quantity of analyte spiked into a sample matrix. The accuracy of an analytical procedure is properly determined by applying the procedure to samples, or to mixtures of excipients (i.e., a suitable placebo), to which known amounts of analyte have been added. The analyte should be spiked into the matrix at concentration values that span the anticipated end result, and spiking levels of 50%, 75%, 100%, 125%, and 150% of the expected concentration are appropriate. The accuracy is calculated from the test results as the percentage of analyte recovered by the assay, and an example of typical accuracy results is given in Table 3.

The "linearity" of an analytical procedure is its ability to yield test results that are directly proportional to the concentration of an analyte in samples within a given range. Linearity is expressed in terms of the variance

**Table 2**  Example of a Precision Data Set

|  | Instrument response (area counts) |
|---|---|
| 1 | 9481 |
| 2 | 9434 |
| 3 | 9416 |
| 4 | 9192 |
| 5 | 9361 |
| 6 | 9224 |
| *Average* | 9351 |
| *Standard deviation* | 1180 |
| *Relative standard deviation* | 1.26% |

**Table 3**   Example of an Accuracy Data Set

| Target concentration | Spiked concentration (mg/mL) | Found concentration (mg/mL) | Percent recovery |
|---|---|---|---|
| 50% | 0.50 | 0.48 | 96.0 |
| 75% | 0.75 | 0.77 | 102.7 |
| 100% | 1.00 | 0.99 | 99.0 |
| 125% | 1.25 | 1.24 | 99.2 |
| 150% | 1.50 | 1.51 | 100.7 |
| *Average recovery* | | 99.5% | |
| *Standard deviation* | | 2.45 | |
| *Relative standard deviation* | | 2.46% | |

around the slope of the line (calculated using standard linear regression) from test results obtained through the analysis of samples containing varying concentrations of analyte. Linearity in a method is typically determined using linear regression analysis to deduce the relation between instrumental response and the known concentration of analyte present in samples within a given interval. For preformulation work, one can typically evaluate linearity by analyzing at least five analyte concentrations, equally spaced throughout the given interval and spanning the intended operating concentration of the assay method, according to the analytical procedure.

The slope of the regression line provides the mathematical relationship between the test results and the analyte concentration. The y-intercept is an estimation of any potential bias in the assay method. For most purposes, the linearity associated with the analytical procedure can be estimated by the correlation coefficient, which should be as close as possible to 1.0000. Any method that has a correlation coefficient less than 0.99 or more than 1.01, may either be insufficiently precise or could be nonlinear. An example of linearity data, and a format for its presentation, is presented in Table 4.

The "limit of detection" of an analytical procedure is the lowest amount of analyte in a sample that can be reported to be present (detected) with a given limit of confidence using the specified experimental procedure. Similarly, the "limit of quantitation" of an analytical procedure is the lowest amount of analyte in a sample that can be quantitatively determined with acceptable precision and accuracy when using the specified experimental procedure. Both quantities are expressed in units of concentration.

The limits of detection and quantitation of a preformulation stage analytical procedure can be approximated from the precision data set. The standard deviation in the analyte response is taken as a measure of the noise associated with the measurement, and one uses the slope from the linearity

**Table 4** Example of a Linearity Data Set

|   | Analyte concentration (mg/mL) | Instrument response |
|---|---|---|
| 1 | 0.089 | 466 |
| 2 | 0.178 | 916 |
| 3 | 0.356 | 1810 |
| 4 | 0.446 | 2268 |
| 5 | 0.535 | 2715 |
| 6 | 0.713 | 3624 |
| 7 | 0.891 | 4510 |
| *Slope* | | 5048 |
| *Intercept* | | 16.3 |
| *Correlation coefficient* | | 0.9999958 |

set to turn this quantity into its concentration equivalent. The concentration equivalent is multiplied by a factor of three to obtain an estimation of the limit of detection, and the limit of quantitation is estimated as the concentration equivalent multiplied by a factor of 10. In the examples used above, the standard deviation from the precision data set was determined to be 118, the slope of the regression line was 5048, and therefore the concentration equivalent is calculated to be 0.023 mg/mL. The limit of detection for this data set is then calculated to be 0.069 mg/mL, while the limit of quantitation is estimated to be 0.23 mg/mL.

## REFERENCES

1.  Cazes J. Ewing's Analytical Instrumentation Handbook. 3rd ed. New York: Marcel Dekker, 2005.
2.  Ahuja S, Scypinski S. Handbook of Modern Pharmaceutical Analysis. San Diego: Academic Press, 2001.
3.  Ahuja S. Impurities Evaluation of Pharmaceuticals. New York: Marcel Dekker, 1998.
4.  Ahuja S, Alsante KM. Handbook of Isolation and Characterization of Impurities in Pharmaceuticals. Amsterdam: Academic-Elsevier Press, 2003.
5.  Karger BL, Snyder LR, Horvath C. An Introduction to Separation Science. New York: John Wiley & Sons, 1973.
6.  Wilson I, Poole C, Cooke M. Encyclopedia of Separation Science. Vol. 1–10. Amsterdam: Elsevier Press, 2000.
7.  Poole CF, Schuette SA. Contemporary Practice of Chromatography. Amsterdam: Elsevier Press, 1984.
8.  Poole CF, Poole SK. Chromatography Today. Amsterdam: Elsevier Press, 1991.

9.  Giddings JC. Unified Separation Science. New York: John Wiley & Sons, 1991.
10. Scott RPW. Techniques and Practice of Chromatography. New York: Marcel Dekker, 1995.
11. Heftmann E. Chromatography. 6th ed. Amsterdam: Elsevier Press, 2004.
12. Miller JM. Chromatography: Concepts and Contrasts. 2nd ed. New York: John Wiley & Sons, 2005.
13. Stahl E. Thin-Layer Chromatography—A Laboratory Handbook. Berlin: Springer-Verlag, 1965.
14. Kirchner JG. Thin-Layer Chromatography. New York: Wiley-Interscience, 1976.
15. Touchstone JC, Rodgers D. Thin-Layer Chromatography—Quantitative Environmental and Clinical Applications. New York: Wiley-Interscience, 1980.
16. Geiss F. Fundamentals of Thin Layer Chromatography. Heidelberg: Verlag, 1987.
17. Fried B, Sherma J. Thin-Layer Chromatography. 4th ed. New York: Marcel Dekker, 1999.
18. Hahn-Deinstrop E. Applied Thin-Layer Chromatography. Weinheim: Wiley-VCH, 2000.
19. Sherma J. Thin layer chromatography. In: Cazes J, ed. Ewing's Analytical Instrumentation Handbook. 3rd ed. New York: Marcel Dekker, 2005: 995–1014.
20. Brittain HG. Nalmefene hydrochloride. In: Brittain HG, ed. Analytical Profiles of Drug Substances and Excipients. Vol. 24. San Diego: Academic Press, 1996:351–95.
21. Kalatzis E. J Pharm Sci 1970; 59:193–6.
22. McErland KM, Wood RJ, Matsui F, Lovering EG. J Pharm Sci 1978; 67: 958–61.
23. Vladimirov S, Fiser Z, Agbaba D, Zivanov-Stakic D. J Pharm Biomed Anal 1995; 13:675–8.
24. Patravale VB, Nair VB, Gore SP. J Pharm Biomed Anal 2000; 23:623–7.
25. Thoppil SO, Cardoza RM, Amin PD. J Pharm Biomed Anal 2001; 25:15–20.
26. Argekar AP, Powar SG. J Pharm Biomed Anal 2000; 21:1137–42.
27. Gorman PM, Jiang H. Isolation methods I: thin-layer chromatography. In: Ahuja S, Alsante KM, eds. Handbook of Isolation and Characterization of Impurities in Pharmaceuticals. Amsterdam: Academic-Elsevier Press, 2003: 203–30.
28. Scott RPW. Instrumentation for high-performance liquid chromatography. In: Cazes J, ed. Ewing's Analytical Instrumentation Handbook. 3rd ed. New York: Marcel Dekker, 2005:687–726.
29. Simpson CF. Practical High Performance Liquid Chromatography. London: Heyden & Son Ltd., 1976.
30. Kucera P. Microcolumn High Performance Liquid Chromatography. Amsterdam: Elsevier Press, 1984.
31. Poppe H. Instrumentation for High Performance Liquid Chromatography. Amsterdam: Elsevier Press, 1978.

32. Kirkland JJ. Modern Practice of Chromatography. New York: John Wiley & Sons, 1971.
33. Browen PR, Hartwick RA. High Performance Liquid Chromatography. New York: John Wiley & Sons, 1989.
34. Meyer VR. Practical High Performance Liquid Chromatography. 3rd ed. Chichester: John Wiley & Sons, 2000.
35. Snyder LR, Kirkland JJ. Introduction to Modern Liquid Chromatography. New York: John Wiley & Sons, 2000.
36. Berridge JC. Techniques for the Automated Optimization of HPLC Separations. New York: John Wiley & Sons, 1985.
37. Snyder LR, Kirkland JJ, Glajch JL. Practical HPLC Method Development. 2nd ed. New York: John Wiley & Sons, 1997.
38. Scott RPW. Small Bore Liquid Chromatography Columns. New York: John Wiley & Sons, 1984.
39. Scott RPW. Silica Gel and Bonded Phases. New York: John Wiley & Sons, 1993.
40. Neue UD. HPLC Columns: Theory, Technology, and Practice. New York: Wiley-VCH, 1997.
41. Sadek PC. The HPLC Solvent Guide. New York: John Wiley & Sons, 1996.
42. Smallwood IM. Handbook of Organic Solvent Properties. New York: Halsted Press, 1996.
43. Brown AC, Wallace DL, Burce GL, Mathes S. Liquid Chromatography Detectors. New York: Basel-Kong, 1983.
44. Parriott D. A Practical Guide to HPLC Detection. San Diego: Academic Press, 1993.
45. Xu QA, Trissel LA. Stability-Indicating HPLC Methods for Drug Analysis. London: Pharmaceutical Press, 2003.
46. Lunn G. HPLC Methods for Recently Approved Pharmaceuticals. New York: Wiley-Interscience, 2005.
47. Bergna HE. J Chromatogr 1991; 549:1.
48. Shoenmakers PJ, Billiet HAH, de Galan L. J Chromatogr 1979; 185:179; ibid 1981; 218:259.
49. King B, Grahm GS. Handbook of Derivatives for Chromatography. Philadelphia: Heyden Press, 1979.
50. Wirth DD, Baertschi SW, Johnson RA, et al. J Pharm Sci 1998; 87:31–9.
51. Lessen T, Zhao DC. J Pharm Sci 1996; 85:326–9.
52. Serrajuddin ATM, Thakur AB, Ghoshal RN, et al. J Pharm Sci 1999; 88: 696–704.
53. Tambwekar KR, Kakariya RB, Garg S. J Pharm Biomed Anal 2003; 32: 441–50.
54. Verma RK, Garg S. J Pharm Biomed Anal 2002; 30:583–91.
55. Shao Y, Alluri R, Mummert M, Koetter U, Lech S. J Pharm Biomed Anal 2004; 35:625–31.
56. Malan CEP, de Villiers MM, Lötter AP. J Pharm Biomed Anal 1997; 15: 549–57.
57. Malan CEP, de Villiers MM, Lötter AP. Drug Dev Indust Pharm 1997; 23: 533–7.

58. Ceshel GC, Badiello R, Ronchi C, Maffei P. J Pharm Biomed Anal 2003; 32: 1067–72.
59. Verma RK, Garg S. J Pharm Biomed Anal 2005; 38:633–44.
60. Kibbey CE, Poole SK, Robinson B, Jackson JD, Durham D. J Pharm Sci 2001; 90:1164–75.
61. Brinkman UATh. Hyphenation: Hype and Fascination. Amsterdam: Elsevier, 1999.
62. Burninsky DJ, Wang F. Mass spectral characterization. In: Ahuja S, Alsante KM, eds. Handbook of Isolation and Characterization of Impurities in Pharmaceuticals. Amsterdam: Academic-Elsevier Press, 2003:249–99.
63. Armentrout PB. The Encyclopedia of Mass Spectrometry. Vol. 1. Theory and Ion Chemistry. Amsterdam: Elsevier, 2003.
64. Gross ML. The Encyclopedia of Mass Spectrometry. Vol. 2. Biological Applications Part A. Amsterdam: Elsevier, 2004.
65. Caprioli RM. The Encyclopedia of Mass Spectrometry. Vol. 3. Biological Applications Part B. Amsterdam: Elsevier, 2004.
66. Nibbering N. The Encyclopedia of Mass Spectrometry. Vol. 4. Fundamentals of and Applications to Organic (and Organometallic) Compounds. Amsterdam: Elsevier, 2005.
67. Shalliker RA, Gray MJ. HPLC-hyphenated techniques. In: Cazes J, ed. Ewing's Analytical Instrumentation Handbook. 3rd ed. New York: Marcel Dekker, 2005:945–94.
68. Yu LR, Conrads TP, Veenstra TD. Mass spectrometry instrumentation. In: Cazes J, ed. Ewing's Analytical Instrumentation Handbook. 3rd ed. New York: Marcel Dekker, 2005:429–43.
69. Niessen WMA, van der Greef J. Liquid Chromatography—Mass Spectrometry. New York: Marcel Dekker, 1992.
70. Chowdhury S. Identification and Quantification of Drugs, Metabolites, and Metabolizing Enzymes by LC-MS. Amsterdam: Elsevier, 2005.
71. Niessen WMA. Liquid Chromatography–Mass Spectrometry. 3rd ed. New York: Taylor & Francis, 2006.
72. Cappiello A. Advances in LC-MS Instrumentation. Amsterdam: Elsevier, 2007.
73. Yu Y, Hwang TL, Algayer K, et al. J Pharm Biomed Anal 2003; 33: 999–1015.
74. Lovdahl MJ, Hurley TR, Tobias B, Priebe SR. J Pharm Biomed Anal 2002; 28:917–24.
75. Brittain HG, Bogdanowich SJ, Bugay DE, DeVincentis J, Lewen G, Newman AW. Pharm Res 1991; 8:963–73.
76. Brittain HG. Physical Characterization of Pharmaceutical Solids. New York: Marcel Dekker, 1995.
77. Robertson JM. Organic Crystals and Molecules. Ithaca: Cornell University Press, 1953.
78. Kitaigorodskii AI. Organic Chemical Crystallography. New York: Consultants Bureau, 1957.
79. Stout GH, Jensen LH. X-Ray Structure Determination: A Practical Guide. New York: Macmillan Co., 1968.

80. Woolfson MM. X-Ray Crystallography. Cambridge: Cambridge University Press, 1970.
81. Rousseau JJ. Basic Crystallography. Chichester: John-Wiley & Sons, 1998.
82. Krawitz AD. Introduction to Diffraction in Materials Science and Engineering. New York: John Wiley & Sons, 2001.
83. Cullity BD, Stock SR. Elements of X-ray Diffraction. 3rd ed. New York: Prentice-Hall, 2001.
84. Suryanarayanan R. X-ray powder diffractometry. In: Brittain HG, ed. Physical Characterization of Pharmaceutical Solids. New York: Marcel Dekker, 1995:187–221.
85. Brittain HG. X-ray diffraction of pharmaceutical materials. In: Brittain HG, ed. Profiles of Drug Substances, Excipients, and Related Methodology. Amsterdam: Elsevier Academic Press, 2003:273–319.
86. Klug HP, Alexander LE. X-Ray Diffraction Procedures for Polycrystalline and Amorphous Materials. 2nd ed. New York: Wiley-Interscience, 1974.
87. Chung FH, Smith DK. Basic Industrial Applications of X-Ray Diffraction. New York: Marcel Dekker, 2000.
88. Roy S, Alexander KS, Riga AT, Chatterjee K. J Pharm Sci 2003; 92:747–59.
89. Yamada T, Saito N, Anraku M, Imai T, Otagiri M. Pharm Dev Tech 2000; 5:443–54.
90. Airaksinen S, Luukkonen P, Jørgensen A, Karjalainen M, Rantanen J, Yliruusi J. J Pharm Sci 2003; 92:516–28.
91. Martinez-Oharriz MC, Martin C, Goni MM, Rodrigues-Espinosa C, Tros-Ilarduya MC, Zornoza A. Eur J Pharm Sci 1999; 8:127–32.
92. Mirza S, Deinamaki J, Miroshnyk I, et al. J Pharm Sci 2006; 95:1723–32.
93. Ford JL, Timmins P. Pharmaceutical Thermal Analysis. Chichester: Ellis Horwood, 1989.
94. McCauley JA, Brittain HG. Thermal methods of analysis. In: Brittain HG, ed. Physical Characterization of Pharmaceutical Solids. New York: Marcel Dekker, 1995:223–51.
95. Craig DQM, Reading M. Thermal Analysis of Pharmaceuticals. Boca Raton: CRC Press, 2007.
96. Giron D. J Pharm Biomed Anal 1986; 4:755–70.
97. Wendlandt WW. Thermal Analysis. 3rd ed. New York: John Wiley & Sons, 1986.
98. Wells JI. Pharmaceutical Preformulation: The Physicochemical Properties of Drug Substances. New York: Halsted Press, 1988.
99. Pope MI, Judd MD. Introduction to Differential Thermal Analysis. London: Heyden, 1977.
100. Brown ME. Introduction to Thermal Analysis: Techniques and Applications. New York: Chapman and Hall, 1998.
101. Alexander KS, Riga AT, Haines PJ. Thermoanalytical instrumentation and applications. In: Cazes J, ed. Ewing's Analytical Instrumentation Handbook. 3rd ed. New York: Marcel Dekker, 2005:445–507.
102. Keattch CJ, Dollimore D. Introduction to Thermogravimetry. 2nd ed. London: Heyden, 1975.
103. Ford JL, Francomb MM. Drug Dev Indust Pharm 1985; 11:1111–22.

104. Durig T, Fassihi AR. Int J Pharm 1993; 97:161–70.
105. Tomassetti M, Catalani A, Rossi V, Vecchio S. J Pharm Biomed Anal 2005; 37:949–55.
106. Mura P, Manderioli A, Bramanti G, Furlanetto S, Pinzauti S. Int J Pharm 1995; 119:71–9.
107. Mura P, Bettinetti GP, Faucci MT, Manderioli A, Parrini PL. Thermochim Acta 1998; 321:59–65.
108. Mura P, Faucci MT, Manderioli A, Furlanetto S, Pinzauti S. Drug Dev Indust Pharm 1998; 24:747–56.
109. Mura P, Faucci MT, Manderioli A, Bramanti G, Ceccarelli L. J Pharm Biomed Anal 1998; 18:151–63.
110. Brittain HG. Molecular motion and vibrational spectroscopy. In: Brittain HG, ed. Spectroscopy of Pharmaceutical Solids. New York: Taylor and Francis, 2006:205–33.
111. Herzberg G. Infrared and Raman Spectra of Polyatomic Molecules. New York, NY: Van Nostrand Reinhold Co., 1945.
112. Herzberg G. Spectra of Diatomic Molecules. 2nd ed. New York, NY: Van Nostrand Reinhold Co., 1950.
113. Pauling L, Wilson EB. Introduction to Quantum Mechanics. New York: McGraw-Hill, 1935.
114. Eyring H, Walter J, Kimball GE. Quantum Chemistry. New York: John Wiley & Sons, 1944.
115. Kauzmann W. Quantum Chemistry. New York: Academic Press, 1957.
116. Davis JC. Advanced Physical Chemistry. New York: Ronald Press, 1965.
117. Levine IN. Quantum Chemistry. Boston: Allyn and Bacon, 1970.
118. Hanna MW. Quantum Mechanics in Chemistry. Menlo Park: Benjamin/Cummings, 1981.
119. Barrow GM. Molecular Spectroscopy. New York: McGraw-Hill, 1962.
120. King GW. Spectroscopy and Molecular Structure. New York: Holt, Rinehart and Winston, 1964.
121. Brittain EFH, George WO, Wells CHJ. Introduction to Molecular Spectroscopy. London: Academic Press, 1970.
122. Guillory WA. Introduction to Molecular Structure and Spectroscopy. Boston: Allyn and Bacon, 1977.
123. McHale JL. Molecular Spectroscopy. Upper Saddle River, NJ: Prentice Hall, 1999.
124. Rao CNR. Chemical Applications of Infrared Spectroscopy. New York: Academic Press, 1963.
125. Kendall DN. Applied Infrared Spectroscopy. New York: Reinhold Pub, 1966.
126. Conley RT. Infrared Spectroscopy. Boston, MA: Allyn and Bacon, 1966.
127. Colthup NB, Daly LH, Wiberley SE. Introduction to Infrared and Raman Spectroscopy. 2nd ed. London: Academic Press, 1975.
128. Nakanishi K, Solomon PH. Infrared Absorption Spectroscopy. San Francisco, CA: Holden-Day, 1977.
129. Bhagavantam S. Scattering of Light and the Raman Effect. New York: Chemical Publishing Co., 1942.

130. Grasselli JG, Snavely MK, Bulkin BJ. Chemical Applications of Raman Spectroscopy. New York: Wiley-Interscience, 1981.
131. Grasselli JG, Bulkin BJ. Analytical Raman Spectroscopy. New York: John Wiley & Sons, 1991.
132. Ferraro JR, Nakamoto K. Introductory Raman Spectroscopy. New York: Academic Press, 1994.
133. Lewis IR, Edwards HGM. Handbook of Raman Spectroscopy. New York: Marcel Dekker, 2001.
134. Wilson EB, Decius JC, Cross PC. Molecular Vibrations: The Theory of Infrared and Raman Vibrational Spectra. New York: McGraw-Hill Book Co., 1955.
135. Fredericks P, Rintoul L, Coates J. Vibrational spectroscopy: instrumentation for infrared and Raman spectroscopy. In: Cazes J, ed. Ewing's Analytical Instrumentation Handbook. 3rd ed. New York: Marcel Dekker, 2005: 163–238.
136. Markovich RJ, Pidgeon C. Pharm Res 1991; 8:663–75.
137. Bugay DE, Williams AC. Vibrational spectroscopy. In: Brittain HG, ed. Physical Characterization of Pharmaceutical Solids. New York: Marcel Dekker, 1995:59–91.
138. Brittain HG. J Pharm Sci 1997; 86:405–12.
139. Bugay DE, Brittain HG. Infrared absorption spectroscopy. In: Brittain HG, ed. Spectroscopy of Pharmaceutical Solids. New York: Taylor and Francis, 2006:235–69.
140. Pivonka DE, Chalmers JM, Griffiths PR. Applications of Vibrational Spectroscopy in Pharmaceutical Research and Development. New York: Wiley, 2007.
141. Bugay DE, Brittain HG. Raman spectroscopy. In: Brittain HG, ed. Spectroscopy of Pharmaceutical Solids. New York: Taylor and Francis, 2006:271–312.
142. Bugay DE, Findlay WP. Pharmaceutical Excipients: Characterization by IR, Raman, and NMR Spectroscopy. New York: Marcel Dekker, 1999.
143. Taylor LS, Langkilde FW. J Pharm Sci 2000; 89:1342–53.
144. Sarisuta N, Kumpugdee M, Müller BW, Puttipipatkhachorn S. Int J Pharm 1999; 186:109–18.
145. Hartauer KJ, Guillory JK. Drug Dev Indust Pharm 1991; 17:617–30.
146. Sekizake H, Danjo K, Eguchi H, Yonezawa Y, Sumada H, Otsuka A. Chem Pharm Bull 1995; 43:988–93.
147. Taylor LS, Zografi G. Pharm Res 1997; 14:1691–8.
148. Martinez-Oharriz MC, Rodriguez-Espinosa C, Martin C, Goni MM, Tros-Ilarduya MC, Sanchez M. Drug Dev Indust Pharm 2002; 28:717–25.
149. Joshi DV, Patil VB, Pokharkar VB. Drug Dev Indust Pharm 2002; 28:687–94.
150. Riley CM, Rosanske TW. Development and Validation of Analytical Methods. Oxford: Pergamon-Elsevier, 1996.
151. Swartz M, Krull IS. Analytical Method Development and Validation. New York: Taylor & Francis, 1997.

152. Miller JM, Crowther JB. Analytical Chemistry in a GMP Environment. New York: John Wiley & Sons, 2000.
153. Chan CC, Lam H, Lee YC, Zhang XM. Analytical Method Validation and Instrument Performance Verification. New York: John Wiley & Sons, 2004.
154. Bliesner DM. Validating Chromatographic Methods. New York: John Wiley & Sons, 2006.
155. United States Pharmacopoeia: General Test <1225>, Validation of Compendial Procedures. United States Pharmacopoeia. 30th ed. Vol. 1. United States Pharmacopoeial Convention, Rockville, MD, 2007:680–3.

# 4.4

# Dissolution Testing

## George Wong

*Global R&D Operations, Johnson & Johnson, Skillman, New Jersey, U.S.A.*

## Charles C. Collins

*College of Pharmacy, East Tennessee State University,*
*Johnson City, Tennessee, U.S.A.*

## PURPOSE OF DISSOLUTION

Dissolution can be defined as a process by which the drug substance in a formulation dissolves into solution. Although dissolution appears to be a simple process, developing a suitable dissolution test requires careful considerations of the physicochemical properties of the drug substance, excipients, dosage form designs, dissolution media, and other important variables.

Since the first publication on the mathematical treatment of dissolution authored by Noyes and Whitney a century ago (1), modeling of dissolution rates from various dosage forms has continued to evolve and has become the research interest of many pharmaceutical scientists. One of the challenges of conducting a dissolution test that is different from many other analytical tests, [such as high performance liquid chromatography (HPLC) assays where data can be obtained with great precision and accuracy], is that dissolution profiles may change significantly upon a slight modification of one of the dissolution parameters. A thorough understanding of the physical process of dissolution has been found to be critical in predicting dissolution rates. In 1897, Noyes and Whitney studied the dissolution in water of two insoluble compounds (benzoic acid and lead chloride) using cylindrical sticks having constant surface areas. They developed an equation to describe dissolution rates using the principles of Fick's second law of diffusion across a thin layer of saturated solution. Later, Brunner and Tolloczko (2) and Nernst and Brunner (3) had incorporated other variables into the Noyes and Whitney equation. Additional parameters included surface area, diffusion coefficient, the thickness of the diffusion layer, and the volume of the dissolution medium. This general "film" theory has remained the basic principle adopted by most pharmaceutical scientists in describing the phenomenon of dissolution.

Up to the early 1970s, scientists have developed other dissolution models and started to standardize the instruments used in dissolution testing. In 1931, Hixson and Crowell developed the "cubic root law" of dissolution, which describes the appearance of a solute in solution (4). Instead of considering the rate of change in concentration as the predicted variable, the cubic root law describes the weight increase of the solute in solution upon its dissolution. Researchers in academia and the pharmaceutical industry have also attempted to understand the source of variability in dissolution by modifying the film theory. Instead of assuming the existence of a stagnant layer and a steady state during dissolution, some scientists incorporated the concepts of continual renewal of the interfacial surface, and the existence of variable diffusion coefficients caused by concentration differences (5,6).

Meanwhile, the design of dissolution apparatus evolved when different instruments were utilized to study theoretical aspects of dissolution. In general, the principle and hydrodynamics of a dissolution apparatus can fall into one of the three categories: (*i*) a beaker-like closed system, (*ii*) a flow-through open system, and (*iii*) two separate compartments based on dialysis. In 1968, Pernarowski et al. developed the rotating basket dissolution apparatus (7), and shortly after that, Poole invented the paddle dissolution method (8). These two dissolution designs have then become USP Apparatus 1 and USP Apparatus 2, respectively, and are still the most commonly used instruments.

## THEORY OF DISSOLUTION TESTING

Most dissolution scientists work in as simplified a fashion as possible, assuming that what happens in a dissolution vessel is not a simulation of what happens in the body. Omission of the absorption step, which would result in the disappearance of drug from the system and thus preventing a buildup of drug concentration, is the principal reason for this difference. Given these specifications, the purpose for a dissolution test environment is one favorable for the dissolving of the drug from a drug product and can be examined within its historical concept.

In 1897, Noyes and Whitney published a paper "The rate of solution of solid substances in their own solution" (1), suggesting that the dissolution rate is controlled by a layer of saturated solution that instantly forms around a solid particle. Their fundamental equation for dissolution is

$$\frac{dc}{dt} = K(c_s - c_t) \tag{1}$$

$dc/dt$ is the dissolution rate of the drug, $K$ is the proportionality (dissolution) constant, $c_s$ is the equilibrium, saturation concentration or maximum solubility, and $c_t$ is the concentration at time $t$.

In 1900, Brunner and Tolloczko (2) presented data that indicated that the dissolution rate depends on the chemical and physical structures of the solid, the surface area exposed to the medium, the agitation speed, the medium temperature, and the overall design of the dissolution apparatus. This resulted in a modification of Equation 1, namely:

$$\frac{dc}{dt} = K_1 S(c_s - c_t) \tag{2}$$

$S$ is the surface area and $K_1$ is the proportionality (dissolution) constant (different than original $K$).

In 1904, Nernst and Brunner (3) used the laws of diffusion to introduce a new relationship between the dissolution rate constant and the diffusion coefficient of the solute by further defining the proportionality constant:

$$\frac{dc}{dt} = K_2 \frac{DS}{vh}(c_s - c_t) \tag{3}$$

$D$ is the diffusion coefficient, $v$ is the volume at dissolution media, $h$ is the thickness of the diffusion layer, and $K_2$ is the proportionality (dissolution) constant (further different than original $K$).

This relationship under sink conditions (i.e., where the amount of drug dissolved creates a concentration in solution, $c_t$, which is so much smaller than the saturation solubility, $c_s$, as to be ignored) results in

$$\frac{dc}{dt} = K_2 \frac{DS}{vh}(c_s) \tag{4}$$

Typically, this condition is met if $c_t$ is $\leq 10\%$ of $c_s$. This very fundamental equation could be considered the basis for the current definition of sink conditions.

In 1931, Hixson and Crowell (4) developed a mathematical model using the original theory of Noyes and Whitney, the volume of the media, the mass of solute (initially, during dissolution, and mass in solution at saturation), which were then incorporated into Fick's first law of diffusion. This yielded

$$V\frac{dw}{dt} = -K_3 S(w_s - w_0 + w) \tag{5}$$

$$w_0^{1/3} - w^{1/3} \left(\frac{4\pi\rho\eta}{3}\right)^{1/3}\left[\frac{Dc_s}{h\rho}\right]t \tag{6}$$

$w_0$ is the initial powder mass, $w$ is the powder mass during dissolution at time $t$, $\rho$ is the particle (powder) density, $\eta$ is the viscosity of the media, $D$ is the diffusion coefficient (diffusivity), $c_s$ is the saturation concentration or maximum solubility, and $h$ is the thickness of the diffusion layer.

Incorporation of all constants on the right of the equation into the constant of proportional yields the relation known as the Hixson and Crowell Cubic Root Law:

$$w_0^{1/3} - w^{1/3} = Kt \tag{7}$$

This relationship was developed for a single spherical particle, but has been modified for multiparticulate systems under nonsink conditions:

$$w_0^{-2/3} - w^{-2/3} = k_4 t \tag{8}$$

The new assumptions include particles of the same size and constant number, thus changing the constant on the right of the equation to $k_4$. Higuchi and Hiestand (9) continued the theoretical development by allowing for a reduction in the radius of the spherical particles to take place during dissolution, resulting in

$$w_0^{2/3} - w^{2/3} = \frac{2Dc_s}{\rho} \left(\frac{4\pi\rho\eta}{3}\right)^{2/3} t = Kt \tag{9}$$

In 1970, the first official dissolution test for a solid dosage form was published in USP XVIII. Since then, the Food and Drug Administration (FDA) has considered dissolution as another test for the quality control of drug products that is separate and distinct from disintegration. The requirement of dissolution has thus created a challenge for scientists who are developing formulations or new dosage forms, but who do not have enough knowledge regarding the impact of their excipients on the dissolution profiles. Substantial debate has taken place over the years on the use of dissolution as a quality control test, including arguments that a drug product could fail the dissolution test while there was no effect on bioavailability or efficacy.

In the last 30 years, the need to establish in vivo/in vitro correlations (IVIVC) has received increasing attention from pharmaceutical scientists. Dissolution has been widely accepted as a useful tool to reduce development costs, a means to screen formulations, and a way to eliminate the conduct of costly clinical trials.

## OFFICIAL DISSOLUTION APPARATUS

For dissolution equipment and methods, the three most referenced official pharmacopoeias are the *European Pharmacopoeia* (EP), the *Japanese Pharmacopoeia* (JP), and the *United States Pharmacopoeia* (USP). A scientist working in this area should always verify that the current version is being referenced, as changes can occur from one edition to another. Additionally, one must check for any supplements that may have been released for the current edition. In the past several editions of the USP (since 1995, or USP 23), seven dissolution testing apparatus have been listed within General Chapters < 711 > and < 724 >.

USP Apparatus 1 is also known as the rotating basket. This system was the original dissolution device that first became official in 1970 (USP 18) and consists of an enclosed basket (Fig 1) into which the drug delivery system is placed. This assembly is immersed into the temperature-controlled media contained in a vessel (Fig 2), and is useful for floating dosage forms, solids, beads, some suppositories, and modified-release preparations.

USP Apparatus 2 is also known as the paddle system. This device was added in 1975 (USP 19) and consists of the same vessel arrangement as for the previous apparatus, except that the drug delivery system should sink to the bottom of the media in the vessel and the media is mixed using a paddle (Fig 3). This apparatus is used for heavier drug delivery systems that spontaneously sink, or those that can be made to sink by attachment to a heavier object or sinker. Apparatus 2 is used for both immediate-release (IR) and modified-release drug delivery systems. However, drug delivery systems

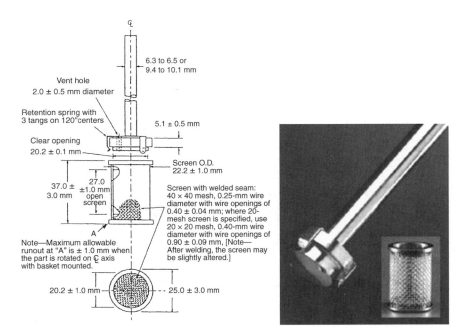

**Figure 1** Rotating basket.

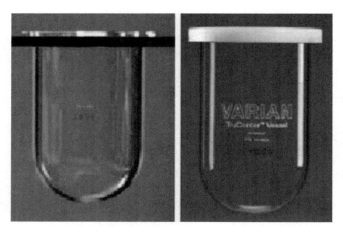

**Figure 2**   Standard 1 L dissolution vessel.

that disintegrate into heavy particles can create a problem (i.e., coning) where reduced mixing dynamics develop at the very bottom of the vessel owing to the inability of the disintegrated powder to mix with the

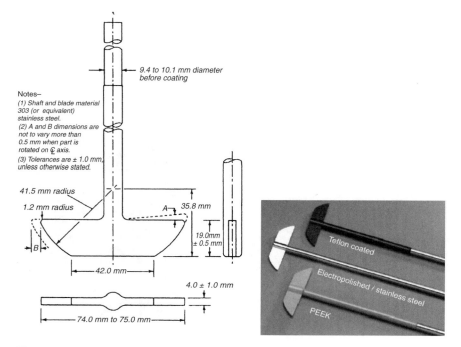

**Figure 3**   Configuration and examples of paddles for Apparatus 2.

dissolution medium. An example of an instrument that can be configured as Apparatus 1 or Apparatus 2 is depicted in Figure 4.

USP Apparatus 3 is an entirely different piece of equipment and is also called the reciprocating cylinder. This device appeared in 1995 (USP 23), and was designed specifically for extended- or modified-release drug delivery systems. It consists of row of smaller vessel containing media (typically 200–300 mL each) within which a glass cylinder moves vertically, has a screen at each end, and contains the drug delivery system (Figs. 5–7). This cylinder moves up and down with net amplitude of 10 cm.

USP Apparatus 4 is the flow-through cell. This also first appeared in 1995 (USP 23) and was designed for nondisintegrating drug delivery systems. It consists of a group of cells, usually six (Figs. 8 and 9) through which media flows. The cells can be of various sizes depending on the drug delivery system. This provides for a perfect sink condition, as fresh media (containing no drug) is continually provided for drug solution.

USP Apparatus 5 was originally introduced in a supplement to USP 22 as Apparatus 3, and is also known as the paddle over disk. This device and the next two listed below were designed for the dissolution testing of transdermal patch drug delivery systems. This device is a simple modification of Apparatus 2, using the same vessel and paddle-stirring element. By attaching the patch to be evaluated to a holder (typically referred to as a disk), the patch is placed into the bottom of the vessel (Figs. 10 and 11). The purpose of the disk is to act as a sinker for the transdermal patch.

USP Apparatus 6, also known as the rotating cylinder, was introduced in USP 22 as Apparatus 4 for the dissolution testing of transdermal patch drug delivery systems. This device uses the same vessel and instrument arrangement as for Apparatus 1, but replaces the basket with a hollow stainless steel cylinder. The transdermal patch is centered on the

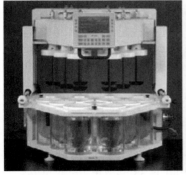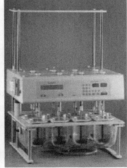

**Figure 4** Instruments that can be configured as Apparatus 1, 2, 5, or 6. *Source:* Courtesy of Varian, Inc.

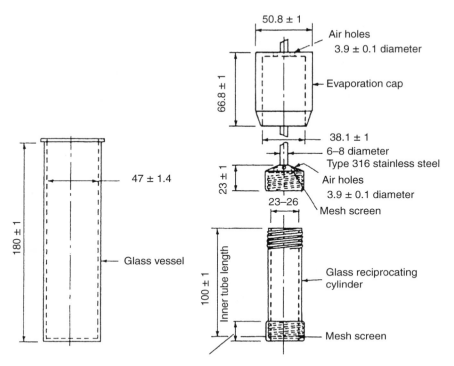

**Figure 5** Schematic of the reciprocating cylinder for Apparatus 3.

circumference of the cylinder, with the drug-release side directed outward (Fig. 12).

USP Apparatus 7 was originally known as Apparatus 5 (or the reciprocating disk) when initially introduced in USP 22. As new ways to use this device were developed, and as it is now used for nondisintegrating drug delivery system dissolution as well as transdermal patches, Apparatus 7 is currently termed the "reciprocating holder." The various transdermal patch holders are illustrated in Figure 13, and other holders can be seen in Figure 14. The instrument is similar in arrangement to Apparatus 3, using rows of media-filled vessels (Fig. 15), but the reciprocating amplitude of each holder is only 2 cm.

The dissolution devices in the EP 4 are identical to three of the USP official apparatuses. In the EP, the paddle apparatus is the same as USP Apparatus 2. The EP basket apparatus is the same as USP Apparatus 1, and the EP flow-through apparatus is the same as USP Apparatus 4. However, the EP contains only one apparatus for transdermal patch drug delivery systems, namely the cell method (Fig. 16) that is similar in many ways to USP Apparatus 5. The patch is loaded into an appropriately sized cell and placed into a vessel, where a paddle is used to mix the media.

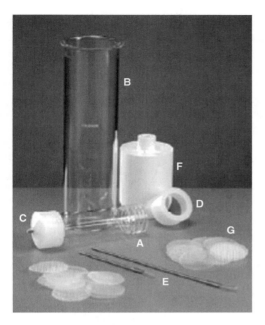

**Figure 6** Pictured are various parts of an Apparatus 3: *A*: internal glass cylinder; *B*: media vessel; *C*: end caps for the glass cylinder; *D*: sampling cannula; *E*: evaporation cover; *F*: screens to be placed in the end caps.

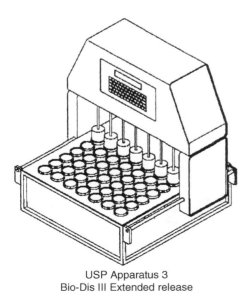

USP Apparatus 3
Bio-Dis III Extended release

**Figure 7** Schematic of USP Apparatus 3 made by Varian, Inc.

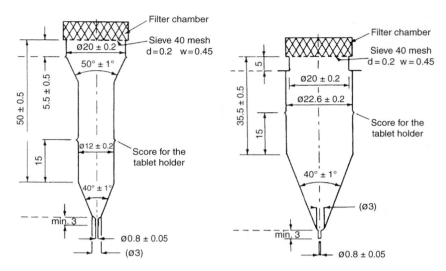

**Figure 8**  Schematic of two sizes of flow-through cells for USP Apparatus 4.

The JP 14 lists three dissolution devices, which at first appear to be identical with their USP counterparts. The JP lists these as Method 1 (the rotatory basket method), Method 2 (the paddle method), and Method 3 (the flow-through cell method). There are no significant differences between JP Method 2 and USP Apparatus 2, and none between JP Method 3 and USP Apparatus 4. In every way but one, JP Apparatus 1 and USP Apparatus 1 are the same, but the one difference can be significant. The description of the wire mesh used in the USP and JP baskets are different, namely a 40-mesh screen for the USP basket and a 36-mesh screen for the JP basket. This

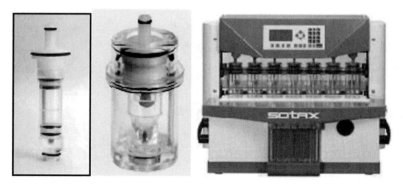

**Figure 9**  Example of flow-through Apparatus 4 manufactured by Sotax.

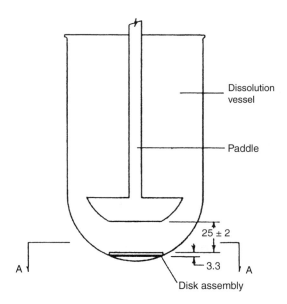

Dissolution
vessel

Paddle

25 ± 2

3.3

A

A

Disk assembly

**Figure 10** Schematic of Apparatus 5, the paddle over disk.

seemingly small difference can result in a significant difference for a dissolution test, as these baskets are not interchangeable.

## APPLICATION AND METHOD DEVELOPMENT

### Formulation Design

In the pharmaceutical industry, the final marketed product is usually a tablet or a capsule oral dosage form. During the development process, this final formulation is often not optimized or developed until the end of

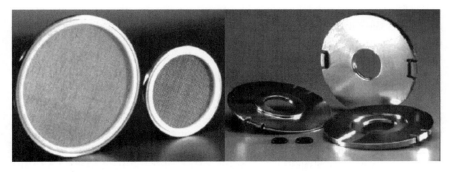

**Figure 11** Parts of disk assembly.

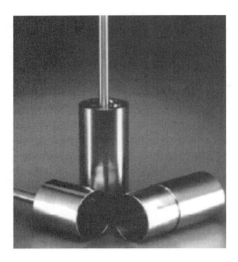

**Figure 12**   USP Apparatus 6 cylinder.

Phase 1 clinical studies. When a drug has showed some promising results in Phase 1 human clinical trials, a formulator will begin collecting the necessary preformulation data, such as excipient compatibility, hygroscopicity, compressibility, etc., in trying to understand the physiochemical properties of the drug substance. Then he or she will select different types or various amounts of diluents, disintegrants, binders, or lubricants in an attempt to manufacture a product having the desirable hardness and disintegrating times. Several probe formulations are often prepared before a final decision is made on the choice of excipients or processing parameters. A brief summary of how the choice of diluent, disintegrant and lubricant, can affect dissolution behavior is described below (10).

### Effect of Diluent

The rate of dissolution can vary depending upon whether a hydrophilic or a hydrophobic diluent is chosen in the formulation. In 1963, Levy et al. (11) examined the amount of starch (a hydrophilic diluent and disintegrant) on the dissolution rates of salicylic acid tablets. When the tablets were manufactured by dry compression, the rate of dissolution was enhanced three times by increasing the amount of starch from 5% to 20% (Fig. 17). Through a study including one hydrophobic and three hydrophilic diluents, Yen (12) further confirmed that a hydrophilic diluent could increase the dissolution rate. When starch, lactose, and glycine were employed as hydrophilic fillers to manufacture triamterene products by wet granulation, the dissolution rates were significantly higher. Both of these studies suggest that drug particles can be surrounded by a thin layer of hydrophilic diluent, and thus wetting of the drug is enhanced and subsequently the dissolution is faster.

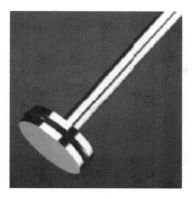

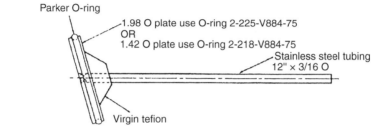

Parker O-ring

1.98 O plate use O-ring 2-225-V884-75
OR
1.42 O plate use O-ring 2-218-V884-75

Stainless steel tubing
12" × 3/16 O

Virgin tefion

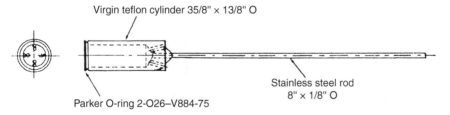

Virgin teflon cylinder 35/8" × 13/8" O

Parker O-ring 2-O26–V884-75

Stainless steel rod
8" × 1/8" O

**Figure 13** Transdermal patch holders for Apparatus 7.

An example showing the importance of physical binding between a hydrophilic diluent and drug particles in dissolution was demonstrated by Ishizaka et al. (13). Indomethacin was studied as a model molecule, where during a dry blending procedure, the drug was hybridized with potato starch. After the blending process, amorphous indomethacin was found to form a layer over the starch surface, as evidenced in the powder X-ray diffraction patterns and the scanning electron microscopy results. Over time, the amorphous indomethacin converted to fine crystalline particles that became firmly bound to the starch particle surfaces. Dissolution of indomethacin in this "hybrid" state was compared with dissolution of granules prepared from a physical mixture, or of granules taken from

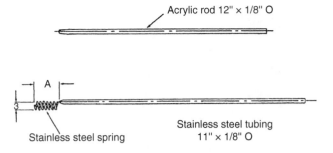

Figure 14   Solid dosage form holders for Apparatus 7.

capsules in a marketed product. The dissolution rate of the hybridized indomethacin was significantly higher in the dissolution medium even at an acidic pH (Fig. 18).

The application of soluble diluents in the encapsulation of tablets for clinical studies was examined by Kleinebudde et al. (14) for sustained-release tablets where dissolution profiles of the original and blinded product could be considered to be equal. Using fast-dissolving tablets as a model, different fillers were found to have an effect on the dissolution rate of the

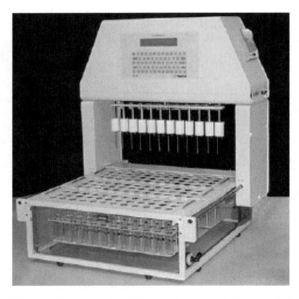

Figure 15   Example of Apparatus 7, with 12 sample locations and 9 rows of tubes. *Source*: Courtesy of Varian, Inc.

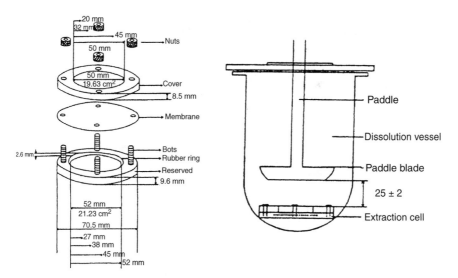

**Figure 16** Diagrams of the extraction cell found in the *European Pharmacopoeia*. Exhibits the same concept for transdermal patches as USP Apparatus 5.

encapsulated tablets. Comparable dissolution rates were found when soluble fillers were used, but dissolution profiles changed when insoluble or swellable diluents were added.

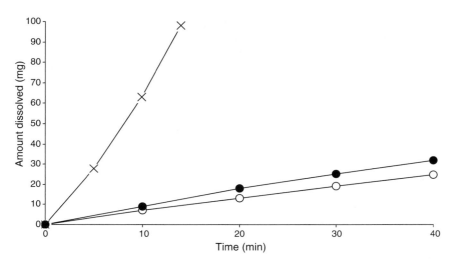

**Figure 17** Effect of starch content of granules on dissolution rate of salicylic acid contained in compressed tablets: (o) 5%; (●) 10%; (x) 20% starch in granules. *Source*: Adapted from Ref. 11.

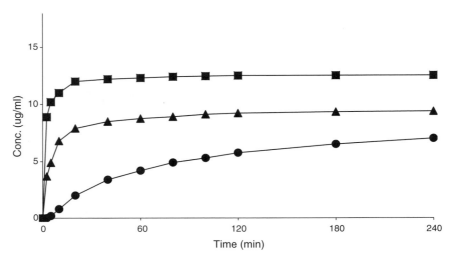

**Figure 18**   Dissolution profiles of indomethacin from the powder samples in pH 4.7 buffer. (●) original indomethacin powder; (▲) physical mixture (5% indomethacin); (■) hybrid powder (4.1% indomethacin) stored for 237 days. *Source:* Adapted from Ref. 13.

Effect of Disintegrants

Since the disintegration of a tablet must occur before drug substance in the inner core can dissolve, the choice of a disintegrant can potentially change the rate of dissolution. The degree of hydrophilicity of a disintegrant is important in determining the initial rate of dissolution, as is the ability of a disintegrant to absorb water and swell (15).

In 1983, Proost et al. (15) compared the swelling capacities of two disintegrants, starch and sodium starch glycolates, and found that the latter has a stronger swelling capacity and is less prone to a decrease in the dissolution rate as would be caused by a hydrophobic lubricant in the formulation. When potato starch was employed as a disintegrant in diazepam tablets, the disintegration times and dissolution rates varied substantially, depending on the mixing time with magnesium stearate. However, when sodium starch glycolate was used as the disintegrant, sufficient swelling of the tablet occurred such that drug substance in the inner of the tablets became exposed and dissolved readily (Fig. 19). As a result, the mixing time with magnesium stearate did not have an effect on dissolution.

The processes of disintegration, wettability, and solubilization during dissolution were investigated by Buckton (16) using compensation analysis. It was proposed that there are basically two mechanisms of disintegration, interfacial and diffusional. When the free energy of the wetting process varied widely, a more reliable enthalpy-free energy compensation plot and the

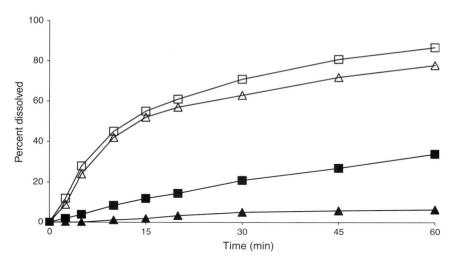

**Figure 19** Dissolution profiles of diazepam with the paddle method at 50 rpm. (■) potato starch, 2 min mixing time for magnesium stearate; (▲) potato starch, 30 min mixing time for magnesium stearate; (□) sodium starch glycolate, 2 min mixing time with magnesium stearate; (△) sodium starch glycolate, 30 min mixing time with magnesium stearate. *Source*: Adapted from Ref. 15.

expansion rate constants could be obtained (Fig. 20). Based on the values of expansion rate constants, disintegrants can be sorted into one of two classes. Examples of interfacial disintegrants include Polyplasdone® XL and Ac-Di-Sol®, while Primojel® and Avicel PH-101 are diffusional disintegrants.

Even though the hydrophilic property of a disintegrant is highly desirable, exposing a tablet formulation to high humidities may have an adverse effect on the dissolution process. Recently Rohrs et al. (17) investigated the reason for the decrease in the dissolution of delavirdine mesylate tablets upon exposure to high humidity (Fig. 21). Croscarmellose sodium was used as the disintegrant in delavirdine tablets, and its carboxyl sites were found by FT-IR to be protonated at high humidity. It was proposed that water had served as a plasticizer as well as a reaction medium for the drug and disintegrant. The protonated carboxyl moieties of croscarmellose sodium reacted with liberated methanesulfonic acid in the solid state. Solid-state NMR spectrometry was used to demonstrate that 30% of the delavirdine mesylate salt had converted to its less soluble free base form.

### Effect of Lubricants

Lubricants are used to improve the processing characteristics of drug powder during compression by improving the flowability of the drug powder and its adhesion onto the surface of the punch and die. Talc,

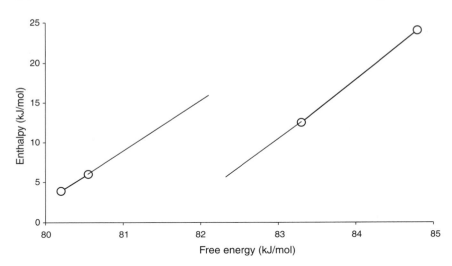

**Figure 20** Free energy–enthalpy compensation plot for the disintegration of four different tablet formulations, two of which have been shown to disintegrate by an interfacial and two by a diffusional mechanism. *Source*: Adapted from Ref. 16.

magnesium stearate, stearic acid, and hydrogenated vegetable oils are commonly used lubricants. In order to be an effective lubricant, a thin coat forms on the drug powder or granulation particles. However, due to the hydrophobic nature of these lubricants, the thin coating outside the drug powder repels water and reduces the rate of dissolution (18). Different lubricant types were investigated by Levy and Gurutow regarding their effects on the dissolution of salicylic acid tablets (19). The authors confirmed that a hydrophobic lubricant such as magnesium stearate could reduce the rate of dissolution, whereas a hydrophilic lubricant such as sodium lauryl sulfate (SLS) drastically increased the dissolution rate (Fig. 22). However, in additional to the hydrophilic property of SLS, its surface-active characteristics and its ability to increase the pH in the microenvironment around a weak acid drug powder were also found to be critical in enhancing the dissolution rates. For example, when Carbowax™ 4000 was used as a water-soluble lubricant to produce sodium salicylate tablets, the rates of dissolution were actually reduced in comparison to tablets that used magnesium stearate as the lubricant (20). It appears that when a hydrophobic lubricant is used in the formulation and it is desirable to increase the dissolution rates, then a hydrophilic lubricant with surfactant characteristics could be included to obtain the appropriate effect.

### Effect of Binders

Binders are excipients used to improve the cohesive properties of drug powders and formulations so that the final tablets will remain intact after

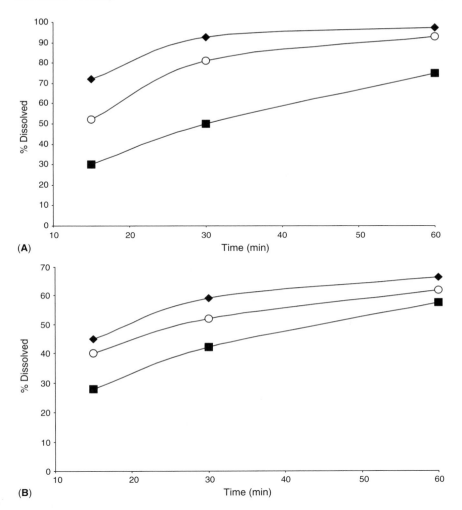

**Figure 21** Dissolution profiles of delavirdine 200 mg tablets (**A**) before and (**B**) after eight weeks of exposure to 40°C/75% RH, at paddle rotation speed of (■) 50 rpm, (○) 75 rpm, and (◆) 100 rpm. *Source*: Adapted from Ref. 17.

compression. During the wet granulation process, a binding agent can be first mixed with the drug as a dry powder before water is added, or it can be added to the drug powder as a solution (which is considered to be a more effective method in coming into contact with and wetting the drug particles). This hydrophilic property of a granulating agent has been shown to be important in enhancing the rates of dissolution of prednisone granules and phenobarbital tablets (Fig. 23). Solvang and Finholta have also reported that gelatin has significantly enhanced the dissolution

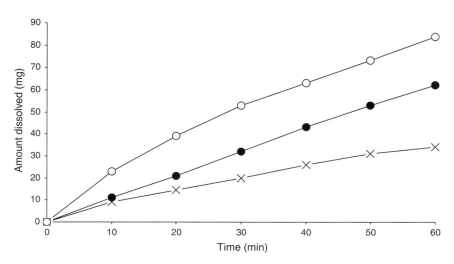

**Figure 22** Effect of lubricant on dissolution rate of salicylic acid contained in compressed tablets. (X) 3% magnesium stearate; (●) no lubricant; (○) 3% sodium lauryl sulfate. *Source*: Adapted from Ref. 19.

of phenobarbital tablets in gastric fluid more than does sodium carboxymethylcellulose or polyethylene glycol 6000 (21). It was proposed that polyethylene glycol can form an insoluble complex with phenobarbital and sodium carboxymethylcellulose, yielding a less soluble cellulose derivative in an acidic environment. Similar results of faster dissolution profiles were found when carboxymethylcellulose, ethylcellulose, and gelatin were used in preparing sulfadiazine and phenacetin in tablets (22,23). However, it should be noted that increasing the amount of gelatin as a binder can result in tablets with greater hardness and slower dissolution rates.

In making a decision regarding the composition of the final formulation, a formulator can compare the probe formulations by examining either the dissolution profiles or the animal bioavailability data. One advantage of utilizing the dissolution data to choose a final formulation is that a dissolution test can be performed in a short period of time and it is much less labor intensive than performing animal studies. However, a desirable dissolution profile is often unknown until the actual dissolution test is performed and some in vivo correlations have been established with the dissolution results. In developing a dissolution method for screening formulations, scientists often need to vary the dissolution media and other dissolution parameters.

After a final formulation has been selected, scaled-up batches will be made and they are often prepared by employing a different manufacturing process or equipment. As such, dissolution testing has been found to be a

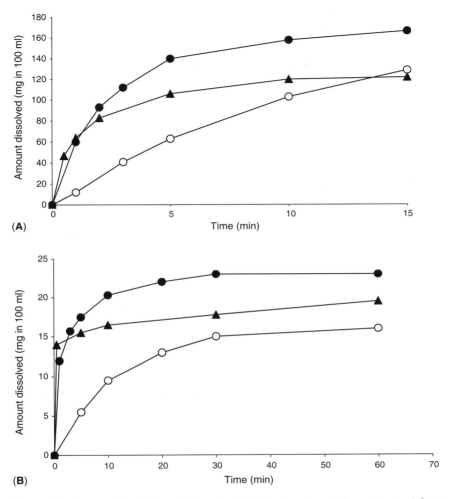

**Figure 23** Rate of dissolution of phenobarbital (*top*) and prednisone (*bottom*) from powder, granules, and tablets in diluted gastric juice. (O) powder; (▲) granules; (●) tablets. *Source*: Adapted from Ref. 21.

quality control tool to ensure that the final products possess the same physicochemical characteristics, bioavailabilities, and efficacies.

## Quality Control

In an effort to ensure that tablets with the same properties can be produced each time, pharmaceutical scientists have utilized in vitro testing as a quality control tool in (a) developing formulations, (b) assessing or modifying a manufacturing process, and (c) assuring the bioequivalency of a marketed product. The batch-to-batch quality of a product is often determined by conducting dissolution tests with defined procedures and the acceptance criteria are based on conclusions drawn from previous experimental data of the same product. Generally, it is expected that the in vivo performance of a product can be predicted and correlated with the in vitro dissolution data generated from an appropriate dissolution method.

The criteria for accepting or failing a batch is often referred to as the "$Q$" value of specification. This $Q$ value is the amount of dissolved active ingredient at a specific time point, expressed as a percentage of the total amount of active in the product. The acceptance criteria of USP dissolution tests on IR oral dosages are summarized in Table 1. A product can be subjected to a total of three stages of testing depending upon the results in stage 1 (S1) and stage 2 (S2) during a dissolution experiment. If a product passes the acceptance criteria at a given stage, there is no need to go to the next stage of testing. However, if a dissolution method possesses the ability to discriminate products with varying physicochemical properties, it is expected that a product may sometimes need to go to S2 or S3 before it passes the set specifications.

Setting the dissolution specifications for extended-release or enteric-coated dosage forms takes into consideration the required in vivo release characteristics suitable for that particular product. For example, an extended-release product is meant to allow the patient to take the medication less frequently (e.g., once or twice a day) by releasing the drug into the gastrointestinal tract for absorption at a constant rate. Thus, an ideal dissolution profile is close to a zero-order release kinetic while the amount of drug dissolved at a given time is within a predetermined range. The acceptance criteria for an extended-release dosage in the USP are listed in Table 2.

The goal of enteric coating is to delay the release of an active ingredient until the oral dosage reaches the intestine. It can serve one of two purposes: (*i*) to protect an acid-labile drug from degrading in the stomach;

**Table 1** Acceptance Criteria of USP Dissolution Test Intended for Immediate-Release Products

| Stage | Number tested | Acceptance criteria |
|---|---|---|
| $S_1$ | 6 | Each unit is not less than $Q + 5\%$ |
| $S_2$ | 6 | Average of 12 units ($S_1 + S_2$) is equal to or greater than $Q$, and no unit is less than $Q - 15\%$ |
| $S_3$ | 12 | Average of 24 units ($S_1 + S_2 + S_3$) is equal to or greater than 0, not more than 2 units are less than $Q - 15\%$, and no unit is less than $Q - 25\%$ |

*Source*: Adapted from USP 30/NF 25, 2007.

**Table 2** Acceptance Criteria of USP Dissolution Test Intended for Extended-Release Products

| Level | Number tested | Acceptance criteria |
|---|---|---|
| $L_1$ | 6 | No individual value lies outside each of the stated ranges and no individual value is less than the stated amount at the final test time |
| $L_2$ | 6 | The average value of the 12 units ($L_1 + L_2$) lies within each of the stated ranges and is not less than the stated amount at the final test time; none is more than 10% of the labeled content outside each of the stated ranges; and none is more than 10% of the labeled content below the stated amount at the final test time |
| $L_3$ | 12 | The average value of the 24 units ($L_1 + L_2 + L_3$) lies within each of the stated ranges and is not less than the stated amount at the final test time; not more than 2 of the 24 units are more than 10% of the labeled content outside each of the stated ranges; not more than 2 of the 24 units are more than 10% of the labeled content below the stated amount at the final test time; and none of the units is more than 20% of the labeled content outside each of the stated ranges or more than 20% of labeled content below the stated amount at the final test time |

*Source*: Adapted from USP 30/NF 25, 2007.

(*ii*) to avoid irritation of the upper gastrointestinal (GI) tract caused by the drug. Dissolution testing of an enteric-coated dosage consists of two phases. First dissolution is performed in an acidic medium (e.g., 0.1N hydrochloric acid) that mimics the conditions in the stomach. Subsequently, the same dosage is taken to a buffered dissolution medium (e.g., pH 6.8 phosphate buffer) to simulate the environment in the intestine. Ideally, an enteric-coated dosage should have a minimal release of the active in the acidic phase and a complete release of the active in the buffer phase. The USP acceptance criteria for the acid and buffer phases are summarized in Tables 3 and 4.

The timing for setting specifications depends on the amount and the quality of available dissolution data on the product. In a recent AAPS/FDA Workshop on dissolution of special dosage forms, it was suggested that setting specifications for dissolution studies as a quality control should be based primarily on data collected after the manufacture of pivotal clinical batches and biobatches. There can be instances where only limited dissolution data are available for setting a specification. An interim specification is found to be suitable in these cases, and the specifications can be finalized after the manufacture of three production batches (24).

**Table 3**  Acceptance Criteria of USP Acid Phase Dissolution Intended for Enteric-Coated Products

| Level | Number tested | Acceptance criteria |
|-------|---------------|---------------------|
| $A_1$ | 6 | No individual value exceeds 10% dissolved. |
| $A_2$ | 6 | Average of the 12 units $(A_1 + A_2)$ is not more than 10% dissolved, and no individual unit is greater than 25% dissolved. |
| $A_3$ | 12 | Average of the 24 units $(A_1 + A_2 + A_3)$ is not more than 10% dissolved, and no individual unit is greater than 25% dissolved. |

*Source*: Adapted from USP 30/NF 25, 2007.

There are cases where it is not completely known if one can predict the in vivo performance of a product from in vitro dissolution data. Investigations of IVIVC between in vitro dissolution and in vivo bioavailability have then become increasingly important and can often be an important part of quality control (25). When certain preapproval and postapproval changes are made in excipients, equipment, manufacturing process, or manufacturing site, IVIVC investigations could lead to an improved product quality by setting more relevant dissolution specifications. A predictive IVIVC can also allow in vitro dissolution to replace expensive biostudies, which are required to demonstrate the bioequivalence of two different formulations.

## FDA Compliance

During the drug approval process, pharmaceutical companies are required to submit to the FDA in vitro dissolution data and related bioavailability results. Before a drug product is approved for use in humans, dissolution

**Table 4**  Acceptance Criteria of USP Buffer Phase Dissolution Intended for Enteric-Coated Products

| Level | Number tested | Acceptance criteria |
|-------|---------------|---------------------|
| $B_1$ | 6 | Each unit is not less than $Q + 5\%$ |
| $B_2$ | 6 | Average of 12 units $(B_1 + B_2)$ is equal to or greater than $Q$, and no unit is less than $Q - 15\%$ |
| $B_3$ | 12 | Average of 24 units $(B_1 + B_2 + B_3)$ is equal to or greater than $Q$, not more than 2 units are less than $Q - 15\%$, and no unit is less than $Q - 25\%$ |

*Source*: Adapted from USP 30/NF 25, 2007.

specifications are established to ensure that all batches produced are bioequivalent. The final dissolution specifications of a new product are then published in the USP as compendial standards as they will become the official specifications for subsequent products containing the same active ingredients. For IR products, the compendial dissolution standards are in general single-point specifications in comparison to profile specifications for modified-release products.

In the New Drug Applications (NDAs), the qualities of the raw drug substance and the final product are described in details in the chemistry, manufacturing, and controls (CMC) section to ensure that the same product can be manufactured each time. Also included in the NDAs are the physicochemical properties and pharmacokinetics data of a drug product as this information is often used in the considerations of defining the dissolution specifications. In August 1997, the FDA published a guidance entitled "Guidance for Industry: Dissolution Testing of Immediate Release Solid Oral Dosage Forms." One of the purposes of this guidance is to set the precedent in defining when dissolution testing can be used to waive certain in vivo bioequivalence studies. It states that for IR products with multiple strengths, biowaivers can be provided for the lower strengths of the same dosage form provided that the pharmacokinetics is linear. In addition, the lower strengths need to be similar in composition within the scope of changes covered under the SUPAC-IR guidance. If these two requirements are met, a bioequivalence study may be performed at the highest strength using a pivotal clinical/ bioequivalence batch, and based on a comparison of the dissolution profiles, in vivo bioequivalence studies can be waived for the lower strengths.

Following the publication of the guidance on IR dosage form, FDA issued another guidance in September 1997, entitled "Guidance for Industry: Extended-Release Oral Dosage Forms—Development, Evaluation and Application of In Vitro/In Vivo Correlations." This guidance has listed the requirements for applying biowaivers of extended-release products. Much emphasis has been put on the methodologies in determining IVIVC, setting dissolution specification based on a predictable IVIVC, documenting when it is necessary to demonstrate bioequivalency during the initial approval process or after certain pre- or postapproval changes are made in the formulation, equipment, process, and manufacturing site changes. Since the publication of this FDA guidance, investigations of IVIVC between in vitro dissolution and in vivo bioavailability have increasingly becoming an integral part of extended-release drug-product development. Furthermore, the principles of IVIVC are considered to be similar for nonoral dosage forms, the guidance for oral extended-release products may be applied for nonoral products as well. Although the principles are likely to be the same, it is interesting to examine alternative dissolution methods for dissolution and IVIVC for special dosage forms such as cream, gel, or liposome formulations (25).

Two important recent regulatory developments in dissolution are the application of the Biopharmaceutics Classification Scheme (26) in granting biowaiver status and the recommendation of a more physiologically relevant dissolution medium by the regulatory agency. In August 2000, a guidance was issued on "Waiver of In Vivo Bioavailability and Bioequivalence Studies for Immediate-Release Solid Oral Dosage Forms Based on a Biopharmaceutics Classification System (BCS)." According to the BCS, drug substances are classified as follows:

Class 1: high solubility, high permeability
Class 2: low solubility, high permeability
Class 3: high solubility, low permeability
Class 4: low solubility, low permeability

The BCS approach for applying biowaivers as described in the guidance is focused on a drug substance with high solubility and high permeability (i.e., class I drug substance). It is accepted that differences observed in the rate and extent of in vivo absorption may be due to a difference in the in vivo dissolution rates. However, when an IR solid oral dosage form has a faster dissolution rate relative to the gastric emptying time, the rate and extent of absorption is not going to be dependent on the dissolution rate and the gastrointestinal transit time. Under such conditions, it may not be necessary to demonstrate in vivo bioequivalency or bioavailability of class I drug substances in IR products, provided rapid in vitro dissolution can be shown using the recommended test methods [21 CFR 320.22(e)]. This is a significant step initiated by the FDA in reducing the number of human clinical studies and burdens on the pharmaceutical companies during the drug approval process while the rationales are based on purely scientific principles.

To develop dissolution tests that better predict the in vivo performance of drug products, a biologically relevant dissolution medium is often suggested by the regulatory agency. Dressman et al. have investigated the physiological conditions of the human gastrointestinal tract (27). The composition, volume, flow rates, and mixing patterns of gastrointestinal fluids have been taken into considerations for the design of a dissolution test. The composition of the dissolution media, the hydrodynamics, and duration of the test are all critical parameters of a predictive dissolution test. As certain medications can be taken with food or in an empty stomach, a physiologically relevant dissolution media will be FeSSIF (fed state simulated intestinal fluid) or FaSSIF (fast state simulated intestinal fluid) under these circumstances.

For example, Galia et al. studied the dissolution behavior of two poorly soluble drugs, GR-92132X and GV-118819X, using a dissolution medium that simulates the fed or fasted states of the gastrointestinal tract

(28). It was shown that the composition of the dissolution medium had a greater effect on the dissolution results than the difference in the formulations. Dissolution profiles using the FaSSIF and FeSSIF have correctly predicted the insignificance of formulation effects, and also the importance of improved absorption when the drug was administered after meals.

A biorelevant dissolution method was explored by Tang et al. to study the effect of surfactant concentrations in the dissolution medium (29). Three formulations of a poorly soluble new chemical entity were designed to enhance bioavailabilities. The dissolution rates were compared to corresponding in vivo bioavailability data in dogs. It was concluded that a nonsink-condition dissolution medium containing 0.25% SLS gave dissolution results with better IVIVC than a dissolution medium with higher SLS concentrations.

The observed difference in dissolution behavior between class I and class II drugs in a physiologically based media was also investigated by Galia et al. (30). Two class I drugs (acetaminophen and metoprolol) and three class II drugs (danazol, mefenamic acid, and ketoconazole) were chosen to predict the trends of in vivo performance using the following dissolution media: water, simulated gastric fluid, milk, simulated intestinal fluid without pancreatin, FaSSIF, and FeSSIF. It was found that all class I drug powders dissolved rapidly in the media tested. On the other hand, dissolution of class II drugs was greatly affected by the choice of medium. For example, dissolution profiles of danazol capsule formulations were found to be highly dependent on the concentration of the solubilizing agent in the dissolution media. There was a 30-fold increase in dissolution at 90 minutes upon changing the dissolution medium from an aqueous medium without surfactants to FaSSIF. The use of FeSSIF or milk as a dissolution medium has given an even higher dissolution rate and the amount dissolved has increased by 100- and 180-fold respectively. As mefenamic acid is a weak acid, dissolution of mefenamic capsule formulations is dependent on both pH and bile salt concentration. Ketoconazole is a weak base and a tablet formulation dissolved completely in simulated gastric fluid without pepsin within 30 minutes (Fig. 24). However, only 6% had dissolved in two hours under the fast state conditions. In summary, dissolution of a class II drug has been shown to be in general much more dependent on the dissolution medium than class I drugs.

## Conditions

A significant portion of method development consists of establishing the conditions of the dissolution test. This would include the selection of a dissolution apparatus and the composition of the solvent contained within the dissolution vessel.

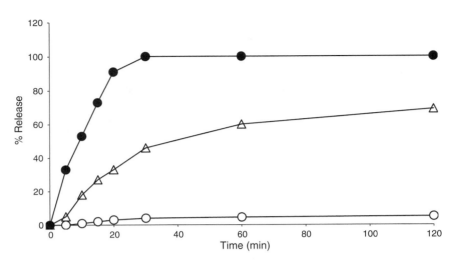

**Figure 24** Mean dissolution profiles of ketoconazole from Nizoral tablets in various media at 100 rpm. (●) simulated gastric fluid; (○) fast state simulated intestinal fluid; (△) fed state simulated intestinal fluid. *Source*: Adapted from Ref. 30.

The standard arrangement for a dissolution tester has six vessels, though most are manufactured with the capability of containing eight vessels. The default standard of testing six dosage units at a time evolved from the original dissolution testing instruments and has proved to be a statistically acceptable number. The additional two vessels, when used, often contain a blank and a standard solution, especially useful for instruments connected to automated sampling devices.

The most frequently used dissolution testing configurations are USP Apparatus 1 and Apparatus 2, more commonly referred to as the paddle and the basket, respectively. Each of these configurations uses the same instrument and vessel arrangement. The principal differences lie with the location of the dissolving dosage unit and the manner of stirring the dissolution media within the vessel. Thus we can examine some common issues with both the basket and the paddle methods. These issues mainly deal with the mechanics of the instrument that provides the base and heating elements for the media in the vessels and the mechanics for attachment and turning of the shafts that are affixed to the baskets and paddles (31).

To maintain maximum reproducibility, the relationship between the shaft and the vessel is to be such that the shaft is to be as close to vertical as possible (to avoid wobble) and is centered within the vessel (within ±2 mm of the center axis of the vessel according to the USP). Each of these mechanical parameters can be tested and measured using commercially available instruments designed for the purpose. Such positions of the shaft relative to the vessels of media are to assure the consistence and reproducibility of mixing. Significant deviations could result in as much as a 25% deviation in dissolution concentration measurements (32).

Another mechanical check involves the stirring speed, typically measured using the revolutions per minutes (rpm) of the shaft. Current requirements state that the actual rpm (or speed) of the shaft is to be within 4% of the desired speed. This would mean within 2 rpm for a shaft set to 50 rpm. The rotational speed can be measured with a commercial tachometer.

The dissolution instrument is to be level in order to maintain the proper vessel orientation and shaft positioning. The typical dissolution testing instrument has adjustable feet used to level the device, which can be verified with a carpenter's level of suitable length. The level should be from front to back as well as from side to side.

There is no mention in the USP of a vibration requirement, except for the statement "No part of the assembly, including the environment in which the assembly is placed, contributes significant motion, agitation, or vibration beyond that due to the smoothly rotating stirring element." Vibration is a complicated concept that can result in the addition of energy to a system. The addition of energy from an external source can alter the results of a dissolution evaluation. Such an alteration is an unacceptable source of error that must be minimized. It can be minimized by eliminating all external sources so that only the tester machinery is left as a potential vibration source that is external to the drug delivery system under evaluation. The energy (vibration) causing movement is an interrelated function involving acceleration, velocity, displacement, and frequency (which can occur in three dimensions). From the available research, the more important of these vectors has been the $z$-axis (i.e., up and down). Most current research has concentrated on the up and down plane, and the value most reported is displacement. The units used for displacement is "mil," which is an English unit that corresponds to 0.001 inch. As a measure of vibration, displacement is often reported, since it is this relative motion that can be sensed by placing a hand on the tester. This is a measure of the up and down motion of the item of interest, in this instance a dissolution tester. How often this up and down motion occurs is of equal importance, and this is the frequency. To measure one without the other does not provide sufficient information concerning the overall vibration. Vibrations of the same displacement but with differing frequency would not input the same amount of energy into a system over a given period of time. Vibrations in the range of 0.1 mil and above in the frequency of 50 to 150 Hz are potentially harmful to dissolution results (33,34).

There are several other operational specifications designed to assure consistency. This includes the location of the basket and paddle within the vessel. Previous mechanical checks included the vertical position and centering of the shaft. The remaining specification is the depth of placement of the basket and paddle within the vessel. The USP requirement is $25 \pm 2$ mm from the curved bottom of the vessel to the bottom of the basket and the paddle. This height can be set and/or checked with commercial, validated instruments. The temperature of the media in each vessel also needs verification prior to each dissolution evaluation. Many modern dissolution testers have validated temperature probes designed to measure and monitor the temperature within each vessel.

Apparatus Selection

Having established that all potential dissolution devices have been mechanically verified, the choice of conditions is the next step in dissolution method development. The choice of conditions would involve selection of the apparatus and its operational conditions, the dissolution medium, selection of the number and timing of samples, and the end point (35,36).

The choice of apparatus is usually restricted to one of the seven USP compendial dissolution devices. Selection may be limited to apparatus design and availability. Most dissolution methods use either Apparatus 1 or Apparatus 2. Apparatus 1 tends to work best for drug delivery systems that float and/or contain small bead-like components that disintegrate slowly and for capsules containing light or fluffy components. Apparatus 2 works best for drug delivery systems that sink on their own, such as compressed tablets and capsules with dense components. Selection of agitation or stirring speed is dependent upon the desired outcome. The speed should be sufficient to assure an even mixture of dissolved drug in the media for sampling, yet allow the test to differentiate between a good product and a bad product. Differences in the dissolution pattern are more likely to be observed at lower (slower) stirring speeds (50–75 rpm for baskets and 25–50 for paddles). However, mixing would be more complete, and even at higher stirring speeds, which for the basket is 75 to 100 rpm and for the paddle is 50 to 75. The ranges are considered roughly equivalent between these two apparatus (31).

As was previously discussed, both Apparatus 3 and Apparatus 4 were designed for modified-release drug delivery systems (its design was based upon the rotating bottle). A distinct advantage of Apparatus 3 is the more vigorous agitation, which is similar to holding and shaking a container. Agitation speed is set as dips per minute (dpm), typically in the range of 5 to 30. As the dosage unit is placed inside a glass cylinder, screens are placed on each end (a variety of micron openings are available) to prevent the escape of any pieces that may have formed during the process. This works well for bead-type systems. As there are several rows of dissolution flasks, a pH gradient can easily be established. Thus this could be useful for delayed-release type systems (such as enteric coated). Evaporation could be an issue for extended-release products, but newer evaporation caps have limited this issue.

The theory behind Apparatus 4 is the best of all compendial devices concerning concentration gradient and sink effect. When used as an open system, there is a perfect sink effect, as fresh media is constantly provided for dissolution of drug from the delivery system. As fractions of sample are collected, drug content can be analyzed immediately, without waiting for the end of the run. This is very convenient for drugs with limited stability in solution. Nondisintegrating drug delivery systems work best, as these minimize the possibility of loss of sample and clogging of filters and sample tubing. This is another environment in which change of pH is extremely easy, simply by changing the source of dissolution media that is being pumped through the cells past the dosage unit. As this set-up is more difficult to use, it has been largely avoided in the United States to this point, though there seems to be an increasing interest. With the many poorly soluble substances being examined, this is a method that could be very beneficial.

Originally designed for transdermal patches, Apparatus 7 has most recently been used to solve specific dissolution method problems. In external appearance, this device can resemble an Apparatus 3. The fundamental difference is mechanical, with a dip having an amplitude of only 2 cm and not the 10 cm found in Apparatus 3. This gentler mixing was sufficient for modified-release, nondisintegrating drug delivery systems in that dosage unit attachment to a holder on Apparatus 7 could guarantee the orientation of delivery systems during dissolution analysis. Specifically, one holder was used for an osmotic delivery system that utilized a laser-drilled hole to expel drug that went into solution. In order to obtain consistent results, the location of the exit for drug solution must be known and constant.

Apparatus 5, 6, and 7 were originally intended for transdermal patch dissolution. Temperature of the receptor media is to be set at 32°C, the average temperature of the surface of the skin. Of these methods, for the first time or novice user, Apparatus 5 would be the method of choice, which presents the least expensive alternative. This apparatus is based upon a standard Apparatus 2, and all that is needed is a patch holder of some type to which the patch is attached and placed in the bottom of the vessel. Thus, it is similar to using a sinker on a dosage form that floats. An agitation rate of 75 to 100 rpm would be typical. Apparatus 6 is more expensive, as six cylinder devices must be purchased, but the mixing action is more uniform for the patch (it is not located in the bottom of the vessel). Stirring rate does not need to be as high as the paddle, but more in the 50 rpm range, since the patch is attached to the stirring device. This would reduce the effect of a diffusion layer forming near the release surface of the patch. Apparatus 7 has the vertical stroke mixing previously described, which can also minimize the diffusion layer effect. The agitation rate would typically be in the 5 to 15 dpm range.

Modifications of these compendial apparatuses would fall in the area of dosage form introduction, effect of entrapped air, and receptor media composition and volume. Depending on the apparatus, a sinker may be needed for a dosage unit that would typically float. Considerations must be made for both the initial unit being introduced and what happens to the unit after introduction into the media, such as disintegration and/or release of small particles or beads. Compendial sinkers include the USP description of a "few twists of wire" and the JP sinker cages. There are various "unofficial" adaptations, including a plastic, three-prong capsule holders, "mini-baskets," paperclips, and others.

Media

Selection of the dissolution, or receptor, media tend to be limited to aqueous-based solutions (37–39). Selections typically include such solutions as water (deaerated), buffered aqueous solution (pH 4–6.8), and dilute acid (0.001–0.1N HCl). The volume selected depends on drug delivery system formulation and choice of apparatus. For Apparatus 1, 2, 5, and 6, typical volume selection is in the range of 500 to 1000 mL (though the USP describes other vessels with volumes of 2000–4000 mL). Smaller vessels in the range of 100 to 200 mL are also available. Apparatus 4 would have a volume dependent upon flow rate, while Apparatus 3 and 7 typically use individual vessel volumes in the 200 to 300 mL range, though a single unit can be exposed to 1500 mL if several rows are utilized during the evaluation. There are also some smaller and larger size vessels available for each of these methods. Selection of receptor volume should include consideration of maintaining a proper "sink effect." This can most easily be described as having sufficient excess volume to limit or prevent a significant change in dissolution rate of active from its solid state as a function of the amount of active in solution. This can be accomplished for most molecules if the volume of solution is no closer than 30% of the volume required to form a saturated solution (in other words, the concentration is 70% of saturation). By comparison, during the development of a new chemical entity, the target is much less, being no closer than 90% of the value for saturation (having a maximum concentration of 10% of saturation). This is commonly referred to as a 10-fold dilution.

Deaeration

Another significant media factor is deaeration. This is a much misunderstood factor, though its effect and subsequent importance is well documented. It is often discussed in the context of the effect of dissolved gas on the dissolution process. However, dissolved gas would have no effect on the dissolution of a drug. It is the existence of excess gas in the solution, in the form of bubbles, which can and often do have a significant adverse effect on the rate of dissolution. Bubbles at an interface (surface of dosage unit, within a screen through which media must flow, within the bulk of the media, and other locations) would decrease the effective contact surface area for dissolving molecule and receptor media, with obvious effect. The common process of "deaeration" cannot remove all dissolved gas, but can remove the excess that contributes to the formation of bubbles. Thus if bubbles are an issue within the media of choice, then this should be incorporated as one of the preparation steps.

To enhance the dissolution of the molecule of interest, other ingredients can be added to the receptor media. Using the fundamental principles of solutions, the addition of electrolytes, surfactants, and other solubility-enhancing agents may be necessary (including various pH values). Cosolvents cannot be routinely used in the dissolution media. Water remains the primary media ingredient. Hydroalcoholic media are generally not permitted, unless the use of such a cosolvent supports a documented IVIVC (50). If the receptor media allows dissolving of drug too easily, the test may experience a "loss of discriminatory power." This is often a difficult distinction.

## New Chemical Entity Dissolution Method Development

The physicochemical properties of the drug substance will determine the dissolution profile characteristics of its products under various conditions. In order to develop a dissolution method that gives relevant physiological meanings with convenient sampling times and enough sink conditions, the aqueous solubilities of the drug substance need to be known ahead of time. This information is becoming increasingly important as many of the new chemical entities in the pharmaceutical industries are poorly soluble, and the solubility values are significantly less than 1 mg/mL. Having to meet the challenges of working with poorly soluble compounds, formulation scientists have developed lipid-based or other surfactant-based drug delivery systems to enhance the solubility of drug substance and the bioavailability of the drug product.

### Information Needed for Dissolution "Solubility"

According to the Noyes–Whitney equation, the saturation solubility of the drug substance is a major factor in determining the dissolution rate. However, the saturation solubilities of a new chemical entity can vary depending upon the conditions in which the solubility experiment is conducted. The following three factors should be considered in setting up a solubility experiment: temperature, pH of the vehicle, and ionization constants of the drug substance.

*Temperature effect—25°C versus 37°C.* Saturation solubility can be defined as the concentration of a dissolved drug substance in a solvent, which is in an equilibrium state with an excess amount of solid in the system. Thus, the solubility is a constant value at a given temperature and pressure, provided the physical form of the drug substance is the same. In the development stage of a product, solubility is often determined at room temperatures or ~25°C. On the other hand, routine dissolution testing is to be performed at 37°C to represent the physiological temperature of the human body. In order to establish a correct assessment of the sink condition provided by a dissolution medium, it is desirable to determine the solubility at different temperatures (40). In general, a linear relationship between temperature and solubility can be expressed by the van't Hoff equation:

$$\ln(S) = \frac{-\Delta H}{RT} + b \qquad (10)$$

where $S$ is the saturation solubility at an absolute temperature $T$, $R$ is the gas constant, $\Delta H$ is the apparent heat of solution, and $b$ is an arbitrary constant (41). The same equation can also be represented in another way by the Hildebrand plot.

$$\ln(S) = \frac{-a' \ln T}{R} + b' \qquad (11)$$

where $S$ is the saturation solubility at an absolute temperature $T$, $R$ is the gas constant, $a'$ is the apparent molar entropy of solution, and $b'$ is an arbitrary constant.

For practical purposes, the van't Hoff equation is often used because the heat of solution, $\Delta H$, of the drug substance can be readily determined by a solution calorimeter. If the solubility is known at 25°C, the constant $b$ can be calculated using the following equation:

$$b = \ln(S_{298}) + \left(\frac{\Delta H}{RT_{298}}\right) \qquad (12)$$

Assuming that $\Delta H$ is independent of temperatures, we can calculate the solubility of the drug substance at 37°C.

$$\ln(S_{310}) = \left(\frac{-\Delta H}{RT_{310}}\right) + \ln(S_{310}) + \left(\frac{\Delta H}{RT_{298}}\right) \qquad (13)$$

*pH effect.* The pH of a solvent has a profound effect on the saturation solubility of a drug substance especially when the drug is an acid or a base. For weak acids and bases, the solubility values are highly dependent on the ionization states of the drug substance because the ionized species of a drug is in general more soluble. In determining the solubility of a drug substance, however, the buffer capacity of the solvent can sometimes be overcome by the dissolved drug. It is often true when the drug is soluble and exists as a salt of a strong acid or a strong base. In these cases, the pH of the solvent will change and it is necessary to report the final pH of the solubility samples.

If a compound is a weak acid, the observed solubility at a given pH can be represented by the following equation:

$$S_{obs} = S_{(HA)} + [A^-] \qquad (14)$$

where HA is the undissociated drug, $A^-$ is the anionic form of the drug, and SHA is the solubility of the free acid. The concentrations of the anionic and undissociated forms are also related to the pH and $pK_a$ of the drug molecule (Eqs. 15 and 16).

$$K_a = [H_3O^+] \otimes \frac{[A^-]}{[HA]} \tag{15}$$

$$pK_a = pH - \log\left(\frac{[A^-]}{[HA]}\right) = pH - \log[A^-] + \log[HA] \tag{16}$$

By rearranging the terms and taking an antilog on both sides of equations,

$$[A^-] = [HA]10^{(pH-pK_a)} \tag{17}$$

Substituting $(A^-)$ from Eq. 17 into Eq. 14:

$$S_{obs} = S_{(HA)}\left(1 + 10^{(pH-pK_a)}\right) \tag{18}$$

Thus, the solubility of the drug substance can be increased dramatically by raising the pH above the $pK_a$ value. Similarly, lowering the pH of the dissolution media can increase the solubility of a basic drug substance. However, limits exist for selecting the pH of a dissolution medium in order for it to be physiologically relevant.

Noory et al. have described three steps in developing a dissolution method for a sparingly water-soluble drug product (42). The first step is an evaluation of dissolution medium pH, followed by an investigation of employing different surfactants, and an examination of the surfactant concentrations. In selecting the choice of aqueous media, 0.1N HCl, pH 4.5 sodium acetate buffer, and pH 6.8 phosphate buffers are recommended. This covers the physiological pH range of the stomach and the small intestine where absorption of most drugs will take place.

As the number of compounds in discovery has increased as a result of combinatorial chemistry and high-throughput screening, methods to determine pH solubilities in a timely manner are needed. A recent advancement in the determination of pH-solubility profile is the use of potentiometric titrations for compounds with ionizable functional groups (43). The theory is based on a three-component model to determine the reactant concentrations at interfacial, diffusion layer, and the bulk water. Ten model drug molecules were selected to demonstrate the usefulness of this titration methodology. The commercially available compounds include cimetidine, diltiazem hydrochloride, enalapril maleate, metoprolol tartrate, nadolol, propoxyphene hydrochloride, quinine hydrochloride, terfenadine, trovafloxacin mesylate, and benzoic acid. Compared to the traditional shake-flask method, the titration method was shown to be faster in determining saturation solubilities.

*Dissociation constant—*$pK_a$. Compounds containing acidic or basic functional groups can become ionized in water depending on the value of the dissociation constant and the pH of dissolution media. As described in the pH section, the solubility of the ionized species is greater than the unionized molecule. Thus, the dissolution behavior can be dramatically different, depending on whether the pH of the dissolution media is above or below the $pK_a$ value of the drug substance.

For example, Parojcic et al. investigated the effect of pH on the dissolution of aspirin, which has an acidic $pK_a$ of 3.5 (44). Dissolution of aspirin tablets was performed at pH values representing the stomach in a fasting state (pH 1.2), and fed states (pH 3.0) and pHs 4.5 and 5.3 (Fig. 25). Based on the $pK_a$ value, the solubility of aspirin increases above pH 3.5 and the dissolution rate is expected to increase at the same time. In fact, a significant effect of pH was observed on the mean dissolution time (MDT) and the amount of drug dissolved after 30 min. A linear relationship between pH and first-order dissolution constant ($k_D$) was found except for one of the formulations, and the agitation speed had a significant effect on the dissolution for all formulations. In comparison to aspirin, paracetamol has a $pK_a$ significantly different from the pH range of the tested dissolution media. Because of this, there was no effect of the pH on the dissolution of paracetamol tablets other than an apparent linear relationship with the dissolution constant, $k_D$, for one of the paracetamol formulations. Use of bioavailability and bioequivalence data from the literature has allowed the authors to calculate and correlate in vivo MDTs with in vitro data. It was shown that the targeted MDT for paracetamol could be achieved regardless of the pH of the medium. For ASA tablets, the targeted MDT would differ depending on the pH of the dissolution media and the agitation speed. In an acidic pH environment, the in vitro agitation speed needs to be higher in order to achieve the same desirable in vivo MDT.

The combination effects of pH and surfactant on the dissolution of piroxicam were investigated by Jinno et al. (45). The intrinsic dissolution rate was measured in the pH range of 4.0 to 7.8 and the surfactant concentration varied from 0%, 0.5% to 2.0% SLS (Fig. 26). A theoretical model was established to predict the dissolution behavior of an ionizable water-insoluble drug as a function of pH and surfactant concentrations. In this model, a simple additive effect was considered based on the ionization equilibrium of the drug and two micellar solubilization equilibria of the surfactant. It was found that the experimental data were well predicted by the proposed model using a nonlinear regression analysis. Also, the mean $pK_a$ value of piroximan, 5.63, estimated from the solubility data, agreed well with the reported value. This established model could be useful in predicting the combined effects of pH and surfactants on the dissolution behavior of other water insolubles.

Polymorph and Salt Screening—Intrinsic Dissolution

Different polymorphic and salt forms of a new chemical entity can have radically different physicochemical properties including aqueous solubilities. During the drug development process, the solid form utilized by the discovery scientists may not have all the desirable characteristics for further development activities such as physical and chemical stabilities. In terms of

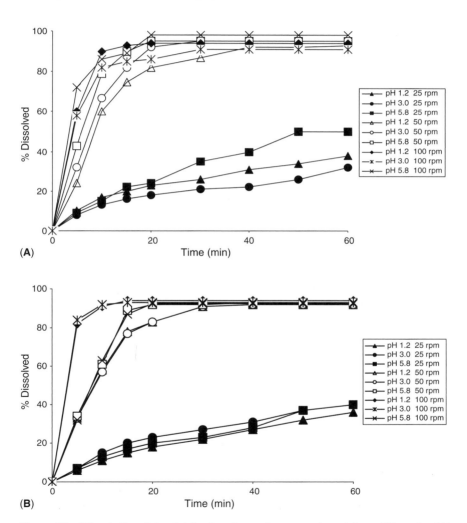

**Figure 25** Dissolution data obtained under various experimental conditions for (**A**) paracetamol immediate-release tablets lot no. 1; (**B**) paracetamol immediate-release tablets lot no. 2; (**C**) aspirin, plain tablets; and (**D**) aspirin, buffered tablets. *Source*: Adapted from Ref. 44.

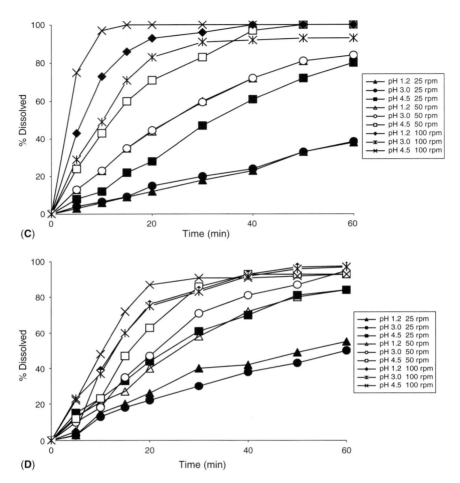

**Figure 25**   (continued).

physical stabilities, an ideal solid-state form should be crystalline and not amorphous. However, crystalline solids are significantly less soluble than the amorphous solid of the same compound. Because of this, it is often needed to produce a crystalline solid or another salt form with better aqueous solubilities. Having a more soluble solid-state form is especially important if the initial solid form has a very poor oral bioavailability. A higher solubility will also help the development scientists in developing an injectable formulation, which is required in order to establish absolute bioavailabilities.

In comparing the solubility characteristics of two different solid-state forms, intrinsic dissolution rates are used to minimize any effect caused by any difference in the particle size distributions of the drug substances.

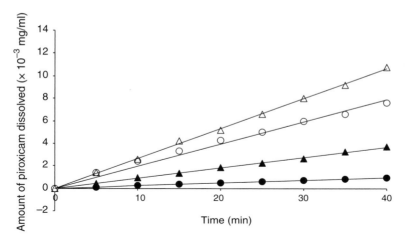

**Figure 26** Dissolution curves of piroxicam from the rotation disk at 50 rpm. (●) pH 4; (○) pH 6; (▲) pH 4 + 2% SLS; (△) pH 6 + 2% SLS. *Abbreviation*: SLS, sodium lauryl sulfate. *Source*: Adapted from Ref. 45.

The most common intrinsic dissolution procedure is the rotating "disc" or "plate" method where the drug powder is compressed into a disc-shaped tablet and only one face is exposed to the dissolution media (46). The experimental set-up is often referred to as the Wood's dissolution apparatus and the factors affecting the flux can be expressed by the Levich's equation (47):

$$\text{Intrinsic dissolution} = \frac{(dM/dt)}{A} = qD^{(2/3)}\omega^{(1/2)}v^{-(1/6)}S \tag{19}$$

where $M$ is the mass, $A$ is the exposed surface area, $q$ is a constant, $D$ is the diffusion constant, $\bar{\omega}$ is the rotational speed, $v$ is the viscosity of the medium, and $S$ is the saturation solubility. The dimension of the intrinsic dissolution rate is in mg/(cm$^2$ sec).

If the "disc" method is not readily available, the intrinsic dissolution rate can be determined by using a "powder" method. In this case, the surface area of the dry powder is first measured via a gas adsorption method and assumed to be equal to the initial wetted surface of the drug in the dissolution experiment.

It should be pointed out that the criteria for selecting a salt form and a polymorphic form during the product development process could be quite different. When several salts are being compared, the salt with the highest intrinsic dissolution rate is preferred. This is an attempt to maximize the in vivo dissolution rate and oral bioavailabilities provided that the selected salt form has comparable stabilities. On the other hand, in selecting polymorphs, the most stable form is often desirable. It means that the ideal polymorph will possess a lower intrinsic dissolution rate. Depending on whether two polymorphs are related monotropically or enantiotropically, the relative intrinsic dissolution rates can differ, depending on the temperature at which the experiment is conducted. An example of demonstrating the enantiotropic behavior of polymorphs is sulfathiazole (48). There are three crystalline forms of sulfathiazole (forms I, II, and III), all of which are kinetically stable at ambient temperatures. The initial intrinsic dissolution rates for these three forms were all different (form II > form I > form III), showing that form III is the most stable form under the experimental conditions (Fig. 27). During dissolution, forms I and II converted to form III, and the final dissolution rates became the same. When the melting points were determined for these three forms, it was found that form I is actually more stable at higher temperatures and has the highest melting point.

Other analytical techniques such as differential scanning calorimetry (DSC) have also been used to correlate the intrinsic dissolution results and polymorph characterizations (49). Two crystalline (forms I and II) and an amorphous form exist for terfenadine. The initial dissolution rates of amorphous, partial crystalline and crystalline samples of terfenadine polymorphs (forms I and II) were first measured using a rotating disk method. In addition, the heats of fusion due to the crystalline fraction of samples were obtained from the DSC data. It was found that the logarithms of initial dissolution rates of samples with different crystallinities were linearly

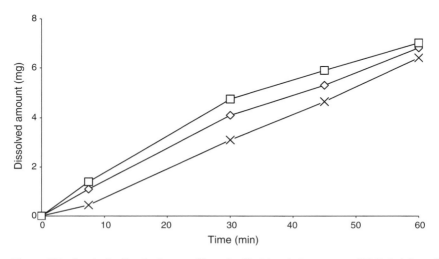

**Figure 27**   Intrinsic dissolution profiles of sulfathiazole in water at 37°C. (◇) form I; (□) form II; (x) form III. *Source*: Adapted from Ref. 48.

correlated with the corrected heats of fusion after the heat capacity of glass transitions was taken into account (Fig. 28).

Terada et al. have examined the use of isothermal microcalorimetry to estimate the initial dissolution rates (83). Different polymorphic forms and a glass of indomethacin were studied together with samples of terfenadine containing various degrees of crystallinities. The initial dissolution rates of these samples were determined by a rotating disk method at 25°C and the heats of solution of the same samples were measured by isothermal microcalorimetry. It was shown that the heats of solution have a linear relationship with the logarithms of initial dissolution rates for both indomethacin and terfenadine (Fig. 29). Also, the degree of crystallinity estimated by isothermal microcalorimetry can be predicted by the initial dissolution rates. The authors presented a theory on the relationship between the heat of solution and dissolution rates based on Gibbs free energy and Noyes–Whitney equation.

The same theory was applied on the characterization of carbamazepine, which can exist as three polymorphic forms (forms I, II, and III) and as a dehydrate (51). In additional to the initial dissolution rates, both the heats of solution and the heats of fusion were determined by microcalorimetry and DSC respectively. It was shown that a similar linear relationship existed between the logarithm of the initial dissolution rate and the heats of fusion or the heats of solutions (Fig. 30). It was proposed that all the three techniques could be applied as a quality control tool to assess the polymorph present in the drug substance.

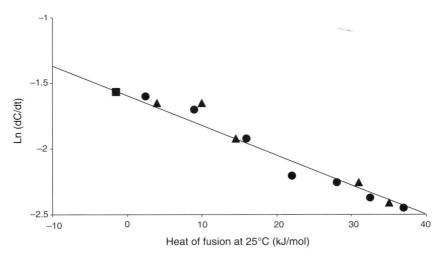

**Figure 28** Relationship between heat of fusion and logarithms of initial dissolution rate of terfenadine. (●) form I; (▲) form II; (■) glass. *Source*: Adapted from Ref. 49.

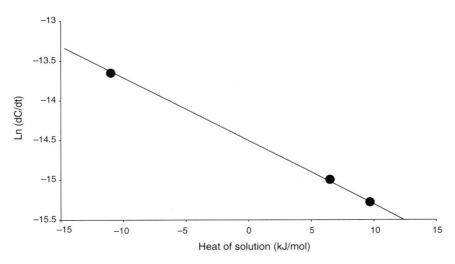

**Figure 29** Relationship between heat of solution and logarithm of initial dissolution rate of indomethacin polymorphs and glass at 25°C. *Source*: Adapted from Ref. 83.

## Drug Delivery System

### Peroral Administration

The dissolution characteristics of an oral formulation depend on the purpose and design of the dosage form. For an IR tablet, it is assumed that a

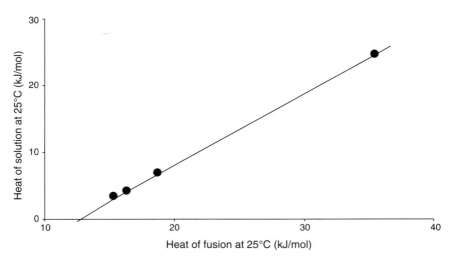

**Figure 30** Relationship between heat of fusion and heat of solution of carbamazepine. *Source*: Adapted from Ref. 51.

more rapidly dissolving formulation is preferred and more bioavailable. On the other hand, a rapid release of drug is not desirable in a modified-release dosage, especially when a large amount of drug is absorbed into the body in a short period of time for an extended-release dosage causing unwanted toxic or side effects. In this section, the dissolution profiles of various oral dosage forms are discussed.

Immediate Release

IR formulations are purposely designed to provide a rapid absorption of drug in the early section of the gastrointestinal tract, allowing for a fast onset of actions, such that sufficient plasma levels are achieved in a short period of time to produce the desired therapeutic effects. For certain categories of drugs, such as the pain medications, a rapid onset of action and relief of symptoms are highly preferred by the patients.

From the regulatory perspective, an IR product is considered to be rapidly dissolving when no less than 85% of the labeled drug substance amount dissolves within 30 minutes using the USP Apparatus 1 at 100 rpm or the Apparatus 2 at 50 rpm in a volume of 900 mL or less in each of the following dissolution media: (*i*) 0.1N HCl or simulated gastric fluid USP without enzymes; (*ii*) at pH 4.5 buffer; and (*iii*) a pH 6.8 buffer or simulated intestinal fluid USP without enzymes (FDA Guidance on "Waivers of In Vivo Bioavailability and Bioequivalence Studies for Immediate Release Solid Oral Dosage Forms based on Biopharmaceutics Classification System," Center for Drug Evaluation and Research, August 2000). This is a requirement that can be difficult to meet because many of the new chemical entities nowadays are poorly soluble and 0.1N HCl, pH 4.5, and pH 6.8 buffers usually cannot provide enough sink conditions for the drug to dissolve completely.

Various techniques have been used to improve the solubility and rates of dissolution of poorly soluble drug products such as varying the amount or choice of excipients, changing the manufacturing process from direct compression to wet granulation, increasing the agitation speed, and modifying the dissolution media. Sometimes, a hydroalcoholic dissolution medium is chosen to improve the solubility of the drug. However, adding an organic solvent to the dissolution medium has created concerns because it has no relevancy to the in vivo system. As the human body produces natural surfactants such as the bile salts, many scientists studied the effect of surfactants in enhancing the solubility of drug substance in the dissolution medium.

Galia et al. investigated the effects of surfactants on the dissolution of BCS class I (highly soluble, highly permeable) and BCS class II (poorly soluble, high permeable) compounds (30). The presence of a surfactant in FaSSIF has proved to give a 30-fold increase in the dissolution of danazol capsules within 30 minutes compared to an aqueous media (Fig. 31). The use of FeSSIF as the dissolution medium has given an even faster dissolution

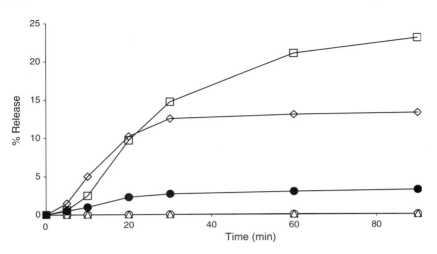

**Figure 31**  Mean dissolution profiles of danazol capsules in various media at 100 rpm. (○) water; (△) SIF; (●) fast state simulated intestinal fluid; (◇) fed state simulated intestinal fluid; (□) milk. *Source*: Adapted from Ref. 30.

rate of 100-fold. It was concluded that the dissolution behavior of class II compounds could be greatly affected by the choice of the dissolution medium.

Tang et al. studied the effect of surfactant concentration and sink conditions in the dissolution of poorly water-soluble compounds (29). Raising the concentration of a surfactant, SLS, could produce an increase in the intrinsic dissolution rate (Fig. 32). Sink conditions could also be achieved by using a high concentration of surfactant (e.g., 1% SLS) in the dissolution medium. However, when the in vivo data were compared to the dissolution result, a lower surfactant concentration was actually found to be better in predicting the in vivo results. As such, it is not desirable to select a very high concentration of surfactant in developing a dissolution method unless it is necessary to solubilize the drug.

The solubilizing effect of a surfactant can be quite different when the drug is ionized (45). For example, piroxicam is a weakly acidic drug with a $pK_a$ of 6.3. At a pH of 6.0, the drug is relatively unionized and the solubility is 0.2 mg/mL (Fig. 33). At a pH of 7.8, the drug becomes ionized and the solubility increases to 4.8 mg/mL. Adding SLS at 0.5% and 2% increases the intrinsic dissolution rate in an approximately additive manner. However, a simple additive model based on ionization equilibrium and two micellar solubilization equilibria demonstrates that SLS improves the solubilization of the unionized species only. The mean micellar solubilization coefficient for the unionized species of piroxicam was 348 L/mol compared to a value close to zero for the ionized species.

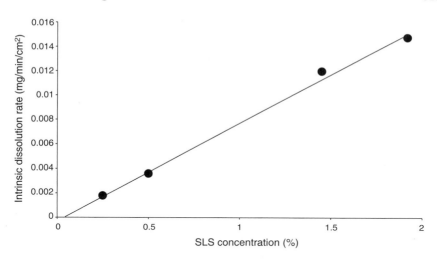

**Figure 32** Relationship between intrinsic dissolution rate and SLS concentration. *Abbreviation*: SLS, sodium lauryl sulfate. *Source*: Adapted from Ref. 29.

Noory et al. summarized the strategies of employing surfactants in developing dissolution methods for poorly soluble drug products (42). This is also a stepwise approach adopted by the FDA field laboratories in dissolution development to evaluate (*i*) the effects of pH, (*ii*) the type of surfactants, and (*iii*) the concentrations of surfactant. First of all, the solubility

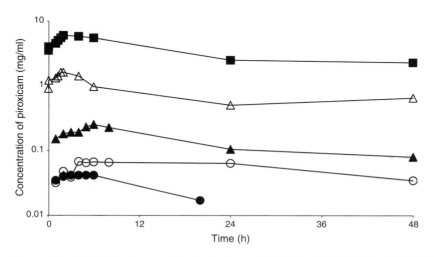

**Figure 33** Solubility time profile of piroxicam: (●) pH 4; (○) pH 5; (3) pH 6; (▲) pH 7; (△) pH 7.8. *Source*: Adapted from Ref. 45.

of the product is determined using standard USP dissolution media such as 0.1N HCl, pH 4.5 sodium acetate buffer, and pH 6.8 phosphate buffer. If none of the aqueous dissolution media provide a sufficient sink condition for the product, the need to use a surfactant in the dissolution media is warranted. In choosing a particular type of surfactant, anionic (e.g., SLS), cationic (e.g., cetyltriammonium bromide, CTAB), and nonionic (e.g., polysorbate or Tween) reagents should all be evaluated, as different drugs may react to the same surfactant differently. It was suggested that a 2% surfactant concentration could be a good starting point for testing the solubilizing effect of a surfactant. After a specific surfactant has been selected, the next step is to determine the lowest amount of surfactant required to provide a sufficient sink condition to solubilize the drug product. In deciding whether a dissolution method is suitable or not, the criteria can be that there is a greater than 85% dissolution in less than 120 minutes. It was noted that according to the experience of the FDA, the surfactant concentration in the dissolution medium does not need to be very high or above the critical micelle concentration to solubilize most drug products.

As discussed above, adding a surfactant in the dissolution media has been found to be useful in improving the dissolution profiles of an IR dosage without modifying the formulations (52). In the next few paragraphs, theories and approaches to improve the dissolution rate are discussed, and they include (*i*) particle size reduction and (*i*) formation of solid dispersion in the formulation.

In the GI tract, the in vivo solubility of a drug is determined by the aqueous solubility property, crystallinity of the drug substance, lipophilicity, native surfactants, and the GI tract pH in relation to the $pK_a$ of the drug (53). Compounds with aqueous solubilies less that 0.1 mg/mL will present dissolution-limited absorption. Consideration of the Noyes–Whitney equation demonstrates that the wetted surface of the drug substance is going to be a critical factor in determining the in vivo dissolution rate. The wetted surface area in turn depends on the particle size of the solid and the ability to be wetted by lumenal fluids. By reducing the particle size via micronization or other techniques, the surface area can be greatly increased.

Johnson and Swindell examined the relationship between particle size and percent absorption and provided guidance in setting the particle size specifications for poorly soluble drugs (54). Using computer simulations of pharmacokinetic models, the percent of dose absorbed was determined as a function of particle size, solubility, dose, and absorption rate constant. The authors found that the greatest effect of particle size was on the absorption of low dose–low solubility drugs. As the solubility or dose increased, the particle size played a lesser role in dissolution. Given a dose between 1 and 250 mg, if the solubility was greater than 1 mg/mL, the particle size did not have an effect on the predicted percent absorption. However, it should be noted that many new drugs being developed are poorly soluble and have solubilities significantly less than 1 mg/mL.

The effect of the particle size of indomethacin, a poorly soluble drug, on the dissolution rate was studied (55). Different size fractions were collected and characterized with respect to solubility, degree of crystallinity, density, specific surface area, and particle size distributions. In determining the particle size distribution, a Coulter Multisizer™ II was used. Also, the size and number of suspended particles were monitored during the dissolution process to evaluate the dissolution behavior. A strong relationship between the dissolution rate and particle size was found, i.e., smaller particle has a higher dissolution rate. The mean particle size of the various indomethacin fractions can be used to predict the MDT (Fig. 34).

There are various methods of reducing the particle size of drug substances. Fluid energy micronization has been used as a technique to reduce the particle size and examine the effects on the dissolution of tablet formulations of two poorly soluble compounds, spironolactone and diethylstilbestrol (56). Samples of both drug substances were micronized using a micron fluid energy mill, and the surface areas as well as the particle size were measured. All tablet formulations have been prepared using 1% magnesium stearate as a lubricant. The dissolution of tablets using unmicronized spironolactone was slower. As the tablet hardness increased, the disintegration time and the percent of drug dissolved at 30 minutes was also reduced. When the surface area of spironolactone was increased threefold, a

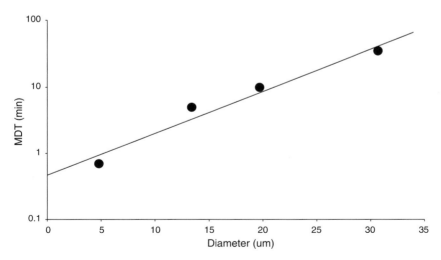

**Figure 34** Relationship between the MDT and the mean particle size for each indomethacin fraction. *Abbreviation*: MDT, mean dissolution time. *Source*: Adapted from Ref. 55.

slight increase of 7% dissolution was observed at 30 minutes. On the other
hand, micronization improved both the dissolution rate and content uniformity of diethylstilbestrol tablets. When the particle size was greater than
40 μm, the dissolution profile did not meet the specifications established by
the standard formulation. The content uniformity of the low-dose formulation, 1 mg tabletalso failed due to the nonhomogeneity of drug powder
mixture during compression.

The particle size of an excipient can also have a profound effect on the
dissolution rate. The ability of calcium carbonate, sodium carbonate, and
sodium citrate dehydrate to enhance the dissolution of indomethacin was
correlated to the particle size distributions (57). Indomethacin is a weakly
acidic compound and the solubility at pH 2 is less than the solubility at pH
7. The effect of adding a buffering agent in the tablet was determined by
blending indomethacin with various amounts and particle sizes of a buffer
(Fig. 35). The three particle size ranges selected were 124 to 129 μm, 105 to
125 μm, and < 74 μm. It was observed that sodium carbonate gave the
highest increase in dissolution rate followed by sodium citrate. When calcium carbonate was used, less than 6% increase in dissolution could be
found under any of the tested conditions. On the other hand, incorporating
sodium carbonate improved the dissolution rates significantly, and more

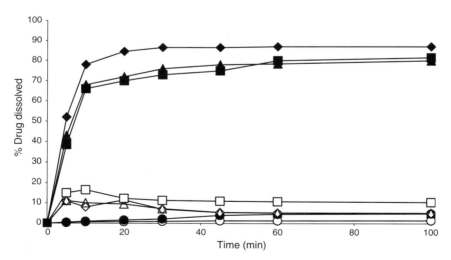

**Figure 35** Dissolution profiles of indomethacin from indomethacin–sodium
carbonate cocompressed tablets with a 25% buffer weight ratio ($n = 3$). (◇) buffer
size < 74 μm at pH 2; (△) buffer size 105–125 μm pH 2; (□) buffer size 125–149 at pH
2; (◆) buffer size < 74 μm at pH 7; (■) buffer size 105–125 μm as pH 7; (▲) buffer size
125–149 μm at pH 7; (○) control at pH 2; (●) control at pH 7. *Source*: Adapted from
Ref. 57.

than 70% of indomethacin has dissolved within 20 minutes in all cases or particle size ranges. When sodium citrate was used, using a lower weight percent increased the dissolution rate better than a larger amount of the buffer. A trend also existed that the dissolution rate was enhanced in the order of decreasing particle size of sodium citrate, i.e., less than 74 μm > 105 to 125 μm > 125 to 149 μm. The results suggested that sodium citrate and sodium carbonate could be used to improve the dissolution of indomethacin and possibly other poorly soluble compounds with similar physicochemical properties.

Another method to enhance the dissolution of hydrophobic drugs is to develop solid dispersions using hydrophilic excipients or employing surface modification agents (58). Poloxamer-407 and Synperonic® F127 was studied by Rouchotas et al. as surface modifiers and as solid-dispersion carriers for preparing phenylbutazone formulations. To modify the surface of phenylbutazone drug substance, an adsorption procedure was followed. In preparing solid dispersions of 10% or 20% w/w of phenylbutazone, untreated and surface-modified drug substances were dissolved in molten poloxamer and filled into capsules. Both the surface-modified and solid-dispersion formulations have improved dissolution rates in pH 6.4 buffer compared to the untreated drug. In addition, a combination of the surface modification and solid-dispersion techniques has enhanced the dissolution rate more than either of the techniques alone (Fig. 36). The amount of phenylbutazone dissolved at 140 minutes was 16.7% for the untreated drug

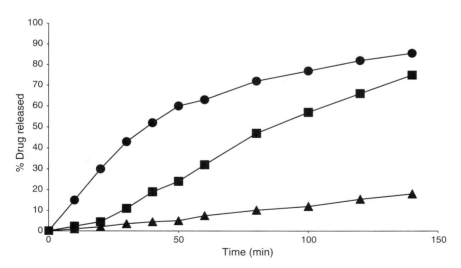

**Figure 36** Dissolution profiles of (▲) phenylbutazone, (■) 20% w/w solid dispersion in F127 with untreated phenylbutazone; (●) phenylbutazone previously modified with Synperonic® F127 in molten P127. *Source*: Adapted from Ref. 58.

substance, 71.4% for the solid dispersion, and 85.6% for the solid dispersion prepared with previously surface-modified phenylbutazone.

Gupta et al. conducted a similar study in the investigations of employing Gelucire® as the solid-dispersion carrier and magnesium aluminum silicate as the surface modifier (59). A poorly soluble drug, BAY 12-9566, was chosen as the model compound. Solid dispersions of Gelucire 50/13 and the drug were prepared by a hot-melt granulation method and the resulting molten mixture was adsorbed to the surface of magnesium aluminum silicate. Various ratios of the drug Gelucire and magnesium aluminum silicate produced solid-dispersion granules or physical mixtures with different dissolution characteristics. The dissolution method was USP paddle at 75 rpm in 0.1N HCl with 1% w/v SLS. In general, the solid-dispersion granules had a higher dissolution rate compared to the physical mixtures (Fig. 37). Also, dissolution was enhanced by raising the amount of Gelucire or magnesium aluminum silicate in the formulations, but decreased with an increase in drug loading. It was noted that the dissolution upon storage at 40°C/75% RH has actually improved over a four-week period. Also, the flow and compressibility properties of the solid-dispersion granules were significantly better than the physical mixtures.

Other methods of producing solid dispersions or mixtures to increase dissolution rates were evaluated using modified gum karaya as a carrier for nimodipine, a poorly soluble compound (60). The order of methods of

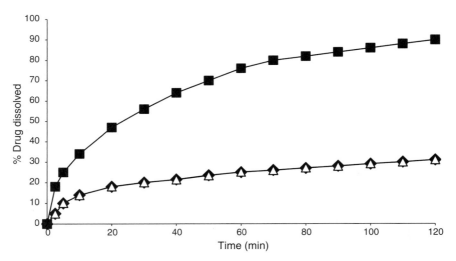

**Figure 37**  Comparison of dissolution profiles of BAY 12-9566 in 0.1N HCl 1% w/v USP Type 2 apparatus at 75 rpm. (■) solid dispersion granules; (△) physical mixture with Gelucire 10/13 and magnesium aluminum silicate; (◆) drug alone. *Source*: Adapted from Ref. 59.

preparation in enhancing dissolution is physical mixture < cogrinding mixture < swollen carrier mixture < kneading mixture (water as kneading agent) < kneading mixture (70% v/v ethanol as kneading agent) < solid dispersion. As the amount of modified gum karaya increased, the dissolution rate increased accordingly, and the optimal ratio of nimodipine/modified gum karaya is 1:9 in weight. It was found that cogrinding at a 1:9 ratio could yield a significant improvement in the dissolution rate without the addition of organic solvent (e.g., in the kneading process) or subjecting the drug to high temperatures (e.g., in the solid-dispersion process). Thus, cogrinding with modified gum karaya can be used as an alternative method to enhance the dissolution rate of IR formulations.

The last topic of this section is on the research of an alternate instrument for the dissolution of IR products. Even though the basket and paddle methods remain the primary apparatuses for testing tablet and capsule formulations, the flow-through instrument and USP Apparatus 3 have been explored in the past few years as possible options to evaluate dissolution profiles of IR formulations (31). Some of the applications were focused on providing a sink condition sufficient for the dissolution of poorly soluble compounds.

In 1993, Mehta reviewed the dissolution methods for oral formulations and the corresponding analytical procedures such as HPLC and UV/VIS spectrometry (61). It was noted that in vitro dissolution of a poorly soluble drug often has to be conducted in a large volume of dissolution medium in order to simulate the in vivo sink condition. Also, the dissolution rates depended on the manufacture method of the dosage form and the pH of the dissolution medium. A flow-through dissolution method could allow dissolution to be performed with a fresh medium so that the drug concentration would remain within 10% to 15% of the maximum solubility.

An automated flow-through dissolution system was later developed for the dissolution of poorly soluble drugs with pH-dependent solubility and chemical stability (62). Uncoated and coated pellets of fenoldopam mesylate were tested with the addition of acids, bases, or buffers to the dissolution medium to ensure the stability of the drug in solution. The developed flow-through system has provided a sufficient sink condition over the entire dissolution time and the pH range of the dissolution medium. The drug-release profiles were the same as the results obtained from a basket method (Fig. 38) while the dissolution rates were slightly lower. Changes in filling volumes and flow rates have been found to be the two parameters that could affect the dissolution profiles significantly. Overall, the developed flow-through method was proved to be a rugged dissolution method in terms of sample weight and mechanical stress.

Another flow-through method was applied on the dissolution of formulations containing two drugs that have significantly different solubility properties (63). Malarone® tablets were made of two compounds,

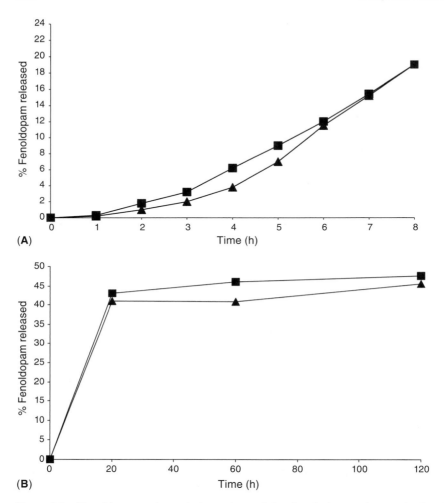

**Figure 38** Fenoldopam release–independent of the dissolution testing method. (**A**) uncoated pellets (50% fenoldopam mesylate, 25% succinic acid) at pH 7.5; (■) flow-through 5 mL/min; (▲) basket 75 rpm; (**B**) coated pellets (34% fenoldopam mesylate, 34% succinic acid, 8% w/w Surelease coat) at pH 1.2 for 2h+ pH 7.5 for six hours; (■) flow-through 5 mL/min; (▲) basket 100 rpm. *Source*: Adapted from Ref. 62.

atovaquone and proguanil hydrochloride. The solubility or dissolution of atovaquone increased slightly with an increase in pH or an increase in the concentration of sodium hydroxide. At the same time, the solubility of atovaquone decreased when proquanil hydrochloride dissolved (Fig. 39). In order to dissolve proguanil and atovaquone simultaneously from a tablet formulation, an optimal concentration of NaOH was needed (Fig. 40).

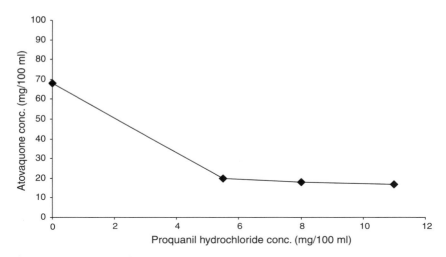

**Figure 39** Solubility of atovaquone in 0.1M sodium hydroxide at 20°C in the presence of proguanil hydrochloride. *Source*: Adapted from Ref. 63.

Using 0.1M NaOH a flow-through method was developed and validated for dissolving formulations containing drugs with different physicochemical properties.

Bhattachar et al. studied the effect of flow rate on the extent and rate of dissolution (64). PD198306 is a Pfizer compound that has poor aqueous solubilities and wettability even in the presence of 0.5% SLS. Micronized

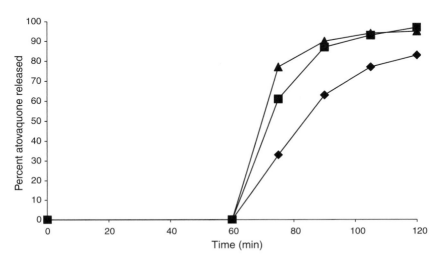

**Figure 40** Atovaquone dissolution profiles in water for one hour, then in (♦) 0.05M, (■) 0.1M and (▲) 0.15M sodium hydroxide. *Source*: Adapted from Ref. 63.

and unmicronized drug powders were loaded into the flow-through dissolution apparatus in the form of a suspension (Fig. 41). By using a 25 mM pH 9 sodium phosphate buffer with 0.5% SLS as the dissolution medium, a suitable dissolution profile can be obtained. A flow rate of 4 mL/min provided a dissolution profile with a desirable dissolution rate and extent of dissolution. Also, this flow-through method could discriminate drug powders of different particle sizes.

USP Apparatus 3 has been evaluated as an alternative instrument to USP Apparatus 2 for the dissolution of immediate-release tablets and capsules of poorly soluble (acyclovir, furosemide) and highly soluble drugs (metoprolol, ranitidine) (65). In comparison to the paddle method, the USP Apparatus 3 can provide a dissolution environment that better simulates the pH changes and mechanical stresses experienced by the drug products along the gastrointestinal tract. It also avoids the possibility of establishing poor hydrodynamics created by the cone formation in the bottom of the dissolution vessel. By varying the agitation speed at 5, 15, and 25 dpm, the dissolution profiles of generic and branded dosage forms were generated and compared to the results obtained from USP Apparatus 2 at 50 rpm. As noted, the agitation rate of Apparatus 3 has a significant effect on the dissolution rate. Similar hydrodynamic conditions and dissolution results using Apparatus 2 at 50 rpm could be provided by a low agitation speed of 5 dpm in Apparatus 3 (Fig. 42). It was found that the dissolution profiles of metoprolol, ranitidine, and acyclovir were similar. Thus, it was concluded that USP Apparatus 3 could be

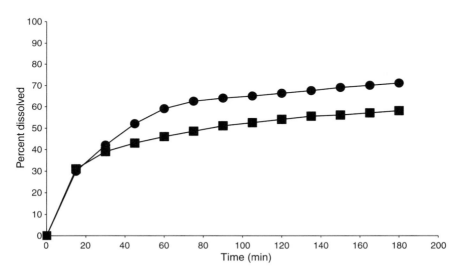

**Figure 41** Dissolution profiles of micronized and unmicronized drug Pd198306 in suspension. (●) unmicronized; (■) micronized. *Source*: Adapted from Ref. 64.

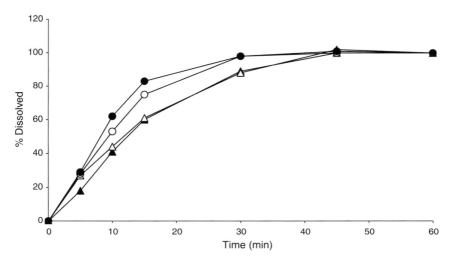

**Figure 42** Dissolution profiles of metoprolol tartrate tablets of generic product. (●) USP 325 dpm; (○) USP 315 dpm; (▲) USP 35 dpm; (△) UPS 250 rpm. *Source*: Adapted from Ref. 65.

extended to dissolve IR products of highly soluble compounds and possibly some poorly soluble compounds such as acyclovir.

In summary, during the process of developing a suitable dissolution method for an IR product, careful consideration should be given to the pH, and the selection and concentration of the solubilizing agent in the dissolution medium so that the dissolution conditions are relevant to the physiological environment. When it is necessary to improve the dissolution rate of a formulation so that the oral bioavailability can be maximized, reducing the drug particle size, preparing a solid dispersion, or employing a surface modifier could be tried. In terms of choosing a suitable dissolution apparatus, besides the paddle or the basket instruments, USP Apparatus 3 and the flow-through apparatus are suitable alternatives.

### Modified Release

Modified-release formulations are designed to achieve drug actions that IR dosage forms could not provide. For example, if an acid-labile drug is formulated in an IR dosage, the drug can decompose quickly in the stomach, resulting in a lack of therapeutic effect. In this case, an enteric-coated dosage can be formulated to protect an unstable drug from degrading in the acidic environment of the stomach. In general, modified-release products can be divided into three classes: delayed, extended/prolonged, and controlled release. Extended- and controlled-release delivery systems are both targeted to release the drug and maintain drug actions for a long period of time. For our discussion, the mechanism of a controlled-release dosage is very specific and inherent in the drug delivery system. In addition, a controlled-release system is often successful at maintaining a constant blood level. Meanwhile, the release mechanism of an extended-release dosage could depend on the environment such as the physiological pH.

Delayed Release

The postponed action of a delayed-release dosage is achieved by an application of a special coating (e.g., an enteric coating) to the surface of the drug powder or formulation. The purpose of the coating is to allow the drug to be released in the lower part of the gastrointestinal tract. For an enteric-coated formulation, the coating allows minimal release of the drug in the stomach. When the dosage reaches the small intestine, an immediate and complete drug release occurs to produce the desired therapeutic actions. For the treatment of inflammatory bowel disease or ulcerative colitis, the drug release is targeted to happen in the distal ileum or large intestine to minimize any systemic side effects.

The USP acceptance criteria for dissolution were discussed earlier for quality control of delayed-release formulations. In selecting a suitable instrument for the dissolution of a delayed-release product, a flow-through system and USP Apparatus 3 have been examined as alternative methods to the paddle and basket apparatuses (66–68). A historical review of the flow-through cell by Langenbucher et al. in 1989 revealed the need for standardization of the general construction, dimensions, flow rate, and degassing of the dissolution medium. It was concluded that different types of formulations could require different flow-cell chambers. Different types of flow-through cells have then been developed by Moeller et al. (67) in the dissolution of enteric-coated diclofenac tablets, chlorthalidone powders, and tablets. The authors have highlighted the advantages of the flow-through method such as the ease of changing the dissolution media and the lack of requirement of maintaining a certain dosage form in position in the dissolution medium.

Klein et al. (68) studied the drug-release characteristics of delayed release products of mesalazine for the treatment of ulcerative colitis. Using USP Apparatus 3, the dissolution profiles were determined at various pH to simulate the passage of the dosage form through the gastrointestinal tract (Fig. 43). Table 5 summarizes the dissolution media and transit times of the formulation in each medium to simulate the physiological environment.

The type and release characteristics of the coating polymer in the formulations are described in Table 6. In simulated gastric fluid, minimal release of the drug was observed from tablets coated with Eudragit L or Eudragit S (i.e., Claversal, Salofalk, and Asacolitin tablets). In comparison, > 50% of the drug was released when the tablets were coated with ethylcellulose (i.e., Pentasa tablet), demonstrating that the release of the drug is

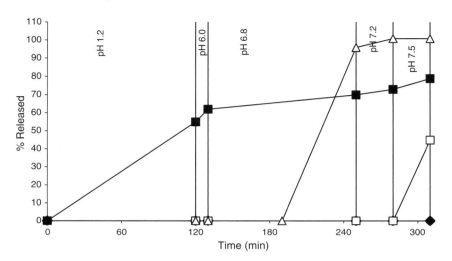

**Figure 43** Dissolution profiles of different mesalazine dosage forms during gastrointestinal passage simulated using a pH-gradient method. (△) Salofalk 250 mg; (□) Claversal 250 mg; (■) Pentasa 500 mg; (◆) Asacolitin 400 mg. *Source*: Adapted from Ref. 68.

diffusion controlled and thus independent of the pH of the dissolution medium.

Even though Salofalk and Claversal tablets used the same type of polymer coating, the lag times were significantly different due to a difference in the film thickness. Salofalk tablets have a ~100 μm coating and started to dissolve at 6.8. On the other hand, a ~250 μm thick film coat of Eudragit L in Claversal tablets prevented it from dissolving until the pH of the dissolution medium reached 7.5. As expected, Asacolitin tablets had the slowest dissolution rate because Eudragit S was used as the enteric coating

**Table 5** Dissolution Media in Studying Delayed Release Products of Mesalazine

| Gastrointestinal segment | Transit time (min) | Medium | pH value |
|---|---|---|---|
| Stomach | 120 | Simulated gastric fluid USP 24 without pepsin | 1.2 |
| Duodenum | 10 | Phosphate buffer Ph Eur 1997 | 6.0 |
| Jejunum | 120 | Simulated intestinal fluid USP 24 without pancreatin | 6.8 |
| Proximal ileum | 30 | Phosphate buffer Ph Eur 1997 | 7.2 |
| Distal ileum | 30 | Simulated intestinal fluid USP 24 without pancreatin | 7.5 |

*Source*: Adapted from Ref. 68.

**Table 6**  Type of Polymer Coating in Mesalazine Products

| Product | Dosage form | Polymer type | Polymer trademark | Release pH |
|---|---|---|---|---|
| Claversal | Coated tablets | MA:MM 1:1 | Eudragit L | >6 |
| Salofalk | Coated tablets | MA:MM 1:1 | Eudragit L | >6 |
| Asacolitin | Coated tablets | MA:MM 1:2 | Eudragit S | >7 |
| Pentasa | Coated microgranules | Ethylcellulose | Surelease | pH independent |

*Abbreviations*: MA, methacrylic acid; MM, methacrylate.
*Source*: Adapted from Ref. 68.

polymer. It was concluded that the proposed pH-gradient method in combination with USP Apparatus 3 could be used to discriminate the drug-release behavior of various delayed-release dosage forms and possibly other modified-release delivery systems.

### Extended and Controlled Release

Conventional or immediate oral dosage forms will not provide an extended duration of action if the drug does not have a long half-life. Multiple dosing of an immediate dosage can sometimes provide a therapeutic blood level for a longer period of time; however, patient noncompliance and fluctuating blood levels could lead to an undesirable outcome and side effect. Extended and controlled-release delivery systems are designed to provide a constant release of drug for absorption. Some examples of these delivery systems include matrix tablets, polymer-coated sugar beads or granules, erosion nondisintegration tablets, pellets with altered densities, and osmotically controlled dosages. Even though the principle of drug-release mechanism is different for each of these delivery systems, the ultimate goal is the same, i.e., to provide a sustained therapeutic plasma level for drug actions.

In developing dissolution methods for an extended-release or a controlled-release oral dosage form, several factors require careful consideration (69). First of all, the dissolution medium should have a pH similar to the physiological pH of the gastrointestinal tract where the drug is exposed and released. Often, the presence of food in the stomach can have a profound effect on the residence time and the rates of dissolution of the drug. In these cases, a dissolution medium that simulates the fed state in the gastrointestinal tract is more appropriate if the medication is going to be taken together with food. Dissolution media containing bile salts, enzymes, and oil have been used to simulate the effects of food on drug absorption.

The pH of the dissolution medium is critical in testing a controlled-release dosage if the drug has an ionizable functional group (70). Sorasuchart et al. have compared the dissolution characteristics of ketoprofen, nicardipine, and acetaminophen by preparing controlled-release formulations of drug-layered beads that were coated with ethylcellulose. Even though the solubility of ethylcellulose is independent of pH, the dissolution profiles in enzyme-free simulated gastric fluid (pH 1.4) and enzyme-free simulated intestinal fluid (pH 7.4) were different for each drug (Figs. 44 and 45). In an acidic environment, the weak acid drug ketoprofen had a slower dissolution rate than the weak basic drug nicardipine. In basic media, the reverse was true: nicardipine dissolved slower than ketoprofen. Meanwhile, acetaminophen dissolved approximately at the same rate in both acid and basic media, because it is not ionized under those conditions. It was suggested that dissolution of controlled-release formulation should be performed in both gastric and intestinal fluid for ionizable drugs.

The choice of the type of dissolution apparatus is also important, because it can influence the dissolution profile and the extent of IVIVC. For example, the flow-through method has been reported to be better than the paddle or basket method in the dissolution of phenylpropanolamine and theophylline matrix tablets (69). The ease of changing the dissolution media is one of the advantages of the flow-through dissolution apparatus as mentioned earlier (67).

USP Apparatus 3 has also been found to be better than the paddle method in the dissolution of a poorly soluble compound in a hydrophilic polymer-based matrix (71). When the paddle method was used to dissolve

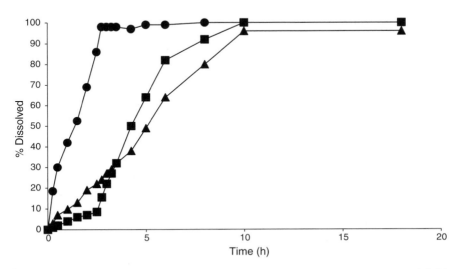

**Figure 44** Dissolution profiles of model drugs in enzyme-free simulated gastric fluid (pH 1.4) for two hours and then in enzyme-free simulated intestinal fluid (pH 7.4) paddle method. (■) I ketoprofen; (●) nicardipine; (▲) acetaminophen. *Source*: Adapted from Ref. 70.

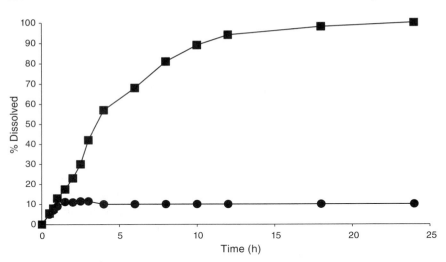

**Figure 45**  Dissolution profiles of ketoprofen and nicardipine HCl in enzyme-free simulated intestinal fluid (pH 4) paddle method. (■) ketoprofen; (●) nicardipine. *Source*: Adapted from Ref. 70.

the formulation, less than 80% of the drug had dissolved over 24 hours in all of the tested media, including the use of PEG, SLS, or Tween-80 as possible solubilizing agents. When Apparatus 3 was tested, 30% PEG in water was initially discovered to be a suitable dissolution medium where an IVIVC could be established. To better simulate the in vivo conditions, the same formulation was exposed to the simulated gastric fluid without enzymes for an hour. This change in the experimental procedure has caused dissolution to fall below 80%. To improve the rate and the extent of dissolution, PEG was replaced by Tween®-80 as the solubilizing agent, and various concentrations of Tween-80 were tested. It was found that concentrations of Tween-80 above 1.0% and agitation rates greater than 20 dpm could cause unacceptable foaming to occur. By maintaining the agitation rate at 20 dpm, greater than 80% dissolution could be achieved at 24 hours using simulated gastric fluid containing 0.25% Tween-80 in the first row of vessels and 10 mM phosphate buffer containing 0.25% Tween-80 in the remaining vessels. It was thus concluded that USP Apparatus 3 could be successfully used in developing dissolution methods for controlled-release formulations.

The position of the dosage in the dissolution apparatus can have an effect on the dissolution profiles and thus the establishment of an IVIVC. Pillay and Fassihi have investigated three controlled-release formulations that are based on a different type of release mechanisms: swellable floatable, swellable sticking, and osmotic pump (72). Each of the delivery systems was evaluated by putting the dosage form in the dissolution vessel in accordance with the USP 23 methods or placing it over/below a designed ring-mesh device for achieving full surface exposure to the dissolution medium. Dissolution results indicate that the overall release profiles of theophylline were sensitive to the dosage positioning in the dissolution vessel, especially from both the sticking and the floatable controlled-delivery systems (Figs. 46 and 47). In contrast, the dissolution profiles of diltiazem were sensitive for the sticking and not the floatable delivery system. This could be explained by the difference in solubilities of the two drugs as theophylline is a sparingly soluble compound and less soluble than diltiazem. It became apparent that for an accurate evaluation of certain types of controlled delivery systems, a full surface exposure during solution would be desirable. This could be provided by a modification of the dissolution method using a ring-mesh assembly. For an osmotically controlled delivery system, the drug-release profiles were found to be identical under all experimental conditions (Fig. 48). These results demonstrate that the release mechanism of an osmotic pump formulation was independent of dosage position in the dissolution apparatus or the hydrodynamic condition in the surroundings.

Transdermal Drug Delivery Systems for Systemic Use

Use of Apparatus 5, 6, or 7 for the dissolution testing of transdermal patch systems is similar to the evaluation of an oral modified-release product. These are also modified release, and as such, would require multiple time-point samples, basically a dissolution profile. As with other MR DDS, the

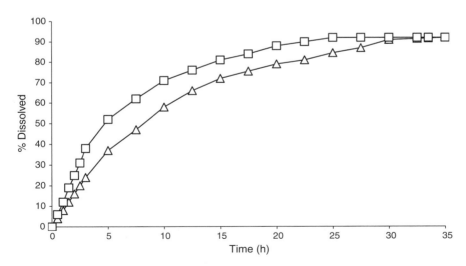

**Figure 46**   Theophylline release from a swellable sticking drug delivery system: (□) delivery system placed over the ring/mesh assembly for full surface exposure to the dissolution medium; (△) delivery system dropped into the vessel with one surface to the bottom of the vessel. *Source*: Adapted from Ref. 72.

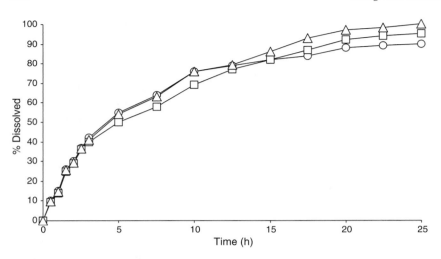

**Figure 47** Theophylline release from a swellable floatable drug delivery system: (□) delivery system placed under the ring/mesh to prevent flotation to the surface of the dissolution medium; (△) delivery system dropped into the vessel and allowed to float at the surface of the dissolution medium; (○) delivery system enclosed within a helical wire sinker to prevent flotation to the surface of the dissolution medium. *Source*: Adapted from Ref. 72.

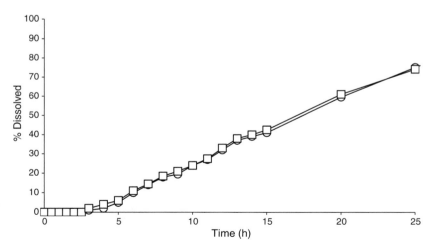

**Figure 48** Nifedipine release from osmotic pump delivery system (Procardia XL® 30 mg tablets); (□) delivery system placed over the ring/mesh assembly for full surface exposure to the dissolution medium; (○) delivery system dropped to the bottom of the vessel. *Source*: Adapted from Ref. 72.

early sample would evaluate for dose-dumping, the late sample for completeness, and the middle sample to assess that the rate is as expected. There the similarity ends, as the drug content of transdermal drug delivery systems (TDDS) is typically far in excess of the labeled amount to be delivered. There can be as much as 300% to 500% of the intended delivery amount contained within the system. This is necessary to maintain a concentration gradient during the entire time of the use of the system, which can be one day to several days, or even a month. This can result in some "out of the ordinary" dissolution values.

As is typical with DDS, the dissolution is calculated as a percentage of the intended-to-be-delivered amount. As this is *not* the content of the patch, and the skin will not be present in the dissolution vessel, the percentage ranges can be in excess of 100%. In addition, the last value of a profile would not be a greater-than or equal-to limit, but would also consist of a range. To obtain compliance with a set of criteria, all observed values should be within the specified ranges. There will be a greater divergence for patch systems that are made without a rate-controlling membrane (usually the skin would control the rate of drug entry into the body) when compared to those made with a rate-controlling membrane.

## Topical Drug Delivery Systems for Local Use

Drug release from semisolid formulations is a property of the dosage form, and with suitable validation, it can be used for the same quality control and product comparisons as for solid drug delivery systems. The current scientific consensus is that in vitro release is an acceptable comparative measure in the presence of certain formulation and manufacturing changes. Such a product evaluation is more reproducible than the typical series of tests used for semisolid preparations, which include evaluations such as particle size determination, viscosity, and other rheological factors. The drug-release evaluation should optimize the test procedure for the product in a manner analogous to the use of in vitro dissolution to assess the quality of extended-release products from batch to batch. This can also be used in a sponsor-specific comparability protocol to allow more extensive post-approval changes in formulation and/or manufacturing. As with any test, the statistical approaches to the documentation of "sameness" in quality attributes must be considered.

The FDA's current position concerning in vitro release testing can be summarized in four points: (*i*) in vitro release testing is a useful test to assess product "sameness"; (*ii*) the development and validation of an in vitro release test are not required for approval of a new drug application (NDA), or abbreviated NDA (ANDA) nor as a routine batch-to-batch quality control test; (*iii*) in vitro release testing is not a surrogate test for in vivo bioavailability or bioequivalence; and (*iv*) the in vitro release rate should not be used for comparing different formulations, either within or between manufacturers.

Drug release is theoretically proportional to the square root of time. The in vitro release method for topical dosage forms is based on a diffusion cell system, using either a vertical diffusion cell with a closed donor compartment (such as the Franz type) or an internal compartment variable-volume diffusion cell (such as the Enhancer™ cell), usually fitted with a synthetic membrane. The test product is placed in the donor chamber of the diffusion cell, and a sampling fluid is placed on the other side of the membrane, which is either a part of the diffusion cell or is within a separate temperature-controlled vessel. The diffusion of the drug from the product through the membrane is monitored by an analysis of sequentially collected samples of the receptor media. Aliquots of these samples would then be properly analyzed using an appropriate technique. Data will be analyzed and represented as a graph of the amount of drug released per unit area ($mcg/cm^2$) as a function of the square root of time. This should yield a straight line, and the slope of this line represents the release rate. This release rate is formulation specific and can be used to monitor product quality. The release rate of the biobatch or currently manufactured batch should be compared with the release rate of the product prepared after a change.

Appropriate inert and commercially available synthetic membranes should be used, as this significantly contributes to reproducibility. The membrane selected should have, in addition to the above criteria, as many of the following ideal characteristics as possible. It should have minimal resistance to drug transport, as well as no significant binding of the drug, so that drug release is more a function of interaction with the product. The membrane should have a relatively high porosity, to allow easy diffusion of media as well as the drug molecule. It should have minimal thickness so as to eliminate the diffusion-distance effect of drug through the membrane. Finally, it should be transparent, for in that way, the researcher can observe the sample and/or the receptor media for the presence of entrapped air, which would significantly alter the results by changing the diffusion surface area. There are a variety of membrane materials, including but not limited to regenerated cellulose (dialysis membrane), cuprophan, polydimethyl siloxane, fluoropore FHLP hydrophobic membrane, ethylene vinyl acetate (Cotrans 9702), carbosil, and polysulfone. The selection of membrane type depends on the physical and chemical properties of the drug.

The receptor medium could be an aqueous buffer for water-soluble drugs or a hydroalcoholic medium for sparingly water-soluble drugs. Other media may be appropriate but would require proper justification. The receptor media volume would depend on the diffusion cell selected. The vertical diffusion cells have chambers that can range from 7 to 45 mL. The variable-volume diffusion cell uses an external vessel as a receptor compartment, and the receptor fluid can be as little as 50 mL, up to the maximum content of the vessel into which it is placed.

As with a standard dissolution test, in vitro evaluations are done in sets of six samples. The sample should be appropriately loaded into the diffusion cell selected (73–77). The amount of the sample should be sufficient to provide a constant concentration gradient and thus a constant value for the release rate during the time interval of the evaluation. Multiple sampling (at least five times) over an appropriate time period (typically four to six hours) is used to generate an adequate release profile to determine the drug-release rate. The sampling times may vary depending on the formulation. Sample points that are too early may not reflect a constant release rate, since equilibration of the product and media may still be occurring. In addition, samples that are too late, evident by the presence of a flattening or a plateau, are to be avoided, since this indicates significant depletion of the drug from the sample. This may also indicate that too little sample was loaded into the diffusion cell.

The data can be expressed as the amount of drug released per unit area on the y-axis and the square root of time on the x-axis. The slope of the best-fit line represents the release rate. This release rate can then be used for comparisons. A statistical test based on a standard confidence interval procedure that is related to the Wilcoxon Rank Sum/Mann-Whitney rank test can be applied to the log slopes. Acceptance criteria will typically use a 90% confidence interval, and the median in vitro release rates for comparing the test with a reference should be within the limits of 75% to 133.33%. References to this confidence interval procedure can be found in the reference section (78,79).

## Computation of Dissolution Measurement Results

Dissolution results depend on the drug delivery system being evaluated. A typical representation involves the cumulative amount of drug released as a function of time, most often expressed as a percentage of the labeled content of the unit. When conducting a search for an IVIVC, this data may be transformed into an amount remaining to be released as a function of time. Although single-point dissolution tests are still very common, it is becoming increasingly desirable to obtain samples at several time points, or a dissolution profile. The desirable characteristics of such a profile include its being completely dissolved (> 80–85%), frequently/adequately sampled, sensitive/discriminatory, and reproducible, and with the possibility of establishing in vitro equivalence. Both the rate and the extent of drug released/dissolved can be determined, whereas USP specifications, when available, tend only to address the extent of drug release/dissolved and not the rate (80).

With determination of profiles, data can more easily be compared. Although there are many statistical techniques that can be used, comparison of profiles can be accomplished through the use of the $f$ factors, $f_1$ and $f_2$

(81,82). The first is the difference factor ($f_1$), which calculates the percent difference between two curves at each time point (a measure of the relative error between the two curves), utilizing the following equation (Eq. 10).

$$f_1 = \left\{ \frac{\left[ \sum_{t=1}^{n} |R_t - T_t| \right]}{\left[ \sum_{t=1}^{n} R_t \right]} \right\} \times 100 \qquad (20)$$

where $n$ is the number of sample time points in a profile, $R_t$ is the dissolution value (% dissolved) of reference at time $t$, and $T_t$ is the dissolution value (% dissolved) of the test batch at time $t$. If these are similar curves (units > 12 each point), then $f_1 = 0$ to 15.

The second is referred to as the similarity factor ($f_2$). This is a logarithmic reciprocal square root transformation of the sum of the squared error and is a measurement of the similarity in the percent dissolution between two curves. Equation 11 is used to determine this value.

$$f_1 = 50 \times \log \left\{ \left[ 1 + (1/n) \sum_{t=1}^{n} (R_t - T_t)^2 \right]^{-0.5} \times 100 \right\} \qquad (21)$$

$n$ is the number of sample time points in a profile, $R_t$ is the dissolution value (% dissolved) of reference at time $t$, and $T_t$ is the dissolution value (% dissolved) of the test batch at time $t$.

If the profiles are to be considered similar curves (units > 12 each point), then the value of $f_2 = 50$ to 100. Each of these methods would require a minimum of three to four points in each profile (more preferred), all time points must be the same (such as 15, 30, 45, and 60 minutes), and only one point after 85% dissolution (or the presence of a plateau, whichever is first) is acceptable.

## Regulatory Applications

Dissolution data are often required for regulatory filings and to serve as a basis for comparing the bioavailabilities and bioequivalence of new products and batches prepared by a new manufacturing process. In 1997, the FDA issued two important guidance documents on developing dissolution methodology, setting specifications, and filing regulatory applications of dissolution testing: (*i*) Dissolution Testing of Immediate Release Solid Oral Dosage Forms (August 1997); (*ii*) Extended-Release Oral Dosage Forms: Development, Evaluation, and Application of In Vitro In Vivo Correlations (September 1997). Both documents highlighted the use of dissolution testing as a surrogate for human bioequivalence studies. One of the advantages of employing dissolution data to prove bioequivalency is that it can reduce the number of costly human clinical studies during the initial drug approval process and when certain postapproval and scale-up changes are made.

In October 2000, the FDA published a more detailed guidance entitled "Bioavailability and Bioequivalence Studies for Orally Administered Drug Products—General Considerations" to address methods acceptable for the documentation of products that are bioequivalent and possess the same bioavailability. A revision of this guidance started in July 2002. The described methods in a descending order of preference are: pharmacokinetic, pharmacodynamic, comparative clinical end-point, and in vitro/dissolution studies. According to the guidance, bioequivalency can be documented using dissolution testing for highly soluble, highly permeable, and rapidly dissolving orally administered products. The following sections describe the roles of dissolution from a regulatory perspective in the investigational NDAs (INDs), NDAs, and ANDAs.

Investigational New Drug

For Phase 1 studies of drugs in the INDs, dissolution testing of the clinical formulation is not required for regulatory filing. One of the reasons is that the formulation tested in Phase 1 is developed as a prototype to prove the concept that the drug molecule is safe and suitable for further development. In most cases, the Phase 1 formulation is not going to be the final dosage form. When Phase 2 studies start, the clinical formulation will be close to or the same as the one that is going into the market.

In April 1999, a guidance on Phase 2 and 3 studies was issued and entitled "INDs for Phase 2 and 3 Studies of Drugs, Including Specified Therapeutic Biotechnology-Derived Products; Chemistry, Manufacturing, and Controls Content and Format". Starting at Phase 2, dissolution is listed in the guidance document as one of the chemical tests required for the drug product. Specification and tentative acceptance criteria need to be set and reported. The analytical procedure (e.g., HPLC) used to perform the assay and support the acceptance criteria should be indicated. The complete description of the dissolution procedure and supporting validation data need to be available upon request.

In Phase 3, dissolution is included as one of the tests for the drug product in the stability protocol. The stability protocol should include a description of the packaging, sampling time points, temperature and humidity conditions, expected duration of the stability program, and the proposed bracketing or matrixing scheme, if applicable. Dissolution data should be generated in physiologically relevant media with reasonable speeds of agitation whenever they are found to be adequate in providing a sink condition or a suitable hydrodynamic environment. The specific analytical procedures can be referenced to the drug product specification section of the IND application and, if possible, the USP.

It should be noted that the bioavailability of the clinical dosage form is normally optimized during the IND period. This is crucial because once the in vivo bioavailability of a formulation is established, biowaivers of subsequent in vivo bioequivalency studies using dissolution data may be possible. Following the Biopharmaceutic Classification System (BCS) category, biowaivers can be applied for a to-be-marketed formulation when changes in components, composition, and/or method of manufacture occur to the clinical trial formulation, provided that the dosage forms have rapid and similar in vitro dissolution profiles.

### Clinical Trials—Pilot Studies

Under certain circumstances, a sponsor company may choose to conduct a pilot study of a prototype formulation in a small number of subjects before proceeding with a full bioequivalence study. In these cases, in vitro dissolution data can be found to be useful for all investigated formulations if in vivo absorption profiles are also being determined. This is because such efforts can lead to the establishment of an IVIVC. When an in vitro/in vivo association is available, the in vitro dissolution test can serve as an indicator of how well a formulation will perform in vivo.

Of course, there are other purposes of a pilot study. It can be used to validate the analytical methodology, assess variability, and optimize sample collection time intervals. For conventional or IR dosages, a pilot study can give valuable information about a suitable time for collecting the sample of the first data point and avoid a subsequent finding in a full-scale study that the first sample collection occurs after the plasma concentration peak. For modified-release dosages, a pilot study can help determine the sampling schedule to assess lag time and dose dumping.

During clinical trials, tablet formulations often have to be reworked or encapsulated in a blind study. There are instances where the only difference is that the tablet or tablet mix is put into a capsule. A biowaiver can be applied based on comparable dissolution profiles in three media: 0.1N HCl, and phosphate buffers 4.5 and 6.8 (84). Kleinebudde et al. studied the effects of fillers and milling on dissolution profiles (14). For IR products, the addition of soluble fillers and milling the tablets led to comparable dissolution profiles, whereas the addition of insoluble or swellable fillers resulted in deviations from the dissolution profile of the original tablets. It is interesting to note that based on an analysis of historical data for sustained-release products, blinding by encapsulation did not have an effect on the dissolution profiles.

### New Drug Application

When an NDA is filed, a validated dissolution method needs to be available and be used as a quality control test for future batches. For an NDA, the dissolution specifications should be based on acceptable clinical, bioavailability, and/or bioequivalence batches. These specifications will be applied in testing formulations when postapproval changes are made.

Another use of a dissolution method in the NDA is to provide evidence of bioavailability or bioequivalence of the drug product. The code of federal regulations CFR 320.24 (4) has stated that either an in vitro test that has been correlated with and is predictive of human bioavailability or a currently available in vitro test that ensures adequate human in vivo bioavailability is acceptable for the evaluation of bioavailability or bioequivalence. Based on this, various types of biowaivers can be granted by performing a comparison of the dissolution profiles.

For IR formulations, both lower and higher strengths of the same dosage form can be given a biowaiver status if the dissolution profiles are comparable and the dosages are proportionally similar in their active and inactive ingredients. To get a waiver for the higher strength, a sponsor also needs to provide clinical safety and efficacy data for the higher dose and prove that the pharmacokinetics is linear over the dose range.

For modified-release formulations, a bioequivlaence study can be performed on the highest strength and a waiver of in vivo studies can be requested for the lower strengths based on dissolution profiles. If the formulation is a beaded capsule, the $f_2$ test (previously discussed) should be used to compare dissolution profiles from different strengths of the same product. An $f_2$ value of $> 50$ means that in vivo studies are not needed for the lower strengths. If the formulation is an extended-release tablet, the active and inactive ingredients in the formulation should be proportionally the same. Dissolution profiles should be similar using the $f_2$ test in at least three dissolution media to apply for a biowaiver status.

### Abbreviated NDA

While an NDA is submitted for regulatory filing of a new molecular entity, a new salt, or other noncovalent derivatives, an ANDA is used for the approval of a previously approved new molecular entity. Also, if a drug was originally formulated as an IR formulation, the first modified-release drug product needs to be submitted as an NDA. However, subsequent filings for similar modified-release formulations that are pharmaceutically equivalent and bioequivalent to the approved drug product in the market can be submitted as ANDAs. In accordance with 21 CFR 320.31, for some products that will be submitted in ANDAs, an IND may be required for conducting bioequivalence studies in order to ensure patient safety.

Overall acceptable bioequivalence data and comparable in vitro dissolution profiles are necessary for the approval of ANDAs (21 CFR 314.94). The dissolution method should be either (*i*) a USP method or (*ii*) the FDA method for the reference drug product if a USP method is not available. If both the USP and FDA methods are not available, a dissolution method development report needs to be submitted. Similar to the requirements in NDAs, the dissolution specifications should be based on the performance of acceptable clinical, bioavailability, and/or bioequivalence batches of the drug product. In the FDA guidance entitled "Bioavailability and Bioequivalence Studies for Orally Administered Drug Products—General Considerations," it recommends that dissolution data from three batches should be used to set dissolution specifications for modified-release dosage forms, including extended-release dosage forms.

Similar to the NDAs, waivers of in vivo bioequivalence studies can be granted based on comparison of dissolution profiles to lower strengths of modified-release products and higher/lower strengths of IR products. In addition, for rapidly dissolving IR products containing highly soluble and highly permeable drug substances, biowaivers can be granted if the reference drug product in the market is also rapidly dissolving and the test product exhibits similar dissolution profiles to the reference drug product. It should be pointed out that the choice of dissolution apparatus (USP Apparatus 1 or 2) should be the same as that established for the reference drug product. This type of biowaiver can be very useful to demonstrate that the test product is therapeutically equivalent when the test and reference dosage forms are pharmaceutical equivalents.

## FDA Guidance

In the 1990s, the FDA issued a number of guidance documents related to dissolution based on scientific principles. Two important areas of interest among the pharmaceutical companies are the roles of the BCS on applying for biowaivers and the functions of dissolution in approving certain scale-up and postapproval changes.

## Biopharmaceutics Classification System

The concept of BCS was introduced in 1995 by Amidon et al. to correlate the in vitro dissolution results with in vivo bioavailabilities (26). According to BCS, a drug can be classified into one of the four categories depending on the values of aqueous solubility and intestinal permeability: Class 1 (high solubility, high permeability), Class 2 (low solubility, high permeability), Class 3 (high solubility, low permeability) and Class 4 (low solubility, low permeability). In combination with the dissolution data to demonstrate whether a drug product is fast or slow dissolving, the BCS category represents three important factors (i.e., solubility, permeability, and rate of dissolution) in determining the rate and extent of oral absorption of IR formulations.

When determining the solubility class, a drug substance is considered "highly soluble" when the highest dose strength is soluble in ≤250 mL of aqueous media over a pH range of 1 to 7.5. For permeability measurement, a drug substance is considered "highly permeable" when the extent of absorption in humans is greater than 90% of an administered dose. The absorption value can be calculated based on mass balance or by comparing with an intravenous reference dose. Other methods of measuring permeability include intestinal perfusion in humans, in vivo/in situ intestinal perfusion studies in animals, in vitro permeation experiments with excised human or animal intestinal tissue, or epithelial cell monolayers. When determining the dissolution rate, a drug product is considered to be "rapidly dissolving" when greater than 85% of the labeled amount of drug substance dissolves within 30 minutes using USP Apparatus 1 or 2 in a volume of less than 900 mL buffer solution.

In August 2000, the FDA published a guidance entitled "Waiver of in Vivo Bioavailability and Bioequivalence Studies for Immediate-Release Solid Oral Dosage Forms Based on a Biopharmaceutics Classification System (BCS)." The scientific principle behind a BCS-based biowaiver is that the rate and extent of drug absorption are not going to be dependent on drug dissolution and gastrointestinal transit time if the in vivo dissolution is rapid and the drug is highly permeable. As a result, in vivo bioavailability or bioequivalence studies do not need to be conducted for products containing Class 1 compounds that exhibit rapid in vitro dissolution. One additional consideration is that absorption of the drug in the formulation is not affected by any excipients or inactive ingredients in the formulation. In summary, for applying for BCS-based biowaivers, (*i*) the drug substance needs to be highly soluble, (*ii*) the drug substance needs to be highly permeable, and (*iii*) the drug product should have a fast dissolution rate.

In September 2002, an AAPS/FDA workshop on BCS was held on the implementation, challenges, and extension opportunities (62). It was discussed that the approach adopted in the current BCS biowaiver guidance is conservative and there are various ways to extend the biowaiver applications.

1. Change the solubility range from pH 1.2 to 7.4 to pH 1.2 to 6.8.
2. Use 500 mL as the average volume for the small intestine to determine solubility.
3. Lower the high permeability cutoff from 90% absorption to 85%.
4. Use acceptable class 1 dissolution rates for class 2 drugs with the use of surfactants or pH 6.8 buffer.
5. Apply the dissolution rate of 85% in 15 minutes for class 3 drugs.

It should be noted that the current BCS-based biowaivers are only intended for bioequivalence studies. They do not apply to food-effect bioavailability studies or other pharmacokinetic studies. In addition, BCS-based biowaivers do not apply to drugs with a narrow therapeutic index, drug products intended for absorption in the oral cavity, and modified-release products. However, there was an effort to extend the BCS biowaiver to fed state studies of Class 1 drugs, and other new regulatory policies based on BCS are expected in the future.

SUPAC (IR, MR, SS)

After a drug product has been approved, a pharmaceutical company sometimes decides to make changes to the formulation or manufacturing processes that may have an effect on oral bioavailabities. Some of these changes can include (*i*) the formulation components or composition, (*ii*) the site of manufacture, (*iii*) the scale-up or scale-down of manufacture, and (*iv*) the manufacturing process and equipment. At times, these changes can happen before a drug product is approved. The FDA has issued three guidance documents on orally administered products to provide recommendations to sponsors on the type of information to be submitted for specific postapproval changes.

1.  Guidance for Industry: Immediate Release Solid Oral Dosage Forms—Scale-Up and Post-Approval Changes: Chemistry, Manufacturing and Controls, In Vitro Dissolution Testing, and In Vivo Bioequivalence Documentation, SUPAC-IR (November 1995).
2.  Guidance for Industry: SUPAC-MR: Modified Release Solid Oral Dosage Forms Scale-Up and Post-Approval Changes: Chemistry, Manufacturing and Controls; In Vitro Dissolution Testing and In Vivo Bioequivalence Documentation (October 1997).
3.  Guidance for Industry: SUPAC-IR/MR: Immediate Release and Modified Release Solid Oral Dosage Forms Manufacturing Equipment Addendum (January 1999).

Three levels of changes are described in these guidance documents based on the probability of causing a significant impact in the formulation performance, and a lower level represents a lower chance to have a significant effect. A level 1 change is considered to be a change that is unlikely to have a detectable effect on the formulation quality or performance. A level 2 change is a change that could have a significant impact on formulation quality and performance. Many level 1 and 2 changes can be approved solely based on a comparison of the dissolution profiles between the initial and the changed formulations. A level 3 change is defined as a change that is likely to have a significant impact on formulation quality or performance.

The types of change that can be approved based on dissolution profiles are summarized in Tables 7 and 8 (84). For all level 1 changes, the dissolution method in the compendium or original application can be used to prove the sameness of formulation quality and performance. On the other

**Table 7** Summary of the In Vitro Dissolution Data for the Manufacturing Changes for Immediate Release Formulations for which In Vivo Bioavailability Waiver Can Be Obtained

| Application/ compendial requirements | Case A | Case B | Case C |
|---|---|---|---|
| Level 1 component and composition | Level 2 component and composition for high-permeability and high-solubility drugs | Level 2 component and composition for low-permeability and high-solubility drugs | Level 2 component and composition for high-permeability and low-solubility drugs |
| Level 1 and 2 site change | | Level 3 site change | Level 2 equipment change |
| Level 1 change in batch size | | Level 2 change in batch size | |
| Level 1 equipment change | | Level 2 and 3 process change | |
| Level 1 process change | | | |

*Source*: Adapted from Ref. 84.

hand, for level 2 and level 3 changes, another dissolution method and additional dissolution media are required to satisfy the conditions for regulatory approval. Three cases of dissolution testing have been defined in the SUPAC-IR guidance.

*Case A*: Dissolution of $Q = 85\%$ in 15 minutes in 900 mL of 0.1 N hydrochloride (HCl), using USP Apparatus 1 at 100 rpm or Apparatus 2 at 50 rpm.

*Case B*: Multipoint dissolution profile in the application/compendial medium at 15, 30, 45, 60, and 120 minutes or until an asymptote is reached for the proposed and currently accepted formulation.

*Case C*: Multipoint dissolution profiles performed in water, 0.1 N HCl, and USP buffer media at pH 4.5, 6.5, and 7.5 (five separate profiles) for the proposed and currently accepted formulations. Adequate sampling should be performed at 15, 30, 45, 60, and 120 minutes until either 90% of drug from the drug product is dissolved or an asymptote is reached. A surfactant may be used with appropriate justification.

**Table 8**  Summary of the In Vitro Dissolution Data for the Manufacturing Changes for Modified-Release Formulations for which In Vivo Bioavailability Waiver Can Be Obtained

| Application/compendial requirements | Application/compendial requirements + 0.1N HCl for 2 hr followed by testing in USP buffer pH 4.5–7.5 under standard conditions + 2 additional agitation speeds using the compendial test apparatus | Application/compendial requirements + 3 additional media such as water, 0.1N HOI and phosphate buffer pH 4.5–7.5 |
|---|---|---|
| Level 1 change in nonrelease-controlling excipients | Level 2 change in nonrelease-controlling excipients for delayed release | Level 2 change in nonrelease-controlling excipients for extended release |
| Level 1 change in release-controlling excipients | Level 2 change in release-controlling excipients for delayed-release nonnarrow therapeutic drug | Level 2 change in release-controlling excipients for extended-release nonnarrow therapeutic drug |
| Level 1 change in batch size | Level 2 site change for delayed release | Level 2 site change for extended release |
| Level 1 site change | Level 2 change in batch for extended release | Level 2 change in batch size for delayed release |
| Level 1 equipment change | Level 2 manufacturing process change for delayed release | Level 2 manufacturing process change for extended release |
| Level 1 manufacturing process change | Level 2 change in equipment for delayed release | Level 2 change in equipment for extended release |

*Source*: Adapted from Ref. 84.

In summary, both the SUPAC guidance and BCS-based biowaiver documents represent significant steps taken by the regulatory agency to reduce the number of in vivo bioavailability and bioequivalence studies based on scientific principles. In vitro dissolution tests that are able to discriminate drug-product release characteristics will continue to be utilized as a surrogate for bioavailability testing. More regulatory guidance and discussion on the role of dissolutions are expected in the future.

## REFERENCES

1. Noyes A, Whitney W. The rate of solution of solid substances in their own solution. J Am Chem Soc 1897; 19:930.

2.  Brunner B, Tolloczko S. Phys Chem 1900; 35:283.
3.  Nemst W, Brunner E. Reaction kinetics in heterogeneous systems. Phys Chem 1904; 47:52–102.
4.  Hixson A, Crowell J. Md Eng Chem 1931; 23:923.
5.  Dankwerts PV. Significance of liquid-film coefficients in gas absorption. Md Eng Chem 1951; 43:1460–7.
6.  Nedich RL, Kildsig DO. J Pharm Sci 1972; 61:214h.
7.  Pernarowski M, Woo W, Searle R. J Pharm Sci 1968; 57:1419.
8.  Poole J. Drug Inform Bull 1969; 3:8.
9.  Higuchi W, Hiestand B. J Pharm Sci 1963; 52:67.
10. Abdou HM. Dissolution, Bioavailability & Bioequivalence. Mack Printing Company, 1989, pp. 73–80.
11. Levy G, Lantkowiak J, Procknal J, White D. Effect of certain tablet formulation factors on dissolution rate of activ ingredient II. J Pharm Sci 1963; 52:1047.
12. Yen J. Can Pharm J 1964; 97:25.
13. Ishizaka T, Honda H, Koishi M. Drug dissolution from indomethacin-starch hybrid powders prepared by the dry impact blending method. J Pharm Pharm 1993; 45(9):770–4.
14. Kleinebudde P, Sieg A, Held K, Redeker U. Dissolution testing of reworked tablets. Pharm Technol Eur 2002; 14(1):20-21 + 24-25.
15. Proost J, Bolhuis G, Lerk C. The effect of swelling capacity of disintegrants on the in vitro and in vivo availability of diazapam tablets containing magnesium stearate as lubricants. Int J Pharm 1983; 13:287.
16. Buckton G. The role of compensation analysis in the study of weftability, solubility, disintegration and dissolution. Int J Pharm 1990; 66(1–3): 175–82.
17. Rohrs BR, Thamann TJ, Gao P, Stelzer DJ, Bergren MS, Chao RS. Tablet dissolution affected by a moisture mediated solid-state interaction between drug and disintegrant. Pharm Res 1999; 16(12):1850–6.
18. Bergman L, Bandeline F. J Pharm Sci 1965; 54:445.
19. Levy G, Gurutow R. Effect of certain tablet formulation factors on dissolution rate of the active ingredient iii—tablet lubricants. J Pharm Sci 1963; 52:1139.
20. Marlowe E, Shangraw R. J Pharm Sci 1967; 56:498.
21. Solvang S, Finholta P. Effect of tablet processing and formulation factors on dissolution rate of the active ingredient in human gastric juice. J Pharm Sci 1970; 59:49.
22. Finholt P, Kristiansen H, Schmidt O, Wold K. Medd Norsk Farm Selsk 1966; 28:17.
23. Jacob J, Plein B. J Pharm Sci 1968; 57:802.
24. Gray V. AAPS/FDA workshop on dissolution/in vitro release testing and specifications for special dosage forms. Dissolution Technol 2002; 9(4):16–8, 26.
25. VR Uppoor. Regulatory perspectives on in vitro (dissolution)/in vivo (bioavailability) correlations. J Control Rel Soc 2001; 72(1–3):127–32.
26. Amidon GL, Lennemas H, Shah VP, Crison JR. A theoretical basis for a biopharmaceutics drug classification: the correlation of in vitro drug product dissolution and in vivo bioavailability. Pharm Res 1995; 12:413–20.

27. Dressman JB, Amidon GL, Reppas C, Shah VP. Dissolution testing as a prognostic tool for oral drug absorption: immediate release dosage forms. Pharm Res 1998; 15(1):11–22.

28. Galia B, Nicolaides B, Efihymiopoulos C, Reppas C, Dressman J. Physiologically based dissolution tests: experience with two poorly soluble Glaxo Wellcome drugs. Pharm Res 1997; 14(11)(Suppl.):S491.

29. Tang L, Khan SU, Muhammad NA. Evaluation and selection of bio-relevant dissolution media for a poorly water-soluble new chemical entity. Pharm Dev Technol 2001; 6(4):531–40.

30. Galia E, Nicolaides E, Horter D, Lobenberg R, Reppas C, Dressman JB. Evaluation of various dissolution media for predicting in vivo performance of class I and II drugs. Pharm Res 1998; 15(5):698–705.

31. Sanghvi PP, Nambiar JS, Shukla AJ, Collins CC. Comparison of three dissolution devices for evaluating drug release. Drug Dev Ind Pharm 1994; 20 (6):961–80.

32. Hanson WA. Handbook of Dissolution Testing, 2nd edn. 1991.

33. Collins CC. Vibration: what is it and how might it affect dissolution testing? Diss Tech 1998; 5(4):November.

34. Kaniwa N, Katori N, Aoyagi N, et al. Collaborative study on the development of a standard for evaluation of vibration levels for dissolution apparatus. Int J Pharm 1998; 175:119–29.

35. Siewert M, Weinandy L, Whiteman D, Judkins C. Typical variability and evaluation of sources of variability in drug dissolution testing. Eur J Pharm Biopharm 2002; 53:9–14.

36. Kukura J, Arratia PB, Szalai ES, Muzzio FJ. Engineering tools for understanding the hydrodynamics of dissolution tests. Drug Dev Ind Pharm 2003; 2(29):231–9.

37. Kostewicz ES, Brauns U, Becker R, Bressman JB. Forecasting the oral absorption behavior of poorly soluble weak bases using solubility and dissolution studies in biorelevant media. Pharm Res 2002; 19(3):345–9.

38. Gray VA. Update on dissolution testing—recent activities and trends. Diss Tech 2002; 9(1):13–28.

39. Amidon GL, Lennemas H, Shah VP, Crison JR. A theoretical basis for a biopharmaceutic drug classification: the correlation of in vitro drug product dissolution and in vivo bioavailability. Pharm Res 1995; 12(3):413–20.

40. Boulle C, Abelli C, Becart A, et al. Dissolution test applied to oral formulations for immediate release. STP Pharm Prat 1999; 9(4):287–93.

41. Alexander KS, Laprade B, Mauger JW, Paruta AN. J Pharm Sci 1978; 67:624.

42. Noory C, Tran N, Ouderkirk L, Shah V. Steps for development of a dissolution test for sparingly water-soluble drug products. Am Pharm Rev 2002; 5(4): 16–20.

43. Avdeef A, Berger CM. pH-metric solubility. 3. Dissolution titration template method for solubility determination. Eur J Pharm Sci 2001; 14(4):281–91.

44. Parojcic J, Duric Z, Jovanovic M, Ibric S, Nikolic L. Influence of pH and agitation intensity on drug dissolution from tablets evaluated by means of factorial design. Pharm Ind 2001; 63(7):774–9.

45. Jinno J, Oh DM, Crison JR, Amidon GL. Dissolution of ionizable water-insoluble drugs: the combined effect of pH and surfactant. J Pharm Sci 2000; 89(2):268–74.

46. Wood JH, Syarto JE, Letterman H. J Pharm Sci 1965; 54:1068.

47. Levich VG. Physicochemical Hydrohynamics. Englewood Cliffs, New Jersey: Prentice Hall, 1962.

48. Lagas M, Lerk CF. The polymorphism of sulphathiazole. Int J Pharm 1981; 8(1):11–24.

49. Yoshihashi Y, Kitano H, Yonemochi B, Terada K. Quantitative correlation between initial dissolution rate and heat of fusion of drug substance. Int J Pharm 2000; 204(1–2):1–6.

50. Rohrs BR. Dissolution assay development for in vitro-in vivo correlations. Am Pharm Review 2003; Spring:8–14.

51. Yoshihashi Y, Yonemochi B, Terada K. Estimation of initial dissolution rate of drug substance by thermal analysis: application for carbamazepine hydrate. Pharm Dev Technol 2002; 7(1):89–95.

52. Chen LR, Wesley JA, Bhaftachar S, Bienvenido R, Bahash K, Babu SR. Dissolution behavior of a poorly water-soluble compound in the presence of Tween 80. Pharm Res 2001; 20(5):797–801.

53. Horter D, Dressman JB. Influence of physicochemical properties on dissolution of drugs in the gastrointestinal tract. Adv Drug Del Rev 2001; 46 (1–3):75–87.

54. Johnson KG, Swindell AC. Guidance in the sefting of drug particle size specifications to minimize variability in absorption. Pharm Res 1996; 13(12): 1795–98.

55. Simoes S, Sousa A, Figueiredo M. Dissolution rate studies of pharmaceutical multisized powders—a practical approach using the Coulter method. Int J Pharm 1996; 127(2):283–91.

56. Sadeghnejad GR, Rajabi Siahboom AR. The influence of particle size on the dissolution of poorly soluble drugs. J Pharm Pharm 1999; 51(Suppl.):273.

57. Preechagoon D, Udomprateep A, Manwiwattanagul G. Improved dissolution rate poorly soluble drug by incorporation of buffers. Drug Dev Ind Pharm 2000; 26(8):891–4.

58. Rouchotas C, Cassidy QE, Rowley G. Comparison of surface modification and solid dispersion techniques for drug dissolution. Int J Pharm 2000; 195(1–2): 106.

59. Gupta MK, Goldman D, Bogner RH, Tseng YC. Enhanced drug dissolution and bulk properties of solid dispersions granulated with a surface adsorbent. Pharm Dev Technol 2001; 6(4):563–72.

60. Murali Mohan Babu GV, Prasad Ch DS, Ramana Murthy KV. Evaluation of modified gum karaya as carrier for the dissolution enhancement of poorly water-soluble drug nimodipine. Int J Pharm 2002; 234(1–2):1–17.

61. Mehta AC. Dissolution testing of tablet and capsule dosage forms. J Clin Pharm Ther 1993; 18(6):415–20.

62. Thoma K, Ziegler I. Development of an automated flow-through dissolution system for poorly soluble drugs with poor chemical stability in dissolution media, Pharmazie 1998; 53(11):784–90.

63. Butler WCG, Bateman SR. A flow-through dissolution method for a two component drug formulation where the actives have markedly differing solubility properties. Int J Pharm 1998; 173(1–2):211–9.
64. Bhattachar Shobha N, Wesley James A, Fioritto A, Martin Peter J, Babu Suresh R. Dissolution testing of a poorly soluble compound using the flow-through cell dissolution apparatus. Int J Pharm 2002; 236(1–2):135–43.
65. Yu LX, Wang JT, Hussain A. Evaluation of USP apparatus 3 for dissolution testing of immediate-release products. AAPS PharmSci 2002; 4(1):E1.
66. Langenbucher F, Benz D, Kueth W, Moeller H, Otz M. Standardized flow-cell method as an alternative to existing pharmacopoeial dissolution testing, PharmInd 1989; 51(11):1276–81.
67. Moeller H, Wirbitzki E. Regulatory aspects of modified release dosage forms: special cases of dissolution testing using the flow-through system. Boll Chim Farm 1993; 132(4):105–15.
68. Klein S, Rudolph MW, Dressman JB. Drug release characteristics of different mesalazine products using USP Apparatus 3 to simulate passage through the GI tract. Dissol Technol 2002; 9(4):6–21, 26.
69. Zahirul M, Rhan I. Dissolution testing for sustained or controlled release oral dosage forms and correlation with in-vivo data: challenges and opportunities. Int J Pharm 1996; 140(2):131–43.
70. Sorasuchart W, Wardrop J, Ayres JW. Drug release from spray layered and coated drug-containing beads: effects of pH and comparison of different dissolution methods. Drug Dev Ind Pharm 1999; 25(10):1093–98.
71. Jorgensen F, Grace C, Giambalvo D, Shlyankevich A, McCall T, Bhagwat D. Development of optimized dissolution test methods for analysis of controlled-release formulations of an insoluble drug. Pharm Res 1997; 14(11) (Suppl.):S121.
72. Pillay V, Fassihi R. Evaluation and comparison of dissolution data derived from different modified release dosage forms: an alternative method. J Control Rel 1998; 55(1):45–55.
73. Li JB, Rahn PC. Automated dissolution testing of semisolids. Pharm Tech 1993; July:44–54.
74. Shah VP, Elkins JS. In vitro release from corticosteroid ointments. J Pharm Sci 1995; 84(9).
75. Sanghvi PP, Collins CC. Comparison of diffusion studies of hydrocortisone between the Franz cell and the Enhancer cell. Drug Dev Ind Pharm 1993; 19(13):1573–85.
76. Rege PR, Vilivalam VD, Collins CC. Development in release testing of topical dosage forms: use of the Enhancer Cell with automated sampling. J Pharm Bio Anal 1998; 17:1225–33.
77. Rapedius M, Blanchard J. Comparison of the Hanson Microefte and the VanKel Apparatus for in vitro release testing of topical semisolid formulations. Pharm Res 2001; 18(10):1440–7.
78. Conover WJ. Practical Nonparametric Statistics, 2nd edn. John Wiley & Sons, 1980, p. 223.
79. Hollander M, Wolfe DA. Nonparametric Statistical Methods. John Wiley & Sons, 1973, p. 78.

80. Hofer JD, Gray VA. Examination of selection of immediate release dissolution acceptance criteria. Diss Tech 2003; 10(1):16–20.
81. Moore JW, Flanner HH. Mathematical comparison of curves with an emphasis on in-vitro dissolution profiles. Pharm Tech 1996; 20(6):64–74.
82. Shah VP, Tsong Y, Sathe P, Liu J-P. In vitro dissolution profile comparison—statistics and analysis of the similarity factor, $f_2$. Pharm Res 1998; 15(6):889–96.
83. Terada K, Kitano H, Yoshihashi Y, Yonemochi B. Quantitative correlation between initial dissolution rate and heat of solution of drug. Pharm Res 2000; 17(8):920–4.
84. Marroum PJ. The role of dissolution from a regulatory prospective. Am Pharm Rev 2002; 5(3):24–8.

*Part 5: Beyond Preformulation*

## 5.1

# Structure, Content, and Format of the Preformulation Report

**Ram N. Gidwani**

*Pharmaceutical Consultant, Milford, New Jersey, U.S.A.*

## INTRODUCTION

Preformulation, the cornerstone of science-based formulation development, should always be an integral part of all new drug development projects to facilitate the progression of formulation optimization on a sound scientific basis precept by precept. Needless to say, as a prelude to formulation, it should pave the way for the formulation scientist to successfully formulate stable dosage forms for clinical trials in record time. In other words, prior to embarking on the product development, the formulator should have a clear understanding of the physicochemical properties of the drug substance under consideration. In short, preformulation is considered as a rate-limiting step in the overall planning of new drug development activities.

Inasmuch as the formulation development and process development go hand in hand, the scope of preformulation studies should not be limited to the drug substance characterization alone. It might as well encompass formulation stability and optimization activities prior to, and beyond, the Phase I and Phase II studies until formulation process development has been fully defined for Phase III pivotal clinical batch scale-ups.

### Historical Perspective

Traditionally, preformulation studies, as a rule of thumb, are usually initiated to primarily characterize the candidate drug substance as much as possible to get a head start in designing physically and chemically stable and optimized delivery systems for Phase I safety and Phase II efficacy studies.

However, based on a critical review of the published literature (1–8) by the author, it appears that there is more to preformulation than meets the eye, since the very nature of preformulation evaluation per se has apparently been underrated. In order to address such visionary concepts, I personally advocate the four-step approach for a holistic preformulation undertaking to:

1.  fully characterize the drug substance under study to establish quality control specifications as acceptance criteria,
2.  screen potential excipients that are both physically and chemically compatible with the drug substance of interest, and select excipient use levels on a rational basis,
3.  assess the accelerated and real-time isothermal stability performance to identify the final prototype formulation, with at least one backup for contingency purposes,
4.  stay focused on optimization studies to zero in on the final formulation for process scale-up of registration batches for stability testing and pivotal batches for Phase III clinical trials.

In the absence of formal FDA guidelines for the preformulation reporting program, an attempt is made in this chapter to present a conceptual framework for the "Structure, Content, and Format" of the Preformulation Report, based on my experience. The lurking expectations and requirements for the preformulation report are hard to predict, and they should be considered on an ad hoc basis as they can vary in the structure, content, and format from one drug candidate to another. Since the onus for the preparation of a submission-ready preformulation report lies on the preformulation scientist, a written strategy in the form of a "Preformulation Study Master Protocol" is invariably warranted. Without further ado, let me begin by giving the reader a bird's-eye view of the salient features of what a typical preformulation report should entail.

## Master Protocol Design

The Master Protocol is the heart of the preformulation report. From a GMP perspective, common sense dictates that prior to the commencement of any preformulation activity, one should have a Preformulation Study Master Protocol in place that complies with industry practice. The challenge should be to develop a protocol that is both comprehensive and flexible in nature from a regulatory standpoint. As an illustration, the basic format of a typical preformulation protocol is presented in Table 1, as food for thought.

## ACTIVE PHARMACEUTICAL INGREDIENTS

For all practical purposes, the most commonly used term "active pharmaceutical ingredient" unequivocally means the drug substance per se. Simply stated, both of these terms are used interchangeably. Traditionally, a drug substance

**Table 1**   Typical Preformulation Study Master Protocol

| Company Name _____ | Page 1 of _____ |
|---|---|
| Department Name _____ | Document # _____ |
| Document Title _____ | Revision Level _____ |
| Effective Date _____ | Supersedes Document _____ |

I.   Purpose

To design ways and means of exploring and analyzing with the intent to fully characterize the drug substance on both a qualitative and quantitative basis, in the form of a readily accessible database source for new product development purposes.

II.   Scope

The background information emanating from such preformulation database can be crucial to the lead formulator in pioneering innovative drug-delivery systems unique in terms of quality, stability, performance, and bioavailability attributes.

III.   Responsibility

It will primarily be the responsibility of the Preformulation Department to execute the protocol with both the cooperation and assistance of the Product Development Department.

IV.   Methodology

This protocol is tailored to address some of the critical issues concerning the influence of such factors as pH, temperature, light, moisture, and crystal habit on the stability and suitability of the optimized formulation for pivotal clinical batch scale-up under OMP conditions.

4.1   Drug Substance Characterization

- Develop an analytical procedure
- Characterize critical physicochemical properties
- Identify degradants and process related impurities
- Establish bulk drug substance release specifications
- Conduct accelerated stability at 40 °C/75 % RH
- Generate dissolution profiles

4.2   Physical Characterization of Excipients

- Characterize at molecular, particulate, and bulk levels
- Establish functionality based acceptance criteria
- Conduct 2 wk drug/excipient compatibility at 75 °C

4.3   Stability

- Develop a stability-indicating analytical procedure
- Conduct accelerated stability at 40 °C/75% RH
- Generate dissolution profiles in distilled water, 0.1N HCI (pH 1.2), buffer solution (pH 4.5) and buffer solution (pH 7.2)

*(Continued)*

**Table 1**  Typical Preformulation Study Master Protocol (*Continued*)

4.4  Process Optimization

- Identify critical and noncritical variables
- Define response variables
- Establish predetermined acceptance criteria
- Optimize the critical factor levels

V.  Recommendations for Solid Oral Dosage Forms

5.1  For drug substances hygroscopic in nature, dosage Forms need to be:

✓  Processed under extremely low humidity conditions
✓  Protected from moisture at temperature not exceeding 30 °C
✓  Stored in tight containers

5.2  In order to optimize stability and minimize exposure to moisture:

✓  Both the drug substance and potential enteric polymer be dissolved in a suitable  solvent and the solution cospray dried with the enteric polymer to encapsulate API crystals with a physical barrier
✓  And, the encapsulated drug substance upon dry blending with suitable excipients be filled into hard-gelatin capsules or directly compressed without the tedium of wet granulation.

VI.  Approvals

Product Development  Analytical Research  Regulatory Affairs

VII.  History of Change

| Revision | Supercedes | Reason for Revision | Effective Date |
|---|---|---|---|
| 00 | None | Original Issue | DD/MM/YY |
| 01 | 00 | Editorial Changes | DD/MM/YY |
| 02 | 01 | Ad hoc Changes | DD/MM/YY |

synthesized by a sequence of chemical reactions is defined by its typical chemical structure and characterized by its unique physicochemical properties. Besides chemical synthesis, other alternate processes including fermentation, recovery from natural materials, recombinant DNA, and monoclonal antibody production are also used in the manufacture of drug substances.

As part of the overall chemical synthesis scheme, the crude form of the synthesized drug substance following the purification step usually undergoes identification, purity assessment, and structure elucidation to characterize the molecule in terms of its molecular weight, molecular formula, and chemical structure by mass spectroscopy and nuclear magnetic resonance.

With regard to the impurity profile, unknown impurities stemming from the drug substance synthesis and degradation at levels above or equal to 0.1% should always be isolated, and if possible, identified and characterized. Typically, impurities occurring at levels greater than 0.5% are considered major, and those occurring below 0.5% are considered minor.

Based on the above discussion related to both chemical synthesis and the impurity profile of the target drug molecule, a suggested preformulation checklist for active pharmaceutical ingredients is presented in Table 2.

**Table 2** Suggested Preformulation Checklist for Active Pharmaceutical Ingredients

| Aspect | Technique | Prospect |
|---|---|---|
| Identification | LC-MS, NMR, IR | Structure confirmation |
| Assay | HPLC, stability indicating | Purity assessment |
| Bulk density | Loose and tapped | Carr's flowability index |
| Particle size | Laser light scattering | Particle size distribution |
| Specific surface area | Multipoint BET method | Dissolution enhancement |
| Crystal morphology | X-ray diffraction, | Define polymorphic, |
| Crystal lattice | SEM, DSC, DTA, | pseudopolymorphic, |
| Crystal habit | and MTDSC | and/or amorphous |
| Melting range | | states |
| Glass transition temperature | | |
| Eutectic temperature | | |
| Polymorphic forms | | |
| Hydrates | | |
| Solvates | | |
| Amorphous form | | |
| Enantiomerism | Polarimeter | Specific optical rotation |
| Loss on drying | NIR, TGA, KF | Moisture content |
| Water adsorption isotherm | Moisture balance | Hygroscopicity profile |
| Aqueous solubility | Equilibrium solubility | Intrinsic solubility |
| Ionization constant, $pK_a$ | Spectrophotometric | pH solubility profile |
| Aqueous solution stability | Spectrophotometric | pH stability range |
| Partition coefficient | Spectrophotometric | Drug lipophilicity |
| Impurity profile | LC-MS, NMR, GC | Molecular weight, |
| Synthesis impurities | | and structure |
| Degradation products | | elucidation |
| Residual solvents | | |

*(Continued)*

**Table 2** Suggested Preformulation Checklist for Active Pharmaceutical Ingredients
(*Continued*)

| Aspect | Technique | Prospect |
|---|---|---|
| Stress testing<br>Acid/base hydrolysis<br>Oxidation<br>Photolysis<br>Thermal/humidity | HPLC, LC-MS, NMR | Degradation pathways, and stability-indicating method validation |
| Intrinsic dissolution<br>Distilled water<br>0.1N HCI (pH 1.2)<br>Buffer solution (pH 4.5)<br>Buffer solution (pH 7.2) | HPLC, UV | pH dissolution profile |
| Formal stability testing<br>25°C/60% RH<br>30°C/60% RH<br>40°C/75% RH | HPLC, stability indicating | Ideal storage conditions, package compatibility, and retest period estimation |
| Process optimization | Pilot batch scale-up | Optimal operating ranges |

*Abbreviations*: BET, Brunauer Emmett Teller; DSC, differential scanning calorimetry; DTA, differential thermal analysis; GC, gas chromatography; HPLC, high performance liquid chromatography; IR, infrared; KF, Karl Fischer; LC-MS, liquid chromatography–mass spectroscopy; MTDSC, modulated temperature DSC; NIR, near infrared; NMR, nuclear magnetic resonance; SEM, scanning electron microscopy; TGA, thermogravimetric analysis; UV, ultraviolet.

## BULK PHARMACEUTICAL EXCIPIENTS

Although excipients, by definition, are considered inactive components that are therapeutically inert in nature, they can, depending on the functionality attributes, influence the overall stability, performance, and manufacture of drug products. Nevertheless, based on a long safe track record, most excipients are generally regarded as safe (GRAS) materials for use in pharmaceutical applications; and as such do not require premarket FDA approval.

There is a whole gamut of excipients available with unique functionality potentials for unique pharmaceutical applications. Notwithstanding their inert physical nature, most excipients are more often than not selected on the basis of their unique functionality for evaluation as potential inactive components of the intended end product under development. In order to characterize excipients adequately, both physical and functionality testing of key excipients is normally conducted at the molecular, particulate, and bulk levels. An ideal functionality test can correlate with or predict finished product performance for the drug candidate.

## Excipients as Adjuvants

A drug-delivery system can be designed into various dosage forms, depending on whether it is intended for the inhalation, nasal, oral, parenteral, topical, transdermal, or transmucosal route of administration. For instance, emulsions have been traditionally used as vehicles for oral, parenteral, and transdermal drug-delivery systems. It is noteworthy that emulsions such as oral dosage forms have been known to enhance drug bioavailability by means of delaying gastric emptying and by-passing the hepatic first-pass drug metabolism as a result of improved absorption through the lymphatic system. Likewise, biodegradable vegetable oil emulsions can be conveniently used to parenterally administer a variety of drugs. Among other countless uses, functional excipients can be used discriminatingly to control, enhance, modify, or optimize the drug release, stability, and bioavailability characteristics of the proposed drug-delivery systems under development.

There are many types of functional excipients on the market. Without going into too much detail, an abbreviated account of some typical examples of the functional excipient systems is presented here for theoretical considerations.

### Cosolvancy

When the drug substance exhibits more solubility in a mixture of two or more mutually miscible solvents than in one primary solvent alone, the phenomenon is referred to as cosolvancy, and the secondary solvents are termed as "cosolvents."

During the initial preformulation phase of formulation development utilizing commercially available pharmaceutical solvents of interest such as cosolvents, ternary phase diagrams for the drug substance, cosolvents, and water system are used to identify apparent miscibility domains representing improved drug solubility. The ternary phase diagrams are normally constructed by titrating known binary mixtures of the drug substance and cosolvent with water, using optical transparency or turbidity as end-points.

### Solid Dispersions

A solid dispersion is defined as a monolithic dispersion of the drug in an inert carrier matrix. Using the solvent evaporation method, solid dispersions can be conveniently prepared by cospray-drying the drug–excipient solution. In contrast to the general tendency of microencapsulated drug substances to rupture and leak when compressed under pressure, solid dispersions by their very nature are amenable to tableting without any problems.

Furthermore, solid dispersions of water-soluble drugs in pH-labile enteric or pH-independent nonerodible matrices impervious to water can be used to create a three to five hour postgastric delay of drug release for colon-targeted delivery systems. By the same token, lipid-based delivery systems including water-in-oil types of emulsions such as semisolid matrices filled in hard gelatin capsules and microemulsions filled in soft gelatin capsules can be used to target the drug to the lymphatics.

Coacervation

When two oppositely charged hydrophilic materials are mixed together, they interact due to electrostatic attraction between them to form a weak complex that separates out as a new phase. The complex formed by phase separation is called coacervate, and the phenomenon is referred to as coacervation.

Since most drug substances are either weak acids or bases, it is reasonable to surmise that acid salts of basic drugs will be cationic in nature and prone to ion exchange with oppositely charged anionic polymers, resulting in the formation of potential drug–polymer coacervates as controlled-release matrices. This concept of coacervation as a means of controlling drug release opens a new window of opportunity, assuming that the drug release in the gastrointestinal (GI) tract will be controlled by the rate at which the coacervate complex exchanges free drug base for other cations in the GI fluids.

Liquid Crystal Phase

Conventional oil-in-water and/or water-in-oil types of emulsions and creams can be stabilized by the formation of anisotropic, birefringent liquid crystals as a third phase at the water–oil interface.

Under the polarized-light microscope, birefringent phases do exhibit the characteristic property of alternately appearing as colored and dark images when rotated between the cross-polarized analyzer and polarizer. The angle through which a birefringent sample is rotated from a brightly colored position to a completely dark position is commonly referred to as the angle of extinction. This measurement of extinction angle for the birefringent liquid crystal phase can easily be used as an in-process control specification.

Based on the above discussion related to both physical and functionality testing issues, a suggested preformulation checklist for inactive functional excipients is presented in Table 3.

## STABILITY

Stability may simply be defined as the extent to which the drug substance or drug product retains, within specified limits throughout its storage period and use, the same properties and characteristics that it possessed at the time of manufacture and packaging. Therefore, the overall stability of both the drug substance and the drug product will depend on the physicochemical nature of the active ingredient alone or in combination with other inactive ingredients such as excipients and packaging components.

**Table 3**  Suggested Preformulation Checklist for Bulk Pharmaceutical Excipients

| Aspect | Technique | Prospect |
|---|---|---|
| Identification | FTIR | Identity verification |
| Loss on drying | NIR, TGA, KF | Moisture content |
| Bulk density | Loose and tapped | Carr's flowability index |
| True density | Helium pyknometer | Functionality correlation |
| Specific surface area | Multipoint BET method | Functionality correlation |
| Particle size distribution | Laser light scattering | Functionality correlation |
| Contact angle | Goniometer | Powder wettability |
| Crystal morphology | X-ray diffraction, SEM, hot | Define crystalline, and |
|   Melting range |   stage microscopy, DSC, |   amorphous states |
|   Glass transition temp |   and DTA | |
|   Eutectic temperature | | |
| Functionality | | |
|   Cosolvancy | Ternary diagram | Solubilization |
|   Solid dispersions | DSC, and DTA | Dissolution enhancement |
|   Coacervation | DSC, and DTA | Controlled release |
|   Liquid crystal phase | Polarized-light microscopy | Absorption enhancement |
| Microbial limits testing | USP method | Bioburden levels for |
|   Total plate count | |   GMP compliance |
|   Yeast | | |
|   Mold | | |
|   Coliform | | |
|   Pathogens | | |
| Compatibility with API | 50/50 binary mixtures | 2-week stability at 75°C |

*Abbreviations*: API, active pharmaceutical ingredient; BET, Brunauer Emmett Teller; DSC, differential scanning calorimetry; DTA, differential thermal analysis; FTIR, Fourier transform infrared; GMP, good manufacturing practices; KF, Karl Fischer; NIR, near infrared; SEM, scanning electron microscopy; USP, US Pharmacopeia.

## Formal Stability Studies

The purpose of formal stability studies is twofold: first, to collect the long-term, intermediate, and accelerated stability data on at least three primary batches of the drug substance under the influence of temperature, humidity, and light as a function of time, and then, to establish the retest period for the drug substance, the shelf-life for the drug product, and the storage conditions. Both the retest period and shelf-life are proposed based on the outcome of these real-time stability studies under long-term testing storage conditions, and are supported by the accelerated stability data.

These formal stability studies should be conducted on the drug sub-stance packaged in the container-closure system that is the same as or simulates the final packaging proposed for warehouse storage, distribution, and subsequent use and handling.

### Accelerated Stability Study

The accelerated stability evaluation should cover a minimum of six months. In addition, a minimum of three time points, including the initial and final time points at zero-, three-, and six-month intervals for the six-month study are normally used.

### Intermediate Stability Study

Initially, a minimum of six-months data from a 12-month study is evaluated. The intermediate stability evaluation, under normal conditions, is not initiated until after significant changes have occurred at any time during six-months testing at the accelerated storage conditions. A minimum of four time points including the initial and final points at 0-, 6-, 9-, and 12-month intervals are normally used.

### Long-Term Stability

The long-term, real-time stability evaluation should cover a minimum of 12 months. However, when the available long-term, real-time stability data do not cover the proposed retest period, the stability studies should continue to firmly establish the retest period. In addition, the frequency of testing should normally be every three months over the first year, every six months over the second year, and annually thereafter through the proposed retest period.

## Stability-Testing Protocol

There is no such thing as one model protocol that will address all types of stability-testing programs. The protocol format and content will vary from product to product, depending on the type of drug substance or drug product used. A well-designed, product-specific protocol will go a long way to getting the stability-testing program on the right track. An example of the typical stability-testing protocol format for the drug substance or drug product storage conditions and testing frequency is presented in Table 4.

## PROCESS OPTIMIZATION

### Design of Experiment (DOE)

It is common knowledge that during the early stages of product development, the formulation scientist is more often than not faced with an uphill battle of exploring all controllable variables that need to be

**Table 4** Typical Stability-Testing Protocol for No Less Than Three Batches of the Drug Substance or Drug Product Packaged in the Proposed Final Container-Closure System

| | Storage conditions | | |
| --- | --- | --- | --- |
| Months | Long-term, 25°C/60% RH | Intermediate, 30°C/60% RH | Accelerated, 40°C/75% RH |
| 0 | Yes | No | No |
| 1 | Yes | Yes | Yes |
| 3 | Yes | Yes | Yes |
| 6 | Yes | Yes[a] | Yes |
| 9 | Yes | Yes[a] | No |
| 12 | Yes | Yes[a] | No |
| 18 | Yes | No | No |
| 24 | Yes | No | No |
| 36 | Yes | No | No |

[a] No testing required if no failures detected under accelerated storage conditions.

factored into the preformulation equation to evaluate all potential factors from a tenable formulation standpoint. Fortunately, the optimization techniques (9,10) allow the formulator to zoom in on the formulation and process variables for the purpose of designing a robust dosage form.

## Hypothetical Three-Level Factorial Experimental Design Model

Using an appropriate factorial experimental design, the formulation scientist can diligently undertake the following steps:

1. Carefully define both the formulation and process factors, levels, and responses

**Table 5** Normal Zero Level Prototype Formulation for Two Treatments Consisting of Lubricant Level and Lubrication Time

| | Composition | | Treatments | |
| --- | --- | --- | --- | --- |
| Components | mg | % | Factor | Range |
| Drug substance | 40 | 20 | | |
| Filler | 150 | 75 | | |
| Glidant | 6 | 3 | | |
| Lubricant level | 4 | 2 | A | 2–6 mg |
| Lubrication time | 5 min | | B | 3–7 min |
| Capsule fill weight | 200 mg | 100 | | |

**Table 6** High (+) and Low (−) Levels for Both the Factor A (Lubricant) and Factor B (Lubrication Time) Corresponding to ±50% and ±40% of the Normal Zero Level (0), Respectively

| | Factors | |
|---|---|---|
| Levels | A (mg) | B (mg) |
| High level (+) | 6 | 7 |
| Zero level (0) | 4 | 5 |
| Low level (−) | 2 | 3 |

**Table 7** Test Matrix for Experimental Formulation Runs

| | Factors and levels | | |
|---|---|---|---|
| Runs | A (mg) | B (min) | Main effects (response variables) |
| 1 | 0 | 0 | Y1 = blend homogeneity |
| 2 | + | + | Y2 = bulk density |
| 3 | + | − | Y3 = tap density |
| 4 | − | + | Y4 = dissolution |
| 5 | − | − | Y5 = accelerated stability |

| | Critical factors | | Noncritical factors | | |
|---|---|---|---|---|---|
| Runs | A (mg) | B (min) | Drug (mg) | Filler (mg) | Glidant (mg) |
| 1 | 4 | 5 | 40 | 150 | 6 |
| 2 | 6 | 7 | 40 | 148 | 6 |
| 3 | 6 | 3 | 40 | 148 | 6 |
| 4 | 2 | 7 | 40 | 152 | 6 |
| 5 | 2 | 3 | 40 | 152 | 6 |

**Table 8** Suggested Structure of Various Sections of a Typical Preformulation Report

| Section | Table of contents |
|---|---|
| I | Objective |
| II | Scope |
| III | Background |
| IV | Active pharmaceutical ingredient (API) update |
| V | Bulk pharmaceutical excipients |
| VI | Results and discussion |
| VII | Summary and conclusion |

**Table 9** Suggested Content and Format of Key Sections of the Preformulation Report

| Section | | Active pharmaceutical ingredient (API) update |
|---|---|---|
| IV | A. | Generic Information Review |
| | | 1. Nomenclature Designations |
| | | 2. Structure Elucidation |
| | | 3. Method of Manufacture |
| | | 4. Process Impurities |
| | | 5. Degradation Products and Pathways |
| | | 6. Reference Standards |
| | | 7. Analytical Methods Validation |
| | | 8. Standards and Specifications |
| | B. | Empirical Data Evaluation |
| | | 1. Physical and Chemical Characterization |
| | |    a. Melting Point and Loss on Drying |
| | |    b. Glass Transition and Eutectic Temperatures |
| | |    c. Polymorphism and Chirality |
| | |    d. Bulk Density and Flowability Index |
| | |    e. Hygroscopicity and Specific Surface Area |
| | |    f. Aqueous Solubility and Partition Coefficient |
| | |    g. $pK_a$, pH-Solubility and pH-Stability Profiles |
| | |    h. Particle Size and Intrinsic Dissolution |
| | | 2. Proposed Container-Closure System |
| | | 3. Photostability Testing |
| | | 4. Formal Stability Studies |
| | |    a. Long-Term (25°C/60% RH) |
| | |    b. Intermediate (30°C/60% RH) |
| | |    c. Accelerated (40°C/75% RH) |
| | | 5. Process Optimization |
| | |    a. Critical Processing Steps Characterization |
| | |    b. Proven Acceptable Ranges (PAR) for Critical Steps |
| V | | Bulk Pharmaceutical Excipients |
| | A. | Vendor Qualification |
| | B. | Physical Characterization |
| | C. | Functionality Correlation |
| | D. | Compatibility with API |

2. Meaningfully evaluate all potential factors to identify a final prototype formulation as a basis for optimization studies
3. Gainfully optimize the critical factor levels of the final prototype formulation to meet the predetermined acceptance criteria for the prototype formulation responses.

As per the hypothetical experimental design depicted in Tables 5 to 7, it will require only five trial runs for the optimization experiment to study the effects of two treatments each at high and low levels, as well as the normal zero level as a reference.

## CONCLUSION

The intent of this refresher is to provide the reader with some general guidance in the preparation of the preformulation report. The suggested structure for the sections of a typical preformulation report as reflected by the Table of Contents is outlined in Table 8. Last but not least, the suggested content and format of each section are delineated in Table 9.

## REFERENCES

1. Akers MJ. Preformulation testing of solid oral dosage form drugs. Can J Pharm Sci 1976; 11:1–10.
2. Greene DS. Preformulation. In: Banker GS, Rhodes CT, eds. Modern Pharmaceutics. New York: Marcel Decker Inc, 1979, pp. 211–25.
3. Fiese EF, Hagen TA. Preformulation. In: Lachman L, Lieberman HA, Kanig JL, eds. The Theory and Practice of Industrial Pharmacy. Philadelphia: Lea & Febiger, 1986, pp. 171–96.
4. Wells JI. Pharmaceutical Preformulation: The Physicochemical Properties of Drug Substances. New York: Halsted Press, 1988.
5. Brittain HG, Sachs CJ, Fiorelli K. Physical characterization of pharmaceutical excipients: practical examples. Pharm Technol 1991; 15:38–52.
6. Motola S, Agharkar SN. Preformulation research of parenteral medications. In: Avis KE, Lachman L, Lieberman HA, eds. Pharmaceutical Dosage Forms: Parentral Medications. New York: Marcel Decker Inc, 1992, pp. 115–72.
7. Chowhan ZT. Excipients and Their Funtionality in Drug Product Development. Pharm Technol 1993; 17:72–82.
8. Radenbough GW, Ravin U. Preformulation. In: Gennaro AR, ed. Remington: The Science and Pharmacy, 9th ed. Easton, PA: Mack Publishing Company, 1995, pp. 1447–62.
9. Renoux R, Demazieres JA, Cardot JM, Aiache JM. Experimentally designed optimization of direct compression tablets. Drug Dev Ind Pharm 1996; 22: 103–9.
10. Hwang R, Gemoules MK, Ramlose DS, Thomasson CE. A systematic formulation optimization process for a generic pharmaceutical tablet. Pharm Technol 1998; 22:48–64.

## 5.2

# Significance of Drug Substance Physicochemical Properties in Regulatory Quality by Design[*]

**Sau Lawrence Lee, Andre S. Raw, and Lawrence Yu**

*Office of Generic Drugs, United States Food and Drug Administration, Rockville, Maryland, U.S.A.*

## INTRODUCTION TO QUALITY BY DESIGN

Due to the growing complexity of drug substances and formulations, developing a quality (1) drug product and a process that manufactures it in a reproducible manner becomes increasingly challenging and costly. Very often, even though a final drug product is successfully manufactured to meet the regulatory specifications, the drug product development is in part based on correlative methods, in which the limits on quality attributes and process parameters are derived empirically to ensure that the produced batches mimic the performance of batches tested clinically. This approach can guarantee consistent high-quality drug products only if the relationship between these limits and the drug performance, as well as the variability within the drug substance, excipient raw materials, and process characteristics, is well understood. Without this knowledge, the restrictions on quality attributes are established mainly based on the so-called zero tolerance criterion, which often leads to overspecification. In the worst-case scenario, other critical attribute(s) may not even be identified, monitored, and controlled. As a result, continuous improvement on product quality

---

[*]The opinions expressed in this chapter by the authors do not necessarily reflect the views or policies of the Food and Drug Administration (FDA).

and process, as well as risk assessment and management (2), would be difficult to carry out under this circumstance.

In order to gain such knowledge, the concept of quality by design (QbD) should be emphasized. In this approach, the design of quality drugs is based on fundamental understanding of the drug substance, formulation, process characteristics, and their relation to the drug product performance. This concept has already been incorporated into the ICH guidance on Pharmaceutical Development (ICHQ8) (3). To achieve the objective of QbD, product and process characteristics that are critical to the desired performance must be derived from experience and experimental assessment during drug product development (4). This information and knowledge could potentially be used to develop a multivariable model that links drug substance, excipient, and process variables with drug product quality attributes and to construct the design space. (The design space is the established range of process parameters that has been demonstrated to provide assurance of quality. In some cases, design space can also be applicable to formulation attributes. Working within the design space is not generally considered as a change of the approved ranges for process parameters and formulation attributes. Movement out of the design space is considered to be a change and would normally initiate a regulatory postapproval change process.)

Consequently, QbD allows pharmaceutical companies to develop their drug products with an enhanced knowledge of product performance over a wider range of material attributes, processing options, and process parameters. These approaches provide a basis for achieving the goals of FDA's cGMPs for the 21st Century Initiative of having (*i*) product quality and performance achieved by the design of effective and efficient manufacturing processes, (*ii*) drug product specifications based on a mechanistic understanding of how formulation and process factors impact drug product performance, (*iii*) manufacturing process improvements that are within the design space described in the original application without further regulatory reviews, and (*iv*) real-time quality assurance that leads to a reduction of end-product release testing. Therefore, by demonstrating a higher degree of understanding of product properties and manufacturing process through QbD, it provides opportunities to develop more flexible regulatory approaches.

## PHYSICOCHEMICAL PROPERTIES OF DRUG SUBSTANCES

As an initial step toward achieving QbD, it is essential, in the early stage of drug product development, to gain a fundamental understanding of drug substance properties that can potentially influence drug product performance and manufacturability. This study of drug substance physicochemical properties is usually conducted in the preformulation stages of development. In general, preformulation work can start as early as during biological screening, in which diverse compounds are screened for the desired activity. An extensive physicochemical characterization of the drug substance, however, usually will not start until one or more potential candidates are identified and taken into clinical testing during the investigational stages. The information and knowledge gained from preformulation studies not only constitute a framework for QbD but also may help to accelerate the introduction of new therapeutic entities for a customer's needs. For instance, the selection of compounds that have physical properties favorable for oral absorption and certain types of process operations can facilitate the rapid progress of these compounds at later stages of drug product development.

Depending on the expertise, equipment, and drug substance availability, the scope of preformulation activities to be carried out can be somewhat different for every company. Not all physicochemical properties are examined extensively for every new compound. Data or information, as they are generated during preformulation studies, must be evaluated carefully to determine what additional studies will be needed in order to have sufficient data available for further development. Nevertheless, preformulation studies, in general, start with an investigation of solubility and permeability and continue to the study of stability, hygroscopicity, particle size, polymorphism, etc. Moreover, since some of these characteristics could be interrelated, their analysis may need to be considered in combination.

These drug substance properties should be emphasized in the pharmaceutical development section of the original new drug applications as well as abbreviated new drug applications. This information provides early insights to both industry and regulators, regarding the potential significance of these physicochemical properties on drug product quality and manufacturing process. Due to the limited space in this review, we will, in this chapter, focus only on some of these physicochemical properties of the drug substance and discuss them in the context of QbD by addressing their potential influence on drug product bioavailability, stability, and manufacturability.

## Solubility and Permeability

One of the primary regulatory concerns with regard to the physicochemical properties of drug substance is their potential effect on drug product bioavailability. This is due to the fact that prior to any drug absorption through the gastrointestinal (GI) membrane, the orally bioavailable drugs must first dissolve in the GI fluids. Since the dissolution rate of a solid is a function of its solubility in the dissolution medium, solubility can have a significant influence on the rate and extent of drug absorption. Thus, the solubility of a candidate drug becomes a critical factor for determining its usefulness and developability. In general, because many candidate drugs are ionizable organic compounds (predominantly weak acids and weak bases), with their solubility depending on the pH of the medium, it is important to ascertain the aqueous solubility of a drug candidate over the physiologically relevant pH range of 1 to 7.5. (The solubility of an acidic or basic compound, at a given pH, is a function of the solubility of the ionized form and the limiting solubility of the corresponding neutral form, and the degree of ionization at a given pH is dictated by the $pK_a$ of the compound). Moreover, although this type of experiments is conceptually simple, such measurements of solubility should be done with caution, particularly where the dissolution of a compound is accompanied by degradation or polymorphic transformation in solvents, or where a candidate drug is poorly soluble. For instance, the solubility of poorly soluble compounds could be overestimated due to the presence of soluble impurities (5). In addition, it is essential to determine pH of the system after equilibration simply because the pH of ionizable compounds in a buffered system may not be the same as that of the starting buffer.

In the case of a poorly soluble drug substance, the solubility can be improved without molecular modifications, as a means of maximizing oral absorption. The most common method of increasing solubility (either a weak acid or a weak base) is to induce salt formation. The solubility enhancement by salt formation is related to several factors including the thermodynamically favored aqueous solvation of cations or anions used to create the salt of the active moiety, the differing energies of the salt crystal lattice, and the ability of the salt to alter the resultant solution pH (6). In addition, even if the salt formation has no significant effect on the solubility, the dissolution rate of the salt will often be enhanced due to the difference in the pH of the thin diffusion layer surrounding the drug particle (7). It is important to emphasize that other factors, in addition to solubility and dissolution rate, should be taken into consideration in a salt selection process. These factors may include the physical and chemical stability of a salt and its in vivo behavior (e.g., some salts of weak acids may precipitate in the stomach in an uncontrollable fashion). When the drug substance under consideration is not amenable to the salt formation, or when the salt form is not a recommended final form due to some stability or safety issues, other means of enhancing solubility can be employed. These include the use of a more soluble metastable polymorph and the utilization of complexation and coprecipitates that are mixtures of solid solutions or dispersions (8,9).

Moreover, permeability is a critical factor for determining the developability of a candidate compound. This is because absorption of drugs administered orally can be viewed as two consecutive steps: dissolution of drugs in the GI fluids and permeation of dissolved drugs through the GI membrane. As mentioned previously, for relatively insoluble compounds, the rate-limiting step is generally the rate of dissolution. In contrast, for relatively soluble drug substances, the permeation across biological membranes may be determinative of the overall rate of absorption. Thus, both solubility and permeability can have a significant effect on bioavailability. In contrast to solubility, which can often be improved by physical intervention or formulation principles [since permeability is a function of molecular weight, relative aqueous and lipid solubility (lipophilicity), number of hydrogen-bonding groups, and number of charges on the drug molecule], permeability in majority of cases can only be enhanced through molecular modifications. Hence, it is difficult to improve permeability, for example, by decreasing the molecular size, without compromising the intrinsic activity of the drug substance. Even though in some cases the extent of drug absorption due to poor permeability (e.g., azithromycin) can be overcome by increasing solubility (10), it is nevertheless important to gain an early knowledge on the absorption potential of candidate drugs. This can be sought, for example, through the measurement of partition coefficients that are usually performed in the octanol–water system and through the in vitro permeability measurement using biological membranes and cultured cells (11). It should be noted that the GI motility and metabolism limitation also play an important role on bioavailability, but these are outside the intended scope of this chapter and hence will not be discussed here.

The importance of solubility and permeability obtained in pre-formulation studies can be further understood in terms of their use in the biopharmaceutic classification system (BCS) (12). According to the BCS, drug compounds are classified as follows:

- *Class I*: high permeability, high solubility
- *Class II*: high permeability, low solubility
- *Class III*: low permeability, high solubility
- *Class IV*: low permeability, low solubility

In this system, a drug substance is considered highly soluble when the highest dose strength is soluble in $\geq 250$ mL water over a range of pH from 1 to 7.5. For a highly permeable drug substance, the extent of absorption in humans is $\geq 90\%$ of an administered dose, based on mass-balance or in comparison to an intravenous reference dose. When $\geq 85\%$ of the label amount of drug substance dissolves within 30 minutes using USP apparatus I or II in a volume of $\leq 900$ mL buffer solutions, a corresponding drug product is considered to be rapidly dissolving.

The BCS contains several implications in drug development, even though it has been developed primarily for regulatory applications and particularly for oral immediate-release products. One obvious advantage of analyzing the solubility and permeability data in the BCS context is that it provides clear and simple guidelines for determining the rate-limiting factor in the GI drug absorption process. Therefore, the BCS framework can be useful in an early selection of candidate drugs for further development. For example, the developability of a new compound into a clinically useful drug product may be limited if this new compound has a very low permeability and/or solubility, which will likely result in low and highly variable bioavailability. The BCS can also provide some guidance on the choice of formulation principles. For instance, drug substances with good permeability (class I and class II drugs) should be more suitable for an oral extended-release administration (13). This is due to the fact that the colon has been shown to have a lower permeability than the small intestine, and a significant amount of the drug substance in the extended-release formulation will be delivered there. This implies that the drug substance needs to have a good permeability in order to ensure drug absorption throughout the entire intestine.

Knowledge of drug substance solubility and permeability is useful not only for evaluating the drug product bioavailability but also in the development of in vitro dissolution and permeation testing. These in vitro tests may be used to complement or replace certain in vivo bioavailability and bioequivalence studies. In addition, solubility data for different dissolution mediums are useful for selecting the appropriate solvent for the unit operations, such as granulation and coating.

## Stability

Another regulatory concern regarding drug substance physicochemical properties is their potential effect on drug product stability. Since a drug substance is an integral part of a drug product, it is apparent that the intrinsic drug substance stability has a direct impact on the overall drug product stability. Moreover, the physical properties of the drug substance, such as crystal form, equilibrium moisture content, and particle size also influence its stability. Thus, it is necessary to gain some basic understanding of the solid- and liquid-state drug substance stability properties in the early stages of drug development.

For small molecules, information on drug substance stability could be first sought through an examination of their chemical structure. The molecular structure or functional groups of a compound may give some indication of its chemical reactivity. For example, compounds that have functional groups such as an ester, amide, and lactam may be susceptible to degradation via hydrolysis (14), whereas compounds that contain electron-rich centers are more vulnerable to photocatalyzed oxidation. This knowledge is potentially useful in designing experiments as leads to further assess drug substance stability.

In general, it is not possible to perform stability studies under normal storage conditions in the early stage of drug development. This is simply due to the fact that there is a time constraint for preformulation studies and most degradation reactions, especially solid-state degradation, are very slow. Therefore, it is customary to use stress conditions in an early investigation of the solid- and liquid-state stability of a drug substance (15). The accelerated stability studies should include an investigation of drug stability at elevated temperatures, under high-humidity conditions (for a drug substance in the solid state), and with enhanced oxygen and light exposure. This is because the major routes of drug degradation in the solid state are via pyrolysis, hydrolysis, oxidation, and photolysis, and the stability of a drug substance with respect to these degradation reactions can be accessed quickly under these stress conditions. It should be noted that some liquid-state stability studies are still necessary even for a drug substance that is expected to be formulated into a solid dosage form. One of the main reasons for having these studies is to ensure that the drug substance does not degrade intolerably when it is exposed to GI fluids prior to drug absorption across the GI membrane. Thus, it is useful to evaluate the drug substance stability in the physiological relevant pH range from 1.0 to 7.5.

The data obtained under these stress conditions are often used to predict long-term stability under normal storage conditions. However, this approach must be applied cautiously, and the stability data must be interpreted carefully. For example, a pharmaceutical solid that is susceptible to hydrolysis may become more stable at elevated temperatures because of the loss of residual water due to evaporation. Moreover, some degradation reactions observed at high temperatures may not occur to any appreciable extend in a low temperature range. Nevertheless, accelerated stability studies do provide an early insight into drug substance stability, including some understanding of reaction kinetics and degradation mechanisms as well as the nature and level of the resulting degradants.

This data derived from solid- and liquid-state stability studies is vital to the formulation design with respect to its stability characteristics. This can be best understood by considering a drug substance that is vulnerable to both hydrolysis and oxidation. In this case, a solid oral dosage form using excipients such as starch that contain a significant amount of free water may not be suitable for this compound, while in comparison, the addition of an antioxidant to the solid formulation would aid in suppressing oxidative degradation and thus extend drug product shelf life. This type of stability data is also useful in the selection of process conditions used to manufacture the drug product. For instance, a nonaqueous solvent should be used if a compound becomes chemically or physically unstable when exposed to moisture. Therefore, understanding the drug substance stability with respect to different stresses and the nature of the resulting degradants, and using this information in the design of the product will lead to an improvement of drug product quality.

In addition, because the drug substance is often in intimate contact with one or more excipients in the formulation, it is also important to gain some early knowledge of drug–excipient compatibility (i.e., the excipient effect on the chemical stability of new candidate drugs), in addition to understanding the intrinsic drug substance stability. These types of studies are critical for avoiding chemical incompatibilities such as the reactions of nucleophilic drugs (e.g., amines) with electrophilic excipients (e.g., esters) or electrophilic drugs (e.g., carboxylic acids) with nucleophilic excipients (e.g., alcohol), which would clearly have an adverse effect on drug product stability. For example, one very common reaction that occurs between drugs and excipients is the Maillard reaction that involves interactions between primary and secondary amine drugs and reducing sugars. Most of these reactions, such as the Maillard reaction, are accelerated by moisture and temperature and have been responsible for several product failures on stability (16). To accentuate drug–excipient interactions, the compatibility screening tests usually involve the use of powder blends of drug and excipients and employ elevated temperature and humidity conditions, allowing a rapid detection of drug–excipient incompatibility. The knowledge gained from these drug–excipient compatibility studies will be helpful in selecting appropriate excipients that are compatible with the drug substance in the formulation design.

## Hygroscopicity

Many drug substances have a tendency to adsorb water. The hygroscopic characteristics of the drug substance are usually assessed by the sorption isotherm, which shows the equilibrium moisture content of the drug substance as a function of the relative vapor pressure. It is usually determined by placing samples in desiccators under different relative humidity (RH) conditions. According to the recent version of European Pharmacopeia (17), the degree of hygroscopicity is defined based on water content measurements after storage at 25°C for 24 hours at 80% RH:

- *Deliquescent*: sufficient water is absorbed to form a liquid
- *Very hygroscopic*: increase in mass is equal to or greater than 15% (w/w)
- *Hygroscopic*: increase in mass is less than 15% (w/w) and equal to or great than 2% (w/w)
- *Slightly hygroscopic*: increase in mass is less than 2% (w/w) and equal to or greater than 0.2% (w/w)

   The principal regulatory concern regarding moisture is its potential effect on drug substance stability. The effect of moisture on stability depends on whether water molecules are in the free or bound state, and in general, this effect arises as a function of free water. In this context, water can increase the chemical reactivity of the drug substance through several possible mechanisms. For instance, water can contribute to the chemical instability by participating in reactions such as hydrolysis (18). It can also serve as a solvent medium through which damaging species (e.g., oxygen) are dissolved in order to react with the drug substance. Furthermore, the presence of free water may increase the reactivity of the drug substance with other excipients, which could lead to chemical degradation such as the Maillard reaction. Water is also a strong plasticizer that depresses the glass transition temperature ($T_g$) of an amorphous solid (19,20). Thus, the addition of water to the amorphous solid causes an increase in free volume and a decrease in viscosity. The resulting enhancement in molecular mobility has significant effects on the rates of diffusion and degradation processes (21). In addition, there may be moisture-induced phase transformation (e.g., hydrates) that could have a direct impact on drug substance stability as well as other physicochemical properties such as solubility. In an analogous fashion, the corresponding stability of the drug product could also be affected by moisture through the same mechanisms, particularly when the drug substance constitutes the major component of the drug product.

Besides its effect on stability, moisture could also change the flow and compression characteristics of drug powders. For instance, powders with high moisture will be difficult to transport since they are more likely to stick on surfaces. Due to the overall impact of moisture on both stability and manufacturing processes, hygroscopicity data help to determine suitable storage conditions as well as the choice of formulations and unit operations for drug substances. In general, when water uptake of drug substances is more than 5% (w/w) at 25°C and 60% RH, formulation development and compound handling will likely become an issue (22).

## Particle Size

From a regulatory perspective, particle size is an important physicochemical parameter primarily due to its effect on biopharmaceutical behavior of the drug substance. For poorly soluble drugs whose bioavailability is limited by the dissolution rate, particle size reduction is a common way to increase the bioavailability through the surface area enhancement. However, very fine particles are often hard to handle. This is possibly due to the manifestation of electrostatic effects and changes in other surface active properties that cause unwarranted stickiness and lack of flowability (23). Particle size can also affect drug substance stability, since fine particles, by virtue of exposing a greater surface to oxygen, light, and humidity, may be more chemically reactive. For example, it has been shown that the reactivity of sulfacetamide increases with reducing particle size (24). It should be noted that drug substance particles may be susceptible to polymorphic and chemical transformation when they undergo size reduction.

Due to the significant effects on drug quality, it is important to control the drug substance particle size within the range that generally yields a good balance of bioavailability and processability. The particle size can be assessed by techniques such as light scattering and optical microscopy, while the surface area of powders is usually determined based on the Brunauer Emmett Teller theory of adsorption (25).

## Crystal Properties (Polymorphism)

Most drug substances can exist in different solid-state forms. This property is known as polymorphism. These differing forms (polymorphs) can be conceptually divided into three distinct classes. The first group includes crystalline phases that have different arrangements and/or conformations of the molecules in the crystal lattice. The second group includes solvates that contain either stoichiometric or nonstoichiometric amounts of a solvent, and sometimes are referred to as pseudopolymorphs in the literature. When the entrapping solvent is water, these solids are referred to as hydrates. The last group includes amorphous solids, which have a liquid-like structure that does not possess a long-range order. They can be often described as a glass. It is important to stress that amorphous solids are nonequilibrium solid phases and hence are generally less stable relative to their corresponding crystalline phases (26).

Different polymorphic forms of a given drug substance usually have different physical and chemical properties, such as solubility, dissolution rate, chemical reactivity, and mechanical properties (27). Some of these effects were already mentioned briefly in previous sections. As will be discussed here, the differences in these properties have potential influence on the drug product bioavailability and stability, as well as on the ability to process and manufacture the drug product.

One of the principal regulatory concerns with regard to drug substance polymorphism is based on the effect that it may have on drug product bioavailability. This is particularly evident with solid oral dosage forms. The differences in solubility among different polymorphic forms are mainly due to the differing lattice energies. When the solubility of the various drug substance polymorphs varies significantly, these differences in solubility may alter drug product in vivo dissolution, thereby affecting drug product bioavailability. A good example demonstrating this point comes from the classic work of Aguiar and others on chloramphenicol palmitate, in which form B was shown to exhibit greater oral absorption than form A because of its enhanced solubility (28,29). As mentioned previously, drug product bioavailability depends on several factors, such as GI motility, drug dissolution, intestinal permeability, and metabolism that control the rate and extent of drug adsorption. Nevertheless, the effect of polymorphism on bioavailability can be assessed in the context of the BCS, which provides a useful scientific framework for regulatory decisions regarding polymorphism (30). In the case where the rate of absorption is limited by the rate of dissolution (class II drugs), large differences in the solubility of various polymorphs are likely to influence bioavailability. On the other hand, when the rate of absorption is controlled by the intestinal permeability (class III drugs), differences in solubility of various polymorphs are unlikely to have a meaningful effect on bioavailability. For drug substances that exhibit high aqueous solubility and high intestinal permeability (class I drugs), polymorphism is generally not a major concern. With all the points stated above, an early knowledge of the solubility as well as the dissolution profile of various polymorphic forms is an important aspect of product design with respect to delivering reproducible drug product bioavailability.

Another regulatory concern regarding polymorphism of drug substance is the effect that it may have on drug product stability. This is due to the fact that various polymeric forms of the drug substance may differ in their physical and chemical reactivity, as well as in their hygroscopicity. These differences are attributed to the differences in thermodynamic stability, molecular environment, and mobility. The change in chemical reactivity as a result of a polymorphic transformation could potentially lead to adverse effects on drug product potency and impurity profile. Examples of this phenomenon have been demonstrated in enalapril maleate (31), indomethacin (32), furosemide (33), and carbamazepine (34). In general, the most stable form of the drug substance should be chosen for development mainly because of its minimal potential for polymorphic transformation and its greater chemical stability. However, in some cases, the metastable form or the amorphous form may be preferred due to, amongst other reasons, bioavailability enhancement as mentioned earlier in this chapter. Thus, knowledge of polymorphic stability for drug substances is useful in the design of a drug product with acceptable stability.

Polymorphism also influences the drug product manufacturability. Polymorphs may exhibit different physical and mechanical properties, including hygroscopicity, particle shape, density, flowability, and compactability. The differences in these drug substance properties could have the potential to affect drug substance processability and drug product manufacturability. Some of these effects have been mentioned previously. It should be emphasized that product manufacturability depends not only on the intrinsic physical and mechanical properties of drug substance polymorphic forms but also on the formulation and manufacturing process. In direct compression, the solid-state properties of a polymorphic solid will likely be critical to drug product manufacturability, particularly when the solid constitutes a majority of the tablet mass. On the contrary, the properties of a polymorphic solid will be often masked by other excipients in the wet granulation. Thus, the original solid-state properties of the solid are less likely to influence drug product manufacturability. In addition, for most injectable solution products, the issues regarding polymorphism become irrelevant, since the memory of solid-state properties is lost on dissolution.

Thus, polymorphism can affect the critical performance quality attributes of the drug product, its safety and efficacy. It is essential, therefore, to define and monitor the solid-state form of drug substance during development. Several methods have been employed for polymorph characterization, including X-ray powder diffraction, microscopy, thermal analysis (e.g., differential scanning calorimetry, thermal gravimetric analysis, hot-stage microscopy), and spectroscopy (e.g., Infrared, Raman, solid-state NMR) (35,36). Thus, based on this knowledge of drug substance polymorphism, formulators will be better able to judiciously select the optimal polymorphic form(s), so as to circumvent potential drug product stability, bioavailability, and processing problems.

## Miscellaneous Properties

In addition to the drug substance properties described above, information related to other properties, such as density, compressibility, compactability, and flowability, is important to the selection of the best candidate drugs for development, since these properties have the potential to affect both the drug product quality and its manufacturability. This information should also be gathered and evaluated as early as possible and used to advantage in the product and process design.

## CONCLUSION

This review provides a concise perspective on some drug substance physicochemical properties in the context of QbD. These drug substance properties include solubility, permeability, hygroscopicity, particle size, polymorphism, and stability. Their importance during drug development is emphasized through a discussion of their potential effects on drug product bioavailability, stability, and manufacturability. Knowledge gained from preformulation studies aids in understanding the potential effects of drug substance properties on drug product performance and constitutes a basis for QbD, which is essential to a design of quality drug products as well as for enabling more flexible regulatory approaches.

## REFERENCES

1. Woodcock J. Ind Pharmacy 2005; 5:6–9.
2. ICH, Q9 Quality Risk Management, ICH, June 2006.
3. ICH, Q8 Pharmaceutical Development, ICH, May 2006.
4. Woodcock J. Am Pharm J Rev 2004; 7:6–9.
5. Higuchi T, Shih FM, Kimura T, Rytting JH. J Pharm Sci 1979; 68:1267–72.
6. Ando HY, Radebaugh GW. Preformulation. In: Gennaro AR, ed. Remington: The Science and Practice of Pharmacy. Maryland: Lippincott Williams & Wilkins, 2000:700–20.
7. Stavchansky R, McGinity J. Bioavailability and tablet technology. In: Lieberman HA, Lachman L, Schwartz JB, eds. Pharmaceutical Dosage Forms: Tablets, Vol. 2. New York: Marcel Dekker, 1989:349–569.
8. Wolf B, Finke I, Schmitz W. Pharmazie 1996; 51:104–12.
9. Loftsson T, Hreinsdóttir D, Másson M. Inter J Pharm 2005; 302:18–28.
10. Curatolo W. Pharm Sci Technol Today 1998; 1:387–93.

11. Avdeef A. Absorption and Drug Development: Solubility, Permeability, and Charge State. New Jersey: Wiley, 2003.
12. Amidon GL, Lennernäs H, Shah VP, Crison JR. Pharm Res 1995; 12:413–9.
13. Corrigan OI. Adv Exp Med Biol 1997; 423:111–28.
14. Stewart PJ, Tucker IG. Aust J Hosp Pharm 1985; 185:11–6.
15. Waterman KC, Adami RC. Inter J Pharm 2005; 293:101–25.
16. Wirth DD, Baertschi SW, John RA, et al. J Pharm Sci 1998; 87:31–9.
17. European Pharmacopeia 5.0. 2005; 5:565.
18. Waterman KC, Adami, RC, Alsante KM, et al. Pharm Dev Tech 2002; 7:1113–46.
19. Orford PD, Parker R, Ring SG. Carbohydr Res 1990; 196:11–8.
20. Roos Y. Carbohydr Res 1993; 238:39–48.
21. Ahlneck C, Zografi G. Inter J Pharm 1990; 62:87–95.
22. Callahan JC, Cleary GW, Elefant M, Kaplan G, Kensler T, Nash RA. Drug Dev Ind Pharm 1982; 8:355–69.
23. Wadke DA, Serajuddin ATM, Jacobson H. Preformulation testing. In: Lieberman HA, Lachman L, Schwartz JB, eds. Pharmaceutical Dosage Forms: Tablets, Vol. 1. New York: Marcel Dekker, 1989:1–71.
24. Weng H, Parrott EL. J Pharm Sci 1984; 73:1059–63.
25. Gregg SJ, Sing KSW. Adsorption, Surface Area, and Porosity. New York: Academic Press, 1967.
26. Yu L. Adv Drug Delivery Rev 2001; 48:27–42.
27. Grant DJW. Theory and origin of polymorphism. In: Brittain HG, ed. Polymorphism in Pharmaceutical Solids. New York: Marcel Dekker 1999; 1–34.
28. Aguiar AJ, Krc J, Kinkel AW, Symyn JC. J Pharm Sci 1967; 56:847–53.
29. Aguiar AJ, Zelmer JE. J Pharma Sci 1969; 58:983–7.
30. Yu LX, Amidon GL, Polli JE, et al. Pharm Res 2002; 19:921–5.
31. Eyjolfsson R. Pharmazie 57:347–8.
32. Chen X, Morris KR, Griesser UJ, Byrn SR, Stowell JG. J Am Chem Soc 2002; 124:15012–9.
33. De Villiers MM, van der Watt JG, Lotter AP. Int J Pharm 1992; 88:275–83.
34. Matsuda Y, Akazawa R, Teraoka R, Otsuka M. J Pharm Phamacol 1993; 46:162–7.
35. Brittain HG, Grant DJW. Methods for the characterization of polymorphs and solvates. In: Brittain HG, ed. Polymorphism in Pharmaceutical Solids. New York: Marcel Dekker, 1999; 227–78.
36. Yu L, Reutzel SM. Pharm Sci Tech 1998; 1:118–27.

# Index